Insurance Handbook for the Medical Office

ELSEVIER

evolve

To access your Student Resources, visit the Web address below:

http://evolve.elsevier.com/Fordney/handbook/

- **WebLinks**
  An exciting resource that lets you link to hundreds of Web sites carefully chosen to supplement the content of the textbook. The WebLinks are regularly updated, with new ones added as they develop.

- **Content Updates**
  The latest content updates from the authors of the textbook to keep you current with recent developments in this area of study.

- **Self-Assessment Quizzes**
  Includes mutiple choice, true/false, fill-in-the-blank, and matching questions with instant scoring and feedback at the click of a button.

Insurance Handbook for the Medical Office

EIGHTH EDITION

Marilyn Takahashi Fordney, CMA-AC, CMT
Formerly Instructor of Medical Insurance, Medical Terminology, Medical Machine
Transcription, and Medical Office Procedures

Ventura College
Ventura, California

Technical Collaborator and Contributing Author:

Steven M. Verno, CMBS
Compliance Director and Instructor

Medical Association of Billers
Las Vegas, Nevada

An Imprint of Elsevier

SAUNDERS
An Imprint of Elsevier

11830 Westline Industrial Drive
St. Louis, Missouri 63146

INSURANCE HANDBOOK FOR THE MEDICAL OFFICE, EDITION 8   ISBN 0-7216-0517-6

Previous editions copyrighted 2002, 1999, 1997, 1995, 1989, 1981, 1977

Library of Congress Cataloging-in-Publication Data

Fordney, Marilyn Takashashi.
  Insurance handbook for the medical office/Marilyn Takahashi Fordney; technical collaborator
and contributing author, Steven M. Verno.– 8th ed.
    p. cm.
  Includes index.
  ISBN 0-7216-0517-6
    1. Insurance, Health–United States–Handbooks, manuals, etc. 2. Medical
offices–Management–Handbooks, manuals, etc. 3. Medical claims processing industry.
  I. Verno, Steven M. II. Title.
HG9396.F67 2003
368.38′0024′61–dc22   2003057102

International Standard Book Number 0-7216-0517-6

Acquisitions Editor:	Susan Cole
Associate Developmental Editor:	Lisa M. Neumann
Publishing Services Manager:	Patricia Tannian
Project Manager:	Sharon Corell
Designer:	Amy Buxton

Printed in the United States of America.

Last digit is the print number: 9   8   7   6   5   4   3   2

This book is dedicated to insurance billing and coding specialists throughout the nation, to insurance billing and coding instructors, and to new and former students who motivate me to continue writing in this challenging and ever-changing career field.

"I hear and I forget, I see and I remember, I do and I understand."

Chinese Proverb

Preface

Welcome to the Eighth Edition. When this book made its first appearance in 1977, few people were aware of how important the subject of health insurance would become. *Insurance Handbook for the Medical Office* now celebrates its 27th year and through the years has gained wide acceptance across the nation. It won a national award, the 2002 William Holmes McGuffey Award, given by the Text and Academic Authors Association. Putting the eighth edition together has been challenging and exciting. Because changes take place in the insurance industry on a regular basis, *Insurance Handbook for the Medical Office* will be revised every two years to keep the information current.

Purpose

The goals of this text are to increase efficiency and streamline administrative procedures for one of the most complex tasks of the physician's business: insurance coding and billing.

In the last decade, community and health care professionals have witnessed the emergence of an administrative medical specialty known as insurance billing specialist, medical biller, or reimbursement specialist. Certification is being offered by several national organizations, and the career is quickly achieving recognition and professionalism. Thus the *Handbook* has been written to address this specialty as another branch of the administrative medical assistant profession. Health care reform is leading to an explosion of jobs in the medical field, especially for those trained in coding and processing insurance claims, manually as well as electronically. Training in this area is necessary because it is common to find medical practices either undercharging or not charging for billable services because of a lack of knowledge among office personnel.

Insurance claims are being submitted for patients on recommendation of management consultants to control cash flow, obtain correct reimbursement amounts, honor insurance contracts, compete with other medical practices, and maintain a good relationship with patients. Even offices that do not routinely complete insurance claims for patients will make exceptions for the aged or those patients who suffer from mental incompetence, illiteracy, diminished eyesight, or a poor command of the English language. When the amount of a bill is hundreds or thousands of dollars or when a surgical report is required, the physician's office should submit the bill to obtain maximum reimbursement. Because of HIPAA, those who administer the federal government's Medicare program now require electronic transmission of insurance claims. The amount of paperwork has increased by leaps and bounds, becoming burdensome and unwieldy. This text addresses all clerical functions of the medical biller, and illustrations throughout the text feature generic forms created to help simplify billing procedures.

A number of schools and colleges have established one-year certificate programs for those interested in a career as an insurance billing specialist, and many existing programs offer medical insurance as a full-semester, 18-week course. Community college extension divisions also offer community service classes and short courses in this subject. Some schools include it as part of a medical assisting program's curriculum so the individual has knowledge of all administrative functions in a physician's office. The text may be used as a learning tool and resource guide in all of those programs as well as in vocational or commercial training institutes and welfare-work programs. It also serves as a text for in-service training in the private medical office. It may be used for independent home study if no formal classes are available in the community. The lay reader not pursuing a career in the medical field will find it useful when working with a claims assistance professional or for billing his or her insurance plans. Insurance companies and their agents have found this a valuable reference book when answering clients' questions.

The text is designed primarily for the student who plans to seek employment in an outpatient setting (physician's office or clinic) or wishes to establish an independent billing business and needs a good understanding of the reimbursement process. Since many types of insurance coverage are available in the United States, those types most commonly encountered in physicians' offices and clinics have been emphasized in this text in simple, nontechnical explanations and tables. Documentation in the medical record is the key to substantiating procedure and diagnostic code selections for proper reimbursement. In recent years, the federal government targeted this issue with the introduction of Medicare compliance policies related to documentation and confidentiality. HIPAA and other compliance regulations are therefore covered to help physicians comply with possible reviews or audits of their billing practices. Finally, this book may be used as a stand-alone reference source or as an educational tool to increase the knowledge of someone currently working as an insurance billing specialist in a private medical office.

Content

New Features

Each chapter has been updated to reflect 2003 policies and procedures.

▶ Chapter 3, Medical Documentation, has been updated and enhanced to address compliance and confidentiality more thoroughly.

▶ The Blue Plans (Blue Cross and Blue Shield) information has been incorporated into Chapter 10, Private Insurance and Managed Care Systems.

▶ HIPAA Compliance Alerts highlight sections throughout the text that help students learn how to comply with governmental privacy regulations.

General Features

The chapters of the previous edition were reviewed by experts so that improvements in content, clarity of topics, and deletions could be considered. A unique color-coded icon feature used throughout the book denotes and clarifies information specific to each type of payer. This system makes the learning process more effective by helping students identify each insurance payer with a specific color and graphic. These icons follow:

 All Payers: All payer guidelines including all private insurance companies and all federal and state programs.

 All Private Payers: All private insurance companies.

 Medicaid: State Medicaid programs.

 Medicare: Federal Medicare programs, Medicare/Medicaid, Medicare/Medigap, and Medicare Secondary Payer (MSP).

 TRICARE: TRICARE Standard (formerly CHAMPUS), TRICARE Prime, TRICARE Extra.

 CHAMPVA: Civilian Health and Medical Program of the Department of Veterans Affairs.

 Workers' Compensation: State workers' compensation programs.

Additional features of this textbook include the following:

▶ Objectives are presented at the beginning of each chapter to guide the instructor in preparing lecture material and inform the reader about what will be presented. By reviewing the key terms introducing each chapter, the student is alerted to important words pertaining to the topic.

▶ Basic health insurance information and coding examples are provided to assist the person who is studying for a certification examination. Special emphasis is placed on correct and incorrect procedural codes and appropriate documentation—the keys to obtaining maximum reimbursement.

▶ Chapter 6, The Health Insurance Claim Form, uses a unique block-by-block approach specific to each different payer, which denotes and clarifies information about the CMS-1500 insurance claim form. The icons and graphics system is used to help the student retain information. Templates illustrate placement of information on the form.

▶ Chapter 7, Electronic Data Interchange (EDI), explains electronic claims transmission and computer claim systems, both carrier direct and clearinghouse. Many specific quick-action solutions to insurance problems and ways to trace delinquent claims and appeal denied claims are mentioned. Thorough up-to-date information is presented for Medicare, Medicaid, TRICARE, private plans, workers' compensation, managed care plans, disability income insurance, and disability benefit programs. Helpful billing tips and guidelines for submitting insurance claims are given for each type of insurance program covered.

▶ Chapter 16, Hospital Billing, is intended especially for those students interested in pursuing a career in the hospital setting. A final chapter provides information pertinent to seeking a position as an insurance billing specialist, a self-employed claims assistance professional, or an electronic claims processor.

▶ Appendix A lists addresses of insurance claims offices and insurance commissioners by state, territory, or Canadian province.

▶ Appendix B is a comprehensive reference resource of available audiotapes, books, newsletters, periodicals, software, and videotapes designed to assist the insurance billing specialist. Addresses, toll-free telephone numbers, and Web sites are listed to assist the reader in locating a special item, if desired.

▶ An extensive glossary of basic medical and insurance terms and abbreviations is included.

Supplemental Material

Workbook

New Features

▶ Patient records and ledgers have been completely updated for technical clinical content and reworded to correspond with the 2003 procedural and diagnostic code books.

▶ The book has been reformatted to ensure easy removal of assignments for completion.

General Features

For the student, the *Workbook* that accompanies the text is a practical approach to learning insurance billing. It progresses from easy to more complex issues within each chapter and advances as new skills are learned and integrated. Chapter outlines serve as a lecture guide. Each chapter has performance objectives for assignments that indicate to students what will be accomplished. Key terms are repeated for quick reference when studying. Patients' medical records, ledgers, and encounter forms are presented as they might appear in the doctor's files, so the student may learn how to abstract information to complete claim forms properly and accurately. Some assignments give students hands-on experience in typing forms for optical character recognition (OCR) computer equipment, which is used in many states for insurance claims processing and payment. Current procedural and diagnostic code exercises are used throughout the *Workbook* to facilitate and enhance coding skills necessary for submitting a claim or posting to a patient's ledger. Critical thinking problems are presented in each chapter. Special appendixes are included at the end of the *Workbook*. The appendixes may be used as reference tools to complete the procedural code problems. These appendixes include the following:

▶ Appendix A details information for a simulated practice, called The College Clinic. Information is provided about the group of physicians, and a mock fee schedule is included with codes and fees (including Medicare)

▶ Appendix B provides an abbreviated Medicare Level II HCPCS alphanumeric code list.

▶ Appendix C provides Medi-Cal information and review questions.

▶ The answers to self-study review questions in each chapter can be found in Appendix D.

Student Software Challenge

Because many medical practices use computer technology to perform financial operations, a user-friendly computer software tutorial program has been developed to accompany the *Handbook* and *Workbook*. The goal is to give students a hands-on, realistic approach, as though they were working in a medical setting, by having them select appropriate patient files and extract specific information to complete the CMS-1500 insurance claim form, financial accounting record, authorization form, and insurance claims tracer. Health Insurance Portability and Accountability Act (HIPAA) compliance requirements are integrated into the software to alert the user to the sensitive nature of health information and the need for confidentiality when handling such records.

Additional features of the tutorial software for the 2004 edition of this text include the following:

▶ Timekeeper tracks time needed to complete a claim form.

▶ Split screen allows student to view source documents while inputting information on other forms.

▶ Weighted scoring feature awards more points for more difficult information. Block values may be found in Block Help.

▶ Block Help provides block values and feedback for the authorization form, insurance claim tracer form.

▶ Complete fee schedule simplifies the insertion of fees on the CMS-1500 claim form or financial accounting record.

▶ Computerized accounting record automatically calculates a running balance for the financial ledger.

▶ Authorization form and Insurance Claim Tracer forms are available and may be completed for any case included on the software or in the *Workbook*.

▶ Claims Management screen allows the student to search for or sort claims by work date, account or case number, patient name, insurance carrier, score, and time needed to complete the claim.

▶ Separate log for "Other Patients" allows individual tracking of all claims completed from *Workbook* cases or those assigned by an instructor.

▶ Electronic submission screens simulate the process of sending electronic claims to insurance carriers.

The instructor may ask the student to work through the first case or basic cases one through four strictly for learning and use case five for testing and grading. The last five cases, which are advanced and insurance specific (e.g., Medicare, TRICARE), may be used for practice or testing. This simulated learning methodology makes possible an easier transition from classroom to workplace.

Instructor's Curriculum Resource

The instructor's manual is now available in printed form, with additional information included on a CD-ROM bound into the book. This resource allows the instructor the flexibility to quickly adapt the textbook for his or her individual classroom needs and to gauge students' understanding. The printed *Instructor's Manual* includes the following:

▶ Guidelines for establishing a medical insurance course
▶ Answer keys to the *Workbook* assignments and tests with rationales, optional codes, and further explanations for the majority of the code problems
▶ Suggested classroom activities
▶ Ideas on how to use the text as an adjunct to a medical office procedures course
▶ Contact information for the author if an instructor is interested in establishing a one-year certificate program for insurance billing specialists or desires further information about this career field

The CD-ROM includes all of the information in the printed *Instructor's Manual*, plus the following:

▶ An image collection of forms from the textbook for use as overheads or in Power Point presentations
▶ An ExamView test bank with more than 1000 questions to assist the instructor in test construction

Evolve Course Management System

Evolve is an interactive learning environment that works in coordination with the main textbook. It provides Internet-based course management tools the instructor can use to reinforce and expand on the concepts delivered in class. It can be used for the following:

▶ Publish the class syllabus, outline, and lecture notes
▶ Set up "virtual office hours" and e-mail communication
▶ Share important dates and information through the online class calendar
▶ Encourage student participation through chat rooms and discussion boards

Evolve also provides online access to free Learning Resources designed specifically to give students and instructors the information they need to quickly and successfully learn the topics covered in this textbook. These Learning Resources include:

▶ Self-assessment quizzes to evaluate the student's mastery through multiple choice, true/false, fill-in-the-blank, and matching questions. Instant scoring and feedback are available at the click of a button.
▶ Weblinks: Hundreds of Web sites have been carefully gathered to supplement the content of the textbook. The Weblinks are regularly updated, with new ones added as they are developed.
▶ Content updates to keep up with changes in government regulations, codes, and other industry changes.

Medical Insurance Online

Medical Insurance Online is an exciting new resource for instructors and students. It offers a simulated, interactive office externship experience with feedback provided throughout. The following list is just a sampling of what students will experience with the innovative Medical Insurance Online program:

▶ It functions as a "virtual externship" in which users go through an office orientation where they meet their virtual office manager and medical staff.
▶ Users gain "on the job" training as they perform a number of true-to-life activities, interacting with virtual patients, troubleshooting claims, maintaining compliance with regulations, meeting insurance payer requirements, and more.
▶ Users fill in specific portions of the insurance claim form and receive immediate feedback.
▶ The program provides direct interaction with and constant access to all paperwork relevant to each patient claim.
▶ After completing each "virtual day," users have a chance to review the material they encountered with the virtual office manager by answering a number of questions and receiving feedback.
▶ Automatically scored quizzes at the end of each phase and an exam at the end of each module allow students to demonstrate their mastery of the content.
▶ By the end of the course, the user has followed claims through their life cycle for each of the various insurance payers, including private commercial carriers, Medicare/Medicaid, Medigap, Managed Care (HMOs), and others.

Summary

The *Handbook* and its ancillaries provide a complete competency-based educational program. *Handbook* learning objectives, *Workbook* performance objectives, assignments, tests, tutorial software and text, the virtual externship available on *Medical Insurance*

Online, and incorporation of classroom activities and suggestions from the *Instructor's Curriculum Resource* ensure students know everything they need to succeed in the workforce.

Escalating costs of medical care, the impact of technology, and the explosion of managed care plans have affected insurance billing procedures and claims processing and have necessitated new legislation for government and state programs. Therefore it is essential that all medical personnel who handle claims continue to update their knowledge. This may be accomplished by reading bulletins from state agencies and regional insurance carriers, speaking with insurance representatives, or attending insurance workshops offered at local colleges or local chapters of professional associations, such as those mentioned in Chapters 1 and 17. It is hoped that this text will resolve any unclear issues pertaining to current methods and become the framework on which the insurance billing specialist builds new knowledge as understanding and appreciation of the profession are attained.

Acknowledgments

During my 14 years as a medical assistant, 19 years of teaching, and 28 years of writing, hundreds of students, physicians, friends, colleagues, and instructors have contributed valuable suggestions and interesting material for this book. I wish to express my thanks to all of them, with special appreciation to the following:

Lois C. Oliver, retired Professor, Pierce College, Woodland Hills, California, helped me organize my first medical insurance class in 1969 and offered assistance and encouragement throughout the preparation of the first edition of the *Handbook*.

Marcia O. "Marcy" Diehl, CMA-A, CMT, retired instructor, Grossmont Community College, El Cajon, California, generously shared her knowledge, ideas, and class materials.

Members of the *California Association of Medical Assistant Instructors* (*CAMAI*) contributed suggestions for improving the text and gave me motivation from time to time to continue the project.

Mary E. Kinn, CPS, CMA-A, author and retired Assistant Professor, Long Beach City College, Long Beach, California, provided a perspective review of my syllabus. Without her positive endorsement, the first edition of this book might not have been published.

Overwhelming thanks to my technical collaborator and contributor, Linda L. French, CMA-C, NCICS, who helped with the tremendous overhaul and restructuring of each chapter and lent technical and editorial assistance for the entire project. Writing has its ups and downs, and she gave me support during many of the difficult periods. Special thanks to the students of Linda's classes at the Simi Valley Adult School and Career Institute in Simi Valley, California, who contributed their criticisms, lent technical subject matter, offered suggestions, and through voluntary participation helped to enhance and create *Workbook* assignments. A note of appreciation to my assistants, Ginger Daughterty and Barbara Evans, who performed many tasks to allow me free time to research and write.

I gratefully acknowledge the assistance of the artist involved with the design, Amy Buxton, Design Department, Elsevier. The photograph for the Preface was taken by Friedman Photography of Ventura, California, whom I wish to acknowledge and thank.

I also wish to thank the Print Shop Staff, Publications Department, Ventura College, Ventura, California, who printed the first California syllabus of this text.

I am indebted to many individuals on the staff at Elsevier for encouragement and guidance. I express particular appreciation to Adrianne Cochran, Senior Acquisitions Editor, and Lisa Neumann, Associate Developmental Editor. Thanks also to Jeanne Genz and Sharon Corell, Project Managers, for expert editing and coordination of the entire project.

Numerous supply companies were kind enough to cooperate by providing forms and descriptive literature of their products, and their names will be found throughout the text and workbook figures.

But colleagues, production staff, and editors working as a team do not quite make a book; there are others to whom I must express overwhelming debt and enduring gratitude, and these are the consultants who reviewed some of the chapters or who provided vital information about private, state, and federal insurance programs. Without the knowledge of these advisers, the massive task of compiling an insurance text truly national in scope might never have been completed. Although the names of all those who graciously assisted me are too numerous to mention, I take great pride in listing my principal consultants for this eighth edition.

Marilyn Takahashi Fordney, CMA-AC, CMT
Oxnard, California

Principal Consultants and Reviewers

Conejo Chapter of the American Association of Professional Coders
Thousand Oaks, California

George S. Conomikes and Staff
President, Conomikes Associates, Inc., Los Angeles, California

Deborah Emmons, CMA
President, S.T.A.T. Transcription Service, Port Hueneme, California

Jane Fether
Former Assistant Supervisor, Accounts Payable, Los Robles Medical Center

Ronna Jurow, MD
Active Staff and Attending Physician in Obstetrics, Gynecology and Infertility, Community Memorial Hospital, Ventura, California

Lucille M. Loignon, MD, FACS
Diplomate, American Board of Ophthalmology, Oxnard, California

Kathy A. McCall, CMA-AC, BS, MA
Retired Professor of Allied Health, Community College of Allegheny County, Pittsburgh, Pennsylvania

Walter A. Shaff
President, CPR, Lake Oswego, Oregon

Griff Stelzner
Assistant Claims Manager, State Compensation Insurance Fund, Oxnard, California

Sue Stratton
Vice President, Health Care Services, Medical Administrative Consultants, Inc., Agoura Hills, California

Carolyn Talesfore
Ad and Promo Manager, Bibbero Systems, Inc., Petaluma, California

Barbara Warfield
Rhino Graphics, Port Hueneme, California

Brief Table of Contents

Contents

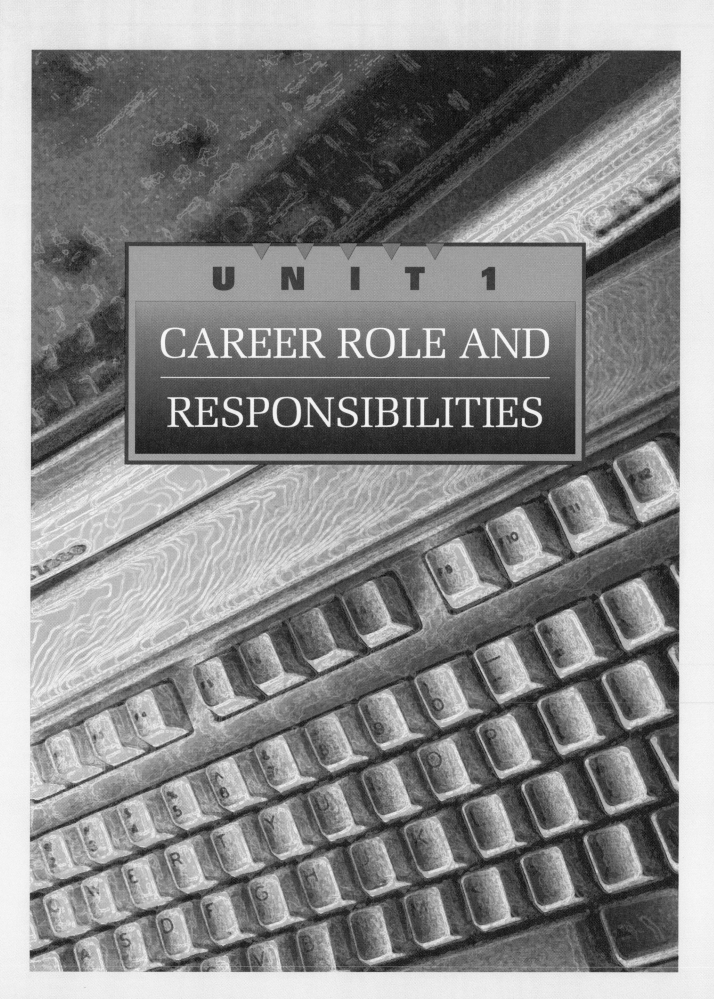

U N I T   1

CAREER ROLE AND

RESPONSIBILITIES

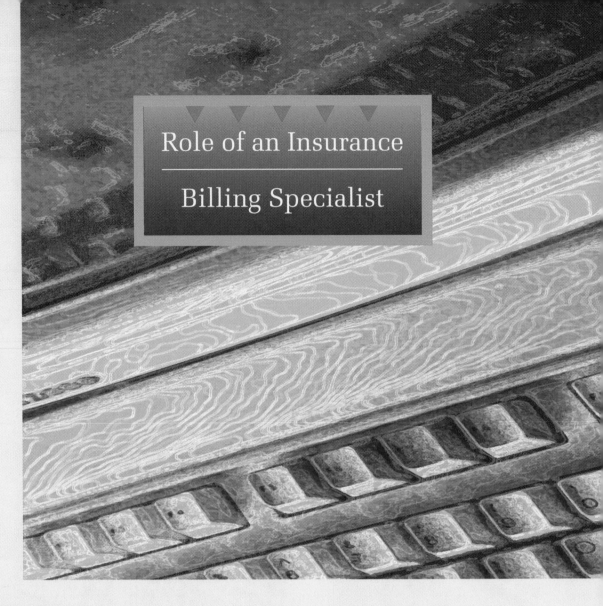

Role of an Insurance Billing Specialist

CHAPTER OUTLINE

- List personal qualifications and skills to be acquired by an insurance billing specialist.
- State the personal image to be projected as an insurance billing specialist.
- Specify the educational requirements for a job as an insurance billing specialist and a coder.
- Explain how insurance knowledge and medical knowledge can be kept current.
- Differentiate between medical ethics and medical etiquette.
- Define confidential communication.
- Illustrate the difference between privileged and nonprivileged information.
- Translate the Latin phrase *respondeat superior*.
- List various types of insurance fraud.
- Define abuse as it relates to the subject of insurance claims.
- State some precautions to take for financial protection.

OBJECTIVES*

After reading this chapter you should be able to:

- Identify the background and importance of insurance claims completion, coding, and billing.
- Name at least three skills possessed by insurance billing specialists.
- Describe the variety of career possibilities and areas of specialization open to those trained as insurance billing specialists.

KEY TERMS

abuse

American Health Information Management Association (AHIMA)

American Medical Association (AMA)

blanket-position bond

bonding

cash flow

churning

claims assistance professional (CAP)

confidential communication

embezzlement

ethics

etiquette

fraud

insurance billing specialist

list service (listserv)

multiskilled health practitioner (MSHP)

nonprivileged information

personal bond

phantom billing

ping-ponging

position-schedule bond

privileged information

reimbursement specialist

respondeat superior

yo-yoing

---

*Performance objectives and exercises for hands-on practical experience for this chapter appear in the *Workbook*.

Role of the Insurance Billing Specialist

Welcome to the world of insurance billing, an exciting, ever-changing, and fast growing career field. To help you focus on important terms and definitions, some of the basic words in this and subsequent chapters appear bold-faced or italicized. See the Glossary at the end of this textbook for a comprehensive list of key terms, with detailed definitions to broaden your knowledge.

In the past, a medical assistant working in a physician's office performed both administrative and clinical duties. Then, as decades passed, he or she performed either one or the other. Now, because of changes in government regulations and standards for the insurance industry, specific medical assisting job tasks have become specialized. In a medical practice, it is commonplace to find administrative duties shared by a number of employees (e.g., administrative medical assistant, bookkeeper, file clerk, insurance billing specialist, office manager, receptionist, or transcriptionist). In some work settings, an **insurance billing specialist** may be known as an electronic claims processor, a medical biller, or a **reimbursement specialist.** In clinics and large practices, it is common to find a billing department made up of many people, and within the department each position is a specialist, such as Medicare billing specialist, Medicaid billing specialist, coding specialist, insurance counselor, collection manager, and medical and financial records manager.

Some medical practices and clinics contract with management services organizations (MSOs), which perform a variety of business functions, such as accounting, billing, coding, collections, computer support, legal advice, marketing, payroll, and management expertise. An insurance billing specialist may find a job working for an MSO as a part of this team.

Cost pressures on health care providers are forcing employers to reduce personnel costs by hiring **multiskilled health practitioners** (MSHPs). An MSHP is a person cross-trained to provide more than one function, often in more than one discipline. Knowledge of insurance claims completion and coding enhances skills so that he or she can offer more flexibility to someone hired in a medical setting.

There are also people called **claims assistance professionals** (CAPs), who work for the consumer and help patients organize, file, and negotiate health insurance claims of all types. A CAP's primary goals are to assist the consumer in obtaining maximum benefits and tell the patient what checks to write to providers to make sure there is no overpayment. A medical insurance billing specialist may also function in this role.

Job Responsibilities

Administrative front office duties have gained in importance for the following reasons. Documentation is vital to good patient care. It must be done comprehensively for proper reimbursement. Diagnostic and procedural coding must be reviewed for its correctness and completeness. Insurance claims must be promptly submitted manually or transmitted electronically (ideally within 48 to 72 hours) to ensure continuous cash flow. **Cash flow** is the amount of actual money available to the medical practice. Without money coming in, overhead expenses cannot be met and a practice will fold. Data required for billing must be collected from hospitals, laboratories, and other physicians involved in a case.

An insurance billing specialist in a large medical practice may act as an insurance counselor, taking the patient to a private area of the office to discuss the practice's financial policies and the patient's insurance coverage, and negotiate a reasonable payment plan. The insurance billing specialist discusses claims processing with contracted and noncontracted carriers, the billing of secondary insurances and patients once the carrier pays its portion, self-pay billing, and time payment plans. The patient may not know it is his or her obligation, rather than the provider's, to send the claim to the insurance carrier. Any copays or deductible amounts should be collected from the patient during this time. Self-pay patients should be reminded that payment is due at the time of service. This is done to ensure that the physician will be paid for services rendered and develop good communication lines. Patients who are informed are patients who pay their bills. The counselor learns the deductible amount and verifies with the insurance company whether any preauthorization, precertification, or second-opinion requirements exist. Counseling helps obtain payment in full when expensive procedures are necessary. In some offices, the insurance biller may act as a collection manager who answers routine inquiries related to account balances and insurance submission dates, assists patients in budgeting, follows up on delinquent accounts, and traces denied, "adjusted," or unpaid claims (Fig. 1–1).

The reason most practices have a large accounts receivable (total amount of money owed for professional services rendered) can be traced to a failure to verify benefits, obtain authorization or precertification, or collect copays and deductibles. The rush to get a claim "out the door" cannot be justified when a practice has thousands or millions of dollars in unpaid or denied claims. Accounts receivables will be low and revenue high if a practice takes the extra time to ensure the claim is 100% accurate, complete, and verified.

Figure I–I. Insurance biller talking to a patient on the telephone about copayment required for an office visit under the patient's insurance plan.

In 1997 the American Association of Medical Assistants (AAMA) developed a role delineation study analyzing the many job functions of the medical assistant. Table 1–1 shows the Medical Assistant Role Delineation Chart, with highlighted areas indicating material covered in this textbook. The topics shown on the role delineation chart must be studied to pass the certification examination offered by the AAMA. Further information about many types of certification and registration are shown in Chapter 17.

Educational and Training Requirements

Generally, a high school diploma or general equivalency diploma (GED) is required for entry into an insurance billing or coding specialist accredited program. The accredited program usually offers additional education in medical terminology, insurance claims completion, procedural and diagnostic coding, anatomy and physiology, computer skills, ethics and medicolegal knowledge, and general office skills. Completion of an accredited program for coding certification or an accredited health information medical record technology program is necessary for a job as a coder.

Experience in coding and insurance claims completion, completion of a 1-year insurance specialist certificate program at a community college, or both usually are required for a job as an insurance billing specialist. The curriculum that might be offered in a 1-year certificate program is shown in Figure 1–2. You might find that the courses in your locale may be labeled with different titles and time frames because the information contained in Figure 1–2 is specifically from a community college in Pennsylvania. Courses should cover medical terminology, anatomy and physiology, introduction to computer technology, procedural and diagnostic coding, and comprehensive medical insurance billing. A 2-year educational course can result in obtaining an associate degree. Training prepares an individual for a wide range of employment opportunities. Knowledge of computer hardware and software, electronic data transmission requirements, and health care claim reimbursement is recommended if you are planning to become an electronic claims processor. Many accredited programs include an externship (on-the-job) period of training that may be paid or unpaid.

The **American Health Information Management Association (AHIMA)** published diagnostic and procedure coding competencies for outpatient services and diagnostic coding and reporting requirements for physician billing. Refer to these competencies for a more inclusive list of educational and training requirements by visiting the Web site listed in the Resources at the end of this chapter.

It is necessary to have a moderate to high degree of knowledge of the health insurance business if your goal is to become a claims assistance professional. In addition to insurance terminology, claims procedures, and coding, you must know commercial insurance carriers' requirements and Medicare policies and regulations. You also need human relations skills and proficiency in running a business, including marketing and sales expertise.

To reach a professional level, certification is available from many national associations, depending on the type of certification desired. Refer to Chapter 17 for more information on this topic.

Career Advantages

Jobs are available in every state, ranging from nonmanagement to management positions. Insurance billing specialists can receive a salary of $8000 part time to $40,000 full time or more per year depending on knowledge, experience, duties, responsibilities, locale, and size of the employing institution. Jobs are available in consulting firms, insurance and managed care companies, clinics, hospitals, multispecialty medical groups, private physicians' practices, and as instructors or lecturers. You can be your own boss by either setting up an in-home billing service or establishing an office service for billing.

Many people establish self-owned and self-operated businesses within their communities as medical insurance billing specialists, coders, claim assistance professionals, or collectors. However, the responsibilities are greater in this area because you have to set up the business, obtain clients, and advertise and market the business (Chapter 17).

Another advantage of this career field is the opportunity to have flexible hours. Most employees in the physician's office must adhere to the physician's schedule. However, the medical insurance billing specialist may want to come in early to transmit electronic claims during nonpeak hours or stay

TABLE 1–1

Medical Assistant Role Delineation Chart

Administrative

Administrative Procedures	**Practice Finances**
Perform basic administrative medical assisting functions	Perform procedural and diagnostic coding
Schedule, coordinate, and monitor appointments	Apply bookkeeping principles
Schedule inpatient/outpatient admissions and procedures	Manage accounts receivable
Understand and apply third-party guidelines	Manage accounts payable
Obtain reimbursement through accurate claims submission	Process payroll
Monitor third-party reimbursement	Document and maintain accounting and banking records
Adhere to HIPAA regulations	Develop and maintain fee schedules*
Understand and adhere to managed care policies and procedures	Manage renewals of business and professional insurance policies*
Negotiate managed care contracts*	Manage personnel benefits and maintain records*
	Perform marketing, financial, and strategic planning

Clinical

Fundamental Principles	
Apply principles of aseptic technique and infection control	Prepare patient for examinations, procedures, and treatments
Comply with quality assurance practices	Assist with examinations, procedures, and treatments
Screen and follow up patient test results	Prepare and administer medications and immunizations
Diagnostic Orders	Maintain medication and immunization records
Collect and process specimens	Recognize and respond to emergencies
Perform diagnostic tests	Coordinate patient care information with other health care providers
Patient Care	Initiate IV and administer IV medications with appropriate training and as permitted by state law
Adhere to established patient screening procedures	
Obtain patient history and vital signs	
Prepare and maintain examination and treatment areas	

General (transdisciplinary)

Professionalism	**Legal Concepts**	**Instruction**
Project a professional manner and image	Perform within legal and ethical boundaries	Instruct individuals according to their needs
Demonstrate initiative and responsibility	Prepare and maintain medical records	Explain office policies and procedures
Work as a member of the health care team	Document accurately	Teach methods of health promotion and disease prevention
Manage time efficiently	Follow employer's established policies dealing with the health care contract	Locate community resources and disseminate information
Prioritize and perform multiple tasks	Maintain awareness of federal and state health care legislation and regulations	Develop educational materials
Adapt to change	Comply with established risk management and safety procedures	Conduct continuing education activities
Promote the CMA credential	Recognize professional credentialing criteria	**Operational Functions**
Enhance skills through continuing education	Develop and maintain personnel, policy, and procedure manuals*	Perform inventory of supplies and equipment
Treat all patients with compassion and empathy		Perform routine maintenance of administrative and clinical equipment
Promote the practice through positive public relations		Apply computer techniques to support office operations
Communication Skills		Perform personnel management functions
Recognize and respect cultural diversity		Negotiate leases and prices for equipment and supply contracts
Adapt communications to individual's ability to understand		
Use professional telephone technique		
Recognize and respond effectively to verbal, nonverbal, and written communications		
Use medical terminology appropriately		
Utilize electronic technology to receive, organize, prioritize, and transmit information		
Serve as liaison		

Green colored blocks represent skills taught in this textbook.
White colored blocks are additional skills an insurance billing specialist may need.
*Denotes advanced skills.
Reprinted by permission of the American Association of Medical Assistants from the AAMA Role Delineation Study. Occupational Analysis of the Medical Assisting Profession, 2003.

MEDICAL INSURANCE SPECIALIST CERTIFICATE PROGRAM

PROGRAM DESCRIPTION: The Medical Insurance program prepares you for employment in the area of medical insurance and health care claims processing. This program also serves the needs of health care personnel interested in upgrading their professional skills. Training in computerized medical billing, CPT-4 and ICD-9-CM coding, and processing medical insurance claims are included in the curriculum. Students may be enrolled on a full-time or part-time basis, and may complete the program by attending either day or evening classes. Accelerated or fasttrack courses are also available for those wishing to complete this program within a short time period. The program graduates students with marketable skills that will be in demand well into the 21st century. They are employed in hospitals, insurance companies, private medical laboratories, billing bureaus, and doctors' offices. Graduates may apply credits toward other certificate or associate degree programs.

The following courses are included in this program:

First Semester

Medical Terminology	3 Credits
Administrative Medical Office Management	4 Credits
Biology	3 Credits
Typewriting I or Keyboarding	3 Credits
Computer I	2 Credits
	TOTAL 15 Credits

Second Semester

Principles and Applications of Medical Insurance	3 Credits
Current Issues of Medical Insurance	3 Credits
Medical Financial Management	3 Credits
Word Processing	3 Credits
Basic Principles of Composition	3 Credits
	TOTAL 15 Credits

Figure 1–2. Example of a 1-year medical insurance specialist certificate program offered at a community college. Basic coding is taught as a part of the course in Administrative Medical Office Management, and advanced coding is covered in Principles and Applications of Medical Insurance. Biology may be titled Anatomy and Physiology in some colleges. (Reprinted with permission from Community College of Allegheny County, Pittsburgh, PA.)

late to make collection calls. It may be advantageous to both the physician and insurance specialist to vary his or her schedule according to the needs of the practice. In-home or office billing services save a medical practice valuable time, money, and overhead costs because the physician does not have to cover benefits or equipment.

A collector of delinquent accounts is a great asset to a medical practice. This job is for individuals who have current knowledge of state and federal collection laws and interact well with people in person and by telephone. This aspect of financial management and other jobs involving telephone communications are an opportunity for someone who is visually impaired because he or she is usually a good listener when properly and specifically trained. However, special equipment may be necessary to enhance job performance (e.g., Braille keyboard, magnified computer screen, audible scanner, tape recorder). You may contact the American Collectors Association (ACA) in Minneapolis, which

has developed a training program for the visually impaired. Chapter 9 is devoted entirely to the topic of collections.

Qualifications

Attributes

There are many characteristics or qualities that an individual should have to function well as an insurance billing specialist. Strong critical thinking and reading skills with good comprehension are a must. It is important to be a logical and practical thinker as well as a creative problem solver. Being meticulous and neat makes it easier to get the job done at the work station. A person with good organizational skills and who is conscientious and loyal is always an asset to the employer. A person with a curious nature will dig deeper into an issue and not be satisfied with an answer unless the whys and whats are defined. This also helps one to grow while on the job and not become stagnant. This list is by no means complete; maybe you can think of additional attributes that might lead to a more successful career.

Skills

Completing insurance claims encompasses many skills; one needs the following to be proficient:

▶ Solid foundation and working knowledge of medical terminology, including anatomy, physiology, disease, and treatment terms, as well as the meaning of abbreviations.
Application: Interpretation of patient's chart notes and code manuals.
Incorrect: Final diagnosis: ASHD.
Correct: Final diagnosis: Arteriosclerotic heart disease.
It is difficult to locate the diagnostic code using an abbreviation; therefore, you must be able to translate it.

▶ Expert use of procedural and diagnostic code books and other related resources.
Application: Code manuals and other reference books are used to assign accurate codes for each case billed.

▶ Precise reading skills.
Application: Differentiate between a technical description of two different but similar procedures.
Procedure (CPT) Code No. 43352 Esophagostomy *(fistulization of esophagus, external; cervical approach).*
Procedure (CPT) Code No. 43020 Esophagotomy *(cervical approach, with removal of foreign body).*
Note that the additional letter "s" to the surgical procedure in the first part of the example changes the entire procedure.

▶ Basic mathematics.
Application: Total fees on the insurance claim forms and adjust and total accounts. It is essential that these figures be accurate.

▶ Knowledge of medicolegal rules and regulations of various insurance programs.
Application: Avoid filing of claims considered fraudulent or abusive because of code selection and program policies.

▶ Basic typing or keyboarding and computer skills.
Application: Good keyboarding skills and knowledge of computer software programs is essential because the industry increasingly involves electronic claims submission; handwritten claims are a format of the past.

▶ Proficiency in accessing information through the Internet.
Application: Obtain federal, state, and commercial insurance regulations and current information as needed through the Internet. Sign on as a member of a **list service (listserv),** which is a service run from a Web site where questions may be posted.

Find one composed of working coders to obtain answers on how to code complex, rare, or difficult medical cases.

▶ Knowledge of billing and collection techniques.
Application: Use latest billing and collection ideas to keep cash flow constant and avoid delinquent accounts.

▶ Expertise in the legalities of collection on accounts.
Application: Avoid lawsuits by knowing state and federal collection laws as they apply to medical collection of accounts receivable.

▶ Generate insurance claims with speed and accuracy.
Application: If you develop your own business as a medical claims and billing specialist, you may be paid according to how many claims you can generate in an hour. You may charge less for claims that can be done quickly and more for claims that take longer to complete. The faster you become, the more money you earn. Therefore accuracy in selecting the correct codes and speed in completing claims also become marketable skills. Measure your claim productivity for speed and time when you complete the insurance claim forms for this course and see how progressively fast you can get.

Personal Image

To project a professional image, be attentive to apparel and grooming (Fig. 1–3). If a person works at home, the tendency is to dress casually (e.g., blue jeans, sneakers, shorts, tank tops). However, in a work setting, a uniform may be required or business attire that is conservative and stylish but not trendy. For women, this includes a business suit, dress, or skirt of appropriate length; slacks; sweaters; blouses; and dress shoes. For men, a business suit, or dress slacks and jacket, shirt, tie (optional), and dress shoes are appropriate.

It is important that hair be clean and in a style that flatters. Fragrances can be offensive or cause allergies to some clients and patients; therefore, they should not be used. Fingernails should be carefully manicured. Long artificial nails are not considered part of a professional image; clear or muted pleasant-colored polish without glued-on designs or rhinestones is acceptable. For a woman, subdued eye makeup is appropriate for day use.

For either gender, jewelry should be simple, and dangling earrings should be avoided. A professional pin is frequently worn in an office setting and at professional functions. Consult the employer for office policy regarding body piercing and tattoos.

Behavior

There are many aspects to what makes an individual a true professional: getting along with people rates high on the list, as does maintaining confidentiality

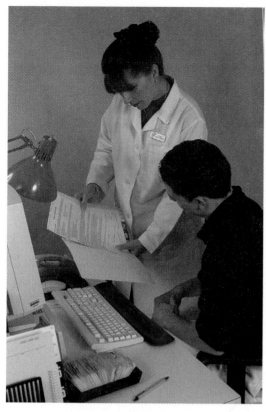

Figure 1-3. Male and female medical personnel who project a clean, fresh, and professional image with appropriate hairstyling.

Figure 1-4. Interaction of insurance billing specialist with patient depicting medical etiquette.

of patients' medical histories and ongoing medical treatment. An insurance billing specialist depends on many co-workers for information needed to bill claims (e.g., the receptionist who collects the patient information). Therefore it is necessary to be a team player and treat patients and co-workers with courtesy and respect. Consider all co-workers' duties as important because they are part of the team helping you obtain the goal of processing the billing and obtaining maximum reimbursement for the patient and physician. Communicate effectively. Be honest, dependable, and on time. Never take part in office gossip or politics. Be willing to do the job and efficient in how you carry it out.

Medical Etiquette

Before beginning work as an insurance billing specialist, it is wise to have a basic knowledge of medical etiquette as it pertains to the medical profession, the insurance industry, and the medical coder (Fig. 1-4). Medical **etiquette** has to do with how medical professionals conduct themselves. Customs, courtesy, and manners of the medical profession can be expressed in three simple words: *consideration for others.*

Several points about medical etiquette bear mentioning:

1. Never keep another physician waiting longer than necessary in the reception room. Usher him or her into the physician's office as soon as it is unoccupied.
2. Always connect another physician who is calling on the telephone to your physician immediately, asking as few questions as possible. The only exception is if you know the physician calling is treating one of your patients and you wish to verify the name to pull the chart for your physician.
3. Follow the basic rules of etiquette with co-workers while working in the office, such as acknowledging people who enter your office or come to your desk by saying, "I'll be with you in a moment."
4. Identify yourself to callers and people you call.
5. Do not use first names until you know it is appropriate to do so.
6. Keep a professional demeanor and maintain a certain amount of formality when interacting with others. Remember to be courteous and always project a professional image.

Medical Ethics

Medical **ethics** are not laws, but standards of conduct generally accepted as moral guides for behavior by which an insurance billing or coding specialist may determine the propriety of his or her conduct in a relationship with patients, the physician, coworkers, the government, and insurance companies. Acting with ethical behavior means carrying out responsibilities with integrity, decency, honesty, competence, consideration, respect, fairness, trust, and courage.

The earliest written code of ethical principles and conduct for the medical profession originated in Babylonia about 2500 BC and is called the Code of Hammurabi. Then about the fifth century BC, Hippocrates, a Greek physician who is known as the Father of Medicine, conceived the Oath of Hippocrates.

In 1980 the **American Medical Association (AMA)** adopted a modern code of ethics called the Principles of Medical Ethics for the benefit of the health professional and to meet the needs of changing times. The Principles of Medical Ethics of the AMA shown in Box 1–1 guide physicians' standards of conduct for honorable behavior in the practice of medicine.

It is the coder's responsibility to inform administration or his or her immediate supervisor if unethical or possibly illegal coding practices are taking place.

Illegal activities are subject to penalties, fines, and/or imprisonment and can result in loss of morale, reputation, and the good will of the community.

Some principles of ethics for the medical assistant and insurance billing specialist are as follows:

▶ Never make critical remarks about a physician to a patient or anyone else.
▶ Maintain dignity; never belittle patients.
▶ Notify your physician if you discover that a patient in your practice may have questionable issues of care, conduct, or treatment with your office or another physician's practice. In certain circumstances, it may be unethical for two physicians to treat the same patient for the same condition.
▶ Maintain a dignified, courteous relationship with all persons in the office: patients, staff, and the physician, as well as with insurance adjusters, pharmaceutical representatives, and others who come into or telephone the office.
▶ Do not make critical statements about the treatment given a patient by another physician.

It is *illegal* to report incorrect information to government-funded programs, such as Medicare, Medicaid, and TRICARE. However, private insurance carriers operate under different laws and it is *unethical, not illegal,* to report incorrect information to private insurance carriers. Incorrect information may damage the individual and the integrity of the database, allow reimbursement for services that should be paid by the patient, or deny payment that should be made by the insurance company.

Some examples of illegal or unethical coding follow:

1. Violating guidelines by using code numbers or modifiers to increase payment when the case documentation does not warrant it.
2. Coding procedures that were not performed for payment.
3. Unbundling services provided into separate codes when one code is available.
4. Failing to code a relevant condition or complication when it is documented in the medical record.
5. Coding a service in such a way that it is paid when usually it is not covered.
6. Coding another condition as the principal diagnosis when the majority of the patient's treatment is for the preexisting condition.

The AAMA has established a code of ethics because some insurance billing specialists also have medical assistant responsibilities. This code is appropriate for all medical assistants, members and nonmembers, regardless of whether they are performing administrative or clinical duties (Fig. 1–5).

In the final analysis, most ethical issues can be reduced to right and wrong with the main focus: to keep in mind the moral dictum to do no harm.

BOX 1–1

Preamble

The medical profession has long subscribed to a body of ethical statements developed primarily for the benefit of the patient.

As a member of the profession, a physician must recognize responsibility not only to patients, but also to society, to other health professionals, and to self. The following Principles adopted by the American Medical Association are not laws, but standards of conduct that define the essentials of honorable behavior for the physician.

   I. A physician shall be dedicated to providing competent medical service with compassion and respect for human dignity.

   II. A physician shall deal honestly with patients and colleagues, and strive to expose those physicians deficient in character or competence, or who engage in fraud or deception.

   III. A physician shall respect the law and also recognize a responsibility to seek changes in those requirements that are contrary to the best interests of the patient.

   IV. A physician shall respect the rights of patients, of colleagues and of other health professionals, and shall safeguard patient confidences within the constraints of the law.

   V. A physician shall continue to study, apply and advance scientific knowledge, make relevant information available to patients, colleagues, and the public, obtain consultation, and use the talents of other health professionals when indicated.

   VI. A physician shall, in the provision of appropriate patient care, except in emergencies, be free to choose whom to serve, with whom to associate, and the environment in which to provide medical services.

   VII. A physician shall recognize a responsibility to participate in activities contributing to an improved community.

AMERICAN ASSOCIATION OF MEDICAL ASSISTANTS, INC. CODE OF ETHICS

The code of ethics of AAMA shall set forth principles of ethical and moral conduct as they relate to the medical profession and the particular practice of medical assisting.

Members of AAMA dedicated to the conscientious pursuit of their profession, and thus desiring to merit the high regard of the entire medical profession and the respect of the general public which they serve, do pledge themselves to strive always to:

A. render service with full respect for the dignity of humanity;

B. respect confidential information obtained through employment unless legally authorized or required by responsible performance of duty to divulge such information;

C. uphold the honor and high principles of the profession and accept its disciplines;

D. seek to continually improve the knowledge and skills of medical assistants for the benefit of patients and professional colleagues;

E. participate in additional service activities aimed toward improving the health and well-being of the community.

Figure 1–5. Code of ethics for medical assistants as established and printed in the bylaws of the American Association of Medical Assistants (AAMA), revised October 2000, Chicago, IL. (Reprinted with permission of the American Association of Medical Assistants.)

HIPAA Compliance Alert

Confidential Communication

The insurance billing specialist must be responsible for maintaining confidentiality of communication when working with patients and their medical records. **Confidential communication** is a privileged communication that may be disclosed only with the patient's permission. Everything you see, hear, or read about patients remains confidential and does not leave the office. Never talk about patients or data contained in medical records where others may overhear. Some employers require employees to sign a confidentiality agreement (Fig. 1–6). Such agreements should be updated periodically to address issues raised by the use of new technologies.

Privileged Information

Privileged information is related to the treatment and progress of the patient. The patient must sign an authorization to release this information or selected facts from the medical record. Some states have passed laws allowing certain test results (e.g., disclosure of the presence of the human immunodeficiency virus [HIV] or alcohol or substance abuse) and other information to be placed separate from the patient's medical record. A special authorization form is used to release this information.

Nonprivileged Information

Nonprivileged information consists of ordinary facts unrelated to treatment of the patient, including the patient's name, city of residence, and dates of admission or discharge. This information must be sensitized against unauthorized disclosure under the Privacy section of the Health Insurance Portability and Accountability Act (HIPAA). The patient's authorization is not needed for the purposes of treatment, payment, or health care operations, unless the record is in a specialty hospital (e.g., alcohol treatment) or a special service unit of a general hospital (e.g., psychiatric unit). Professional judgment is required. The information is disclosed on a legitimate need-to-know basis, meaning that the medical data should be revealed to the attending physician because the information may have some effect on the treatment of the patient.

Right to Privacy

All patients have a right to privacy. It is important never to discuss patient information other than with the physician, an insurance company, or individual who has been authorized by the patient. If a telephone inquiry is made about a patient, ask the caller to put the request in writing and include the patient's signed authorization. If the caller refuses, have the physician return the call. If a relative telephones asking about a patient, have the physician return the call. When you telephone a patient about an insurance matter and reach voice mail, use care in the choice of words when leaving the message in the event the call was inadvertently received at the wrong number. Leave your name, the office name, and return telephone number. Never attempt to interpret a report or provide information about the outcome of laboratory or other diagnostic tests to the patient. Let the physician do it (Fig. 1–7).

Do not discuss a patient with acquaintances, yours or the patient's. Do not leave patients' records or appointment books exposed on your desk. If confidential documents are on your desk that patients can easily see as they walk by, either turn the documents over or lock them in a secure drawer when you leave your desk, even if you are gone for only a few moments. If patient information is on your computer, either turn the screen off or save it on disk, lock the disk in a secure

place, and clear the information from the screen. Never leave a computer screen with patient information visible, even for a moment, if another patient may see the data. Properly dispose of notes, papers, and memos by using a shredding device. Be careful when using the copying machine because it is easy to forget to remove the original insurance claim or medical record from the document glass. Use common sense and follow the guidelines mentioned in this chapter to help you keep your professional credibility and integrity.

Exceptions to the Right to Privacy

The few exceptions to the right of privacy and privileged communication are patient records of industrial cases (e.g., workers' compensation), reports of communicable diseases, child abuse,

---

EMPLOYEE CONFIDENTIALITY STATEMENT

As an employee of <u>ABC Clinic, Inc.</u> (employer), having been trained as an insurance billing specialist with employee responsibilities and authorization to access personal medical and health information, and as a condition of my employment, I agree to the following:

A. I recognize that I am responsible for complying with the Health Insurance Portability and Accountability Act (HIPAA) of 1996 policies regarding confidentiality of patients' information, which, if I violate, may lead to immediate dismissal from employment and, depending on state laws, criminal prosecution.

B. I will treat all information received during the course of my employment, which relates to the patients, as confidential and privileged information.

C. I will not access patient information unless I must obtain the information to perform my job duties.

D. I will not disclose information regarding my employer's patients to any person or entity, other than that necessary to perform my job duties, and as permitted under the employer's HIPAA policies.

E. I will not access any of my employer's computer systems that currently exist or may exist in the future using a password other than my own.

F. I will safeguard my computer password and will not show it in public.

G. I will not allow anyone, including other employees, to use my password to access computer files.

H. I will log off of the computer immediately after I finish using it.

I. I will not use e-mail to transmit patient information unless instructed to do so by my employer's HIPAA privacy officer.

J. I will not take patient information from my employer's premises in hard copy or electronic form without permission from my employer's HIPAA privacy officer.

K. Upon termination of my employment, I agree to continue to maintain the confidentiality of any information learned while an employee and agree to relinquish office keys, access cards, or any other device that provides access to the provider or its information.

Mary Doe
Signature

Mary Doe
Print name

September 14, 20XX
Date

Brenda Shield
Witness

Figure 1–6.   An example of an employee confidentiality agreement that may be used by an employer when he or she is hiring an insurance billing specialist.

litigation by the state or federal government. An insurance biller always should check with his or her physician–employer to see whether he or she is included in the medical professional liability insurance policy otherwise known as malpractice insurance. If not included, he or she could be sued as individuals. It is the physician's responsibility to make certain all staff members are protected.

Figure 1–7. Insurance billing specialist consulting with the supervisor/office manager about office policies regarding release of a patient's medical record.

gunshot wounds and stabbings resulting from criminal actions, and diseases and ailments of newborns and infants. Also, any medical information obtained by a Medicare insurance carrier is subject to disclosure to the beneficiary to whom that information pertains. Medical information cannot be accepted by a Medicare insurance carrier from physicians on a confidential basis without the patient's knowledge, either expressed or implied. Expressed and implied contracts are defined in detail in the next chapter. Even if medical information is marked "Confidential," the Medicare insurance carrier must still disclose it to the beneficiary or his or her representative on request, either directly or through designated professional medical personnel.

Professional Liability

Employer Liability

As mentioned, insurance billing specialists can be either self-employed or employed by physicians, clinics, or hospitals. Physicians are legally responsible for their own conduct and any actions of their employees performed within the context of their employment. This is referred to as vicarious liability, also known as **respondeat superior,** which literally means "let the master answer." However, this does not mean that an employee cannot be sued or brought to trial. Actions of the insurance biller may have a definite legal ramification on the employer, depending on the situation. For example, if an employee knowingly submits a fraudulent Medicare or Medicaid claim at the direction of the employer and subsequently the business is audited, both the employer and employee can be brought into

HIPAA Compliance Alert

Fraud is knowing and intentional deception (lying) or misrepresentation that could result in some unauthorized benefit to the deceiver or some other person. It is a felony, and if detected, financial or prison penalties can be imposed, depending on the laws of the state. It is important to tell the patient how services will be billed to avoid possible fraud and abuse audits. For example, a hospitalized patient is not always aware that the attending physician has requested a consultation, which will result in a separate bill, or that a simple invasive procedure done in the physician's office may be referred to as a surgical procedure on the monthly statement because the code number is obtained from the surgical section of the procedure code book. If a Medicare or TRICARE case is involved, then fraud becomes a federal offense and federal laws apply. TRICARE is a three-option managed health care program offered to spouses and dependents of service personnel with uniform benefits and fees implemented nationwide by the federal government. Claims are audited by state and federal agencies as well as private insurance companies.

Fraud usually involves careful planning. Some examples are shown in Box 1–2. Two types of intent must be proved: intent to agree to practice a fraudulent act and intent to commit a major offense. When an insurance billing specialist completes the insurance claim form with billing information that does not reflect the true situation, he or she may be found guilty of conspiring to commit fraud. It is not necessary to receive monetary profit from a fraudulent act to be judged guilty in participating in a criminal conspiracy.

Unintentional fraud may occur when completing the CMS-1500 insurance claim form. For example, in a Medicare case, if benefits are assigned to the physician and the statement "signature on file" is inserted in Block 12 and the records do not contain the patient's authorization to file the claim on his or her behalf, this is a federal violation. The insurance billing specialist must verify that the authorization is for the insurance company in question. To prevent this

Examples of Fraud

Bill for services or supplies not provided (**phantom billing** or invoice ghosting) or for an office visit if a patient fails to keep an appointment and is not notified ahead of time that this is office policy.

- Alter fees on a claim form to obtain higher payment.
- Forgive the deductible or copayment.
- Alter medical records to generate fraudulent payments.
- Leave relevant information off a claim (e.g., failing to reveal whether a spouse has health insurance coverage through an employer).
- Upcode (e.g., submitting a code for a complex fracture when the patient had a simple fracture).
- Shorten (e.g., dispensing less medication than billed for).
- Split billing schemes (e.g., billing procedures over a period of days when all treatment occurred during one visit).
- Use another person's insurance card in obtaining medical care.
- Change a date of service.
- Post adjustments to generate fraudulent payments.
- Solicit, offer, or receive a kickback, bribe, or rebate in return for referring a patient to a physician, physical therapist, or pharmacy or for referring a patient to obtain any item or service that may be paid for in full or in part by Medicare or Medicaid.
- Restate the diagnosis to obtain insurance benefits or better payment.
- Apply deliberately for duplicate payment (e.g., billing Medicare twice, billing Medicare and the beneficiary for the same service, or billing Medicare and another insurer in an attempt to get paid twice).
- Unbundle or explode charge (e.g., billing a multichannel laboratory test as if individual tests were performed).
- Collusion between a physician and a carrier employee when the claim is assigned (if the physician deliberately overbilled for services, overpayments could be generated with little awareness on the part of the Medicare beneficiary).
- Bills based on gang visits (e.g., a physician visits nursing home and bills for 20 visits without furnishing any specific service to, or on behalf of, individual patients).
- Knowingly bill for the same item or service more than once or when another party bills the federal health care program for an item or service also billed by the physician.

3. Send a memorandum to the office manager or employer stating your concern if no change is made.
4. Maintain a written audit trail with dated memoranda.
5. Do not discuss the problem with anyone who is not immediately involved.

Abuse

Abuse means incidents or practices by physicians, not usually considered fraudulent, which are inconsistent with accepted sound medical business or fiscal practices. Some examples are shown in Box 1–3.

In subsequent chapters about various insurance programs, additional information about fraud and abuse pertinent to each program is given.

Employee Liability

Errors and omissions insurance is protection against loss of monies caused by failure through error or unintentional omission on the part of the individual or service submitting the insurance claim. Some physicians contract with a billing service to handle

Examples of Medical Billing Abuse

- Refer excessively to other providers for unnecessary services, also called **ping-ponging**
- Charge excessively for services or supplies.
- Perform a battery of diagnostic tests when only a few are required for services, also called **churning.**
- Violate Medicare's physician participating agreement.
- Call patients back for repeated and unnecessary follow-up visits, also called **yo-yoing.**
- Bill Medicare beneficiaries at a higher rate than other patients.
- Submit bills to Medicare instead of to third party payers (e.g., claims for injury from an automobile accident, in a store, or the workplace).
- Breach assignment agreement.
- Fail to make required refunds when services are not reasonable and necessary.
- Require patients to contract to pay their physician's full charges, in excess of the Medicare charge limits.
- Require a patient to waive rights to have the physician submit claims to Medicare and obligate a patient to pay privately for Medicare-covered services.
- Require patients to pay for services not previously billed, including telephone calls with the physician, prescription refills, and medical conferences with other professionals.
- Require patients to sign a global waiver agreeing to pay privately for all services that Medicare will not cover, and using these waivers to obligate patients to pay separately for a service that Medicare covers as part of a package or related procedures.

problem from occurring in Medicare cases, obtain lifetime authorizations for the Medicare fiscal intermediary and for the patient's supplemental (Medigap) insurance company.

A coder or biller who has knowledge of fraud or abuse should take the following measures:

1. Notify the provider both personally and with a dated, written memorandum.
2. Document the false statement or representation of the material fact.

Figure 1–8. Explanation of an audit trail to review monies received by a medical practice and monies deposited into a bank account.

claims submission, and some agreements contain a clause stating that the physician will hold the company harmless from "liability resulting from claims submitted by the service for any account." This means the physician is responsible for mistakes made by the billing service. Thus errors and omissions insurance would not be needed in this instance. If a physician asks the insurance biller to do something that is the least bit questionable, such as write off patient balances for certain patients automatically, then make sure you have a legal document or signed waiver of liability relieving you of the responsibility for such actions.

Scope of Practice

An individual who works as a CAP acts as an informal representative of patients (policyholders and Medicare beneficiaries), helping to obtain insurance reimbursement. A CAP reviews and analyzes existing or potential policies; renders advice; and offers counseling, recommendations, and information. A CAP may not interpret insurance policies or act as an attorney. The legal ability of a CAP to represent a policyholder is limited. When a claim cannot be resolved after a denied claim has been appealed to the insurance company, the CAP must be careful in rendering a personal opinion or advising clients that they have a right to pursue legal action. In some states, a CAP could be acting outside the scope of the law (scope of practice) by giving advice to clients on legal issues, even if licensed as an attorney but not practicing law full time. If the client wishes to take legal action, it is his or her responsibility to find a competent attorney specializing in contract law and insurance. In some states, giving an insured client advice on purchase or discontinuance of insurance policies is construed as being an insurance agent.

A number of states require CAPs to be licensed, depending on the services rendered to clients. CAPs who perform only the clerical function of filing health insurance claims do not have to be licensed. Check with your state's Department of Insurance and insurance commissioner (see Chapter 8 and Appendix A) to determine whether you should be licensed.

If working as a CAP who does not handle checks or cash, inquire about an errors and omissions insurance policy by contacting the Alliance of Claims Assistance Professionals (ACAP).* When employed as a medical assistant who is submitting insurance claims, information on professional liability insurance may be obtained from the American Association of Medical Assistants, Inc.†

Embezzlement

Embezzlement means stealing money that has been entrusted in one's care. In many cases of insurance claims embezzlement, the physician is held as the guilty party and has to pay huge sums of money to the insurance carrier when false claims are submitted by an employee. If an undiscovered embezzler leaves the employer and you are hired to replace that person, you could be accused some months down the line of doing something that you did not do. Take precautions as an employee to protect the medical practice.

Precautions for Financial Protection

To prevent stealing from a medical practice, these office policies should be routinely practiced. Ask the physician or supervisor to initial all entries about adjustments, discounts, and write-offs on either the ledger cards or day sheets. If a patient owes money to the physician that is uncollectable and adjusted off, be sure the physician dates and initials the ledger that shows the closed account. Ask the physician to occasionally check an entire day's records (the patient sign-in log and appointment schedule) with the day sheet, ledger cards, encounter forms, and cash receipt slips. A daily trial balance of accounts receivable including daily deposit of checks and cash can assist in reviewing monthly income and aid in discovering embezzlement. Review the monthly bank statement to verify that all deposits tally with the receipts for each business day (Fig. 1–8). If poor

---

*ACAP, 873 Brentwood Drive, West Chicago, IL 60185-3743.
†20 North Wacker Drive, Ste. 1575, Chicago, IL 60606.

bookkeeping and record keeping are noticed, bring this to your employer's attention.

All insurance payment checks should be immediately stamped within the endorsement area on the back "For Deposit Only," called a *restrictive endorsement*. The bank should be given instructions never to cash a check made payable to the physician.

Encounter forms, transaction slips, and cash receipts should be prenumbered. If a mistake is made when completing one, void it and keep the slip as part of the financial records. It is especially imperative to have prenumbered insurance forms if the physician's practice allows the use of a signature stamp when submitting claims. Thus filing of fictitious insurance claims can be totally eliminated.

As a precautionary measure, always type your initials at the bottom left or top right corner of the insurance claim forms that you submit. This will indicate to office personnel who did the work. Always retain the Explanation of Benefits or Remittance Advice documents that accompany checks from insurance companies.

Only a few of the many precautions for protection are mentioned here. Embezzlement can occur in accounts receivable or accounts payable, with petty cash or use of computers, and in various other aspects of a medical practice.

Bonding

Insurance billers, CAPs, or anyone who handles checks or cash should be bonded or insured. A practice that carries a fidelity or *honesty bond* means that an insurance company will prosecute any guilty employees. **Bonding** is an insurance contract by which a bonding agency guarantees payment of a certain sum to a physician in case of a financial loss caused by an employee or some contingency over which the payee has no control. Bonding methods for a practice with three or more office employees are:

▶ A **position-schedule bond** covers a designated position, such as a bookkeeper or nurse, rather than a named individual. If one employee in a category leaves, the replacement is automatically covered.

▶ A **blanket-position bond** provides coverage for all employees regardless of job title.

▶ A **personal bond** provides coverage for those who handle large sums of money. A thorough background investigation is required.

Such bonding contracts may be obtained from a casualty insurance agent or broker. Bond coverage should be reviewed periodically with the insurance agent to ensure that coverage is keeping pace with the expansion of the business.

Future Challenges

As you begin your study to become an insurance billing specialist remember that you are expected to profitably manage a medical practice's financial affairs or patient accounts; otherwise, you will not be considered qualified for this position. In subsequent chapters you will learn the important information and skills to help you achieve this goal. You will be expected to:

▶ Know billing regulations for each insurance program and managed care plan in which the practice is a participant.

▶ State various insurance rules about treatment and referral of patients.

▶ Become proficient in computer skills and various medical software.

▶ Learn electronic billing software and the variances of each payer.

▶ Develop diagnostic and procedural coding expertise.

▶ Know how to interpret remittance advice summary reports, explanation of benefit documents, or both.

▶ Attain bookkeeping skills necessary to post, interpret, and manage patient accounts.

▶ Stay up-to-date by reading the latest journals and newsletters and attending seminars on billing and coding.

▶ Cross-train so you become familiar with other aspects of the medical practice.

| RESOURCES ON THE INTERNET |

 For a list of educational and training requirements of the AHIMA diagnostic and procedure coding competencies for outpatient services and diagnostic coding and reporting requirements for physician billing visit the Web site:

http://www.ahima.org

For up-to-date information on fraud alerts, visit the Office of the Inspector General and Federal Bureau of Investigation Web site:

http://www.cms.gov

The national hotline of the Office of the Inspector General is 1-800-HHS-TIPS. To obtain current information on fraud in the Medicaid program, visit the Web sites:

http://www.cms.hhs.gov/providers/fraud
http://www.cms.hhs.gov/states/fraud

STUDENT ASSIGNMENT LIST

✔ Read Introduction in the *Workbook*, which explains how you will be working as an insurance billing specialist during this course.

✔ Study Chapter 1.

✔ Answer the review questions in the *Workbook* to reinforce the theory learned in this chapter and help prepare for a future test.

✔ Complete the assignments in the *Workbook* to help develop critical thinking and writing skills. As you proceed through the assignments in the *Workbook*, you will broaden your knowledge of medical terminology as well as gain an entry-level skill in diagnostic and procedural coding and insurance claim completion.

✔ Turn to the Glossary at the end of this textbook for a further understanding of the Key Terms used in this chapter.

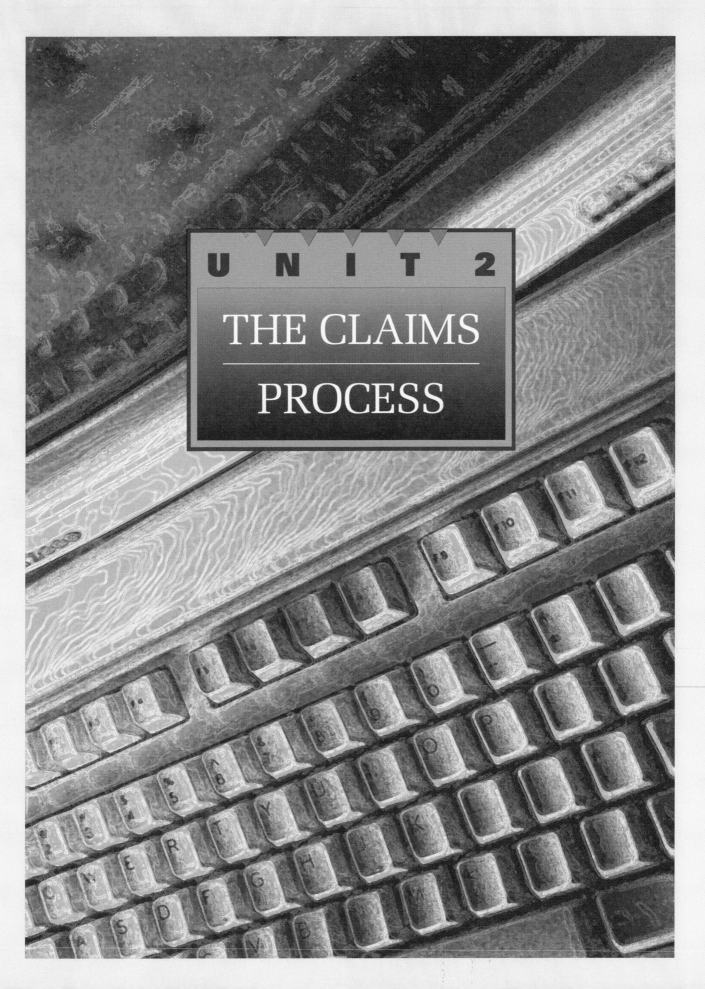

UNIT 2

THE CLAIMS

PROCESS

Basics of Health
Insurance

2

CHAPTER OUTLINE

Determine Fees

Bookkeeping—Financial
  Accounting Record

Insurance Form

Provider's Handwritten
  Signature

Office Pending File and
  Insurance Claims Register

Mailing the Claim Form

Insurance Payments

Monthly Statement

*Procedure: Posting to a
  Patient's Financial
  Accounting Record*

Keeping Up to Date

OBJECTIVES*

After reading this chapter you
should be able to:

- Describe the history of
  insurance in the United
  States.
- Distinguish among the three
  major classes of health
  insurance contracts.
- State four concepts of a
  valid insurance contract.
- Explain the difference
  between an implied and an
  expressed physician–
  patient contract.
- Describe in general terms
  the important federal, state,
  and private health
  insurance plans.
- Define common insurance
  terms.
- List four actions to prevent
  problems when given
  signature authorization for
  insurance claims.
- Handle insurance claims in
  the physician's office to
  obtain payment and
  minimize their rejection by
  insurance carriers.
- Explain the process of a
  physician-based insurance
  claim from obtaining
  patient data, claim form
  completion, insurance
  carrier processing, and
  payment received.
- Establish an insurance
  claims register or log.
- Determine the appropriate
  questions to ask a patient
  for a complete patient
  record.
- List the functions of a
  tickler file.
- Record proper information
  and post to the patient's
  ledger after claims submission and payment received.

KEY TERMS

applicant

assignment

blanket contract

capitation

The Civilian Health and
  Medical Program of the
  Department of Veterans
  Affairs (CHAMPVA)

claim

coinsurance

Competitive Medical Plan

conditionally renewable

contract

daysheet

deductible

disability income insurance

electronic signature

eligibility

emancipated minor

encounter form

exclusions

exclusive provider
  organization (EPO)

expressed contract

extended

financial accounting record

foundation for medical care
  (FMC)

guaranteed renewable

guarantor

health insurance

health maintenance
  organization (HMO)

high risk

implied contract

indemnity

independent or individual
  practice association (IPA)

Continued.

---

*Performance objectives and exercises for hands-on practical experience for this chapter
  appear in the *Workbook*.

KEY TERMS—cont'd

insured

major medical

Maternal and Child Health
   Program (MCHP)

Medicaid (MCD)

Medicare (M)

Medicare/Medicaid
   (Medi-Medi)

member

noncancelable policy

nonparticipating provider
   (nonpar)

optionally renewable

participating provider (par)

patient registration form

personal insurance

point-of-service (POS) plan

post

preauthorization

precertification

predetermination

preferred provider
   organization (PPO)

premium

running balance

State Disability Insurance
   (SDI)

subscriber

TRICARE

Unemployment
   Compensation
   Disability (UCD) or State
   Disability Insurance (SDI)

Veterans Affairs (VA)
   outpatient clinic

Workers' compensation
   (WC) insurance

History

The insurance industry is among the world's largest businesses. In the 1800s, life insurance came to be widely offered. Health insurance began to be available in the early part of this century because anyone can have an accident or become ill unexpectedly, leading to large expenses. **Health insurance** is a contract between a policyholder and an insurance carrier or government program to reimburse the policyholder for all or a portion of the cost of medically necessary treatment or preventive care rendered by health care professionals. Its main purpose was to help offset some of the high costs accrued during sickness or when an injury occurred.

During the Renaissance, when Italian traders insured valuable cargo to be shipped across the Mediterranean, they recorded the insurance agreement on a piece of folded paper called a *polizza*. English merchants adapted the term to their insurance practices, modifying the pronunciation to suit the Anglo-Saxon tongue, resulting in the word "policy."

Insurance in the United States

In 1850 the Franklin Health Assurance Company of Massachusetts began offering insurance for nonfatal injury. About 10 years later, the Travelers Insurance Company of Hartford marketed a plan that is similar to today's health insurance. Many other companies began writing health insurance policies, and in 1911 Montgomery Ward and Company offered benefits to its ill or injured employees. This was the first group plan. These commercial plans paid only when an individual was sick or received an injury.

By the 1960s, most private insurance companies sold policies that included hospital care, surgical fees, and physicians' services. In addition to those benefits, many plans now offer catastrophic health insurance coverage, preventive care, dental insurance, disability income insurance, and long-term care and home health care insurance for the chronically ill, disabled, and developmentally disabled. State insurance laws regulate the way policies are written and minimum requirements of coverage.

In the past decade, medical care costs have escalated, forcing insurance companies to reduce their forms of coverage and the federal government to adopt cost-containment policies for the Medicare, Medicaid, and TRICARE programs (TRICARE is a three-option managed health care program offered to spouses and dependents of service personnel with uniform benefits and fees implemented nationwide by the federal government). Although managed care began in the 1930s when Kaiser Industries provided health care to their employees, it was not until the 1980s that many types of plans sprung up across the nation to control the cost of medical care and help those who could not afford health insurance. Because individual needs vary, each patient may have a different type of health insurance policy with various benefits. Patients may be covered under different types of private, state, or federal programs.

Legal Principles of Insurance

The role of a medical insurance billing specialist is to complete the insurance claim accurately and facilitate claims submission so that reimbursement is received quickly. However, before developing the skill of coding and completing insurance claim forms, it is necessary to know frequently encountered legal problems and how to handle them. Legal situations occur daily in the performance of these job duties and involve confidentiality of medical records, accurate insurance claim completion, fraud and abuse issues, credit and collection laws, and so on. An insurance biller cannot escape liability by pleading ignorance. It cannot be overemphasized that keeping up to date on health care plan policies and procedures is essential. Most legal issues of health insurance claims fall under civil law. Insurance is regulated by state laws and is not considered a federally regulated industry.

It is important for an insurance billing specialist to know some basic insurance terms, understand basic insurance concepts, and have a working knowledge of medical terminology.

Insurance Contracts

The first legal item in the business of handling medical insurance is the insurance contract (also known as a policy). There is no standard health insurance contract. Individuals who take out a policy receive an original document composed by the insuring company.

There are four considerations involved in drawing up a valid insurance contract:

1. The person must be a mentally competent adult and not under the influence of drugs or alcohol.
2. The insurance company must make an offer (the signed application), and the person must accept the offer (issuance of the policy), without concealment or misrepresentation of facts on the application.
3. An exchange of value (the first premium payment) submitted with the application, known as a *consideration,* must be present.
4. A legal purpose must exist, which is an insurable interest in the case of a health insurance policy. This means that the policyholder expects to continue in good health, but that the insurance policy will provide something of value if an accident or illness strikes.

A policy can be challenged when a fraudulent statement is made by the subscriber. A *challenged policy* means that coverage may not be in effect. After a policy has been in force for 2 years (3 years in some states), a policy becomes *incontestable* (may not be challenged). If the time limit has passed and a policy is guaranteed renewable, the policy becomes incontestable even if false statements were made on the application. Further information and additional insurance terminology concerning contracts is provided in detail in Chapter 3.

Physician–Patient Contracts and Financial Obligation

Implied or Expressed Contracts

A physician and his or her staff must be aware of the physician's obligations to each patient, and his or her liabilities in regard to service, and the patient's obligations to the physician. The physician–patient contract begins when the physician accepts the patient and agrees to treat him or her. This action can be either an implied or expressed contract. An **implied contract** is defined as not manifested by direct words but implied or deduced from the circumstance, the general language, or the conduct of the patient. For example, if Mary Johnson goes to Dr. Doe's office and Dr. Doe gives Ms. Johnson professional services that she accepts, this is an implied contract. If the patient is unconscious when treatment is rendered, treatment is based on an implied-in-fact contract. An **expressed contract** can be verbal or written. However, most physician–patient contracts are implied.

Private Patients

Although a patient carries medical insurance, the contract for treatment is between the physician and the patient. The patient is liable for the entire bill. The insurance is meant to help offset the expense.

Guarantor

A **guarantor** is an individual who promises to pay the medical bill by signing a form agreeing to pay or who accepts treatment, which constitutes an expressed promise. Usually, a patient is the guarantor and must be of legal age (18 or 21 years, depending on state law). Most laws governing financial responsibility state that a husband is responsible for his wife's debts; a wife is not always responsible for her husband's debts. However, this always depends on the way the contractual application reads and individual state laws. A father is ordinarily responsible for his children's debts if they are minors and are not emancipated (Fig. 2–1). Children may or may not be responsible for the debts of their parents, depending on the circumstances.

Emancipated Minor

An **emancipated minor** is a person younger than 18 years of age who lives independently, is totally self-supporting, is married or divorced, is a parent even if not married, or is in the military and possesses decision-making rights. College students living away from home even when financially dependent on

Figure 2–1. Receptionist explaining where a guarantor's signature goes on a patient registration form for the medical services rendered to a family member.

their parents are considered emancipated. Parents are not liable for the medical expenses incurred by an emancipated minor. The patient record should contain the minor's signed statement that he or she is on his or her own.

Managed Care Patients

A physician under contract to a managed care plan may or may not periodically receive an updated list of current enrollees. The physician is obligated to see those individuals who are enrolled should one of them call for an appointment. However, the contract for treatment occurs when the patient is first seen. If the physician no longer wishes to treat a patient on a managed care plan, termination is handled according to the same method used when discharging patients who are insured under private insurance or state or government programs. The method of how to do this is explained in the next chapter.

An insurance specialist should be able to read and interpret managed care plan contracts, but if the specialist is unable to interpret these matters, professional assistance from the physician's attorney, the medical practice's accountant, or the managed care plan should be sought. He or she should understand billing and collection requirements and track payments made by the managed care plan.

Employment and Disability Examinations

Courts in most jurisdictions have ruled that there is no physician–patient relationship in an employment or disability examination and the doctor does not owe a duty of care to the person being examined, mainly because the insurance company is requesting the examination and the patient is not seeking the medical services of the physician.

Workers' Compensation Patients

Workers' compensation cases involve a person being injured on the job. These cases may be referred to as industrial accidents or illnesses. In these types of cases, the contract exists between the physician and the insurance company. When there is a dispute as to whether the injured party was hurt at work, a Patient Agreement form (Chapter 14, Fig. 14–17) must be signed by the patient who agrees to pay the physician's fees if the case is declared to be non-work-related.

The Insurance Policy

Insurance policies are complex and contain a great deal of technical jargon. This can cause misunderstanding by patients or anyone trying to obtain information from the policy. Basic health insurance coverage includes benefits for hospital, surgical, and other medical expenses. **Major medical** or *extended benefits* contracts are designed to offset large medical expenses caused by prolonged illness or serious injury. Some of these policies include coverage for *extended care* or *skilled nursing facility* benefits. The **insured** is known as a **subscriber** or, in some insurance programs, a **member**, *policyholder,* or *recipient* and may not necessarily be the patient seen for the medical service. The insured is the individual (enrollee) or organization protected in case of loss under the terms of an insurance policy. In group insurance, the employer is considered the insured, and the employees are the risks. However, when completing an insurance claim form, the covered employee is listed as the insured. A policy might also include *dependents* of the insured. Generally, this term refers to the spouse and children of the insured, but under some contracts, parents, other family members, and domestic partners may be covered as dependents.

Policy Application

Before a policy is issued, the insurance company decides whether it will enter into a contract with the **applicant** who is applying for the insurance coverage. Information is obtained about the applicant so the company can decide whether to accept the risk. Generally, the application form has two sections: part one contains basic information about the application, and part two concerns the health of the individual.

An insurance policy is a legally enforceable agreement, or **contract**. If a policy is issued, the applicant becomes part of the insurance contract or plan. The policy becomes effective only after the company offers the policy and the person accepts it and then pays the initial premium (Fig. 2–2). If a premium is

Figure 2–2. Insurance billing specialist searching in an index file for an insurance company's telephone number to inquire about a patient's coverage under an insurance policy.

paid at the time the application is submitted, then the insurance coverage can be put into force before the policy is delivered. Depending on the laws in some states, the applicant also can have temporary conditional insurance if the agent issues a specific type of receipt.

Policy Renewal Provisions

Health insurance policies may have renewal provisions written into the policy stating the circumstances when the company may refuse to renew, may cancel coverage, or may increase the premium. There are five classifications: (1) cancelable, (2) optionally renewable, (3) conditionally renewable, (4) guaranteed renewable, and (5) noncancelable.

▶ A renewable provision in a *cancelable* policy grants the insurer the right to cancel the policy at any time and for any reason. The company notifies the insured that the policy is canceled and refunds any advance premium the policyholder has paid. In some states, this type of policy is illegal.

▶ In an **optionally renewable** policy, the insurer has the right to refuse to renew the policy on a date (premium due or anniversary date) specified in the contract and may add coverage limitations or increase premium rates.

▶ **Conditionally renewable** policies grant the insurer a limited right to refuse to renew a health insurance policy at the end of a premium payment period. Reasons stated in the policy may be due to age, employment status, or both but not because of the insured's health status.

▶ The **guaranteed renewable** classification is desirable because the insurer is required to renew the policy as long as premium payments are made. However, these policies may have age limits of 60, 65, or 70 years, or they may be renewable for life.

▶ In a **noncancelable policy,** the insurer cannot increase premium rates and must renew the policy until the insured reaches the age specified in the contract. Some disability income policies have noncancelable terms.

Policy Terms

To keep the insurance in force, a person must pay a monthly, quarterly, or annual fee called a **premium.** If the premium is not paid, a *grace period* of 10 to 30 days is usually given before insurance coverage ceases. Many states have laws that allow the insurance company to apply the provider's payment to the patient's insurance premium. This forces the provider to recoup payment from the patient. In addition, usually a **deductible** (a specific amount of money) must be paid each year before the policy benefits begin. The higher the deductible is, the lower the cost of the policy. Most policies have a **coinsurance** or *cost-sharing* requirement, which means the insured will assume a percentage of the fee (e.g., 20%) or pay a specific dollar amount (e.g., $5 or $10) for covered services. Managed care plans and state and federal programs refer to this as *copayment* (copay). It is not advisable to routinely waive copayments because most insurance companies do not tolerate this practice. If the provider is audited, the federal government can assess penalties for not collecting copayments for patients seen under the Medicare program. However, if copayments are waived on a case-by-case basis, as in a courtesy discount, there should not be any problems with commercial insurance carriers or Medicare. Generally, deductibles and copayments should be collected at the time of service with the exception of the Medicare program, which does not recommend collecting the deductible in advance from the beneficiary.

Health insurance policies consider an *accident* to be an unforeseen and unintended event. Some policies cover accidents occurring from the first day the policy is in force. Others may contain an *elimination period* or a *waiting period* before benefits for sickness or accident become payable.

It is the patient's responsibility to give a written notice of **claim** to the insurance company within a certain number of days, known as a *time limit.* However, in most cases, the claim is filed for the patient by the provider of professional services. The insurance billing specialist must be able to abstract proper information from the patient record, which is used to code the diagnoses and services rendered; to complete an insurance claim form; to make entries (post) to a patient's financial accounting record (ledger); and to follow up on unpaid claims. If any one of these procedures is not done properly, correct reimbursement or payment (also called **indemnity**) from the insurance *carrier* will not be generated. Follow-up on unpaid claims is made by contacting the claims representative, called an *adjuster.* If the payment is to go directly from the insurance company to the physician, then the patient must sign a document granting permission.

Coordination of Benefits

A *coordination of benefits* statement is included in most policies and contracts with providers.

When the patient has more than one insurance policy, this clause requires insurance companies to coordinate the reimbursement of benefits to determine which carrier is going to be primary and which secondary, thus preventing the duplication or overlapping of payments for the same medical expense. The combination of payments from the primary and secondary carrier cannot be more that the amount of the provider's charges (Example 2–1).

Most state legislatures have adopted the *birthday law,* which is a change in the order of determination of coordination of benefits regarding primary and secondary carriers for dependent children. Rather than the father's insurance being primary, the father's *or* mother's carrier may be primary. The health plan of the person whose birthday (month and day, *not* year) falls earlier in the calendar year pays first, and the plan of the other person covering the dependent is the secondary payer. If both mother and father have the same birthday, the plan of the person who has had coverage longer is the primary payer. If one of the two plans has not adopted this birthday rule (i.e., if one plan is in another state), the rules of the plan without the birthday rule determine which plan is primary and which secondary. In cases of divorce, the plan of the parent with custody of the children is the primary payer unless the court determines differently and it is so stated in the divorce settlement.

Sometimes the mother brings the child for treatment and tells you the divorce decree states that the father has to pay for the medical bills. Remember that you are not an enforcer of court laws. The divorce decree is between the parents of the child. Have the mother pay the bill at the time of service. She can be reimbursed by the father. If he does not, she can go back to court for resolution.

Unions and companies that self-insure their employees do not fall under this birthday law. The states that do not have birthday laws are Georgia, Hawaii, Idaho, Massachusetts, Mississippi, Vermont, Virginia, and Washington, DC.

Finally, a carrier may delay a claim, stating they are attempting to coordinate benefits with the other carrier. This may take 90 days or more to resolve and may be a stall tactic. The provider should contact the carrier to demand payment or bill the patient if allowed.

General Policy Limitations

Health insurance policies contain **exclusions**—some more than others. If a person has an injury or illness that is excluded in his or her policy, then there is no insurance coverage for that injury or illness. These exclusions or limitations of the policy could be such factors as losses resulting from military service, attempted suicide, or self-inflicted injuries; losses caused by an injury on the job; pregnancy; and so on. Be aware that some insurance policies may state that a procedure or service is not covered (excluded) when the state law says the procedure is a "mandated benefit." Some examples are reconstructive breast surgery after mastectomy, surgical procedures affecting the upper and lower jawbones, and infertility coverage under group policies. Thus further investigation is necessary beyond reading the policy.

Many policies do not provide benefits for conditions that existed and were treated before the policy was issued; these are called *preexisting conditions.* In some instances, such conditions might be covered after a specified period of time after the issuance of the policy. Some policies have a *waiver* or *rider,* which is an attachment to a policy that modifies clauses and provisions of the policy by either adding coverage or excluding certain illnesses or disabilities that would otherwise be covered. Generally, waivers are used to eliminate benefits for specific preexisting conditions.

Case Management Requirements

Preapproval

Many private insurance carriers and prepaid health plans have certain requirements that must be met before they approve hospital admissions, inpatient or outpatient surgeries, and elective procedures. First, **eligibility** requirements must be obtained.

> **EXAMPLE 2–1**
>
> Mr. Smith has Insurance A and Insurance B. The claim is for $100. The claim is sent to Insurance A. Insurance A allows $80 for the procedure and pays $80. The claim is then sent to Insurance B. Insurance B also allows $80 for the procedure. The claim that was sent to Insurance B was not for $100, but for the remaining $20. The $20 is within the amount allowed by Insurance B; therefore, Insurance B pays the $20. Some carriers try to play by their own rules by stating that because Insurance A paid $80 and the $80 equals the amount Insurance B pays, Insurance B will pay no more for the claim. These rules were established by the National Association of Insurance Commissioners and approved by every State Insurance Commissioner. Therefore be observant of insurance claims like this.

These are conditions or qualifying factors that must be met before the patient receives benefits (medical services) under a specified insurance plan, government program, or managed care plan. The carrier can refuse to pay part or the entire fee if these requirements are not met. **Precertification** refers to discovering whether a treatment (surgery, hospitalization, tests) is covered under a patient's contract. **Preauthorization** relates not only to whether a service or procedure is covered, but also to finding out whether it is medically necessary. **Predetermination** means discovering the maximum dollar amount that the carrier will pay for surgery, consulting services, radiology procedures, and so on.

Obtain precertification or predetermination when a procedure is tentatively scheduled. The information that may be required to obtain precertification approval by fax or telephone is shown in Fig. 2–3. Use the form shown in Fig. 2–4 to obtain predetermination by mail. See Chapter 10, Fig. 10–1 for an example of a preauthorization form. This form also can be used to document the information received when verifying the patient's insurance coverage by telephone. It should become part of the patient's record and used for reference when billing future insurance claims.

After the information is received from the insurance carrier, give the patient an estimate of fees for

Figure 2–3. Insurance precertification form. This form can be faxed to the insurance company or used when telephoning to obtain approval for hospitalization under a patient's insurance policy or managed care plan.

COLLEGE CLINIC
4567 Broad Avenue
Woodland Hills, XY 12345-0000

Phone: 555/486-9002   Fax: 555/590-2189

Insurance Precertification Form

Date: 5/4/XX

To: Insurance Carrier ___Cal-Net Care___   From: ___Janet___ Office Mgr.
    Address ___9900 Baker Street___
            ___Los Angeles, CA 90067___

Check those that apply: Admission certification ✔   Outpatient___ Inpatient ✔
                           Surgery certification ✔   Emergency situation ✔

Patient's name ___Ronald Stranton___   Date of Birth: ___4-14-49___
Patient's address ___639 Cedar Street___   Sex: Male ✔ Female ___
                  ___Woodland Hills, XY 12345___   Social Security No. ___527-XX-7250___
Insured's Name ___Same___   Policy Group ID No. ___A59___
Insured's Address _____   Employer: ___Aerostar Aviation___

Treating physician ___Clarence Cutler, M.D.___   NPI #: ___430 500 47XX___
Primary Care Physician ___Gerald Practon, M.D.___ NPI #: ___462 7889 7XX___

Name of Hospital ___College Hospital___   Admission Date: ___5/4/XX___
                                                   Estimated Length of Stay: ___3-5 d___
Admitting Diagnosis ___Volvulus___   Diagnosis Code: ___560.2___
Complicating conditions to substantiate need for inpatient hospitalization_____
                        ___Complete bowel obstruction_____
Date current illness or injury began ___5/2/XX___
Procedure/surgery to be done ___Reduction of Volvulus___ Procedure code ___44050___

Second opinion needed   Yes ___ No ✔ Date performed _____

Telephone precertification: ___Emergency Cert. 5/4/XX___
Name of representative certifying___McKenzie Kwan___
Direct-dial telephone number of representative ___1-800-463-9000 ext. 227___

Reason(s) for denial _____
Certification approved   Yes ✔ No___ Certification approval No. ___69874___
Authorization for services Yes ✔ No___ Authorization No. ___69874E___

Note: The information contained in this facsimile message is confidential and privileged information intended only for the use of the individual or entity named above. If the reader of this message is not the intended recipient, you are hereby notified that any dissemination, distribution, or copying of this communication is strictly prohibited. If you have received this communication in error, please immediately notify me by telephone and return the original facsimile to me via the U.S. Postal Service. Thank you.

COLLEGE CLINIC
4567 Broad Avenue
Woodland Hills, XY 12345-0001

Phone: 555/486-9002   Fax: 555/487-8976

INSURANCE PREDETERMINATION FORM

Perry Cardi, MD
Physician

Patient: __Leslee Austin__   Telephone # __(555) 486-8452__
Address: __209 Refugio Road__   Date of Birth __04-07-44__
City __Woodland Hills__   State __XY__   ZIP __12345-0001__
Social Security # __629-XX-9260__   Accident   Yes ____ No __X__
Insurance Company __American Insurance__   Member # __Am 45692__
Insurance Co. Address __4040 Broadway Ave__   Group # __123P__
__Valley Vista, XY 12345__   Telephone # __(555) 238-5000__
Policy holder __Leslee Austin__
Relationship to insured: Self __X__ Spouse ____ Child ____ Other ____
Type of coverage: HMO __X__ PPO ____ 80/20 ____ 70/30 ____ Other: ____
Procedure/Service __Cardioversion (CPT 92960)__
Diagnosis __Atrial fibrillation (ICD–9–CM 427.31)__

- -

BENEFITS:
Coverage effective date: From __02/01/XX__ To __01/31/XX__   Maximum benefit or benefit limitation: __$1,000,000 lifetime__
Pre-existing exclusions: __Lupus erythematosus__   Second opinion requirements: Yes ____ No __X__
Major medical   Yes __X__ No ____   Precertification/Preauthorization Yes __X__ No ____
Deductible   Yes ____ No __X__ Amount $ _____   Reference # __432786__
  Per family: Yes ____ No __X__ Amount $ _____   Authorized by: __Lucille Vasquez__
  Deductible paid to date: Amount $ _____
Out of pocket expense limit: Amount $ _____
                              Per: _____

- -

COVERAGE: COVERAGE DETAILS AND LIMITS
  Procedures/Services
    Office visits   YES __X__ NO _____   __Physical exam; one per year__
    Consultations   YES __X__ NO _____
    ER visits   YES __X__ NO _____
    X-ray   YES __X__ NO _____
    Laboratory   YES __X__ NO _____   __Need authorization__
    Office surgery   YES __X__ NO _____   __Need authorization__
    Hospital surgery   YES __X__ NO _____
    Anesthesia   YES X   NO   __Need authorization__
  DME
    Physician payment schedule: RVS ____ RBRVS ____ UCR ____ Other __X__

- -

  Payment sent to: Provider __X__ Patient _____ Time limit after submission? __30 days__
  Verification by: __Karen Reynolds__   Date: __07-14-XX__

Figure 2–4. Insurance predetermination form. This form can be sent to the insurance company to find out the maximum dollar amount that will be paid for primary surgery, consulting services, postoperative care, and so on.

the proposed surgery. An example of suggested wording for a letter is given in Fig. 2–5. This written estimate makes collection quicker and easier.

Choice of Health Insurance

There are three ways in which a person can obtain health insurance: (1) take out insurance through a group plan (contract or policy), (2) pay the premium on an individual basis, or (3) enroll in a prepaid health plan.

Group Contract

A *group contract* is any insurance plan by which a group of employees (and their eligible dependents) or other homogeneous group is insured under a single policy issued to their employer or leader, with individual certificates given to each insured individual or family unit. A group policy usually provides better benefits and offers lower premiums. However, the coverage for each person in the group is the same. If a new employee declines enrollment, he or she must sign a waiver stating this fact.

COLLEGE CLINIC
4567 Broad Avenue
Woodland Hills, XY 12345-0000

Phone: 555/486-9002   Fax: 555/487-8976

Current date

Patient's name
Address
City, State, ZIP code

Dear

This letter gives you an estimate of the fees for your proposed surgery. Verification of coverage and benefit information has been obtained from your insurance company. Listed are your benefits for the proposed surgical expenses and the estimated balance after your insurance carrier pays.

Surgical procedure	Craniotomy		
Date of surgery	February 21, 20XX		
Name of hospital	College Hospital		
Hospital address	4500 Broad Ave., Woodland Hills, XY 12345		

		Insurance pays	Estimated balance
Surgeon's fee	2548.09	1344.24	1203.85
Preoperative visit			
Preoperative tests			

You have a policy deductible of $1000   which___ has ✓ has not been met.

The surgery requires the use of an anesthesiologist, assistant surgeon, and a pathologist. These physicians will bill you separately for their services. The hospital will also bill you separately.

This office will file your insurance claim for the surgical procedure, so the insurance payment should come directly to us. If the insurance carrier sends you the payment, then you are responsible to get the payment to this office within five days. Your balance after surgery should be approximately $1203.85. You are responsible for any remaining balance after our office receives the insurance payment.

Thank you for choosing our medical practice. If you have any questions, please call me.

Sincerely,

Karen Martinez, CMA
Administrative Medical Assistant

Figure 2–5. Sample letter to a patient supplying an estimate of the fees for proposed surgery.

Conversion Privilege

Many physicians can obtain comprehensive group coverage through plans sponsored by the professional organizations to which they belong. Sometimes this is called a **blanket contract.** If the person leaves the employer or organization or the group contract is terminated, the insured may continue the same or lesser coverage under an individual policy if the group contract has a *conversion privilege.*

Usually, conversion from a group policy to an individual policy increases the premium and reduces the benefits. However, if the person has a condition that would make him or her ineligible for coverage or is a case considered at **high risk,** it is advantageous to convert to an individual policy because no physical examination is required; therefore a preexisting condition cannot be excluded.

Income Continuation Benefits

According to the Consolidated Omnibus Budget Reconciliation Act of 1985 (COBRA), when an employee is laid off from a company with 20 or more workers, federal law requires that the group health insurance coverage be extended to the employee and his or her dependents at group rates for up to 18 months. This also applies to those workers who lose coverage because of reduced work hours. In the case of death of a covered employee, divorced or widowed spouse, or employee entitled to Medicare, the extension of coverage may be for 36 months. However, the employee must pay for the group policy; this is known as *income continuation benefits.* See the section on COBRA in Chapter 11 for additional information on this topic.

Medical Savings Accounts

The Health Insurance Portability and Accountability Act (HIPAA) of 1996 was federal legislation created to: (1) expand efforts to combat fraud and abuse, as learned in the previous chapter, (2) protect workers and their families so they can obtain and maintain health insurance if they change or lose their jobs, and (3) establish a medical savings account pilot project. A *medical savings account* (MSA) is a type of tax-free savings account that allows individuals and their employers to set aside money to pay for health care expenses. An employer can set up an MSA for his or her employees and make an annual contribution to the MSA, which is tax-deductible for both employer and employee. MSA balances accumulate from year to year tax free, but unused funds may not be carried over in a flex account (another type of MSA). Earned interest is not taxed. MSAs are portable, allowing individuals to take their MSA with them when they change jobs or relocate. When health care services are provided, the patient files a claim to receive reimbursement from these funds and uses the explanation of benefits (EOB) from the insurance company as documentation. Processing of insurance claims with large deductibles (e.g.., over $1,000), even though you know the insurance company will not be paying for the services, is necessary so that the patient/employee may submit documentation and recoup funds from the MSA. It also may be necessary to provide EOB documents from the insurance company to patients who do not receive them for this same purpose.

Individual Contract

Any insurance plan issued to an individual (and dependents) is called an *individual contract.* Usually, this type of policy has a higher premium, and often the benefits are less than those obtainable under a group health insurance plan. Sometimes this is called **personal insurance**.

Prepaid Health Plan

This is a program of health care in which a specified set of health benefits is provided for a subscriber or enrolled group of subscribers who pay a yearly fee or fixed periodic payments. Providers of services are paid by capitation. **Capitation** is a system of payment used by managed care plans in which physicians and hospitals are paid a fixed, per capita amount for each patient enrolled over a stated period of time, regardless of the type and number of services provided. For additional information on this topic, refer to Chapter 10.

Types of Health Insurance Coverage

Many forms of health insurance coverage are currently in effect in the United States. These are referred to as third party payers (private insurance, government plans, managed care contracts, and workers' compensation). A brief explanation of the programs to be discussed in this text is given here, but for an in-depth study, refer to the appropriate chapters that follow.

The Civilian Health and Medical Program of the Department of Veterans Affairs (CHAMPVA)

The **Civilian Health and Medical Program of the Department of Veterans Affairs (CHAMPVA),** administered by the Department of Veterans Affairs, shares the medical bills of spouses and children of veterans with total, permanent, service-connected disabilities or of the surviving spouses and children of veterans who died as a result of service-connected disabilities (Chapter 13).

Competitive Medical Plan

Competitive Medical Plan (CMP) is a type of managed care organization created by the 1982 Tax Equity and Fiscal Responsibility Act (TEFRA). This federal legislation allows for enrollment of Medicare beneficiaries into managed care plans (Chapter 11).

Disability Income Insurance

Disability income insurance is a form of health insurance that provides periodic payments to replace income when the insured is unable to work as a result of illness, injury, or disease (Chapter 15). This type of insurance should not be confused with workers' compensation, because those injuries must be work related.

Exclusive Provider Organization

An **exclusive provider organization (EPO)** is a type of managed health care plan in whic subscriber members are eligible for benefits only when they use the services of a limited network of providers. EPOs combine features of both HMOs and PPOs. Employers agree not to enter into an agreement with any other plan for coverage of eligible employees. EPOs are regulated under state health insurance laws (Chapter 10).

Foundation for Medical Care

A **foundation for medical care (FMC)** is an organization of physicians, sponsored by a state or local medical association, concerned with the development and delivery of medical services and the cost of health care (Chapter 10).

Health Maintenance Organization

A **health maintenance organization (HMO)** is an organization that provides a wide range of comprehensive health care services for a specified group at a fixed periodic payment. The emphasis is on preventive care. Physicians are reimbursed by capitation. An HMO can be sponsored by the government, medical schools, hospitals, employers, labor unions, consumer groups, insurance companies, or hospital medical plans (Chapter 10).

Independent or Individual Practice Association

An **independent or individual practice association (IPA)** is a type of managed care plan in which a program administrator contracts with a number of physicians who agree to provide treatment to subscribers in their own offices or clinics for a fixed capitation payment per month. Subscribers to IPA plans have limited or no choice of physician. IPA physicians continue to see their fee-for-service patients (Chapter 10).

Maternal and Child Health Program

A **maternal and child health program (MCHP)** is a state and federal program for children who are younger than 21 years of age and have special health care needs. It assists parents with financial planning and may assume part or all of the costs of treatment, depending on the child's condition and the family's resources (Chapter 12).

Medicaid

Medicaid (MCD) is a program sponsored jointly by federal, state, and local governments to provide health care benefits to indigent persons on welfare (public assistance), aged individuals who meet certain financial requirements, and the disabled. Some states have expanded coverage for other medically needy individuals who meet special state-determined criteria. Coverage and benefits vary widely from state to state. In California, this program is known as *Medi-Cal* (Chapter 12 and Appendix C).

Medicare

Medicare (M) is a hospital insurance system (Part A), supplementary medical insurance (Part B), and Medicare Plus (+) Choice Program (Part C) for those at 65 years of age, created by the 1965 Amendments to the Social Security Act and operated under the provisions of the act. Benefits are also extended to certain disabled people (e.g., totally disabled or blind) and coverage and payment are provided for those requiring kidney dialysis and kidney transplant services (Chapters 11 and 12).

Medicare/Medicaid

 Medicare/Medicaid is a program that covers those persons eligible for both Medicare and Medicaid (Chapters 11 and 12). In some regions, this program is referred to as Medi-Medi.

Point-of-Service Plan

A **point-of-service (POS) plan** is a managed care plan consisting of a network of physicians and hospitals that provides an insurance company or employer with discounts on its services. Patients can refer themselves to a specialist or see a nonprogram provider for a higher copayment (Chapter 10).

Preferred Provider Organization

A variation of a managed care plan is a **preferred provider organization (PPO).** This is a form of contract medicine by which a large employer (e.g., hospitals or physicians) or any organization that can produce a large number of patients (e.g., union trusts or insurance companies) contracts with a hospital or a group of physicians to offer medical care at a reduced rate (Chapter 10).

TRICARE

A government-sponsored program called **TRICARE** provides non–military hospital and medical services for spouses of active service personnel, dependents of active service personnel, retired service personnel and their dependents, and dependents of members who died on active duty. Active duty service members (ADSMs) are not eligible for TRICARE, but they have benefits such as TRICARE Prime in which the Department of Defense (DoD) covers all allowable charges for medically necessary care (Chapter 13).

Unemployment Compensation Disability

Unemployment Compensation Disability (UCD) or State Disability Insurance (SDI) is insurance that covers off-the-job injury or sickness and is paid for by deductions from a person's paycheck. This program is administered by a state agency in only five states and Puerto Rico (Chapter 15).

Veterans Affairs Outpatient Clinic

 Veterans Affairs (VA) outpatient clinic is where medical and dental services are rendered to a veteran who has a service-related disability (Chapter 13).

Workers' Compensation Insurance

 Workers' compensation (WC) insurance is a contract that insures a person against on-the-job injury or illness. The employer pays the premium for his or her employees (Chapter 14).

Examples of Insurance Billing

Sometimes, it is difficult to comprehend the full scale of insurance billing. As an example of total medical billing, six cases are presented to help you understand the entire billing picture from simple to complex.

Case 1: A new patient comes in with complaints of a sore throat and an infected nail. Evaluation and management (E/M) services are discussed in detail in Chapter 5.

The physician's office bills for:

Evaluation and management services

Penicillin injection

Office surgery for infected nail

Sterile surgical tray (may or may not be billed depending on insurance carrier)

Case 2: A patient comes in because of an accident and has complaints that require evaluation and management services, x-ray films, and laboratory studies (urinalysis) performed in the physician's office.

The physician's office bills for:

Evaluation and management services

X-ray studies (including interpretation) and laboratory tests (urinalysis; including interpretation)

Case 3: A patient is seen by the family physician after office hours in the hospital emergency department.

The physician's office bills for evaluation and management services.

The hospital bills for hospital (outpatient) emergency department services (use and supplies).

Case 4: A physician sends a patient's Papanicolaou smear to a private clinical laboratory.

The physician's office bills for evaluation and management services.

The laboratory bills for the Papanicolaou smear.

Case 5: A patient is sent to a local hospital for an upper gastrointestinal radiographic series. An x-ray technician takes the films in the hospital, and a privately owned radiologic group does the interpretation.

The hospital bills for the technical component of the upper gastrointestinal x-ray series (use of equipment).

The radiologic group bills for the professional component of the upper gastrointestinal x-ray series (the interpretation).

Case 6: A patient is seen in the office and is immediately hospitalized for surgery.

The physician's office bills for initial hospital admission (evaluation and management services) and surgical procedure (e.g., hysterectomy). (The physician is a surgeon.)

The assistant surgeon bills for assisting the surgeon during hysterectomy. (Some insurance carriers do not allow payment.)

The anesthesiologist bills for anesthesia administered during hysterectomy.

The hospital (inpatient) bills for hospital room, operating room, anesthesia supplies, medications, x-ray films, laboratory tests, and medical and surgical supplies (dressings, intravenous lines). The hospital (inpatient) might also bill for blood for transfusions, electrocardiogram, radiation therapy, and respiratory therapy.

A medical assistant or insurance billing specialist in the offices of the attending physician, assistant surgeon, anesthesiologist, radiologic group, and private clinical laboratory submits an itemized statement and/or insurance claim form or gives the patient the necessary information to submit his or her own claim to the insurance company. *Exception:* Generally, Medicare patients may not submit their own claims for physician or hospital services. Exceptions are mentioned in Chapter 11.

In the hospital and hospital emergency department, a member of the hospital staff inputs services into a central computer system that produces an itemized statement and completed insurance claim form via computer to be submitted to the insurance carrier. Hospital billing is explained in Chapter 16.

P R O C E D U R E : Handling and Processing Insurance Claims

You must be friendly and courteous when handling insurance claims in order to maintain a harmonious physician–patient relationship. Collections often can be significantly improved and simplified if the patient feels free to discuss personal financial problems at any time and is educated regarding the physician's fees.

There are four basic methods of processing insurance claims for a medical practice: (1) manually preparing claims for submission, (2) in-office electronic filing by fax or computer, (3) contracting with an outside service bureau to prepare and submit the claims manually or electronically, or (4) use of a telecommunications networking system. The fourth method is a system in which a computer is networked to another computer at another site so that the patient's insurance information is available to generate the insurance claim. This method may be used by an outside billing service or may be used when a medical practice has two or three offices and all billing is accomplished at one site.

In the use of any of these methods, the basic steps (Fig. 2–6, *A* and *B*) in handling and processing insurance claims are as follows:

1. Preregistration—Patient Registration Form: Some medical practices either preregister a new patient during the initial telephone call or a designated staff member may contact the patient before the appointment time. It is a good idea to give instructions on how to get to the office and ask the patient to arrive early. This allows time to collect vital statistics and insurance information and discuss the patient's responsibility with respect to payment policies. The patient may be sent an informative brochure with a patient registration form and a letter confirming the appointment. A patient registration form also may be called a *patient information form* or *intake sheet* (Figs. 2–7 and 2–8). It may be developed by the physician and personalized for his or her own use or may be a generic form purchased from a medical supply company.

If the patient has a medical problem that makes it difficult to complete the form, such as rheumatoid arthritis of the hands or limited vision, then the

Figure 2–6. A, Basic steps in handling an insurance claim.

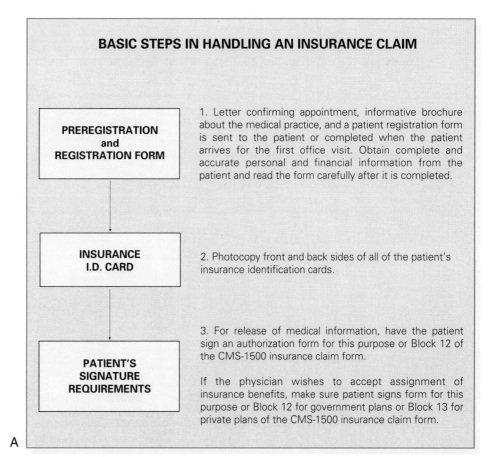

BASIC STEPS IN HANDLING AN INSURANCE CLAIM

PREREGISTRATION and REGISTRATION FORM

1. Letter confirming appointment, informative brochure about the medical practice, and a patient registration form is sent to the patient or completed when the patient arrives for the first office visit. Obtain complete and accurate personal and financial information from the patient and read the form carefully after it is completed.

INSURANCE I.D. CARD

2. Photocopy front and back sides of all of the patient's insurance identification cards.

PATIENT'S SIGNATURE REQUIREMENTS

3. For release of medical information, have the patient sign an authorization form for this purpose or Block 12 of the CMS-1500 insurance claim form.

If the physician wishes to accept assignment of insurance benefits, make sure patient signs form for this purpose or Block 12 for government plans or Block 13 for private plans of the CMS-1500 insurance claim form.

A

Continued.

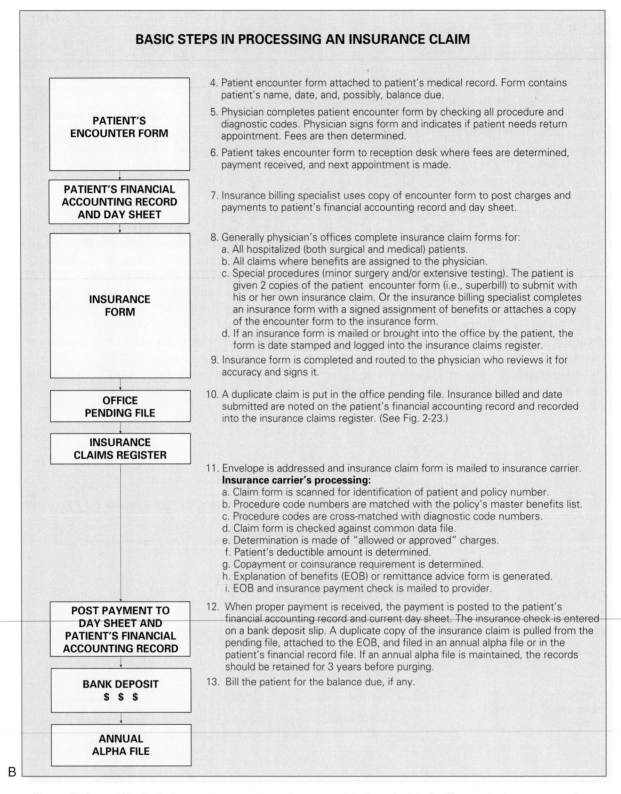

BASIC STEPS IN PROCESSING AN INSURANCE CLAIM

PATIENT'S ENCOUNTER FORM

4. Patient encounter form attached to patient's medical record. Form contains patient's name, date, and, possibly, balance due.

5. Physician completes patient encounter form by checking all procedure and diagnostic codes. Physician signs form and indicates if patient needs return appointment. Fees are then determined.

6. Patient takes encounter form to reception desk where fees are determined, payment received, and next appointment is made.

PATIENT'S FINANCIAL ACCOUNTING RECORD AND DAY SHEET

7. Insurance billing specialist uses copy of encounter form to post charges and payments to patient's financial accounting record and day sheet.

INSURANCE FORM

8. Generally physician's offices complete insurance claim forms for:
   a. All hospitalized (both surgical and medical) patients.
   b. All claims where benefits are assigned to the physician.
   c. Special procedures (minor surgery and/or extensive testing). The patient is given 2 copies of the patient encounter form (i.e., superbill) to submit with his or her own insurance claim. Or the insurance billing specialist completes an insurance form with a signed assignment of benefits or attaches a copy of the encounter form to the insurance form.
   d. If an insurance form is mailed or brought into the office by the patient, the form is date stamped and logged into the insurance claims register.

9. Insurance form is completed and routed to the physician who reviews it for accuracy and signs it.

OFFICE PENDING FILE

10. A duplicate claim is put in the office pending file. Insurance billed and date submitted are noted on the patient's financial accounting record and recorded into the insurance claims register. (See Fig. 2-23.)

INSURANCE CLAIMS REGISTER

11. Envelope is addressed and insurance claim form is mailed to insurance carrier. **Insurance carrier's processing:**
    a. Claim form is scanned for identification of patient and policy number.
    b. Procedure code numbers are matched with the policy's master benefits list.
    c. Procedure codes are cross-matched with diagnostic code numbers.
    d. Claim form is checked against common data file.
    e. Determination is made of "allowed or approved" charges.
    f. Patient's deductible amount is determined.
    g. Copayment or coinsurance requirement is determined.
    h. Explanation of benefits (EOB) or remittance advice form is generated.
    i. EOB and insurance payment check is mailed to provider.

POST PAYMENT TO DAY SHEET AND PATIENT'S FINANCIAL ACCOUNTING RECORD

12. When proper payment is received, the payment is posted to the patient's financial accounting record and current day sheet. The insurance check is entered on a bank deposit slip. A duplicate copy of the insurance claim is pulled from the pending file, attached to the EOB, and filed in an annual alpha file or in the patient's financial record file. If an annual alpha file is maintained, the records should be retained for 3 years before purging.

BANK DEPOSIT $ $ $

13. Bill the patient for the balance due, if any.

ANNUAL ALPHA FILE

B

Figure 2–6, cont'd. B, Basic steps in processing an insurance claim in a physician's office, to the insurance carrier, by the insurance company, and after payment is received.

insurance billing specialist may have to interview the patient and fill in the necessary data. Obtain *complete* information on a new patient by using a form that contains information pertinent to credit and collections. This information must be *accurate.* Instruct the patient to fill in all spaces and indicate N/A (not applicable) if an item does not apply. If the form is returned with blank spaces, assist the patient in completing them. Verify insurance and all other information that may have changed at each visit,

Insurance cards copied ☒
Date: Jan. 20, 20XX

Patient Registration Information

Account #: 84516
Insurance #: H-550-64-5172-02
Co-Payment : $OV $10 ER $50

Please PRINT AND complete ALL sections below!

Is your condition the result of a work injury? YES (NO) An auto accident? YES (NO)
Date of injury: _____

PATIENT'S PERSONAL INFORMATION Marital status ☐ Single ☒ Married ☐ Divorced ☐ Widowed
Sex: ☐ Male ☒ Female
Name: _____ FUHR _____ LINDA _____ L.
    last name   first name   initial
Street Address: 3070 Tipper Street ___ (Apt # 4) City: Oxnard ___ State: CA Zip: 93030
Home phone:(555)276-0101 Work phone:(555)372-1151 Social Security # 550-XX-5172
Date of Birth: 11 /05 /65 Driver's License: (State & Number) G0075012
Employer/Name of School Electronic Data Systems ___ ☒Full Time ☐Part Time
Spouse's Name: FUHR ___ GERALD ___ T. ___ Spouse's Work phone:(555) 921-0075
    last name   first name   initial
How do you wish to be addressed? LINDA ___ Social Security # ___ 545-XX-2771

PATIENT'S/ RESPONSIBLE PARTY INFORMATION
Responsible party: GERALD T. FUHR ___ Date of Birth: 06-15-64
Relationship to patient: ☐ Self ☒Spouse ☐Other ___ Social Security # 545-XX-2771
Responsible party's home phone:(555) 276-0101 ___ Work phone:(555)921-0075
    Address: 3070 Tipper Street ___ (Apt # 4) City: Oxnard ___ State: CA Zip: 93030
Employer's Name: General Electric ___ Phone number:(555) 485-0121
    Address: 317 East Main ___ City: Oxnard ___ State: CA Zip: 93030
    Your occupation: Technician
Spouse's Employer's Name: Electronic Data Systems ___ Spouse's Work phone:(555)372-1151
    Address: 2700 West 5th Street ___ City: Oxnard ___ State: CA Zip: 93030

PATIENT'S INSURANCE INFORMATION Please present insurance cards to receptionist.
PRIMARY insurance company's name: ABC Insurance Company
Insurance address: P.O. Box 12340 ___ City: Fresno ___ State: CA Zip: 93765
Name of insured: Linda L. Fuhr ___ Date of Birth:11/05/65 Relationship to insured: ☒Self ☐Spouse ☐Other ☐Child
Insurance ID number: H-550-XX-5172-02 ___ Group number: 17098-020-00004
SECONDARY insurance company's name: None
Insurance address: ___ City: ___ State: ___ Zip: ___
Name of insured: ___ Date of Birth: ___ Relationship to insured: ☐Self ☐Spouse ☐Other ☐Child
Insurance ID number: ___ Group number: ___
Check if appropriate: ☐Medigap policy ☐Retiree coverage

PATIENT'S REFERRAL INFORMATION   (Please circle one)
Referred by: Margaret Taylor (Mrs. W. T.) If referred by a friend, may we thank her or him?(Yes) No
Name(s) of other physician(s) who care for you: Jason Smythe, MD

EMERGENCY CONTACT
Name of person not living with you:Hannah Gildea ___ Relationship: Aunt
Address: 4621 Lucretia Avenue ___ City: Oxnard ___ State: CA Zip: 93030
Phone number (home):(555) 274-0132 ___ Phone number (work):(___) ___

Assignment of Benefits • Financial Agreement

I hereby give lifetime authorization for payment of insurance benefits be made directly to Gerald Practon, MD, and any assisting physicians, for services rendered. I understand that I am financially responsible for all charges whether or not they are covered by insurance. In the event of default, I agree to pay all costs of collection, and reasonable attorney's fees. I hereby authorize this healthcare provider to release all information necessary to secure the payment of benefits.
I further agree that a photocopy of this agreement shall be as valid as the original.
Date: Jan 20, 20XX Your signature: *Linda L Fuhr*
Method of payment: ☐ Cash ☒ Check ☐Credit Card

Figure 2–7. Patient registration information form showing a comprehensive listing of personal and financial information obtained from the patient on his or her first visit to the office. (Courtesy of Bibbero Systems, Inc., Petaluma, CA.
Phone: 800-242-2376;
Fax: 800-242-9330;
www.bibbero.com.)

because patients may transfer from one insurance plan to another, move, or change jobs. This may be done by giving the patient either an update form or a copy of the previously completed patient registration form and asking him or her to correct any incorrect data in red (Fig. 2–9). Established patients may have changed employers or gotten married or divorced.

The following facts should be recorded:
◗ Name: first, middle initial, and last. The name should be identical to the one on the insurance identification card. (Some pediatric patients do not have the same last name as their parents or stepparents. An insurance check usually is received with the policyholder's name, and it is time-consuming to find

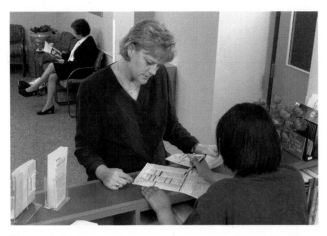

Figure 2–8. Receptionist giving instructions to a patient on how to complete the patient registration form.

and give credit to the patient's account. If a computer system is used, cross-reference the name or Social Security number so that when you call up the policyholder's name, the patient's name also appears. If a manual system is used, keep an alphabetical card index of parental or billing names that also lists each patient's name.)

❱ Street address, including apartment number, ZIP code, and telephone number with area code.

❱ Business address, telephone number with extension, and occupation.

❱ Date of birth (recorded on insurance forms as eight digits, e.g., January 2, 1936 is written as 01-02-1936).

❱ Person responsible for account (guarantor) or insured's name.

Figure 2–9. Patient information update form showing questions to ask the patient for updating a previous patient registration information form. (Courtesy of Professional Filing Systems, Inc., Atlanta, GA.)

PATIENT INFORMATION UPDATE

Welcome, we are delighted to see you again!
Please take a few minutes to help us update our records.

Name __Linda__   __L.__   __Fuhr__   Today's Date __6-30-XX__
           FIRST   MIDDLE   LAST

1. Has your name changed since your last visit here? ___Yes __X__ No
   If yes, what was your old name? __N/A__
   What name do you use for health insurance if different from above?__N/A__

2. If you have a new or different address since your initial visit here, please indicate below:
   __2201 West Klein Street__
   __Oxnard, CA 93033__

3. Has your marital status changed? ___Yes __X__ No

4. Has your telephone number changed?__X__Yes
   Please indicate your correct telephone number ____555-401-7600____

5. Has your employment changed? ___Yes __X__ No
   Please indicate your new employer name and address:
   __N/A__

   New employer telephone #:_____

6. Have you changed health insurance companies? ___Yes __X__ No
   If yes, please indicate your new health insurance carrier and address.
   Primary _____N/A_____   Secondary _____N/A_____

   Group Nos. _____   Group Nos. _____
   Subscriber Nos. _____   Subscriber nos. _____

7. Who is responsible for this bill? __Gerald T. Fuhr__

8. Please note any change in your health since your last visit?
   Illness _____
   Accident _____
   Allergies _____
   Medications being taken __Thyroid__

   Other _____

9. Signature __Linda L Fuhr__

PATIENT INFORMATION UPDATE

▶ Social Security number.

▶ Spouse's name and occupation.

▶ Referring physician's name or other referral source.

▶ Driver's license number.

▶ Emergency contact (close relative or friend with name, address, and telephone number).

▶ Insurance billing information: All insurance company names, addresses, and policy and group numbers. This is important because of the coordination of benefits clause written into some health insurance policies. Elderly patients are given the option of joining managed care programs and are allowed to switch every 30 days. Always ask each elderly patient whether he or she is covered by traditional Medicare or a Medicare HMO. A good patient information sheet has space where this information can be written in by the patient.

2. Insurance Identification Card: Always copy front and back sides of the patient's insurance card and date the photocopy (Fig. 2–10). Sometimes the reverse

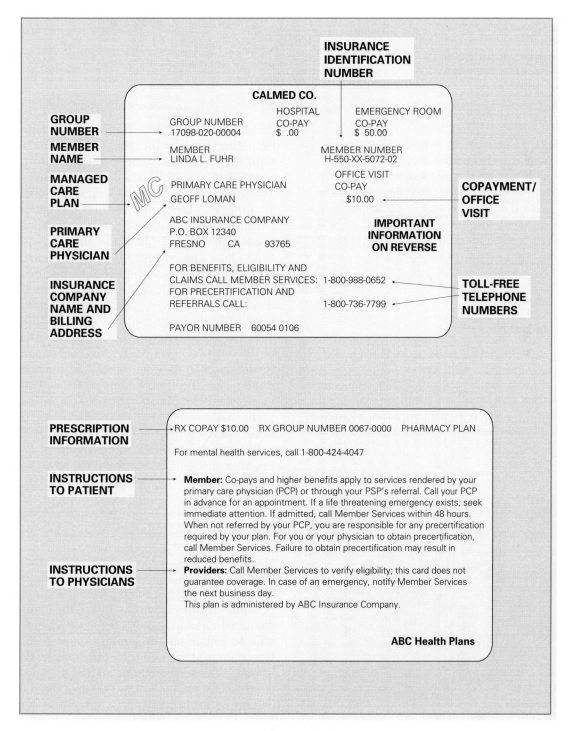

Figure 2–10. Front *(top)* and back *(bottom)* sides of an insurance card.

side of the card provides information, such as deductible, copayment, preapproval provisions, and insurance company address and telephone number. A copy produces error-free insurance data and can be used in lieu of completing the insurance section of the patient registration form. On a return visit, ask to see the card and check it with the data on file (Fig. 2–11). If it differs, photocopy both sides and write the date on the copy, using this as the base for revising data on file.

3. Patient's Signature Requirements

HIPAA Compliance Alert

RELEASE OF INFORMATION

If the physician is submitting an insurance claim for the patient, the patient must sign a release of information form (also known as an authorization or consent form) before information can be given to an insurance company, attorney, or other third party (Fig. 2–12). This often appears on the bottom portion of the patient registration form and may be worded to include an annual or lifetime authorization depending on the type of insurance or federal program.

ASSIGNMENT OF BENEFITS

If the physician wishes to receive the check by accepting assignment, the patient must sign an assignment of benefits form for each insurance company. However, before explaining an assignment, it is important to define the difference between

Figure 2–12. Insurance billing specialist obtaining the patient's signature on a release of information form.

participating and nonparticipating providers. A **participating provider (par)** has a contractual agreement with an insurance plan to render care to eligible beneficiaries and bills the insurance carrier directly. The insurance carrier pays its portion of the allowed amount, and the provider bills the patient for the balance not paid by the insurer after the disallowed portion is adjusted off of the account. However, in Blue Plans, the provider is referred to as a *member physician* and may accept the payment as *payment in full* or may bill the patient for any unpaid balance, depending on the contract. Managed care plans also refer to participating providers as member physicians. A **nonparticipating provider (nonpar)** is a physician without a contractual agreement with an insurance plan to accept an allowed amount and to render care to eligible beneficiaries. The provider may or may not file an insurance claim as a courtesy to the patient and usually expects full payment at the time of service.

The general definition of **assignment** is the transfer, after an event insured against, of an individual's legal right to collect an amount payable under an insurance contract. Most of the time an agreement is obtained by having the patient sign an assignment of insurance benefits document directing payment to the physician. However, many health insurance claim forms (e.g., CMS-1500 form) contain a provision that, when signed by the insured, directs the insurance company to pay benefits directly to the provider of care on whose charge the claim is based. An assignment of benefits becomes a legally enforceable document but must refer to specific hospitalization, course of treatment, or office visits. Each course of treatment needs to have an assignment document executed by the patient unless an annual or lifetime signature authorization is accepted and in the patient's financial file, except when automobile or homeowners' liability insurance is involved.

Figure 2–11. Patient presenting an insurance identification card to the receptionist for photocopying.

Private Carriers

For private insurance companies with whom the provider does not have a contractual agreement, accepting assignment means that the insurance check will be directed to the provider's office instead of to the patient. Because there is no signed agreement with the carrier, the difference between the billed amount and the carrier's allowed amount is not written off but collected from the patient as well as any copayment or deductible. In private third-party liability cases, the physician needs to negotiate with the insurance company to make sure benefits are paid to him or her directly.

Managed Care

In managed care plans, a participating provider (also called a *preferred provider*) is a physician who has contracted with a plan to provide medical services to plan members. A nonparticipating provider refers to a physician who has not contracted with a managed care plan to provide medical services to plan members. The assignment is automatic for individuals who have signed with managed care contracts.

Medicaid

For Medicaid cases, there is no assignment unless the patient has other insurance in addition to Medicaid.

Medicare

The words participating, nonparticipating, and assignment have slightly different meanings in the Medicare program. A physician who accepts assignment on Medicare claims is called a *participating (par) physician* and may not bill, or accept payment for, the amount of the difference between the submitted charge and the Medicare allowed amount. However, an attempt must be made to collect 20% of the allowed charge (coinsurance) and any amount applied to the deductible. A physician who does not participate is called a *nonparticipating* (nonpar) physician and has an option regarding assignment. The physician may not accept assignment for all services or has the option of accepting assignment for some services and collecting from the patient for other services performed at the same time and place. The physician collects the fee from the patient but may bill no more than the Medicare limiting charge. The check is sent to the patient. When treating federal or state government employees or a Medicare recipient, the physician may lose the fee if government guidelines are not followed.

TRICARE

A provider who accepts TRICARE standard assignment (participates) agrees to accept the allowable charge as the full fee and cannot charge the patient the difference between the provider's charge and the allowable charge. The exception to this is when the provider does not accept assignment on the claim. A provider that participates or does not participate with TRICARE can submit a claim and not accept assignment on a claim-by-claim basis. In the event the provider does not accept assignment, TRICARE sends the sponsor all payments. TRICARE does not communicate with the provider if the provider has questions about the claim. It is up to the provider to bill the sponsor for payment. The provider can collect 115% of the TRICARE allowable from the patient when a CMS-1500 claim form is marked "no" in the accepting assignment block.

Workers' Compensation

There is no assignment for industrial cases. The workers' compensation carrier pays the fee for services rendered according to its fee schedule and the check automatically goes to the physician. The patient is not responsible for payment of services for any work-related injury or illness.

SIGNATURE GUIDELINES

Most patient registration forms include a statement to sign regarding these two authorizations (bottom of Fig. 2–7). Also many private insurance forms contain blocks for the patient's signature with authorization for release of information and assignment of benefits. These two requirements are included in Blocks 12 and 13 of the CMS-1500 insurance claim form (Fig. 2–13). If these signature requirements are obtained separately, they may be filed in the patient's medical record and the abbreviation "SOF" (signature on file) may be used on the insurance claim form.

When using an insurance claim with no printed assignment, attach a signed patient authorization form with "SOF" typed in the appropriate place. Because attachments to insurance forms may be lost after their arrival at the insurance company, it is wise to make two copies of the assignment (one for the insurance company and one for the patient's file in the physician's office).

For a patient on a federal program such as Medicare or TRICARE (Chapters 11 and 13), acceptance of assignment means not only that the check will come to the physician but also that the physician will accept what the federal program designates as the "allowed amount." The federal program pays a percentage of the allowed amount, and the patient pays a remaining coinsurance (cost-sharing) percentage.

Figure 2–13. Sections 12 and 13 from the health insurance claim form CMS-1500, illustrating authorization for release of information and assignment of benefits.

Figure 2–14. Encounter form: procedural codes for professional services are taken from the Current Procedural Terminology (CPT) book, and diagnostic codes are taken from the International Classification of Diseases, 9th revision, Clinical Modification (ICD-9-CM) book. (Courtesy of Bibbero Systems, Inc., Petaluma, CA. Phone: 800-242-2376; Fax: 800-242-9330; www.bibbero.com.)

4. Encounter Form: An **encounter form** (also called a charge slip, communicator, fee ticket, multipurpose billing form, patient service slip, routing form, superbill, or transaction slip) is attached to the patient's medical record during the visit (Fig. 2–14). This contains the patient's name, the date, and, in some instances, the previous balance due. It also contains the procedural and diagnostic codes and the date the patient should return for an appointment. This two- or three-part form is a combination bill, insurance form, and routing document used in both computer and pegboard systems. This also can be a computerized multipurpose billing form that may be scanned to input charges and diagnoses into the patient's computerized account. Time is saved and fewer errors occur because no keystrokes are involved. Medical practices use the encounter form as a communications tool (routing sheet) and as an invoice to the patient. When used as a routing sheet, it becomes a source document for insurance claim data. The encounter form's procedure and diagnostic code sections should be updated annually with correct descriptions because changes, additions, and deletions occur. Remove all codes not used or seldom used and revise and add current valid commonly used codes for the practice. Do not print large quantities because codes change annually. Some practices develop encounter forms for different services (e.g., surgical services, office services [within the facility], and out-of-office service [hospital visits, emergency, outpatient facility, nursing home, or house calls]). Examples of encounter forms are shown in Chapter 7, Fig. 7–9 and Chapter 9, Fig. 9–7.

5. Physician's Signature: After examination and treatment, the physician completes the encounter form by checking off the procedure (services and treatments) codes and diagnostic code(s) (Fig. 2–15). The physician signs the form and indicates whether the patient needs another appointment.

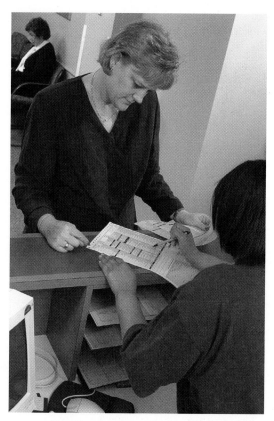

Figure 2–16. Patient carrying the encounter form to the medical office's check-up station.

6. Determine Fees: The patient carries the encounter form to the reception desk where fees are determined and input for billing (Fig. 2–16). He or she is given the opportunity to pay and make a future appointment.

7. Bookkeeping—Financial Accounting Record: The value of maintaining careful records of all insurance matters cannot be overemphasized. A **financial accounting record** or ledger card is maintained for each patient who receives professional services (Fig. 2–17). The medical assistant or insurance billing specialist may use a copy of the encounter form to daily **post** (record) professional fees (charges), payments (cash, check, or credit card), adjustments, and balance due to the patient's ledger card and to the daysheet (Fig. 2–18). A **daysheet,** or daily record sheet, is a register for recording daily business transactions. All patients seen on 1 day have their charges (debits) recorded on the daysheet, along with all payments and adjustments (credits). Each day the totals are carried forward and a new daysheet is set up to receive posting for that day. The ledger card should show an entry of the date an insurance claim is sent, including the date of services that were billed. Each service must be posted on a single line, and a **running balance** is calculated in the right column. When the ledger is completely filled up, the account balance is brought forward (also known as **extended**) to a new

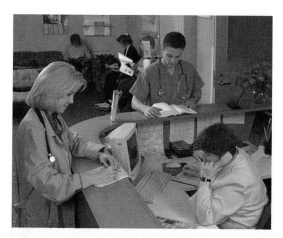

Figure 2–15. Physician checking off procedures on the encounter form at the conclusion of a patient's office visit.

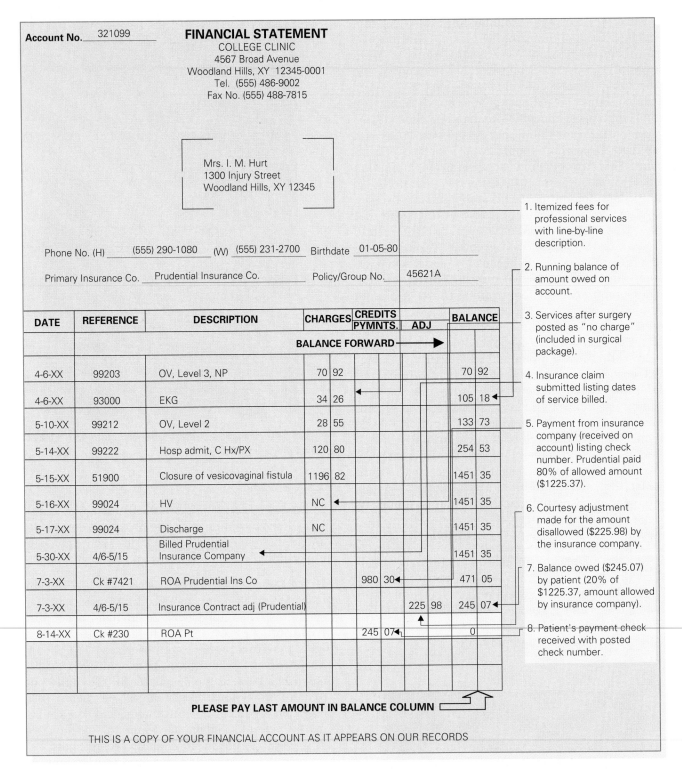

Figure 2–17. Financial accounting record illustrating posting of professional service descriptions, fees, payments, adjustments, and balance due.

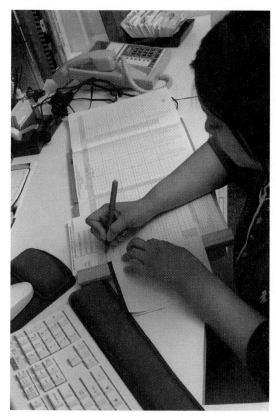

Figure 2–18. Medical office employee posting to a patient's financial accounting record or daysheet.

card. If a practice is computerized, all financial transactions are executed using billing software. Patients who are private 1 month and on the Medicaid program the next may require two ledgers to keep private and state records separate. An established private patient who is injured on the job requires two ledgers, one for private care and one for posting workers' compensation insurance.

Step-by-step instructions for completing a ledger card are given at the end of this chapter in the procedure "Posting to a Patient's Financial Accounting Record."

8. Insurance Form: Generally, the insurance billing specialist in the physician's office completes the insurance claim forms for the following cases: (1) all hospitalized (both surgical and medical) patients, (2) all claims in which the benefits are assigned to the physician, and (3) special procedures (minor surgery or extensive testing). In these cases, the insurance billing specialist completes the CMS-1500 insurance claim form with accurate procedural and diagnostic codes, including any appropriate documents (operative report or invoice), and mails it to the correct insurance carrier.

The minimum information required by third-party payers is:

▶ What was done? (services and procedures using procedure codes discussed in Chapter 5)

▶ Why was it done? (diagnoses using diagnostic codes discussed in Chapter 4)
▶ When was it performed? (date of service [DOS])
▶ Where was it received? (place of service [POS])
▶ Who did it? (provider name and identifying number)

A helpful hint is to group together all ledgers and charts from patients who have the same type of insurance and bill them all at one time. This cuts down on errors and makes it easier to complete the forms.

Submit claims as soon as possible after professional services are rendered except for patients receiving care over a continuing period of time when billing is to be sent in at the end of the treatment. There are time limits (30 days to $1\frac{1}{2}$ years) for filing an insurance claim from the date of service. This can vary depending on the commercial carrier, federal or state program, or whether the claim is for an illness or accident. Claims filed after the time limit will be denied. This topic is discussed further within the chapters on Medicare, Medicaid, TRICARE, and workers' compensation.

Financial losses from delay can occur in the following instances. If a patient has had a long-term illness, insurance benefits can expire before a claim is processed. If several physicians treat the same patient, some insurance companies pay only one of the physicians. (Typically, whoever files the claim first is paid first.) In this scenario, the other physicians may have to wait for disbursement by the physician who received the check. Submit hospitalized patients' insurance claim forms twice a month (on the 15th and 30th) regardless of the discharge date.

If a private insurance claim form is mailed or brought in by the patient at the time of the office visit, that form is date-stamped and reviewed to be sure the patient has signed the release of information statement. Patients who submit their own insurance claims are given two copies of the encounter form. The patient retains one copy for personal records and attaches the second copy to the insurance claim form and forwards it to the insurance company.

9. Provider's Handwritten Signature: The completed insurance form is reviewed for accuracy and routed to the provider (physician). A provider refers to any individual or organization that provides health care services. Providers may be physicians, hospitals, physical therapists, medical equipment suppliers, and pharmacies. Generally when submitting insurance claims, the provider must hand write his or her name attesting to the document. However, there are some exceptions in that most private payers accept a completed insurance claim with no signature as long as the physician's name is preprinted on the form. In addition, some insurance companies require that the provider have a notarized authorization on file before they will accept a claim form without the provider's signature. However, when a signature is required, it can be accepted in several formats—handwritten, facsimile stamp, and electronic signature. State and government programs require a signature.

PHYSICIAN'S REPRESENTATIVE

Sometimes a physician gives signature authorization to one person on the staff to sign insurance claims, who then becomes known as the physician's representative, referred to in Fig. 2–19 as the "attorney-in-fact." For an authorization of this type, a document should be typed and signed before a notary. This means that whoever signs the form is attesting to it because it is a legal document. If the medical practice is ever audited and fraud or embezzlement is discovered, then the person who had signature authorization can be brought into the case as well as the physician. The federal government will prosecute if this involves a Medicare patient. The state will prosecute if a Medicaid patient is involved.

SIGNATURE STAMP

Some medical practices use a facsimile signature stamp so the staff can process insurance forms and other paperwork without interrupting the physician by waiting for her or his signature. For an authorization of this type, a document should be typed and signed before a notary (Fig. 2–20).

However, use of this stamp can lead to problems, because it is possible to stamp unauthorized checks, transcribed medical reports, prescriptions, or credit card charge slips. Discontinue the practice if such a stamp is used infrequently. If one is used regularly, prevent problems by doing the following:

▶ Make only one stamp.
▶ Allow only long-term, trusted, bonded staff members to have access to the stamp.
▶ Keep the stamp in a location with a secure lock.
▶ Limit access to the stamp.

Figure 2–19. Example of a provider's signature authorization form that can be completed, notarized, and sent to the insurance carrier after a copy is retained for the physician's records.

PROVIDER'S NOTARIZED SIGNATURE AUTHORIZATION

State of ____Iowa_____)
)ss
County of _Des Moines____)

Know all persons by these presents:

That I, _John Doe, MD_ have made, constituted, and appointed and by these presents do make, constitute and appoint _Mary Coleman_____ my true and lawful attorney-in-fact for me and in my name place and stead to sign my name on claims, for payment for services provided by me submitted to the _Blue Cross and Blue Shield of Iowa_. My signature by my said attorney-in-fact includes my agreement to abide by the full payment concept and the remainder of the certification appearing on all _CMS-1500_ claim forms. I hereby ratify and confirm all that my said attorney-in-fact shall lawfully do or cause to be done by virtue of the power generated herein.

In witness whereof I have hereunto set my hand this __20th__ day of _January__ 20_XX_.

_____John Doe, MD_____
(Signature)

Subscribed and sworn to before me this_20th_ day of _January_ 20 XX

_____
Notary Public

My commission expires _____.

PROVIDER'S NOTARIZED FACSIMILE OR STAMP SIGNATURE AUTHORIZATION

State of ___Florida___)
)ss
County of ___Jacksonville___)

___John Doe, MD___ being first duty sworn, deposes and says:

I hereby authorize the ___Blue Cross of Florida___
                                         (Name of Fiscal Administrator)
to accept my facsimile or stamp signature shown below

_____ *John Doe, MD* _____
                    (Facsimile or Stamp Signature)

as my true signature for all purposes under the ___Medicare___
                                                                        (Name of Insurance Program)
in the same manner as if it were my actual signature, including
my agreeing to abide by the full payment concept and the
remainder of the certification normally signed by the source of
care as it appears on all __CMS-1500__ claim forms.

                                    _____ *John Doe, MD* _____
                                                         (Signature)

Subscribed and sworn to before me this _3rd_ day
of __January__ 20XX.

                                    _____
                                    Notary Public in and for
_____ County, State of_____
(SEAL)
My commission expires _____ .

Figure 2–20. Example of a provider's facsimile or stamp signature authorization form that can be completed, notarized, and sent to the insurance carrier after a copy is retained for the physician's records.

For information on state laws, contact your state legislature at your state capitol. For data about signatures on hospital medical records, see Chapter 16.

COMPUTERIZED SIGNATURES

There are two types of computerized signatures, electronic and digital. An **electronic signature** looks like the signer's handwritten signature. The signer authenticates the document by key entry or with a pen pad using a stylus to capture the live signature.

E X A M P L E : David Smith, MD

It also can be defined as an individualized computer access and identification system (e.g., a series of numbers, letters, electronic writing, voice, computer key, and fingerprint transmission [biometric system]).

A *digital signature* may be lines of text or a text box stating the signer's name, date, and time and a statement indicating a signature has been attached from within the software application.

**E X A M P L E : Electronically signed:
David Smith, MD**
07/12/2000   10:30:08

---

10. Office Pending File and Insurance Claims Register: A duplicate of the claim is retained in the office pending file in the event payment is not received and the claim must be followed up. This file also may be referred to as a suspense, follow-up, or tickler file (Figs. 2–21 and 2–22). The term "tickler" came into existence because it tickles or jogs the memory at certain dates in the future.

Establish an insurance claims register (tracing file) to keep track of the status of each case that has been billed (Fig. 2–23). Record to whom the claim was sent and the submission date on the insurance claims register and the patient's ledger card. The insurance billing specialist handling the insurance forms can see at a glance which claims are becoming delinquent and the amounts owed to the physician. This is an efficient method used for 30- to 60-day follow-up.

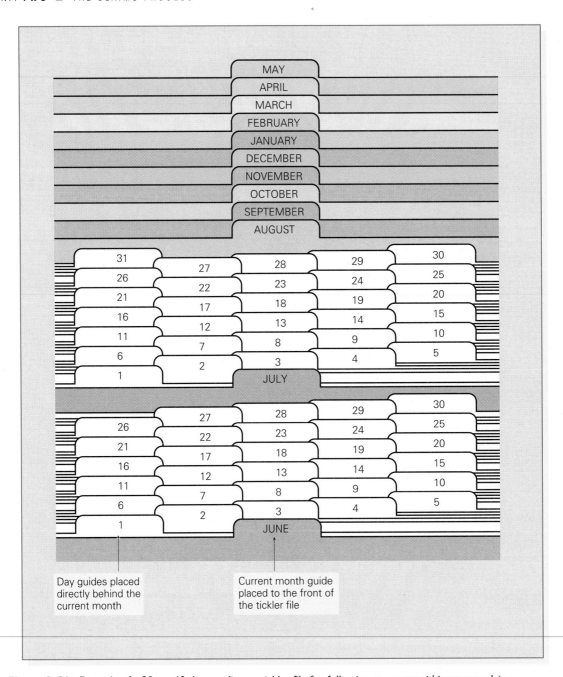

MAY
APRIL
MARCH
FEBRUARY
JANUARY
DECEMBER
NOVEMBER
OCTOBER
SEPTEMBER
AUGUST

31		28	29	30
26	27	23	24	25
21	22	18	19	20
16	17	13	14	15
11	12	8	9	10
6	7	3	4	5
1	2			

JULY

		28	29	30
26	27	23	24	25
21	22	18	19	20
16	17	13	14	15
11	12	8	9	10
6	7	3	4	5
1	2			

JUNE

Day guides placed directly behind the current month

Current month guide placed to the front of the tickler file

Figure 2–21. Example of a 30- to 60-day pending or tickler file for following up on unpaid insurance claims.

Keep two copies of each claim for the physician's records, one to be filed by patient name and the other by carrier name. *Or* simply record the name of the insurance company on each patient's ledger card and keep a file for each carrier by date of service. Filing by carrier allows all inquiries to be included in a single letter to the insurance company to eliminate having to write to the same company three or four times.

In a computerized accounting system, patient's accounts are referred to as financial accounting records. In a manual bookkeeping system they are more commonly referred to as ledger cards and are always kept separate from the medical record. For easy and quick access, some practices prefer to keep additional financial records also separate from the patient's medical records. The financial record should contain all billing information, a copy of the completed patient information form, patient authorization or signature-on-file form, copies of insurance identification cards, responsible-party authorization, insurance correspondence, explanation of benefits or remittance advice documents, and a log of all telephone conversations and actions taken regarding insurance disputes or collection activities.

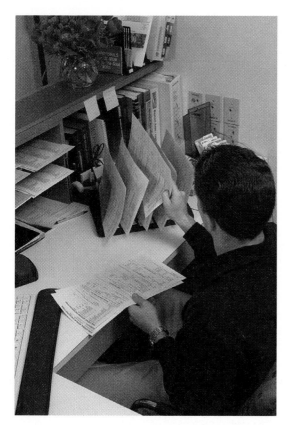

Figure 2–22. Insurance billing specialist using a desk sorter to alphabetize insurance claims to make filing easier in the tickler file.

11. Mailing the Claim Form: A large manila envelope is addressed, and the claim form is mailed to the insurance carrier. Mail claims in batches to each carrier to save on postage. Refer to Fig. 2–6, *B* for the nine phases of processing by the insurance carrier of a claim form for payment.

12. Insurance Payments

BANK DEPOSIT AND ANNUAL ALPHA FILE

A payment (check) from the insurance carrier should be received in 2 to 8 weeks, accompanied by an explanation of benefits/remittance advice document. The duplicate claim form is pulled from the file to verify the payment received against the amount billed. The payment is posted (credited) to the patient's ledger card and current daysheet indicating the date of posting, name of insurance company, check or voucher number, amount received, and contracted adjustment. The check is then entered on a bank deposit slip and may be deposited at the bank. After proper payment is received, the duplicate copy of the insurance claim is attached to the explanation of benefits form. These are filed in an annual alpha file according to insurance type, date of service, or patients' names. A date file using the posting date as reference is another option. Some medical practices file claim forms at the back

section of the patient's medical record after payment is received and accepted; however, this is an optional but not preferred system.

If an annual alpha file is maintained, the records should be retained for 3 years before purging to meet the requirements of the Internal Revenue Service. The Internal Revenue Service can request tax records for the 3 years preceding an audit. The audit can include records for the previous 6 years if taxpayers fail to report more than 25% of their gross income. There are no time limitations if taxpayers file a fraudulent return or fail to file a return.

For further information on improper payments received and tracing delinquent claims, see Chapter 8.

13. Monthly Statement: The patient who has insurance should be sent a monthly statement for all outstanding charges. A note stating "Your insurance has been billed" should appear on the itemized statement. The patient should always be billed the same fee as that submitted to the insurance company. After the insurance plan has paid, a message should appear on the statement indicating the amount the patient owes.

PROCEDURE: Posting to a Patient's Financial Accounting Record

Follow these steps to post charges, payments, adjustments, and balances to a patient's ledger/account (Fig. 2–17).

1. Insert the patient's name and address to prepare the ledger card. Some ledgers may require additional information (attending physician's name, type of insurance, patient's telephone number), depending on the style of card chosen for a medical practice.

2. Post the DOS in the date column, description of the services in the professional service description column, and charge amount in the charge column. The posting date is the actual date the transaction is recorded. If the DOS differs from the posting date, reference the DOS in the description column.

3. Add the charge to the running current balance, and enter the current balance in the right column.

4. Enter a notation each time an insurance claim has been submitted listing the date billed, name of the insurance plan, and the inclusive from and to dates of service covered by the claim submission (e.g., Billed Prudential Insurance Company 4–6 through 5–15).

| INSURANCE CLAIMS REGISTER | | Claim Submitted | | Follow-Up | | Claim Paid | | Page No. ___ |
Patient's Name Group/policy No.	Name of Insurance Company	Date	Amount	Date	Date	Date	Amt	Difference
Davis, Bob	BC/BS	1-7-XX	319.37			2/28/XX	294.82	24.55
Cash, David	BC	1-8-XX	268.08	2-10-XX	3-10-XX			
Smythe, Jan	Medicaid	1-9-XX	146.15	2-10-XX				
Phillips, Emma	Medicare	1-10-XX	96.28	2-10-XX				
Perez, Jose	Medi-Medi	1-10-XX	647.09	2-10-XX				
Amato, Joe	Tricare	2-1-XX	134.78	3-10-XX				
Rubin, Billy	Aetna	2-4-XX	607.67	3-10-XX				
Pfeifer, Renee	Travelers	2-10-XX	564.55	3-10-XX				
Tam, Chang	Prudential	2-15-XX	1515.79					
Brown, Harry	Allstate	2-21-XX	121.21					
Park, James	BC	2-24-XX	124.99					

Figure 2–23. Insurance claims register. This is an example of how a form can be set up to establish an easy way to follow up on insurance claims.

5. Post all amounts paid for each date of service in the payment column, referencing that it was received on account (ROA). List the payer (patient [pt] or name of the insurance company) and check/voucher number (e.g., ROA pt ck #230 or ROA Prudential Ins ck #7421).

6. Subtract the payment received from the amount in the running current balance column and enter the current balance.

7. Post the contracted insurance plan discount in the "Adjustment" column by referencing the DOS, insurance company name, and type of contract discount (e.g., HealthNet PPO discount or Medicare courtesy adjustment).

8. Subtract the adjustment amount from the running balance and enter the current balance as shown in Fig. 2–17. Optional: Post the adjustment on the same line as the payment.

Date	Description	Charge	Payment	Adjustment	Balance
					1346.17
7-3-xx	ROA Prudential Ins #7421		980.30	120.80	245.07

9. Submit an itemized billing statement to the patient for the balance due.

Keeping Up to Date

▶ Make a folder or binder of pertinent insurance information. Obtain information booklets and manuals from the local offices of the various insurance companies. Obtain sample copies of all the forms required for the insurance plans most used in your physician's office. Keep samples of completed claim forms.

▶ Changes occur daily and monthly so keep well informed by reading your Medicaid, Medicare, TRICARE, and local medical society bulletins. Maintain a chronologic file on each of these bulletins for easy reference, always keeping the latest bulletin on top.

▶ Attend any workshops offered in your area on insurance in the medical practice. Network with other insurance specialists to compare policies and discuss common problems. The American Association of Medical Assistants has chapters in many states that feature educational workshops and lectures.

▶ Become a member of the American Academy of Professional Coders, American Association of Medical Billers, Medical Association of Billers, and/or American Health Information Management Association. Each of these associations distributes journals or newsletters on a monthly basis featuring current information.

For addresses of the professional associations mentioned in this chapter, refer to Chapter 17, Table 17–1.

STUDENT ASSIGNMENT LIST

✔ Study Chapter 2.
✔ Answer the review questions in the *Workbook* to reinforce the theory learned in this chapter and to help prepare you for a future test.
✔ Complete the assignments in the *Workbook* to help reinforce the basic steps in submitting an insurance claim form.
✔ Turn to the Glossary at the end of this textbook for a further understanding of the Key Terms used in this chapter.

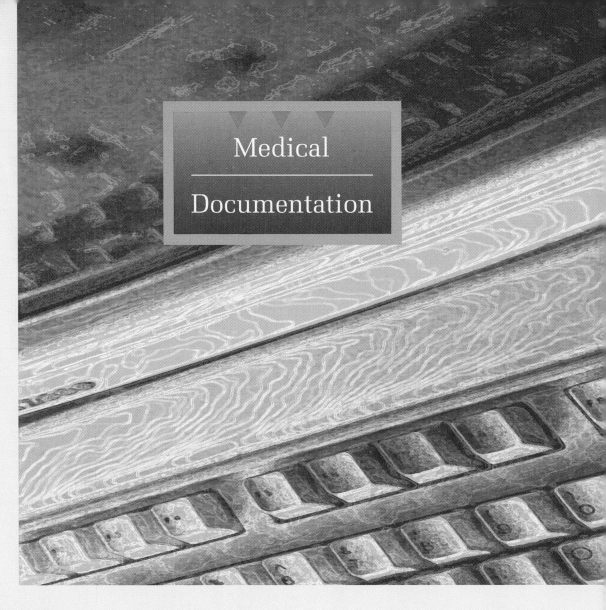

Medical Documentation

3

CHAPTER OUTLINE

- State reasons why an insurance company may decide to perform an external audit of medical records.
- Identify principles for release and retention of medical records.
- Explain techniques used for fax confidentiality.
- Respond appropriately to the subpoena of a witness and records.
- Formulate a procedure for termination of a case.
- Prepare legally correct medicolegal forms and letters.

OBJECTIVES*

After reading this chapter you should be able to:

- Name steps in the documentation process.
- Explain reasons medical documentation is required.
- Identify principles of documentation.
- State contents of a medical report.
- Define common medical, diagnostic, and legal terms.
- List documents required for an internal review of medical records.
- Describe the difference between prospective and retrospective review of records.

*Performance objectives and exercises for hands-on practical experience for this chapter appear in the *Workbook*.

KEY TERMS

acute

attending physician

breach of confidential communication

chief complaint (CC)

chronic

comorbidity

compliance program

comprehensive (C)

concurrent care

consultation

consulting physician

continuity of care

counseling

critical care

detailed (D)

documentation

emergency care

eponym

established patient

expanded problem focused (EPF)

external audit

facsimile (fax)

family history (FH)

high complexity (HC)

history of present illness (HPI)

internal review

low complexity (LC)

medical necessity

medical record

medical report

moderate complexity (MC)

Continued.

KEY TERMS—cont'd

new patient (NP)

ordering physician

past history (PH)

physical examination (PE)

problem focused (PF)

prospective review

referral

referring physician

retrospective review

review of systems (ROS)

social history (SH)

straightforward (SF)

subpoena

subpoena duces tecum

treating or performing
  physician

treating practitioner

The Documentation Process

Medical Record

The connection between insurance billing and the medical record should be explained to better understand the importance of the medical record, the foremost tool of clinical care and communication. A **medical record** can be defined as written or graphic information documenting facts and events during the rendering of patient care. A **medical report** is part of the medical record and is a permanent legal document that formally states the consequences of the patient's examination or treatment in letter or report form. It is this record that provides the information needed to complete the insurance claim form. When billing the insurance company, the DOS, POS, type of service (TOS), diagnosis (dx or Dx), and procedures must be recorded. These data are transferred as codes on the claim form for interpretation by the insurance company.

The key to substantiating procedure and diagnostic code selections for appropriate reimbursement is supporting documentation in the medical record. Proper documentation can prevent penalties and refund requests should the physician's practice be reviewed or audited. Some states or facilities use different terminology when referring to the medical record, such as medical information, health record, progress or chart note, hospital record, or health care record.

Documenters

All individuals providing health care services may be referred to as documenters because they chronologically record pertinent facts and observations about the patient's health. This process is called **documentation** (charting) and may be handwritten or dictated. It is the physician's responsibility to either hand write the medical information or dictate it for transcription. The receptionist obtains the first document completed by the patient, called the patient registration information form, as shown in Chapter 2, Fig. 2–7. The medical assistant is often the one to record entries for no-show appointments, prescription refills, and telephone calls in the patients' medical records. The insurance billing specialist uses the information in the medical record for billing purposes, and it is his or her responsibility to bring any substandard documentation to the physician's attention.

When referring to guidelines for documentation of the medical record and completion of the insurance claim form, a physician's title may change depending on the circumstances of each patient encounter. This can get confusing at times, so to clarify the physician's various roles and the roles of the practitioners who work for the physician, some of these titles are defined as follows:

▶ **Attending physician** refers to the medical staff member who is legally responsible for the care and treatment given to a patient.
▶ **Consulting physician** is a provider whose opinion or advice regarding evaluation or management of a specific problem is requested by another physician.
▶ **Ordering physician** is the individual directing the selection, preparation, or administration of tests, medication, or treatment.
▶ **Referring physician** is a provider who sends the patient for tests or treatment.
▶ **Treating or performing physician** is the provider who renders a service to a patient. In the Medicare program the definition of a treating physician is a physician who furnishes a consultation or treats a

beneficiary for a specific medical problem, and who uses the results of a diagnostic test in the management of the beneficiary's specific medical problem. A radiologist performing a therapeutic intervention procedure is considered a treating physician. A radiologist performing a diagnostic intervention or diagnostic procedure is not considered a treating physician.

▶ **Treating practitioner** is a nurse practitioner, clinical nurse specialist, or physician assistant who furnishes a consultation or treats a Medicare beneficiary for a specific medical problem, pursuant to state law, and who uses the results of a diagnostic test in the management of the beneficiary's specific medical problem.

Reasons for Documentation

It is important that every patient seen by the physician has comprehensive legible documentation about what occurred during the visit for the following reasons:

1. Avoidance of denied or delayed payments by insurance carriers investigating the medical necessity of services.
2. Enforcement of medical record-keeping rules by insurance carriers requiring accurate documentation that supports procedure and diagnostic codes.
3. Subpoena of medical records by state investigators or the court for review.
4. Defense of a professional liability claim.

General Principles of Medical Record Documentation

In the early 1990s the American Medical Association (AMA) decided to eliminate the terminology "office visits" when coding for those services and adopted the phrase "evaluation and management." This term better reflects the components involved when performing an office visit. The AMA and Centers for Medicaid and Medicare Services (CMS) then developed documentation guidelines for CPT E/M services. These were released to Medicare carriers by CMS in 1995 and then modified and released again in 1997. The guidelines were developed because Medicare has an obligation to those enrolled to ensure that services paid for have been provided and are medically necessary. It was discovered during audits that some medical practices should improve their quality of documentation.

Physicians are not required to use these guidelines but are encouraged to for the four reasons stated. Some physicians have adopted the 1995 guidelines, and others use those introduced in 1997. A modification of the 1997 guidelines is under consideration but has not been released as of this edition. Insurance claims processors and auditors may use the 1995 or 1997 guidelines when doing an internal or external chart audit to determine whether the reported services were actually rendered and the level of service was warranted. A variety of formats of documentation are accepted by Medicare fiscal intermediaries (claims processors) as long as the information is discernible. When significant irregular reporting patterns are detected, a review is conducted.

Medical Necessity

Payment may be delayed if the medical necessity of a treatment is questioned. As a rule, **medical necessity** is a criterion used by insurance companies when making decisions to limit or deny payment in which medical services or procedures must be justified by the patient's symptoms and diagnosis. This must be done in accordance with standards of good medical practice, and the proper level of care provided in the most appropriate setting. However, insurers differ on this definition and may or may not cover the services, depending on the benefits of the plan. Inform the patient of this situation with a letter, as shown in Figure 3–1.

External Audit Point System

A point system is used while reviewing each patient's medical record during the performance of an audit. Points are awarded only if documentation is present for elements required in the medical record. Because every medical record is documented differently by each provider of service, a patient's history may contain details for more than one body area. Thus when gathering points, it is possible the auditor may shift the points from the history of present illness to those required for the review of the patient's body systems. In addition, when sufficient points have been reached within a section for the level of code used in billing, no further documentation is counted for audit purposes, even though there may be additional comments for other body systems. This point system is used to show where deficiencies occur in medical record documentation. It is also used to evaluate and substantiate proper use of diagnostic and procedural codes.

HMOs, PPOs, and all private carriers have the right to claim refunds in the event of accidental (or intentional) miscoding. However, Medicare has the power to levy fines and penalties and exclude providers from the Medicare program. If improper coding patterns exist and are not corrected, then the provider of service will be penalized. Insurance carriers go by the rule, "If it is not documented, then it was not performed," and they have the right to deny reimbursement.

COLLEGE CLINIC
4567 Broad Avenue
Woodland Hills, XY 12345-0001
Phone: 555/486-90020
Fax: 555/487-8976

September 20, 20XX

Dear ABC Managed Care Plan Participant:

This is a quick fact sheet to help our patients understand that some services may not be paid by ABC Managed Care Plan unless there is a *medical* reason to perform them.

The coverage provided by ABC Managed Care Plan, in most instances, includes payment for medically necessary services provided to treat a problem or illness. However, patients who wish their health care providers to perform services outside of those considered a "medical necessity" will be responsible for paying for those services out-of-pocket.

For example, many patients come to our office for the purpose of removing noncancerous facial moles. Although this procedure may be desired by the patient, ABC Managed Care Plan will not pay for the removal without a medical reason for it.

The patient's cost for noncancerous facial mole removal at our practice is approximately $75.

Please understand that, legally, we are required to submit our bill to ABC Managed Care Plan using accurate information about all of the services you received. Using a false medical reason to try to get insurance to pay for a service it otherwise would not cover is considered fraud, and our doctors will not do this. We regret that ABC Managed Care Plan may not wish to pay for a service you desire, but we must follow insurance regulations.

If you would like additional information about payment coverage for these services, you may refer to your ABC Managed Care Plan benefits handbook or call your ABC Managed Care Plan customer service representative at 555-271-0311.

Thank you for choosing us to assist you with your health care needs. As always, providing high-quality health care to you is and remains our primary purpose. If you have any questions about this information, please do not hesitate to telephone and ask our front office staff for more information.

Sincerely,

Mary Anne Mason, CPC

Figure 3–1. Letter to a patient who is a member of a managed care plan that provides important information about medical procedures or services that are not covered for payment unless there is a medical necessity.

Enforcement of Medical Record Keeping

Insurance carriers have become stricter in enforcing accurate coding substantiated by documentation. It is not uncommon for prepayment and postpayment random audits or reviews by Medicare carriers to occur that monitor the accuracy of physicians' use of evaluation and management services and procedure codes. Medicare fiscal intermediaries have "walk-in rights" (access to a medical practice without an appointment or search warrant) that they may invoke to conduct documentation reviews, audits, and evaluations. Billing patterns that may draw attention to a medical practice for possible audit are:

▶ Billing intentionally for unnecessary services.
▶ Billing incorrectly for services of *physician extenders* (e.g., nurse practitioner, midwife, physician assistant).
▶ Billing for diagnostic tests without a separate report in the medical record.
▶ Changing dates of service on insurance claims to comply with policy coverage dates.
▶ Waiving copayments or deductibles or allowing other illegal discounts.
▶ Ordering excessive diagnostic tests (e.g., laboratory tests, x-ray studies).
▶ Using two different provider numbers to bill the same services for the same patient.
▶ Misusing provider identification numbers, resulting in incorrect billing.

▶ Using improper modifiers for financial gain.
▶ Failing to return overpayments made by the Medicare program.

Documentation Guidelines for Evaluation and Management Services

The following is a brief overview of documentation guidelines regarding evaluation and management services.

1. The medical record should be accurate, complete (detailed), and legible.
2. The documentation of each patient encounter should include or provide reference to:
   a. Chief complaint or reason for the encounter.
   b. Relevant history.
   c. Examination.
   d. Findings.
   e. Prior diagnostic test results.
   f. Assessment, clinical impression, or diagnosis.
   g. Plan for care.
   h. Date and legible identity of the health care professional.
3. The reason for the encounter or chief complaint should be stated, and the rationale should be documented or inferred for ordering diagnostic and other ancillary services.
4. Past and present diagnoses, including those in the prenatal and intrapartum period that affect the newborn, should be accessible to the treating or consulting physician.
5. Appropriate health risk factors should be identified.
6. The patient's progress, response to and changes in treatment, planned follow-up care and instructions, and diagnosis should be documented.
7. Patient refusal to follow medical advice should be documented and a letter sent to the patient about this noncompliance. Information on termination of a case is found at the end of this chapter.
8. Procedure and diagnostic codes reported on the health insurance claim form or billing statement should be supported by the documentation in the medical record and be at a level sufficient for a clinical peer to determine whether services have been coded accurately.
9. The confidentiality of the medical record should be fully maintained consistent with the requirements of medical ethics and the law. An authorization form signed by the patient must be obtained to release information to the insurance carrier.
10. Each chart entry should be dated and signed, including the title or position of the person signing. If a signature log has been established, then initials are acceptable, because these would be defined in the log (Fig. 3–2). A *signature log* is a list of all staff members' names, job titles, signatures, and initials. In regard to paperless documents, if passwords are used for restricted access, electronic or digital signatures may be acceptable.
11. Charting procedures for progress notes should be standardized. Many physicians use either a method called the SOAP style (Fig. 3–3) or the CHEDDAR style (Fig. 3–4). However, whatever method is used, make sure it is detailed enough to support current documentation requirements (Fig. 3–5).
12. Treatment plans should be written. Include patient/family education and specific instructions for follow-up. Treatment must be consistent with the working diagnosis.
13. Medications prescribed and taken should be listed, specifying frequency and dosage.
14. *Request* for a consultation from the attending or treating physician and the *need* for consultation must be documented. The consultant's opinion and any services ordered or performed must be documented and communicated to the requesting physician. Remember the three Rs: There must be a *requesting* physician, and the consultant must *render* an opinion and send a *report*.

Figure 3–2. Example of a signature log.

SIGNATURE LOG		
Name	Position	Signature or Initials
Ann M. Arch	Receptionist	*Ann M. Arch* AMA
John Bortolonni	Office manager	*John Bortolonni* JB
Gerald Practon, MD	Provider	*Gerald Practon, MD* GP
Rachel Vasquez, CPC	Insurance billing specialist	*Rachel Vasquez, CPC* RV
Mary Ann Worth	Clinical medical assistant	*Mary Ann Worth* MAW

S	**Subjective** statements of symptoms and complaints in the patient's own words	= chief complaint (CC) *reason for the encounter*
O	**Objective** findings	= data from physical examination, x-rays, laboratory, and other diagnostic tests *facts and findings*
A	**Assessment** of subjective and objective findings	= medical decision making *putting all the facts together to obtain a diagnosis*
P	**Plan** of treatment	= documenting a plan for care to be put into action *recommendations, instructions, further testing, medication*

Figure 3–3. Explanation of the acronym "SOAP" used as a format for progress notes defining subjective and objective information, the assessment, and the treatment plan.

15. Record a patient's failure to return for needed treatment by noting it in the medical record, in the appointment book, and on the financial record or ledger card. Follow up with a telephone call or send a letter to the patient advising him or her that further treatment is indicated.

16. Use a permanent, not water-soluble, ink pen (legal copy pen) to cross out an incorrect entry on a patient's record. Mark it with a single line and write the correct information, then date and initial the entry. Never erase, white out, or use self-adhesive paper over any information recorded on a patient record (Example 3–1). Maintain the original entry in the electronic file if correcting a computerized document. Note that the section is in error with the date and time and enter the correct information with a notation. Never delete or key over incorrect data in a

C	**Chief complaint**	Stated by the patient as the main reason for seeing the doctor; usually a subjective statement
H	**History of the present illness**	Includes social history and physical symptoms as well as contributing factors
E	**Examination**	Performed by the physician
D	**Details**	List of complaints and problems
D	**Drugs and dosages**	List of the current medications the patient is taking
A	**Assessment**	The diagnostic process and the impression (diagnosis) made by the physician
R	**Return visit information or referral**	Information about return visits or specialists to see for additional tests

Figure 3–4. Explanation of the acronym, "CHEDDAR," used as a format for progress notes.

Figure 3–5. Physician dictating chart notes. (From Diehl MO, Fordney MT: Diehl and Fordney's Medical Transcribing Techniques and Procedures, 5th ed. Philadelphia, Saunders, 2003.)

computerized file. Another method for correcting a medical record is to create an addendum either typed as a separate document or for a chart note inserted below in the next space available. This is discussed later in this chapter.

17. Document all laboratory tests ordered in the medical record. When the report is received, the physician should initial the report, indicating that it has been read. Each of these documentations is considered an element and allows a point should the record undergo an external audit.

18. Ask the physician for approval for a different code(s) before submitting the claim to the insurance carrier if the insurance biller questions any procedure or diagnostic codes marked on the encounter form (Fig. 3–6).

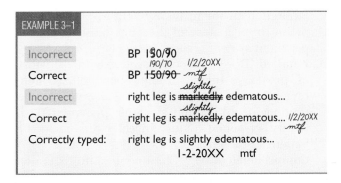

EXAMPLE 3–1	
Incorrect	BP 190/90
Correct	BP 150/90
Incorrect	right leg is markedly edematous...
Correct	right leg is markedly edematous...
Correctly typed:	right leg is slightly edematous...
	1-2-20XX mtf

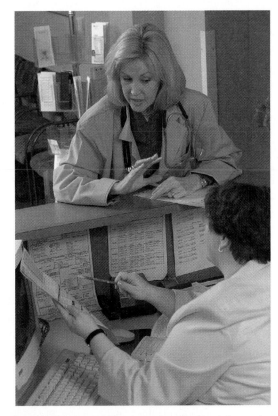

Figure 3–6. Insurance billing specialist checking information with physician before recording it on the insurance claim.

19. Retain all records until you are positive they are no longer needed by conforming to federal and state laws as well as the physician's wishes. Retention of records is discussed at the end of the chapter and shown in Table 3–4.

Contents of a Medical Report

The degree of documentation depends on the complexity of the service and the specialty of the physician. For example, a "normal chest examination" may have a different meaning to a cardiologist than it does to a family physician as far as the details of the examination and documentation.

The first time a new patient is seen, a family and social history is taken. When a new or an established patient comes to see the physician with a new injury or illness, the documentation should also include the patient's health history, the physical examination, results from any tests that are performed, the medical decision-making process, the diagnosis, and the treatment plan.

Documentation of History

The following documentation information for the history and physical examination are based on the 1997 Medicare guidelines.

The history includes the chief complaint (CC); history of present illness (HPI); review of systems (ROS); and past history, family, or social history (PFSH).* The extent of the history is dependent on clinical judgment and on the nature of the presenting problem(s). Each history includes some or all of the following elements (Fig. 3–7).

Chief Complaint

The **chief complaint (CC)** is a concise statement describing the symptom, problem, condition, diagnosis, physician-recommended return, or other factor that is the *reason* for the encounter. *The CC is a requirement for all levels of history*: problem focused, expanded problem focused, detailed, and comprehensive; these are described at the end of the section on history of present illness.

History of Present Illness

The **history of present illness (HPI)** is a chronologic description of the development of the patient's present illness from the first sign or symptom or from the previous encounter to the present. If the physician is unable to obtain a sufficient diagnosis for the patient's condition, the medical record documentation must reflect this. The history may include one or more of the eight descriptive elements:

1. **Location**—Area of the body where the symptom is occurring.
2. **Quality**—Character of the symptom/pain (burning, gnawing, stabbing, fullness).
3. **Severity**—Degree of symptom or pain on a scale from 1 to 10. Severity also can be described with terms such as severe, slight, and persistent.
4. **Duration**—How long the symptom/pain has been present and how long it lasts when the patient has it.
5. **Timing**—When the pain/symptom occurs (e.g., morning, evening, after or before meals).
6. **Context**—The situation associated with the pain/symptom (e.g., dairy products, big meals, activity).
7. **Modifying factors**—Things done to make the symptom/pain worse or better (e.g., "If I eat spicy foods I get heartburn, but if I drink milk afterward the pain is not as bad.").
8. **Associated signs and symptoms**—The symptom/pain and other things that happen when the symptom/pain occurs (e.g., chest pain leads to shortness of breath).

The documented elements are counted and totaled (Fig. 3–8, *A*). The medical record should describe one to three elements of the present illness for a *brief level* of HPI. At least four elements of the HPI or the status of at least three chronic or inactive conditions is required for the *extended level* of HPI. Only two of three history elements are required for certain types of cases, such as newborns or subsequent hospital care. Figure 3–8, *B* shows Section I of the review/audit sheet that depicts the history containing the HPI, ROS, and PFSH. The check marks and circled element in the HPI (Section I) of the figure relate to the case illustrated.

The types of evaluation and management services for the history are based on four levels of history. However, the ROS and PFSH must be totaled before the final decision on the level of service is assigned. The four levels of history may be defined as follows:

1. **Problem focused (PF)**—Chief complaint; brief history of present illness or problem.
2. **Expanded problem focused (EPF)**—Chief complaint; brief history of present illness; problem-pertinent system review.
3. **Detailed (D)**—Chief complaint; extended history of present illness; problem-pertinent system review extended to include a review of a limited number of additional systems; *pertinent* past, family, or social history directly related to the patient's problems.
4. **Comprehensive (C)**—Chief complaint; extended history of present illness; review of systems that is

---

*These abbreviations in the history portion of the report may vary depending on the physician who is dictating (i.e., PI for present illness, PH for past history, FH for family history, and SH for social history).

Figure 3–7. Example of a medical report done in modified block format showing the six components of a history.

```
                                                          Hospital number: 00-83-06

      Scott, Aimee

      Rex Rumsey, MD                           HISTORY


          CHIEF COMPLAINT:        Pain and bleeding after each bowel movement
                                  for the past 3 to 4 months.

          PRESENT ILLNESS:        This 68-year-old white female says she usually has three
                                  bowel movements a day in small amounts, and there
                                  has been a change in the last 3 to 4 months in frequency, size,
                                  and type of bowel movement. She has slight burning pain
                                  and irritation in the rectal area after bowel movements. The
                                  pain lasts for several minutes, then decreases in intensity. She
                                  has had no previous anorectal surgery or rectal infection.
                                  She denies any blood in the stool itself or associated
                                  symptoms. Bright red blood occurs after stools have passed.

            PAST HISTORY:
               ILLNESSES:         The patient had polio at age 8 from which she has made a
                                  remarkable recovery. Apparently, she was paralyzed in both
                                  lower extremities and now has adequate use of these. She
                                  has no other serious illnesses.

                ALLERGIES:        ALLERGIC TO PENICILLIN. She denies any other drug
                                  or food allergies.
              MEDICATIONS:        None.
               OPERATIONS:        Right inguinal herniorrhaphy 25 years ago.

           SOCIAL HISTORY:        She does not smoke or drink. She lives with her husband
                                  who is an invalid and for whom she cares. She is a retired
                                  former municipal court judge.

           FAMILY HISTORY:        One brother died of cancer of the throat (age 59),and
                                  another has cancer of the kidney (age 63).

      REVIEW OF SYSTEMS:
                     SKIN:        No rashes or jaundice.
                    HEENT:        Head normocephalic. Normal TMs. Normal hearing. Pupils
                                  equal, round, reactive to light. Deviated septum. Oropharynx
                                  clear.
                       CR:        No history of chest pain, shortness of breath, or pedal
                                  edema. She has had some mild hypertension in the past but
                                  is not under any medical supervision nor is she taking any
                                  medication for this.
                       GI:        Weight is stable. See present illness.
                  OB-GYN:         Gravida II Para II. Climacteric at age 46, no sequelae.
               EXTREMITIES:       No edema.
               NEUROLOGIC:        Unremarkable.


                       mtf                        _____
                 D: 5-17-20XX                          Rex Rumsey, MD
                 T: 5-20-20XX
```

directly related to the problem(s) identified in the history of the present illness plus a review of all additional body systems; *complete* past, family, and social history.

Review of Systems

A **review of systems (ROS)** is an inventory of body systems obtained through a series of questions that is used to identify signs or symptoms that the patient might be experiencing or has experienced. Checklists are permitted, but if a body system is not considered, then it should be crossed out. For an ROS, the following systems are recognized: constitutional symptoms (e.g., fever, weight loss), eyes, ears, nose, mouth, throat, cardiovascular, respiratory, gastro-intestinal, genitourinary, musculoskeletal, integu-mentary (skin or breast), neurologic, psychiatric, endocrine, hematologic/lymphatic, and allergic/immunologic.

10-21-20XX

Location — HISTORY OF PRESENT ILLNESS: This new patient is an 80-year-old white male who has had problems with voiding difficulty since 9-5-2000. During the night, the patient had only 50 cc output and was **Severity** — catheterized this morning because of his poor urinary output (200 cc). He was thought to have a distended bladder. He has not had any **Genitourinary (ROS)** — gross hematuria. He has voiding difficulty, especially when lying down and voiding in the supine position. His voiding pattern is improved while standing and sitting; however, the patient has developed a **Integumentary (ROS)** — wound to his left lateral malleolus and is only able to ambulate with assistance.

Location
Duration
Context
Genitourinary (ROS)
Modifying factor

Notice that there is no family or social history for this new patient.

PAST MEDICAL HISTORY: Unremarkable. He does have some slowing of his urinary stream and nocturia three to five times.

MEDICATIONS: He was on amitriptyline, which may affect his bladder.

ALLERGIES: He has no known allergies.

Notice that the examination of the wound is missing.

PHYSICAL EXAMINATION: Shows the abdomen to be soft, nontender, and not distended. His bladder was nonpalpable and nondistended.

GENITOURINARY: Normal penis. Testes descended bilaterally. His prostate is 10 g and benign in feeling.

IMPRESSION: Benign prostatic hypertrophy with some mild voiding difficulty exacerbated by the patient's poor ambulatory status.

I suspect that as his ambulatory status improves, his voiding pattern will also improve. I will try him on Hytrin 5 mg/day by mouth. I will follow him as needed.

mtf   Gene Ulibarri, MD

A

SECTION I

CHIEF COMPLAINT:

			Brief 1–3 elements	Brief	Extended ≥ 4 elements or status of ≥ 3 chronic or inactive conditions	Extended
HPI (history of present illness) ☑ Location ☑ Severity ☐ Timing ☐ Modifying factors ☐ Quality ☑ Duration ☑ Context ☐ Associated signs and symptoms						

Descriptive elements of history

Systems of history

ROS (review of systems)	None	Pertinent to problem 1 system	Extended 2–9 systems	Complete ≥ 10 systems, or some systems with statement "all others negative"
☐ Constitutional (wt loss, etc) ☐ Ears, nose, mouth, throat ☐ GI ☑ Integumentary (skin, breast) ☐ Endo ☐ Eyes ☐ Card/vasc ☑ GU ☐ Neuro ☐ Hem/lymph ☐ Resp ☐ Musculo ☐ Psych ☐ All/imm ☐ "All others negative"				

Review of history

PFSH (past family and social history) ☑ Past medical history ☐ Family history ☐ Social history	Established/ subsequent	None	None	One history area	Two or three history areas
No PFSH required: 99231–33, 99261–63, 99311–33	New/ Initial	None	None	One or two history area(s)	Three history areas

Circle the entry farthest to the right for each history area. To determine history level, draw a line down the column with the circle farthest to the left.

| PROBLEM FOCUSED | EXP. PROB. FOCUSED | DETAILED | COMPREHENSIVE |

Levels of history

B

Figure 3–8. A, Documentation from a medical record highlighting elements required for the history. **B,** Review/audit sheet Section I with check marks and circled elements to show how the history in the example is declared as detailed. This shows two of three history components (*arrow*) used for the purpose of determining the assignment of a procedure code at the appropriate level of service. (From the Iowa Medical Society, IMS Services, West Des Moines, IA, 1998.)

The body systems are counted and totaled. The medical record should describe one system of the ROS for a *pertinent to problem level.* For an *extended level,* two to nine systems are required. For a *complete level,* at least 10 organ systems must be reviewed and documented. Refer to Figure 3–8, *B* for a visual understanding of Section I of the review/audit sheet. The check marks and circled element in the ROS (Section I) of the figure relate to the case illustrated.

Past, Family, and Social Histories

The past, family, and social histories (PFSH) consists of a review of three areas:

1. **Past History (PH)**—The patient's past experiences with illnesses, operations, injuries, and treatments.
2. **Family History (FH)**—A review of medical events in the patient's family, including diseases that may be hereditary or place the patient at risk.

3. **Social History (SH)**—An age-appropriate review of past and current activities.

The PFSH review areas are counted and totaled. The medical record must contain at least one history area for a *detailed extended level* and specific items from two of the three history areas for a *comprehensive level* of PFSH. Refer to Figure 3–8, *B* for a visual guide of the PFSH in Section I of the review/audit sheet. Note the difference in the number of required elements for new versus established patients and the circled element for the case in question.

A vertical line is drawn down the right four columns that contain the most elements to determine whether the history is a PF, EPF, D, or C level.

Documentation of Examination

Physical Examination

The **physical examination** (PE or PX) is objective in nature; that is, it consists of the physician's findings by examination or test results. Figure 3–9 is an illustration of a single organ system examination that shows the details (elements) of examination for each body area within the genitourinary system. The three circled elements of the genitourinary system and one circled element of the gastrointestinal system relate to the case in question. For purposes of examination, the following body areas and organ systems are recognized.

Organ Systems/Body Areas—Elements of Examination

Constitutional (vital signs, general appearance)

Eyes

Ears, nose, mouth, and throat

Neck

Respiratory

Cardiovascular

Chest, including breasts and axillae

Gastrointestinal (abdomen)

Genitourinary (male)

Genitourinary (female)

Lymphatic

Musculoskeletal

Skin

Neurologic

Psychiatric

Note: In addition, any reasons for not examining a particular body area or system should be listed.

Types of Physical Examination

When performing an internal review of a patient's medical record, the number of elements identified by bullets are counted for each system and a total is obtained. The total is circled on Section II of the review/audit sheet as shown for the case illustrated (Fig. 3–10).

The levels of evaluation and management services are based on four types of physical examination (PE), as follows:

1. **Problem focused (PF)**—A limited examination of the affected body area or organ system. The medical record should describe one to five elements identified by a bullet for a *problem-focused level* of PE.

2. **Expanded problem focused (EPF)**—A limited examination of the affected body area or organ system and other symptomatic or related organ system(s). At least six elements identified by a bullet are required for an *expanded problem-focused level* of PE.

3. **Detailed (D)**—An extended examination of the affected body area(s) and other symptomatic or related organ system(s). At least two elements identified by a bullet from each of six areas/body systems OR at least 12 elements identified by a bullet in two or more areas/body systems are required for a *detailed level* of PE.

4. **Comprehensive (C)**—A general multisystem examination or complete examination of a single organ system. For a *comprehensive level* of PE, all elements must be identified by a bullet and documentation must be present for at least two elements identified by a bullet from each of nine areas/body systems.

The extent of the examination and what is documented depend on clinical judgment and the nature of the presenting problem(s). They range from limited examinations of single body areas to general multisystem or complete single-organ system examinations.

Documentation of Medical Decision-Making Complexity

In the medical decision-making process the physician must look at the number of diagnoses or treatment options, the amount or complexity of data to be reviewed, and the risk of complications or morbidity or mortality. *Morbidity* is a diseased condition or state, whereas *mortality* has to do with the number of deaths in a given time or place.

▶ *Number of Diagnoses or Management Options.* This is based on the number and types of problems addressed during the visit, the complexity of establishing a diagnosis, and the number of management options that must be considered by the physician. For the case illustrated, the number of problems is 1, which equals 3 points (Fig. 3–11, top section).

▶ *Amount or Complexity of Data to be Reviewed.* This is based on the types of diagnostic tests

MULTIORGAN SYSTEM EXAMINATION REQUIREMENTS (SHADED)
CONTENT and DOCUMENTATION

Level of Exam	Perform and Document
Problem focused	One to five elements identified by a bullet.
Expanded Problem Focused	At least six elements identified by a bullet.
Detailed	At least twelve elements identified by a bullet.
Comprehensive	Perform all elements identified by a bullet; document every element in every shaded box and at least one element in every unshaded box.

Genitourinary

System/Body Area	Elements of Examination
Constitutional	• Measurement of **any three of the following seven** vital signs: 1) sitting or standing blood pressure, 2) supine blood pressure, 3) pulse rate and regularity, 4) respiration, 5) temperature, 6) height, 7) weight (may be measured and recorded by ancillary staff) • General appearance of patient *e.g. development, nutrition, body habitus, deformities, attention to grooming*
Neck	• Examination of neck *e.g. masses, overall appearance, symmetry, tracheal position, crepitus* • Examination of thyroid *e.g. enlargement, tenderness, mass*
Respiratory	• Assessment of respiratory effect *e.g. intercostal retractions, use of accessory muscles, diaphragmatic movement* • Auscultation of lungs *e.g. breath sounds, adventitious sounds, rubs*
Cardiovascular	• Auscultation of heart with notation of abnormal sounds and murmurs • Examination of peripheral vascular system by observation *e.g. swelling, varicosities* and palpation *e.g. pulses, temperature, edema, tenderness*
Chest (breasts)	See genitourinary (female)
Gastrointestinal (abdomen)	⊙Examination of abdomen with notation of presence of masses or tenderness • Examination for presence or absence of hernia • Examination of liver and spleen • Obtain stool sample for occult blood test when indicated
Genitourinary (male)	• Inspection of anus and perineum Examination (with or without specimen collection for smears and cultures) of genitalia including: • Scrotum *e.g. lesions, cysts, rashes* • Epididymides *e.g. size, symmetry, masses* ⊙Testes *e.g. size, symmetry, masses* • Urethral meatus *e.g. size, location, lesions, discharge* ⊙Penis *e.g. lesions, presence or absence of foreskin, foreskin retractability, plaque, masses, scarring, deformities* Digital rectal examination including: ⊙Prostate gland *e.g. size, symmetry, nodularity, tenderness* • Seminal vesicles *e.g. symmetry, tenderness, masses, enlargement* • Sphincter tone, presence of hemorrhoids, rectal masses
Genitourinary (female) Includes at least seven of the eleven elements to the right identified by bullets:	• Inspection and palpation of breasts *e.g. masses or lumps, tenderness, symmetry, nipple discharge* • Digital rectal examination including sphincter tone, presence of hemorrhoids, rectal masses Pelvic examination (with or without specimen collection for smears and cultures) including: • External genitalia *e.g. general appearance, hair distribution, lesions* • Urethral meatus *e.g. size, location, lesions, prolapse* • Urethra *e.g. masses, tenderness, scarring* • Bladder *e.g. fullness, masses, tenderness* • Vagina *e.g. general appearance, estrogen effect, discharge, lesions, pelvic support, cystocele, rectocele* • Cervix *e.g. general appearance, lesions, discharge* • Uterus *e.g. size, contour, position, mobility, tenderness, descent or support* • Adnexa/parametria *e.g. masses, tenderness, organomegaly, nodularity* • Anus and perineum

Genitourinary (continued)

System/Body Area	Elements of Examination
Lymphatic	• Palpation of lymph nodes in neck, axillae, groin and/or other location
Skin	• Inspection and/or palpation of skin and subcutaneous tissue *e.g. rashes, lesions, ulcers*
Neurological/ psychiatric	Brief assessment of mental status including: • Orientation to time, place and person • Mood and affect *e.g. depression, anxiety, agitation*

Skin

System/Body Area	Elements of Examination
Constitutional	• Measurement of **any three of the following seven** vital signs: 1) sitting or standing blood pressure, 2) supine blood pressure, 3) pulse rate and regularity, 4) respiration, 5) temperature, 6) height, 7) weight (may be measured and recorded by ancillary staff) • General appearance of patient *e.g. development, nutrition, body habitus, deformities, attention to grooming*
Eyes	• Inspection of conjuctivae and lids
Ears, nose, mouth and throat	• Inspection of lips, teeth and gums • Examination of oropharynx *e.g. oral mucosa, hard and soft palates, tongue, tonsils, and posterior pharynx*
Neck	• Examination of thyroid *e.g. enlargement, tenderness, mass*
Gastrointestinal (abdomen)	• Examination of liver and spleen • Examination of anus for condyloma and other lesions
Lymphatic	• Palpation of lymph nodes in neck, axillae, groin and/or other location
Extremities	• Inspection and palpation of digits and nails *e.g. clubbing, cyanosis, inflammation, petechiae, ischemia, infections, nodes*
Skin	• Palpation of scalp and inspection of hair of scalp, eyebrows, face, chest, pubic area (when indicated) and extremities • Inspection and/or palpation of skin and subcutaneous tissue *e.g. rashes, lesions, ulcers, susceptibility in and presence of photo damage* in **eight of the following ten areas:** 1) head including face, 2) neck, 3) chest including breasts and axilla, 4) abdomen, 5) genitalia, groin, buttocks, 6) back, 7) right upper extremity, 8) left upper extremity, 9) right lower extremity, 10) left lower extremity Note: For the comprehensive level, the examination of all eight anatomic areas must be performed and documented. For the three lower levels of examination, each body area is counted separately. For example, inspection and/or palpation of the skin and subcutaneous tissue of the head and neck extremities constitutes two areas. • Inspection of eccrine and apocrine glands of skin and subcutaneous tissue with identification and location of any hyperhidrosis, chromhidrosis or bromhidrosis
Neurological/ psychiatric	Brief assessment of mental status including: • Orientation to time, place and person • Mood and affect *e.g. depression, anxiety, agitation*

Figure 3–9. Review/audit worksheet of a general multiorgan system physical examination that shows the details (elements) of examination for each body area/system. Circled bullets relate to the example case shown in Figure 3–8, A. (From the Iowa Medical Society, IMS Services, West Des Moines, IA, 1998.)

SECTION II

Four elements identified

	General Multisystem Exam		Single Organ System Exam
E X A M	1-5 elements identified by •	⟨PROBLEM FOCUSED⟩	1-5 elements identified by •
	≥6 elements identified by •	EXPANDED PROBLEM FOCUSED	≥6 elements identified by •
	≥2 elements identified by • from 6 areas/ systems OR ≥12 elements identified by • from at least 2 areas/systems	DETAILED	≥12 elements identified by • EXCEPT ≥ 9 elements identified by • for eye and psychiatric exams
	≥2 elements identified by • from 9 areas/ systems	COMPREHENSIVE	Perform all elements identified by • ; document all elements in shaded boxes; document ≥ 1 element in unshaded boxes.

Figure 3–10. Review/audit worksheet Section II for a general multisystem physical examination and single organ system examination. The circled item relates to a problem-focused examination for the example case (Fig. 3–8, A) for the purpose of coding. (From the Iowa Medical Society, IMS Services, West Des Moines, IA, 1998.)

ordered or reviewed. A decision to obtain and review old medical records or obtain history from sources other than the patient increases the amount and complexity of data to be analyzed. For the case illustrated, no points apply (Fig. 3–11, middle section).

▶ *Risk of Complications, Morbidity, or Mortality.* This is based on other conditions associated with the presenting problem(s) known as the risk of complications, morbidity, or mortality, as well as comorbidities, the diagnostic procedure(s), or the possible management options (treatment rendered—surgery, therapy, drug management, services, and supplies). **Comorbidity** means underlying disease or other conditions present at the time of the visit.

To discover whether the *level of risk* is minimal, low, moderate, or high, bulleted elements are marked on the review/audit sheet (Fig. 3–12, Section III, Part C). For the case illustrated, the elements fall within the moderate level of risk category.

To conclude the internal review of a patient's medical record, a level from one of four types of medical decision making: **straightforward (SF), low complexity (LC), moderate complexity (MC), and high complexity (HC)** must be determined. The bottom portion of Figure 3–11, Section III, shows the results obtained from Parts A, B, and C circled. For the case illustrated, the number of diagnoses is declared *multiple,* there are *no data reviewed,* and the risk of complications is *moderate;* therefore a *moderately complex* level of decision making has been assigned to be used for coding and billing purposes.

Documentation Terminology

Terminology for Evaluation and Management Services

While learning the complexities of medical documentation and how important it is as it relates to coding and billing, you have discovered that you must have a good foundation of medical terminology. To use the diagnostic and procedure code books efficiently, you must become familiar with their language, abbreviations, and symbols. The first terms introduced are most commonly used for evaluation and management services.

New Versus Established Patient

In procedure coding, two categories of patients are considered: the new patient and the established patient. A **new patient** is one who *has not received* any professional services from the physician or another physician of the same specialty who belongs to the same group practice *within the past 3 years.* An **established patient** is one who *has received* professional services from the physician or another physician of the same specialty who belongs to the same group practice *within the past 3 years.* Medicare policies regarding the definition of new and established patients may have different requirements and are discussed in Chapter 11.

A physician may provide several types of services to evaluate and manage a patient who is seeking medical care (i.e., consultation, referral, concurrent care, continuity of care, critical care, emergency care, or counseling).

SECTION III A AND B

A | NUMBER OF DIAGNOSES OR TREATMENT OPTIONS

Problems to exam physician	Number X points = Result		
Self-limited or minor (stable, improved or worsening)	Max = 2	1	
Est. problem (to examiner); stable, improved		1	
Est. problem (to examiner); worsening		2	
New problem (to examiner); no additional workup planned	Max = 1 1	3	3
New prob. (to examiner); add. workup planned		4	
		TOTAL	3

Bring total to line A in final result for complexity

B | AMOUNT AND/OR COMPLEXITY OF DATA TO BE REVIEWED

Data to be reviewed	Points
Review and/or order of clinical lab tests	1
Review and/or order of tests in the radiology section of CPT	1
Review and/or order of tests in the medicine section of CPT	1
Discussion of test results with performing physician	1
Decision to obtain old records and/or obtain history from someone other than patient	1
Review and summarization of old records and/or obtaining history from someone other than patient and/or discussion of case with another health care provider	2
Independent visualization of image, tracing or specimen itself (not simply review of report)	2
TOTAL	0

Bring total to line B in final result for complexity

Draw a line down the column with 2 or 3 circles and circle decision making level OR draw a line down the column with the center circle and circle the decision making level.

A	Number diagnoses or treatment options	≤ 1 Minimal	2 Limited	3 Multiple	≥ 4 Extensive
B	Amount and complexity of data	≤ 1 Minimal or low	2 Limited	3 Moderate	≥ 4 Extensive
C	Highest risk	Minimal	Low	Moderate	High
	Type of decision making	Straight-foward	Low complex	Moderate complex	High complex

Note: The wound was not a considering factor in the medical decision making.

Figure 3–11. Section III of the review/audit worksheet. Part A: Number of diagnoses or treatment options. Part B: Amount or complexity of data to be reviewed. Lower one third: Used to compile the results obtained from Parts A, B, and C (Fig. 3–10) to determine the level of medical decision making. Circled points and words relate to a moderately complex level of decision making for the example case (Fig. 3–8, A) for the purpose of coding and billing. (From the Iowa Medical Society, IMS Services, West Des Moines, IA, 1998.)

SECTION III

C

RISK OF COMPLICATIONS AND/OR MORBIDITY OR MORTALITY

Level of risk	Presenting problem(s)	Diagnostic procedure(s) ordered	Management options selected
MINIMAL	• One self-limited or minor problem *e.g. cold, insect bite tinea corporis*	• Laboratory tests requiring venipuncture • Chest x-rays • KOH prep • EKG/EEG • Urinalysis • Ultrasound *e.g. echo*	• Rest • Gargles • Elastic bandages • Superficial dressings
LOW	• Two or more self-limited or minor problems • One stable chronic illness *e.g. well controlled hypertension, non-insulin dependent diabetes, cataract, BPH* • Acute uncomplicated illness or injury *e.g. cystitis, allergic rhinitis, simple sprain*	• Physiologic test not under stress *e.g. pulm. function tests* • Non-cardiovascular imaging studies with contrast *e.g. barium enema* • Superficial needle biopsies • Clinical laboratory tests requiring arterial puncture • Skin biopsies	• Over-the-counter drugs • Minor surgery with no identified risk factors • Physical therapy • Occupational therapy • IV fluids without additives
MODERATE	• One or more chronic illnesses with mild exacerbation, progression or side effects of treatment • Two or more stable chronic illnesses • Undiagnosed new problem with uncertain prognosis *e.g. lump in breast* • Acute illness with systemic symptoms *e.g. pyelonephritis, pneumonitis, colitis* • Acute complicated injury *e.g. head injury with brief loss of consciousness*	• Physiologic test under stress *e.g. cardiac stress test, fetal contraction stress test* • Diagnostic endoscopies with no identified risk factors • Deep needle or incisional biopsy • Cardiovascular imaging studies with contrast and no identified risk factors *e.g. arteriogram, cardiac cath* • Obtain fluid from body cavity *e.g. lumbar puncture, thorocentesis culdocentesis*	• Minor surgery with identified risk factors • Elective major surgery (open percutaneous or endoscopic) with no identified risk factors • Prescription drug management • Therapeutic nuclear medicine • IV fluids with additives • Closed treatment of fracture or dislocation without manipulation
HIGH	• One or more chronic illnesses with severe exacerbation, progression or side effects of tx • Acute or chronic illnesses or injuries that may pose a threat to life or bodily function *e.g. multiple trauma, acute MI, pulmonary embolus, severe respiratory distress, progressive severe rheumatoid arthritis, psychiatric illness w/ potential threat to self or others, peritonitis, acute renal failure* • An abrupt change in neurological status *e.g. seizure, TIA, weakness, sensory loss*	• Cardiovascular imaging studies with contrast with identified risk factors • Cardiac electrophysiological tests • Diagnostic endoscopies with identified risk factors • Discography	• Elective major surgery (open, percutaneous or endoscopic) with identified risk factor • Emergency major surgery (open, percutaneous or endoscopic) • Parenteral controlled substances • Drug therapy requiring intensive monitoring for toxicity • Decision not to resuscitate or de-escalate care because of poor prognosis

Figure 3–12. Section III, Part C of the review/audit worksheet used for determining the level of risk. The highlighted areas relate to a moderate level of risk for the example case (Fig. 3–8, *A*) for the purpose of coding. (From the Iowa Medical Society, IMS Services, West Des Moines, Iowa, 1998.)

Consultation

A **consultation** includes services rendered by a physician whose opinion or advice is requested by another physician or agency in the evaluation or treatment of a patient's illness or a suspected problem. The request must be documented in the patient's medical record (e.g., "Patient is seen at the request of Dr. John Doe for a . . . reason."). Consultations may occur in a home, office, hospital, extended care facility, and other locations. A physician consultant recommends diagnostic or therapeutic services and may initiate these services if requested by the referring physician. The opinion must be in writing, documented in a consultation report, and communicated to the referring physician. The consultant may order a diagnostic or therapeutic service to formulate the opinion at an initial or subsequent visit. Reimbursement is significantly more than for an equivalent office visit.

Referral

A **referral** is the transfer of the total or specific care of a patient from one physician to another for known problems. It is *not* a consultation. For example, a patient is sent by a primary case physician to an orthopedist for care of a fracture.

However, when dealing with managed care plans, the term "referral" is also used when requesting an authorization for the patient to receive services elsewhere (e.g., referral for laboratory tests, radiology procedures, specialty care). As a courtesy, the physician may send a thank-you note to the referring physician with comments about the patient's condition.

Concurrent Care

Concurrent care is the providing of similar services (e.g., hospital visits) to the same patient by more than one physician on the same day. Usually, such cases involve the presence of a physical disorder (e.g., diabetes) at the same time as the primary admitting diagnosis, and this may alter the course of treatment or lengthen recovery time for the primary condition. For example, two internists (a general internist and a cardiologist) see the same patient in the hospital on the same day. The general internist admitted the patient for diabetes and requested that the cardiologist also follow the patient's periodic chest pain and arrhythmia. If the second doctor is not identified in carrier records as a cardiologist, the claim may be denied. This is because the services appear to be duplicated by physicians of the same specialty. When billing insurance companies, physicians providing concurrent care may be cross referenced on the claim form. Medicare has a list that includes 62 specialties and subspecialties to help carriers more accurately judge whether concurrent care is necessary. Periodically, the physician should check with the carrier's provider service representative to see if the provider has updated its subspecialty status so that claims for concurrent care are not denied.

Continuity of Care

If a case involves **continuity of care** (e.g., a patient who has received treatment for a condition and is then referred by the physician to a second physician for treatment for the same condition), both physicians are responsible to provide arrangements for the patient's continuing care. In such a case, records must be provided by the referring physician and the insurance billing specialist must obtain summaries or records of the patient's previous treatment. Obtain hospital reports before coding if the patient was seen in the hospital, emergency department, or outpatient department. Contact the hospital's medical record department for copies of reports after outpatient treatment or after a patient's discharge. In some cases, coding from hospital reports can increase reimbursement but can delay submission of claims because reports may not be available in a timely manner.

Critical Care

Critical care means the intensive care provided in a variety of acute life-threatening conditions requiring constant bedside "full attention" by a physician. A critical illness or injury acutely impairs one or more vital organ systems such that there is a high probability of imminent or life-threatening deterioration in the patient's condition. Examples of vital organ system failure include, but are not limited to, central nervous system failure, circulatory failure, shock, and renal, hepatic, metabolic, or respiratory failure. Critical care may sometimes, but not always, be rendered in a critical care area, such as a coronary care unit (CCU), intensive care unit (ICU), respiratory care unit (RCU), or emergency department (ED), also called the emergency room (ER).

Emergency Care

Emergency care differs from critical care in that it is given by the physician in a hospital emergency department. Advanced life support may be required and the physician may spend several hours attending to a patient. Office services also may be provided on an emergency basis.

In the Medicare program, an emergency medical condition is currently defined as a medical condition manifesting itself by acute symptoms of sufficient severity (including severe pain) such that the absence of immediate medical attention could reasonably be expected to result in placing the patient's health in serious jeopardy, serious impairment to body functions, or serious dysfunction of any body organ or part.

Many states have adopted the prudent lay person definition of an emergency as defined in the Balanced Budget Act of 1996. This is similarly stated as "any medical condition of recent onset and severity, including but not limited to severe pain, that would lead to a prudent lay person, possessing an average knowledge of medicine and health, to believe that his or her condition, sickness, or injury is of such a nature that failure to obtain immediate medical care could result in placing the patient's health in serious jeopardy, serious impairment to bodily functions, or serious dysfunction of bodily organ or part."

Counseling

Counseling is a discussion with a patient, family, or both concerning one or more of the following: diagnostic results, impressions, or recommended diagnostic studies; prognosis; risks and benefits of treatment options; instructions for treatment or follow-up; importance of compliance with chosen treatment options; risk factor reduction; and patient and family education.

Diagnostic Terminology and Abbreviations

When completing the medical record, some physicians write "imp" (impression) or "Dx" (diagnosis), which usually serves as the diagnosis when completing the claim. If the diagnosis is not in the chart note and there is doubt about the diagnosis, always pull the chart and request that the physician review it. Attach a note to the insurance claim for the physician to read before signing the form. If the patient has been in the hospital, request a copy of the discharge summary, which contains the admitting and discharge diagnoses.

Official American Hospital Association policy states that "abbreviations should be totally eliminated from the more vital sections of the medical record, such as final diagnosis, operative notes, discharge summaries, and descriptions of special procedures." Many physicians are not aware of this policy, and the final diagnosis may appear as an abbreviation on the patient's record. Frequently, an abbreviation translates to several meanings. Use your medical dictionary (most list abbreviations alphabetically with the unabbreviated words) to interpret the abbreviation or ask the physician if clarification is needed. (If you are using the *Student Workbook for the Insurance Handbook for the Medical Office,* refer to the detailed list of common medical abbreviations in Appendix A.)

If a lay term appears on a patient record, the correct medical term should be substituted to locate the correct diagnostic code (e.g., "bruise" is known as "contusion").

An **eponym** (term including the name of a person) should not be used when a comparable anatomic term can be used in its place (Example 3–2).

The word "**acute**" refers to a condition that runs a short but relatively severe course. The word "**chronic**" means a condition persisting over a long period of time. However, the word "recurrent" is preferable for certain conditions and should be used instead of "chronic." For example, if "chronic asthma" is charted, it should be coded as "recurrent asthma." For proper documentation to support chronic conditions, two criteria are that the documentation actually states something about the chronic condition and that the conditions are pertinent to the patient's current treatment. For example, if a physician states "controlled diabetes"; this is a fact. If the physician asks the patient about his or her sugar level and diet and documents the findings, then something specific has been identified about

EXAMPLE 3–2	
Eponym	**Comparable Medical Term**
Buerger's disease	thromboangiitis obliterans
Graves' disease	exophthalmic goiter
Wilks syndrome	myasthenia gravis

the chronic condition and this would pass an audit for correct documentation.

Whenever the words "question of," "suspected," "rule out," or the abbreviation "R/O" are used in connection with a disease or illness, substitute the words "possible" or "probable" when trying to locate the appropriate diagnostic code number. These are only a few of the many terms used in documentation. See Table 3–1 for a comprehensive reference list of correct symptomatic and diagnostic terms with their lay equivalents.

An abnormal or unexpected finding without elaboration in the medical record is insufficient documentation and should be described. Commonly used phrases or abbreviations that may not support billing of services are "WNL" (within normal limits), "noncontributory," "negative/normal," "other than the above all systems were normal," and so on. For example, phrases used to document findings, such as "all extremities are within normal limits," do not indicate how many extremities or which ones were examined. Documentation must indicate exactly what limb was examined, and abbreviated wording would not pass an external audit. If it is determined such phrases are canned notes that can mean no assessment was actually performed, then this is fraud.

Another phrase commonly used when examining a patient and the findings are within normal limits is the word, "negative" (e.g., "ears, nose, and throat negative" or "chest x-rays negative"). The physician needs to document that there were no abnormalities in the system being examined. Detailed documentation justifies billed services by providing verification and allows points when an external audit is performed. Thus it should be dictated "Chest film (or report) was reviewed." or "Chest x-ray report was read."

Directional Terms

Some terms commonly used to describe location of pain and injuries to areas of the abdomen as shown in Figure 3–13, *A* (four quadrants) and *B* (nine regions), are:

Right upper quadrant (RUQ) or right hypochondriac: liver (right lobe), gallbladder, part of the pancreas, parts of the small and large intestines

TABLE 3–1	Medical Terminology	

Lay Term	Medical Term	Pronunciation
Acute	Use "acute" when referring to a condition that runs a short but relatively severe course	ah-KŪT
Allergy	Allergic asthma	ah-LER-jik AZ-ma
	Allergic bronchitis	ah-LER-jik brong-KĪ-tis
	Bronchial asthma	BRONG-kē-al AZ-ma
Appetite loss (abnormal)	Anorexia nervosa	an"o-REK-sē-ah ner-VŌ-sa
Athlete's foot	Pedal epidermophytosis	PED-al ep"i-der"mō-fī-TŌ-sis
	Tinea pedis	TIN-e-ah PED-is
Bad breath	Halitosis	hal-i-TŌ-sis
Balance, sense of	Equilibrium	Ē-kwi-LIB-rē-um
Baldness	Alopecia	al" ō-PĒ-shē-ah
Bedsore	Decubitus ulcer	de-KŪ-bi-tus UL-ser
Bed-wetting	Enuresis	en"ū-RĒ-sis
Belching	Eructation	ē-ruk-TĀ-shun
Bleeder's disease	Hemophilia	hē"-mo-FIL-ē-ah
Bleeding	Hemorrhage	HEM-or-ij
Blood blister	Hematoma	hēm"ah-TŌ-mah
Blood clot	Thrombus	THROM-bus
Blood, in stools	Melena	MEL-e-nah or me-LĒ-nah
Blood, in urine	Hematuria	hēm"ah-TŪ-rē-ah
Blood poisoning	Septicemia	sep"ti-SĒ-mē-ah
Blood, spitting up of	Hemoptysis	hē-MOP-ti-sis
Bloody vomitus	Hematemesis	hēm"ah-TEM-ĕ-sis
Blue skin	Cyanosis	sī"ah-NŌ-sis
Boil	Furuncle	FU-rung-k'l
Bowel movement	Defecation	def"e-KĀ-shun
Bowleg	Genu varum	JE-nū VA-rum
Breathing, cessation of	Apnea	AP-nē-ah
Breathing, difficult	Dyspnea	DISP-nē-ah or disp-NĒ-ah
Breathing, normal	Eupnea	youp-NĒ-ah
Breathing, rapid	Tachypnea	tak"ip-NĒ-ah
Breathing, slow	Bradypnea	brad"ip-NĒ-ah or brad"IP-nē-ah
Breathing, upright position only	Orthopnea	or"thop-NĒ-ah
Bruise or injury not involving sutures	Contusion	kon-TOO-zhun
	Ecchymosis(ses)	ek"i-MO-sis(sēz)
	Hematoma	hēm"ah-TŌ-mah
	Extravasation	eks-trav"ah-SĀ-shun
Bulging of eyes	Exophthalmos	ek"-sof-THAL-mōs
Burning or cauterizing	Use "surgical removal of"	
Canker sore	Aphthous stomatitis	AF-thus stō-mah TĪ-tis
Cardiac arrest	Cardiac asystole	KAR-dē-ak ah-SIS-tō-le
	Cardiac standstill	KAR-dē-ak STAND-stil
Chafing	Intertrigo	in"ter-TRĪ-gō
Change of life	Menopause	MEN-ō-pawz
	Climacteric	kli"MAK-ter-ik
Chest pain with ECG but not cardiac case	Intercostal neuritis	in"ter-KOS-tal noo-RĪ-tis
	Neurasthenia	nūr"as-THĒ-nē-ah
Chickenpox	Varicella	var"i-SEL-ah
	Variola crystallina	vah-RĪ-ō-lah kris"tah-LĪ-nah
Chronic	Use "recurrent"	
Clubfoot	Talipes	TAL-i-pēz
Cold	Coryza	ko-RĪ-zah
Cold sore; fever blisters on lips	Herpes simplex	HER-pēz-SIM-plex
Cold with runny nose	Coryza with motor rhinitis	rī-NĪ-tis

TABLE 3-1	Medical Terminology—cont'd	

Lay Term	Medical Term	Pronunciation
Collapsed lung	Pneumothorax	nū"mō-THOR-aks
Corn	Clavus	KLĀ-vus
	Heloma molle	he-LŌ-mah MŌL-le
Cross-eye	Convergent strabismus	kon-VER-jent strah BIZ-mus
	Esotropia	os"ō-TRŌ-pō-ah
Cut	Laceration (give location, length, depth)	las"er-Ā-shun
Cutting into	Incision of	in-SIZH-un
Cutting out	Excision of	ek-SIZH-un
Dandruff	Seborrhea capitis	seb"o-RĒ-ah CAP-i-tis
Degenerative joint disease	Osteoarthritis	os"tē-ō-ar-THRI-tis
Dim vision	Amblyopia	am"blē-Ō-pē-ah
Dizziness	Vertigo	VER-ti-go or ver-TI-go
Dog bite	Dog bite (one or more abrasions, give location and description)	
Double vision	Diplopia	di-PLŌ-pē-ah
Drooping eyelids	Ptosis	TŌ-sis
	Blepharoptosis	blef"ah-rō-TŌ-sis
Ear discharge	Otorrhea	o"to-RĒ-ah
Ear procedure involving opening of ear	Myringotomy	mir"in-GOT-ō-mē
Earache	Acute otitis	ah-KŪT-ō-TĪ-tis
	Otitis media	ō-TĪ-tis MĒ-dia
	Otalgia	ō-TAL-jē-ah
	Neuralgic pain in ear (left or right)	nū-RAL-jik
Eardrum	Tympanic membrane	tim-PAN-ik MEM-brān
Earwax removal	Cerumen syringed	see-ROO-men si-RINJD
Enlarged heart	Cardiomegaly	kar"dē-ō-MEG-ah-lē
Excessive eating	Polyphagia	pol"ē-FĀ-je-ah
Excessive thirst	Polydipsia	pol"ē DIP-sē-ah
Eye examination if more than just a check for eyeglasses	Refraction and eye examination	rē-FRAK-shun
Fainting	Syncope	SIN-ko-pē
Farsightedness	Hyperopia	hi"per-Ō-pe-ah
Fat	Obese	o-BĒS
	Exogenous obesity	eks-OJ-e-nus-ō-BĒS-i-tē
Felon	Paronychia	par"ō-NIK-ē-ah
Fever	Pyrexia	pi-REK-se-ah
Fever blister	Lesion of herpes simplex	HER-pēz SIM-plex
Fibroid of uterus	Leiomyoma	li"o-mī-Ō-mah
Fit	Convulsion	kon-VUL-shun
Flatfeet	Pes planus	pes PLA-nus
Flu	Influenza	in"floo-EN-zah
	La grippe	lah GRIP
Freckle	Lentigo	len-TĪ-go
	Ephelis	e-FĒ-lis
Gallstone	Cholelithiasis	kō"le-li-THĪ-ah-sis
Gas pain	Borborygmus	bor"bo-RIG-mus
Gas, passing	Flatulence	FLAT-ū-lens
Gastrointestinal case that is not a duodenal ulcer	Gastroenteritis	gas"trō-en-ter-Ī-tus
German measles	Rubella	roo-BEL-ah
Glands, swollen	Diffuse lymphadenitis	dif-FŪS lim-fad"e-NĪ-tis
Grippe; flu	Influenza	in"floo-EN-zah
	La grippe	lah GRIP
Hammer toe	Hallux malleus	HAL-uks MAL-lē-us
Hangnail	Agnail	AG-nāl

Continued.

TABLE 3-1	**Medical Terminology—cont'd**	
Lay Term	**Medical Term**	**Pronunciation**
Hardening of the arteries	Arteriosclerosis	ar-tē"-rē-ō-skle-RŌ-sis
Harelip	Cleft palate	kleft PAL-at
	Cleft lip	kleft lip
Hay fever	Allergic rhinitis	ah-LER-jik rī-NĪ-tis
	Rhinallergosis	rīn"al-er-GŌ-sis
Headache	Acute cephalalgia	ah-KŪT sef"ah-LAL-jē-ah
	Cephalgia	se-FAL-jē-ah
Heart attack	Coronary thrombosis	KOR-ŏ-nā-rē throm-BŌ-sis
	Coronary occlusion	KOR-ŏ-na-re ŏ-KLOO-zhun
Heart wave (tracing)	Electrocardiogram (ECG), (EKG)	e-lek"tro-KAR-dē-o-gram
Heartbum	Pyrosis	pī-RŌ-sis
Hiccough; hiccup	Singultus	sing-GUL-tus
High blood pressure	Hypertension	hī"per-TEN-shun
Hives	Urticaria	ur"ti-KĀ-rē-ah
Hoarseness	Laryngitis	lar"in-JĪ-tis
	Dysphonia	dis-FŌ-nē-ah
Housemaid's knee	Prepatellar bursitis	prē"pah-TEL-ar bar-SĪ-tis
Humpback; hunchback	Kyphosis	ki-FŌ-sis
Incontinence of urine	Enuresis	en"ū-RĒ-sis
Indigestion	Dyspepsia	dis-PEP-sē-ah
Injury	Trauma	TRAW-mah
Itching	Pruritus	proo-RĪ-tus
Jaundice	Icterus	IK-ter-us
Kidney stone	Nephrolithiasis	ne-frō-li-THĪ-ah-sis
	Renal calculus	RĒ-nal KAL-kū-lus
Knock knees	Genu valgum	JE-nū VAL-gum
Lockjaw	Tetanus	TET-ah-nus
Loss of appetite	Anorexia	an"ō-REK-sē-ah
Loss of hearing	Deafness	DEF-nes
Loss of voice	Aphonia	ah-FŌ-nē-ah
Low blood pressure	Hypotension	hī"pō-TEN-shun
Malnutrition, general ill health	Cachexia	kah-KEK-sē-ah
Marble bones	Osteosclerosis	os"tē-ō-skle-RŌ-sis
Measles	Rubeola	roo-BĒ-ō-lah
Measles, German	Rubella	roo-BEL-ah
Milk leg	Phlebitis	fle-BĪ-tis
Miscarriage	Abortion (AB)	ah-BOR-shun
Mole(s)	Nevus(i)	NĒ-vus(ī)
Mongolism	Down syndrome	down SIN-drŏm
Monthly period	Menses	MEN-sēz
	Menstruation	men"stroo-Ā-shun
Mumps	Contagious parotitis	kon-TĀ-jus par"ō-TĪ-tis
Muscle wasting	Muscular atrophy	MUS-kū-lar AT-rō-fē
Muscular weakness	Atony	AT-ō-nē
Nearsightedness	Myopia	mī-Ō-pē-ah
Nosebleed	Epistaxis	ep"i-STAK-sis
	Rhinorrhagia	rī"no-RĀ-jē-ah
Overweight	Exogenous obesity	eks-OJ-e-nus ō-BĒS-i-tē
Painful periods	Dysmenorrhea	dis"men-o-RĒ-ah
Painful urination	Dysuria	dis-Ū-rē-ah
Pap smear	Papanicolaou smear	pap"ah-nik"-ō-LĀ-ōō-smēr
Piles	Hemorrhoids	HEM-o-roids
Pinkeye	Acute contagious conjunctivitis	ah-KŪT kon-TĀ-jus kon-junk"ti-VĪ-tis
Pneumonia	If both lungs are involved, use "bilateral pneumonitis"	bī-LAT-er-al nū"mō-NĪ-tis

TABLE 3–1	Medical Terminology—cont'd	
Lay Term	**Medical Term**	**Pronunciation**
Poison ivy; poison oak	*Rhus* 'oxicodendron sensitivity	rus tok"si-kō-DEN-dron sen"si-TIV-i-tē
	Rhus dermatitis	rus der"mah-TĪ-tis
Postnasal drip (PND)	Catarrh	kah-TAHR
Protrusion of eyeballs	Exophthalmos	ek"sof-THAL-mos
Pus, full of	Purulent	PŪ-roo-lent or PUR-ū-lent
Pus, in urine	Pyuria	pi-Ū-rē-ah
Question of	Use "possible" or "probable"	
Rabies	Hydrophobia	hi"drō-FŌ-bē-ah
Residual inquiry(ies)	Sequela(ae)	se-KWE-lah(ē)
Ringing in ears	Tinnitus	TIN-Ī-tus
Rule out (R/O)	Use "possible" or "probable"	
Ruptured spleen	Splenorrhexis	sple"no-REK-sis
St Vitus' dance	Chorea	kō-RĒ-ah
Scar	Cicatrix	sik-A-triks, SIK-ah-triks
Sciatica	Sciatic neuritis	sī-AT-ik nū-RĪ-tis
Scraping of uterus	Dilatation and curettage (D & C)	dil-ah-TĀ-shun and kū"rĕ-TAHZH
Sebaceous cyst	Steatoma	ste"ah-TŌ-mah
	Wen	wen
Shingles	Herpes zoster	HER-pēz-ZOS-ter
Sleeping sickness	Encephalitis	en"sef-ah-LĪ-tis
Slipped disk	Herniated intervertebral disk	HER-nē-āt"ed in"ter-VER-te-bral disc
Slow heart rate	Sinus bradycardia	SĪ-nus brad"ē-KAR-dē-ah
Smallpox	Variola	vah-RI-ō-lah
Sore throat	Laryngitis	lar"in-JĪ-tis
	Pharyngitis	far"in-JĪ-tis
	Tonsillitis	ton"si-LĪ-tis
	Alpha-hemolytic streptococcus (milder strep)	AL-fah hē"mō-LIT-ik strep"tō-KOK-us
	Beta-hemolytic streptococcus (real strep throat)	BĀ-tah hē"mō-LIT-ik strep"to-KOK-us
	Acute sore throat for any kind of sore throat unless it is strep	ah-KŪT sor thrōt
Speaking difficulty	Dysphonia	dis-FŌ-nē-ah
Spinal fusion	Arthrodesis	ar"thrō-DĒ-sis
Squint	Strabismus	strah-BIZ-mus
Stiff joint	Ankylosis	ang"ki-LŌ-sis
Stiff neck; wryneck	Torticollis	tor"ti-KOL-is
Stomach ache	Tonic abdominal spasm	TON-ik ab-DOM-i-nal spazm
	Gastritis	gas-TRĪ-tis
	Gastroenteritis	gas"trō-en-ter-Ī-tis
Stone(s)	Calculus(i)	KAL-kū-lus(Ī)
Stroke	Apoplexy	AP-ō-plek"se
	Cerebral hemorrhage	SER-e-bral HEM-or-ij
Stye	Hordeolum	hor-DĒ-o-lum
Swallowing difficulty	Dysphagia	dis-FĀ-je-ah
Swayback	Lordosis	lor-DŌ-sis
Tarry stool	Melena	me-LE-nah
Tennis elbow	Radiohumeral bursitis	ra"dē-ō-HŪ-mer-al ber-SĪ-tis
Tic douloureux	Trigeminal neuralgia	tri-JEM-i-nal nū-RAL-jē-ah
Tongue tie	Ankyloglossia	ang"ki-lo-GLOS-ē-ah
Trench mouth	Acute necrotizing ulcerative infection	ah-KŪT nek-ro-TĪ-zing UL-ser-ah-tiv in-FEK-shun
	Vincent's angina	VIN-sents an-JĪ-nah

Continued.

TABLE 3-1	Medical Terminology—cont'd	
Lay Term	**Medical Term**	**Pronunciation**
Undescended testicle	Cryptorchism	krip-TŌR-kizm
	Cryptorchidism	krip-TŌR-kĪ-dizm
Undulant fever	Brucellosis	broo"sel-LO-sis
Urination, excessive	Nocturia (nighttime)	nok-TŪ-rē-ah
	Polyuria	pol"ē-Ū-rē-ah
Urination, involuntary	Enuresis (bed-wetting)	en"ū-RĒ-sis
Urination, painful	Dysuria	dis-Ū-rē-ah
Urine, scanty	Oliguria	ol"i-GŪ-rē-ah
Urine, sugar in	Glycosuria	gli"kō-SŪ-rē-ah
Vomiting of blood	Hematemesis	hem"-ah-TEM-e-sis
Wall eye	Divergent strabismus	di-VER-jent strah-BIZ-mus
	Exotropia	ek"so-TRŌ-pē-ah
Wart(s)	Verruca(ae)	ve-ROO-kah(sē)
Water on the brain	Hydrocephalus	hĪ-drō-SEF-ah-lus
Water on the knee	Prepatellar bursitis	prē-pah-TEL-ar bur-SĪ-tis
Wen	Sebaceous cyst	sē-BĀ-shus sist
	Steatoma	stē"ah-TŌ-mah
Whooping cough	Pertussis	per-TUS-is
Womb	Uterus	Ū-ter-us
Wristdrop	Carpoptosis	kar"po-TŌ-sis
Writer's cramp	Graphospasm	GRAF-ō-spazm
Wryneck	Torticollis	tor"ti-KOL-is

Epigastric: upper middle region above the stomach

Left upper quadrant (LUQ) or left hypochondriac: liver (left lobe), stomach, spleen, part of the pancreas, parts of the small and large intestines

Right and left lumbar: middle, right, and left regions of the waist

Umbilical: central region near the navel

Right lower quadrant (RLQ) or right inguinal: parts of the small and large intestines, right ovary, right uterine (fallopian) tube, appendix, and right ureter.

Hypogastric: middle region below the umbilical region contains urinary bladder and female uterus.

Left lower quadrant (LLQ) or left inguinal: parts of the small and large intestines, left ovary, left uterine tube, and left ureter.

Surgical Terminology

Surgical procedures of the integumentary system, such as repair of lacerations, are listed in the procedure code book as *simple, intermediate,* or *complex* repairs. Simple lacerations are superficial, requiring one-layer closure. Intermediate lacerations require layered closure of one or more of the deeper layers of the skin and tissues. Complex lacerations require more than layered closure and may require reconstructive surgery.

Documentation should list the length (in centimeters) of all incisions and layers of involved tissues (subcutaneous, fascia, muscle, and grafts) so that correct procedure codes for excision of lesions and type of repair can be determined.

Documentation should list the length of time spent on the procedure, especially if of unusual duration. This should be stated somewhere in the report.

If state-of-the-art instruments or equipment are used, document the equipment as well as the time spent using it.

Therapeutic or cosmetic surgical procedures should be broken down into two categories—state how much of the procedure was functional and how much was cosmetic or therapeutic. Generally, the insurance carrier pays for the functional portion of the procedure even if there is no coverage for cosmetic or therapeutic procedures.

If you type reports to be submitted with insurance claims to help justify the claim, you should also become familiar with the terms for various operational incisions (Fig. 3–14). Terms such as *undermining* (cut in a horizontal fashion), *take down* (to take apart), or *lysis of adhesions* (destruction of scar tissue) appear in many operations but should not be coded separately. Note the *position* (e.g., lithotomy, dorsal) of the patient during the operation and the *surgical approach* (e.g., vaginal, abdominal). These help to determine the proper code selection. Major errors can occur when an insurance biller is not familiar

Figure 3–13. Regions of the abdomen. **A,** Four quadrants. **B,** Nine regions (From Herlihy B, Maebius NK: The Human Body in Health and Illness, 2nd ed. Philadelphia, Saunders, 2003.)

with the medical terms being used. Ask the physician to clarify the case if there is a question, because medical terminology is very technical and can puzzle even the most knowledgeable insurance billing specialist. Additional key words to look for that may affect code selection and reimbursement besides terminology shown in Table 3–2 are listed here along with brief definitions:

bilateral: pertaining to both sides

blood loss of over 600 mL: severe bleeding

complete or total: entire or whole

complicated by: involved with other situations at the same time

hemorrhage: escape of blood from vessels; bleeding

initial: first procedure or service

multiple: affecting many parts of the body at the same time

partial: only a part, not complete

prolonged procedure due to: series of steps extended in time to get desired result

simple: single and not compound or complex

subsequent: second or more procedures or services

surgical: pertaining to surgery

uncomplicated: not intricately involved; straightforward (procedure)

unilateral: pertaining to one side

unusual findings or circumstances: rare or not usual conclusion

very difficult: hard to do, requiring extra effort and skill

Additional words used to detail accidents and injuries are shown in Chapter 14, Figures 14–5 through 14–9.

If you would like a more thorough discussion of medical terminology, many good books are available.*

---

*Chabner DE: *The Language of Medicine,* 6th ed. Philadelphia, Saunders, 2001; Leonard PC: *Building a Medical Vocabulary.* Philadelphia, Saunders, 1997.

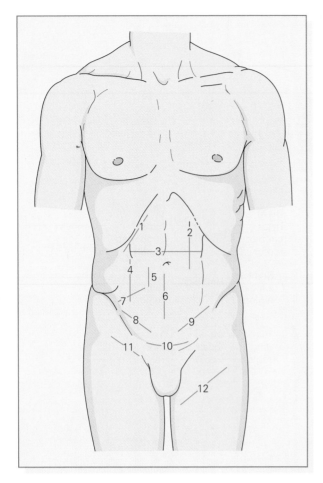

Figure 3–14. Operational incisions. Anterior *(front)* view: *1,* subcostal incision; *2,* paramedian incision; *3,* transverse incision; *4,* upper right rectus incision; *5,* midrectus incision; *6,* midline incision; *7,* lower right rectus incision; *8,* McBurney or right iliac incision; *9,* left iliac incision; *10,* suprapubic incision; *11,* hernia incision; and *12,* femoral incision.

Review and Audit of Medical Records

Internal Reviews

Prospective Review

There are two types of **internal review.** The first type is **prospective review,** which is done *before* billing is submitted. This may be done by some medical practices daily, weekly, or monthly.

▶ Stage one of a prospective review is done to verify that completed encounter forms match patients seen according to the appointment schedule and have been posted on the daysheet. A prospective review is begun by obtaining the encounter form(s) and locating the dates in question for the review in the appointment schedule, printing the schedule as verification. The appointment schedule is then compared to the encounter forms to match patients for the date in question. Next check to

see if all charges (procedures or services) have been posted on the daysheet or daily transaction register.

▶ Stage two of a prospective review is done to verify that all procedures or services and diagnoses listed on the encounter form match data on the insurance claim form. To perform this stage, use the completed claim form or print an insurance billing worksheet. Match the information on the claim or worksheet with the date of service, procedure or service, and diagnosis on the encounter form. It is possible that one or more diagnoses may not match. A common reason this may occur is because an active diagnosis has not been entered into the computer system and the computer defaults to the last diagnosis given for an established patient. Another problem occurs when the diagnosis is not linked to the procedure. Such problems must be found prior to billing and corrected before claims are printed.

Retrospective Review

The second type of internal review is called **retrospective review,** which is done *after* billing insurance carriers. A coder or insurance biller may be asked to perform a retrospective review to determine whether there is a lack of documentation. To accomplish this, pull 15 to 20 medical records from the last 2 to 4 months at random. Recommended internal audit tools are:

pencil

internal record review worksheets

procedure code book

diagnostic code book

HCPCS code book

medical dictionary

abbreviation reference book

drug reference book (i.e., *Physicians' Desk Reference*)

laboratory reference book

provider's manual for insurance program or plan

insurance carrier's newsletters

Forms similar to the Internal Record Review Form shown in Figures 3–8 through 3–12 may be used as tools to gather information from the patient's record, laboratory reports, pathology reports, radiology reports, operative reports, and other diagnostic tests. If the physician's documentation is inadequate, errors or deficiencies will appear as the review is being conducted. You will discover that doing an internal review of this type is not an exact science and critical thinking skills are put into use. Because documentation guidelines and code policies are updated and refined periodically, it is extremely important to read and keep bulletins from all insurance carriers,

TABLE 3–2	Terminology Used in Coding Procedures

Medical Term	Definition
Ablation	Surgical removal of a body part, as by incision.
Acquired	Condition or disorder contracted after birth; not hereditary or innate.
Amputation	Removal of a body part, limb, or organ.
Anastomosis	Surgical or pathologic connection of two tubular structures.
Anomaly	Congenital or developmental defect; deviation from normal.
Arthrocentesis	Surgical puncture of a joint to remove fluid.
Arthrodesis	To surgically immobilize a joint; fusion.
Aspiration	To draw in by inhaling or draw out by suction.
Biopsy	Removal of living tissue for microscopic examination.
Cauterization	Means of destroying tissue, treating infectious wounds, or stopping bleeding with use of chemicals (silver nitrate), heat, freezing, or electrical current.
Chemosurgery	Use of chemicals to destroy tissue.
Chemotherapy	Use of chemicals to treat disease.
Closed treatment	To treat a condition (e.g., a fracture) without surgically opening the location closure to bring together the edges of a wound.
Congenital	Condition present from birth; believed to be inherited.
Curettage	Scraping of a cavity to remove tissue, growths, or debris.
Débridement	Excision of dead or damaged tissue and foreign matter from a wound.
Decompression	Removal of pressure.
Decortication	Removal of external layer (beneath the capsule) from any organ or structure.
Defect	Imperfection, malformation, dysfunction, or absence.
Destructive	Causing ruin; opposite of constructive.
Dialysis	To separate from the blood harmful waste products normally secreted in the urine.
Dilation	Enlargement of a hollow structure or opening.
Discission	Incision or cutting into.
Dissection	Cutting of parts for the purpose of separation and study.
Drainage	Continuous withdrawal of fluid from a wound, sore, or cavity.
Endoscopy	Visual examination of the interior of a canal or hollow internal organ by means of a special instrument.
Evacuation	Removal of waste material.
Excision	The act of cutting out.
Exploration	An active examination, usually involving endoscopy or a surgical procedure, to aid in diagnosis.
Fixation	The act of holding or fastening; immobilize; make rigid.
Foreign body	Any substance or particle in the body that does not appear, form, or grow naturally.
Fulguration	Destruction by means of high-frequency electric sparks.
Graft	Any organ, tissue, or object used for implanting or transplanting to encourage healing, improve function, safeguard against infection, improve appearance, or replace a diseased body organ.
Immunoassay	Any of several methods used for measuring chemical substances such as hormones, drugs, and specific proteins.
Implant	Tissue or substance inserted or grafted into body.
Incision	To cut into.
Indwelling	Located or implanted inside the body, such as a catheter or tube for drainage or administration of drugs.
In situ	Localized; in one specific location without disturbing or invading surrounding tissue.
Instrumentation	Application or use of instruments or tools.
Internal	Within the body.
Insertion	To place or implant; site of attachment.
Introduction	Device for controlling and directing; to insert into the body via tube, needle, oral, or anal entrance.
Ligation	The process of binding or tying a body structure.
Lysis	Destruction, decomposition, breakdown, or separation.
Manipulation	Use of hands to produce a desired movement or effect in the body.
Marsupialization	Surgical conversion of a closed cavity (abscess or cyst) into an open pouch to allow healing.
Obstruction	Blockage of a structure that prevents it from functioning normally.
Occlusion	Blockage of any passage, canal, opening, or vessel in the body; acquired or congenital.
Open treatment	To lay open internal parts to administer treatment.
Paring	Surgical removal of foreign material or dead or damaged tissue by cutting or scraping.
Percutaneous	Through the skin.
Qualitative	Referring to the quality, value, or nature of something.
Quantitative	A measurable amount or portion.
Radical	Extreme or drastic treatment or surgery aimed at eliminating a major disease by removing all affected tissue and any surrounding tissue that might be diseased.

Continued.

TABLE 3–2	**Terminology Used in Coding Procedures—cont'd**
Medical Term	**Definition**
Reconstitution	Returning a substance that has been changed to its original state for preservation and storage.
Reconstruction	Repair, mold, change, or alter to affect recovery.
Reduction	To restore to a normal position.
Repair	To remedy, replace, or heal; restore to a healthy state.
Replantation	Surgical replacement of a body part.
Revision	To amend or alter; to correct or improve.
Resection	Partial excision of a body structure.
Shunt	An artificial passage constructed to divert flow from one route to another.
Suture	Material (wire, thread, or staples) used in closing or attaching body tissue; to unite body tissue by stitching together; the seam formed by stitching body tissue together; line of union (border or joint) such as between the skull bones.
Therapy	Treatment of disease or pathologic conditions.
Transection	A cross section; division by cutting transversely.
Transposition	Displacement of an organ from one side of the body to the other; congenital anomaly in which a part of the body normally appearing on the right side is located on the left side of the body.
Traumatic	Physical or psychological wound or injury.

especially from the local fiscal Medicare intermediary. Advise the physician of any new requirements. This resource may be the only notification of changes unless you routinely attend local or national workshops.

HIPAA Compliance Alert

External Audit

An **external audit** is a retrospective review of medical and financial records by an insurance company or Medicare representative to investigate suspected fraud or abusive billing practices. Government officials discovered deficiencies in medical documentation as a result of external audits conducted by Medicare officials.

In 1984, Michigan signed into law the Health Care Claim Act with felony penalties ranging to 10 years in prison and fines of up to $50,000 per count for attempting to defraud an insurance company. Other states are following suit in establishing such laws.

Most insurance companies perform routine audits on unusual billing patterns. Insurance companies have computer software programs capable of editing and screening insurance claims to identify billing excesses or potential abuses before payment is rendered. Insurance carriers hire undercover agents who visit physicians' offices if overuse and abuse of procedure codes are suspected. Physicians who charge excessive fees are routinely audited by most carriers. Carriers spot check by sending questionnaires to patients and asking them if they received medical care from Dr. Doe to verify the services rendered. The answers are then compared with what the physician billed. Many insurance companies have installed antifraud telephone hotlines or billing question telephone lines for patients. Investigations can result from such calls, depending on the circumstances. Tips also come from peer review organizations, state licensing boards, whistle-blowing physicians, ex-staff members, and patients. If there is any suspicion of fraud, the insurance company notifies the medical practice, specifies a date and time they will come to the office, and indicates which records they wish to audit (Fig. 3–15). Investigators question the patient, look at the documentation in the medical record, and interview the staff and all physicians who have participated in the care of the patient. Points are awarded if documentation is present. Auditors also look at appointment books and add up the hours the physician sees patients on any given day when a medical practice uses time-based procedure codes when submitting insurance claims.

Audit Prevention

Health Insurance Portability and Accountability Act Compliance Program

As mentioned in Chapters 1 and 2, the Health Insurance Portability and Accountability Act (HIPAA) was created in 1996 and 1997 by the Department of Health and Human Services (HHS) Office of the Inspector General (OIG) to combat

Figure 3–15. Insurance billing specialist searching for a patient's chart in the files to pull records for an external audit.

▶ investigation and remediation plan for problems that develop

▶ a response plan for improper or illegal activities

A compliance program must be tailored to fit the needs of each medical practice depending on its corporate structure, mission, size, and employee composition. The statutes, regulations, and guidelines of the federal and state health insurance programs, as well as the policies and procedures of the private health plans, should be integrated into every medical practice's compliance program. The ultimate goals are to improve quality of services and control of claims submission, and also to reduce fraud, waste, abuse, and the cost of health care to federal, state, and private health insurers.

fraud and abuse, protect workers so they can obtain and maintain health insurance if changing or losing a job, and establish a medical savings account. The act also developed the concept of compliance planning as related to clinical documentation. OIG and HHS as well as the Health Care Compliance Association (HCCA) and many other health care agencies have asked physicians to voluntarily develop and implement compliance programs. OIG published guidelines to assist a physician and his or her staff in establishing a medical practice's compliance program to enhance documentation for Medicare cases as well as all patients seen by the physician. Purposes of a compliance program are to reduce fraudulent insurance claims and provide quality care to patients. A **compliance program** is composed of policies and procedures to accomplish uniformity, consistency, and conformity in medical record keeping that fulfills official requirements. If a medical practice experiences an external Medicare audit, HHS OIG and the Department of Justice consider that the medical practice made a reasonable effort to avoid and detect misbehavior if a compliance plan has been in place. When errors are found and a determination is made as to whether there was intent to commit health care fraud, a compliance plan provides evidence that any errors made were inadvertent. There is no single best compliance program because every medical practice is different. However, some elements lead to a successful compliance program. These are:

▶ written standards of conduct

▶ written policies and procedures

▶ compliance officer or committee to operate and monitor the program

▶ training program for all affected employees

▶ process to give complaints anonymously

▶ routine internal audit

Edit Checks

An *edit check* is a good audit prevention measure to have in place because the software program automatically screens transmitted insurance claims and electronically examines them for errors or conflicting code entries. Carriers accept a variety of levels of service; however, if only one or two levels are consistently listed, this is usually not realistic and will attract attention and, possibly, an audit. If services are downcoded and the physician neglected to document the correct level of services performed, an addendum to a medical record must be made to justify the level of service reported (Fig. 3–16). Amended chart notes must be labeled "Addendum" or "Late entry," dated on the day of the amendment, and signed by the physician.

It is vital to be as correct as possible in your choice of diagnostic and procedural codes with modifiers. If the diagnosis does not match the service provided, the claim will be thrown out by the edit check of the computer program. It is equally important that everything involved in patient care be well documented and that records be complete (Fig. 3–17).

In subsequent chapters, you will obtain further knowledge on what needs to be documented in relationship to diagnostic and procedure codes. Information on the Civil Monetary Penalties Law to prosecute cases of Medicare and Medicaid fraud can be found in Chapter 11.

Once an individual has been found guilty of committing a Medicare or Medicaid program-related crime, 5 to 15 years or lifetime exclusion from program participation is mandatory under Sec. 1128(a) of the Social Security Act. An individual can be anyone who participates in fraud or abuse, including the physician, nurse, home health aide, insurance billing specialist, claims assistance professional, electronic claims processor, or medical assistants. If you are ever

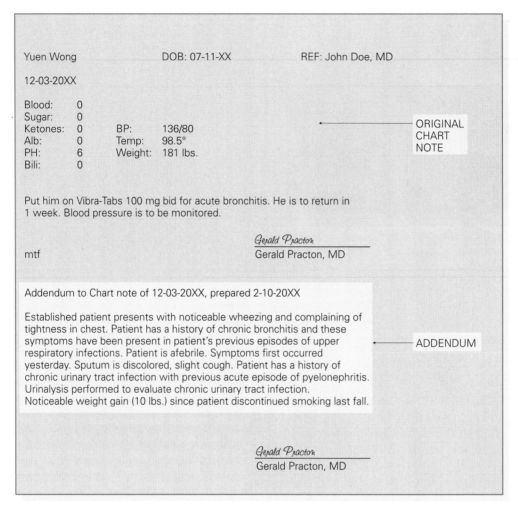

Yuen Wong   DOB: 07-11-XX   REF: John Doe, MD

12-03-20XX

Blood: 0
Sugar: 0
Ketones: 0   BP: 136/80   ORIGINAL
Alb: 0   Temp: 98.5°   CHART
PH: 6   Weight: 181 lbs.   NOTE
Bili: 0

Put him on Vibra-Tabs 100 mg bid for acute bronchitis. He is to return in
1 week. Blood pressure is to be monitored.

                              Gerald Practon
mtf   Gerald Practon, MD

Addendum to Chart note of 12-03-20XX, prepared 2-10-20XX

Established patient presents with noticeable wheezing and complaining of
tightness in chest. Patient has a history of chronic bronchitis and these
symptoms have been present in patient's previous episodes of upper   ADDENDUM
respiratory infections. Patient is afebrile. Symptoms first occurred
yesterday. Sputum is discolored, slight cough. Patient has a history of
chronic urinary tract infection with previous acute episode of pyelonephritis.
Urinalysis performed to evaluate chronic urinary tract infection.
Noticeable weight gain (10 lbs.) since patient discontinued smoking last fall.

                              Gerald Practon
                              Gerald Practon, MD

Figure 3–16. Example of an addendum to a patient's medical record to justify the level of service reported. The insurance carrier downcoded the services from level 99213 to 99212.

suspended from the Medicare program, make sure to obtain a reinstatement letter, because this will be needed when applying for a future position in the medical field.

HIPAA Compliance Alert

Legalities of Medical Records

The basics of confidential communication were provided in Chapter 1, where privileged and nonprivileged information and the right to privacy were discussed. In this chapter, confidentiality is presented as it relates to the medical record and the law.

Patient Confidentiality

The patient record and any photographs taken are confidential documents and require an authorization form that must be signed by the patient to release information (Figs. 3–18 through 3–21). If the form is a photocopy, it is necessary to state that the photocopy is approved by the patient or write to the patient and obtain an original signed document.

Unauthorized release of information is called **breach of confidential communication.**

Confidentiality between the physician and patient is automatically waived in the following situations:

▶ When the patient is a member of a managed care organization (MCO) and the physician has signed a contract with the MCO that has a clause that says "for quality care purposes, the MCO has a right to access the medical records of their patients, and for utilization management purposes, the MCO has a right to audit those patients' financial records." Other managed care providers need to know about the patients if involved in the care and treatment of members of the MCO.

▶ When the physician examines a patient at the request of a third party who is paying the bill, as in workers' compensation cases.

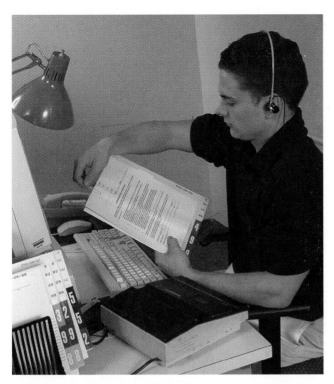

Figure 3–17. Medical transcriptionist inserting a transcribed chart note into a patient's medical record.

▶ When the patient is suing someone, such as an employer, and wishes to protect herself or himself.

▶ When the patient's records are subpoenaed or there is a search warrant.

▶ Other exceptions to the confidentiality requirement include when state law requires the release of information that is for the good of society, such as cases of child or, in some states, elder abuse, certain highly contagious or infectious diseases, and gunshot wounds.

For information on confidentiality as it relates to computer use, refer to Chapter 7.

Principles for Release of Information

Some situations require the insurance billing specialist to release medical information to or for a patient, such as when a patient is seeking a second medical opinion, wishes to acquire insurance, needs it for personal record keeping or upcoming surgery, is transferring to another physician, or is relocating to another city. Some general guidelines are shown in Table 3–3.

To avoid misunderstanding of technical terms, it is preferable not to allow lay persons to examine records without the presence of the physician. If a patient requests to view his or her medical record, inform the physician so that he or she can help interpret the language and abbreviations used in

the record. When working in a hospital, the insurance billing specialist should check with the supervisor at all times to make sure his or her actions conform to hospital policy. If employed by a health facility that has a policy manual, familiarize yourself with its rules regarding release of information. Regardless of the work setting, when in doubt about the release of any information, ask the physician or office manager for guidance and make sure you have obtained the patient's authorization in writing.

Faxing Documents

The common term *fax* is derived from the word **facsimile,** which means transmission of written and graphic matter by electronic means. Faxes have become an important communication tool. Fax transmission is a system of sending and receiving copies of information instantly over telephone lines. It is used to transmit insurance claims data directly to an electronic claims processor, resubmit an unpaid insurance claim, send further documentation on a claim to insurance carriers, obtain preauthorization for surgery on a patient, network with other insurance billers, and send medical reports between offices and to other medical facilities across the country. Unless otherwise prohibited by state law, information that is transmitted by fax is acceptable and may be included in the patient's medical record. Documents to be faxed can be a graphic illustration, typewritten, or handwritten with pen. Pencil does not fax through clearly to the recipient. To prevent deterioration of documents faxed on thermal paper (when the machine is not a plain paper fax), photocopy the document onto regular paper before it is filed in medical records.

Sensitive Information

From the legal standpoint, protecting the patient's confidentiality in the fax process is critical. If, owing to circumstances, medical records or a report must be faxed, you should have the patient sign an authorization to release information via facsimile equipment. The American Health Information Management Association (AHIMA) advises that fax machines should not be used for *routine* transmission of patient information. AHIMA recommends that documents should be faxed *only* when (1) hand or mail delivery does not meet the needs of immediate patient care, or (2) a fax is required by a third party for ongoing certification of payment for a hospitalized patient.

Documents containing information on sexually transmitted diseases, drug or alcohol treatment,

AUTHORIZATION FOR RELEASE OF INFORMATION

Section A: Must be completed for all authorizations.

I hereby authorize the use or disclosure of my individually identifiable health information as described below.

I understand that this authorization is voluntary. I understand that if the organization authorized to receive the information is not a health plan or health care provider, the released information may no longer be protected by federal privacy regulations.

Patient name: _____Chloe E. Levy_____   ID Number: _____3075_____

Persons/organizations providing information: **Persons/organizations receiving information:**

College Clinic, Gerald Practon, MD   Margaret L. Lee, M.D.
4567 Broad Avenue   328 Seward Street
Woodland Hills, XY 12345-0001   Anytown, XY 45601-0731

Specific description of information [including date(s)]: Initial history and physical
and complete medical records for last 3 years

Section B: Must be completed only if a health plan or a health care provider has requested the authorization.

1. The health plan or health care provider must complete the following:
   a. What is the purpose of the use or disclosure? Patient relocating to another city

   b. Will the health plan or health care provider requesting the authorization receive financial or in-kind compensation in exchange for using or disclosing the health information described above? Yes ____ No _X_

2. The patient or the patient's representative must read and initial the following statements:
   a. I understand that my health care and the payment for my health care will not be affected if I do not sign this form.   Initials: _cel_
   b. I understand that I may see and copy the information described on this form if I ask for it, and that I get a copy of this form after I sign it.   Initials: _cel_

Section C: Must be completed for all authorizations.

The patient or the patient's representative must read and initial the following statements:

1. I understand that this form will expire on 09 / 01 /20XX (DD/MM/YR).
   Initials _cel_

2. I understand that I may revoke this authorization at any time by notifying the providing organization in writing , but if I do not it will not have any effect on any actions they took before they received the revocation.
   Initials: _cel_

_____Chloe E. Levy_____   June 1, 20XX
Signature of patient or patient's representative   **Date**
(Form MUST be completed before signing)

Printed name of patient's representative: _____

Relationship to the patient: _____

YOU MAY REFUSE TO SIGN THIS AUTHORIZATION
You may not use this form to release information for treatment or payment
except when the information to be released is psychotherapy notes or
certain research information.

*Labels in left margin:*

Identification of person (or class) authorized to request

Identification of person (or class) to whom covered entity is to use/disclosure

Description of information to be released with specificity to allow entity to know which information the authorization references

Expiration date, time period, or event

Statement that is revocable by written request

Individual's (patient's) signature and date

Statement of representative's authority

Figure 3–18. Completed Authorization for Release of Information form for a patient relocating to another city. *Note:* This form is used on a one-time basis for reasons other than treatment, payment, or health care operations. When the patient arrives at the new physician's office, a consent for treatment, payment, and health care operations form will need to be signed. (From Federal Register, Vol. 64, No. 212, Appendix to Subpart E of Part 164: Model Authorization Form, November 3, 1999.)

NAME OF FACILITY
Consent for Release of Information

Date May 16, 20XX

1. I hereby authorize College Hospital to release the following information from the
   Name of Institution
   health record(s) of Martha T. Jacobson
   Patient name

   52 East Rugby Street, Woodland Hills, XY 12345
   Address

   covering the period(s) of hospitalization from:
   Date of Admission   January 3, 20XX
   Date of Discharge   January 5, 20XX
   Hospital # ___278-1200___   Birthdate ___June 27, 1960___

2. Information to be released:
   ☐ Copy of (complete) health record(s)   ☑ Discharge summary
   ☐ History and physical   ☐ Operative report
   ☐ Other _____

3. Information is to be released to: ___Michael Hotta, MD___
   260 West Main Street, Woodland Hills, XY 12345

4. Purpose of disclosure   June 14, 20XX consultation

5. I understand this consent can be revoked at any time except to the extent that disclosure made in good faith has already occurred in reliance to this consent.

6. Specification of the date, event, or condition upon which this consent expires:
   December 31, 20XX

7. The facility, its employees and officers, and attending physician are released from legal responsibility or liability for the release of the above information to the extent indicated and authorized herein.

Signed _Martha T. Jacobson_
                    (Patient or Representative)

_____
                    (Relationship to Patient)

May 16, 20XX
                    (Date of Signature)

Figure 3–19. Consent for Release of Information form to a hospital. (From the American Health Information Management Association, Chicago, IL.)

or human immunodeficiency virus (HIV) status should not be faxed. Psychiatric records should not be faxed except for emergency requests.

Fax machines should be located in secure or restricted access areas. Do not fax to machines in mail rooms, office lobbies, or other open areas unless they are secured with passwords. To ensure protection, a cover sheet should be used for all transmissions. This can be a half sheet, full sheet, or small self-adhesive form attached to the top of the first page. It should contain the following information:

▶ Name of recipient
▶ Name of sender
▶ Date
▶ Total number of pages, including the cover sheet
▶ Fax and telephone numbers of recipient and sender in case of transmittal problems (e.g., lost page or dropped line)
▶ A statement that it is personal, privileged, and confidential medical information intended for the named recipient only (Fig. 3–22).

Transmittal Destination

Noise or interference from telephone lines can be severe enough to distort a fax message; therefore verify the receipt when necessary. There are a number of ways to ensure that a faxed document has reached the correct destination.

▶ Place a telephone call to the requesting physician's office 10 to 15 minutes after faxing patient records to verify their receipt.
▶ Request that the authorized receiver sign and return an attached receipt form at the bottom of the cover sheet on receipt of the faxed information.
▶ Make arrangements with the recipient for a scheduled time for transmission.
▶ Send the fax to a coded mail box. Coded mail boxes require the sender to punch in a code indicating the individual to whom the fax is addressed and the receiver to then punch in his or her own code to activate the printer.
▶ Ask the receiving party for a patient reference number (e.g., the patient's Social Security number). Blank out the patient's name and

COLLEGE CLINIC
4567 Broad Avenue
Woodland Hills, XY 12345-0001
Phone: 555/486-9002
Fax: 555/487-8976

CONSENT TO THE USE AND DISCLOSURE OF HEALTH INFORMATION

I understand that this organization originates and maintains health records which describe my health history, symptoms, examination, test results, diagnoses, treatment, and any plans for future care or treatment. I understand that this information is used to:

- plan my care and treatment
- communicate among health professionals who contribute to my care
- apply my diagnosis and services, procedures, and surgical information to my bill
- verify services billed by third-party payers
- assess quality of care and review the competence of healthcare professionals in routine healthcare operations

I further understand that:

- a complete description of information uses and disclosures is included in a *Notice of Information Practices* which has been provided to me
- I have a right to review the notice prior to signing this consent
- the organization reserves the right to change their notice and practices
- any revised notice will be mailed to the address I have provided prior to implementation
- I have the right to object to the use of my health information for directory purposes
- I have the right to request restrictions as to how my health information may be used or disclosed to carry out treatment, payment, or health care operations
- the organization is not required to agree to the restrictions requested
- I may revoke this consent in writing, except to the extent that the organization has already taken action in reliance thereon.

☐ I request the following restrictions to the use or disclosure of my health information.

_____

_____   _____
Date   Notice Effective Date

_____   _____
Signature of Patient or Legal Representative   Witness

_____   _____
Signature   Title

Date _____   __ Accepted __ Rejected

Figure 3–20. An example of a consent form used to disclose and use health information for treatment, payment, or health care operations. (From Fordney MT, French L: *Medical Insurance Billing and Coding: A Worktext.* Philadelphia, Saunders, 2003.)

write in the reference number on the document before faxing it. Also ask other providers to fax records by reference number rather than patient name.

To safeguard against a fax sent to the wrong destination, telephone or fax a request to destroy misdirected information. Note the incident, along with the misdialed number, in the patient's medical record. Program frequently used numbers into the fax machine to avoid misdirecting faxed communications. Edit your release of records authorization form to allow for fax transmission because it is acceptable to honor an authorization sent via this method.

Medicare Guidelines

Check with the Medicare fiscal intermediary to find out whether faxing of claims and documents is acceptable for Medicare patients. The use of a

Figure 3–21. Patient signing a consent form.

fax transmittal system requires that the physician retain the original facsimile with the signature on it. Further information on digital fax may be found in Chapter 7.

Financial Data

Never fax a patient's financial data. In court, faxing medical information can be justified on the basis of medical necessity, but faxing financial information cannot be justified.

Legal Documents

Consult an attorney to make sure that documents (e.g., contracts, proposals, and insurance claims) requiring signatures are legally binding if faxed. To ensure legality do the following:

▶ Transmit the entire document (front and back) to be signed, not only the page to be signed, so the receiver has full disclosure of the agreement.

▶ Obtain confirmation that the receiver is in receipt of all pages sent, because an incomplete document may be invalid.

▶ Insert a clause in the contract stating that faxed signatures will be treated as originals.

▶ Follow up and obtain the original signature in hard copy form as soon as possible.

Subpoena

Subpoena literally means "under penalty." In legal language, it is a writ requiring the appearance of a witness at a trial or other proceeding. Strictly defined, a **subpoena duces tecum** requires the witness to appear and to bring or send certain records "in his possession." Frequently, however, only the records may be sent, and the physician is not required to appear in court.

A subpoena is a legal document signed by a judge or an attorney in the name of a judge. In cases in

which a pretrial of evidence or deposition is set up, the subpoena may be issued by a notary public, in which event it is called a *notary subpoena.* If an attorney signs it, he or she must attest it in the name of a judge, the court clerk, or other proper officer.

It is possible for a state investigator to subpoena patient records and then file administrative charges against the physician, not because of the practice of shoddy medicine but rather because the case was inadequately documented for the treatment provided. Medical records also may be subpoenaed as proof in a medical malpractice case. Complete documentation and well-organized patient records help establish a strong defense in a medical professional liability claim.

The Subpoena Process

A subpoena must be personally served or handed to the prospective witness or keeper of the medical records. Neither civil nor criminal subpoenas can be served via the telecopier (fax) machine. The acceptance of a document by someone authorized to accept it is the equivalent of personal service. The subpoena cannot be left on a counter or desk. In a state civil case, a "witness fee" and payment for travel to and from court are given, if demanded, at the time a subpoena is served. The fee is discretionary in criminal cases. In some states, provision is made for substitute service by mail or through newspaper advertisements. This is permitted only after all reasonable efforts to effect personal service have failed.

Never accept a subpoena or give records to anyone without the physician's prior authorization. The medical office should designate one person as keeper of the medical records. If the subpoena is only for medical records or financial data, the representative for the specific doctor then can usually accept it, and the physician will not be called to court.

If a physician is on vacation and there is no designated keeper of the records, tell the deputy that the physician is not in and cannot be served. Suggest the deputy contact the physician's attorney and relay this information.

When the "witness fee" has been received and the subpoena has been served, pull the chart and place it and the subpoena on the physician's desk for review. Willful disregard of a subpoena is punishable as contempt of court.

The medical office is given a prescribed time in which to produce the records. It is not necessary to show them at the time the subpoena is served unless the court order so states. The attorney usually employs a person or copy service to copy records that are under subpoena. At the time the subpoena is served, a date is usually agreed upon in which the representative will return and copy the portion of the record that is named in the subpoena. Often only

HIPAA Compliance Alert

TABLE 3–2   **Principles for Release of Information**

Request From or For	Policy
Physicians involved with patient care	Consent form signed by the patient.
Physician referring a patient to another doctor for consultation	Referring physician sends summary of case or copies of patient's records without signed authorization.
Patient moving to a new location or being released from medical care and transferred to another physician	Letter should be directed to the patient offering to transfer the patient's records with signed authorization to new physician.
Managed care patient seen by different physicians at each office visit	Patient's records may be read by all physicians involved with the case without a separate signed authorization.
Insurance companies and others concerned from a financial point of view	Consent form signed by the patient.
Attorney in litigation case	Records may be released if subpoenaed; otherwise must have written authorization of the patient.
Any party in workers' compensation case	Insurance claims examiner can give patient copy of his or her records but physician cannot release record unless authorized by claims examiner. Authorization must be signed by employer and insurance company.
Any party via telephone	Either ask the caller to put the request in writing and to include the patient's signed authorization, or obtain the name and telephone number of the caller and relationship to the patient and have the physician return the call.
Government and state agencies	Records may be reviewed without patient's consent to verify billing information and determine if services were medically necessary. Data in the records may be used only for audit and may not be released.
Employer	Written consent of patient. Special care should be exercised and the attending physician consulted before release of any information.
For psychiatric records	Consult psychiatrist or attending physician concerned with the case before records are released. If patient has threatened to harm himself or herself or someone else, the patient may lose the confidentiality privilege when he or she files litigation in which mental distress is claimed.
For publication	Written authorization of patient. Care must be exercised in release of any information for publication because this constitutes an invasion of the patient's right to privacy and can result in legal action against the physician releasing such information.
For medical information in an acquired immunodeficiency syndrome (AIDS) or human immunodeficiency virus (HIV) infection	Seek legal counsel and/or learn the state laws before releasing any information. A specific authorization usually is required. Stamp all information released about a patient who has an HIV infection case with a statement prohibiting redisclosure of the data to another party without prior consent of the patient. The party receiving the data should be requested to destroy the information after the stated need is fulfilled.
For medical information on a minor	If a minor patient is legally capable of consenting to medical treatment, only the minor patient may sign a consent form for disclosure. In all other cases, the consent form must be signed by the minor's parent, guardian, or other legal representative.
For medical information on a minor who has received alcohol and/or drug abuse treatment	Where state law permits the minor to apply for and obtain alcohol or drug abuse treatment, the minor may authorize disclosure.

the portion of the medical record requested is removed from the original chart and put in a copy folder. Items such as the patient registration information sheet, encounter form, and explanation of benefits should not be included. You may also telephone the attorney who sent the subpoena and ask if the records can be mailed. If so, mail them by registered mail with return receipt requested. Retain a copy of the records released. You will have to appear in court if specified in the subpoena. Verify with the court

that the case is actually on the calendar. If you do not appear, you are in contempt of court and subject to a penalty, such as several days in jail.

If original records are requested, move them to a safe place, preferably under lock and key, so that they cannot be taken away or tampered with before the trial date. Make photocopies of the original records because this will prevent total loss of the records and facilitate discovery of any altering or tampering while they are out of your custody.

FAX TRANSMITTAL SHEET

To: _____College Hospital (outpatient surgery)_____ Date _10-21-20XX_

Fax Number: _(555) 486 8900_ Telephone Number _(555) 487 6789_ Time _10:00 a.m._

Number of pages (including this one): _3_

From: _Raymond Skeleton, MD_   Phone _(555) 486 9002_

Note: This transmittal is intended only for the use of the individual or entity to which it is addressed, and may contain information that is privileged, confidential, and exempt from disclosure under applicable law. If you are not the intended recipient, any dissemination, distribution, or photocopying of this communication is strictly prohibited. If you have received this communication in error, please notify this office immediately by telephone and return the original FAX to us at the address below by U.S. Postal Service. Thank you.

Remarks:___Enclosed are Margaret Yont's radiology reports on her____
_____L. tibia/fibula and L. foot fractures_____

If you cannot read this FAX or if pages are missing, please contact:

COLLEGE CLINIC
4567 Broad Avenue
Woodland Hills, XY 12345-0001
Phone: 555/486-9002
Fax: 555/487-8976

INSTRUCTIONS TO THE AUTHORIZED RECEIVER: PLEASE COMPLETE THIS STATEMENT OF RECEIPT AND RETURN TO SENDER VIA THE ABOVE FAX NUMBER.

I, _Cheryl Watson, CMA_, verify that I have received   _3_
                                                  (no. of pages including cover sheet)

from _Raymond Skeleton, MD_
       (sending facility's name)

Figure 3–22. Example of a fax cover sheet for medical document transmission.

Number the pages of the records so you will know if a page is missing.

On the day of your court appearance, comply with all instructions given by the court. *Do not* give up possession of the records unless instructed to do so by the judge. *Do not* permit examination of the records by anyone before their identification in court. *Do not* leave the chart in the court unless it is in the possession of the judge or jury and a receipt for it has been obtained.

When you have questions, call the physician's attorney or the court's information and assistance staff.

Retention of Records

Today, most medical records are either stored in color-coded file folders containing a collection of paper documents or reside in multiple electronic databases displayed in a variety of formats via computer access. Regardless of the system used, there are general guidelines that must be followed to record information correctly, use it according to law, and retain it.

Medical Records

Preservation of medical records is governed by state and local laws. Individual states generally set a minimum of 7 to 10 years for keeping records, but it is the policy of most physicians to retain medical records of all living patients indefinitely. Proof materials for the establishment of evidence, such as x-ray films, laboratory reports, and pathologic specimens probably should be kept indefinitely. Calendars, appointment books, and telephone logs also should be filed and stored. Cases that involve radiologic injury claims (e.g., leukemia from radiation) may begin running the statute of limitations after discovery of the injury, which may occur 20 or 30 years after radiation exposure. Recommended retention periods

TABLE 3-4	Records Retention Schedule		
Temporary Record		**Retention Period (yr)**	**Permanent Record**
Appointment sheets		1	Accounts payable records
Bank deposit slip (duplicate)		1	Bills of sale for important purchases (or until you no longer own them)
Bank statements and canceled checks		7	Capital asset records
Billing records (for outside service)		7	Certified financial statements
Cash receipt records		10	Contracts
Contracts (expired)		7	Credit history
Correspondence, general		1–5	Deeds
Daysheets (balance sheets and journals)		5	Equipment guarantees and records (or until you no longer own them)
Employee contracts		6	Income tax returns
Employee time records		5	Insurance policies and records
Employment applications		3	Leases
Insurance claim forms (paid)		3	Legal correspondence
Invoices		7	Medical records (active patients)
Medical records (expired patients)		5	Medical records (inactive patients)
Remittance advice documents		7	Mortgages
Payroll records		7	Property appraisals and records
Petty cash vouchers		3	Telephone records
Postal and meter records		1	X-ray films
Tax worksheets and supporting documents		7	Year-end balance sheets and general ledgers

for paper files are shown in Table 3–4. Electronic health records may have different retention periods depending on state law.

A person's medical record may be of value not only to himself or herself in later years but also to the person's children. In some states a minor may file suit, after he or she has attained legal age, for any act performed during childhood that the person believes to be wrong or harmful. Sometimes a suit may be permitted even 2 to 3 years after the child has reached legal age. Thus it is important to keep records until patients are 3 to 4 years beyond the age of majority.

Deceased patients' charts should be kept for at least 5 years. Shred documents that are no longer needed. Some practices prefer to use medical record storage companies, which may put records on microfilm before disposal. If records are disposed of by a professional company, be sure to obtain a document verifying method of disposal. Maintain a log of destroyed records showing the patient's name, Social Security number, date of last visit, and treatment.

Financial Documents

According to income tax regulations on record retention, accounting records should be kept a minimum of 4 years (following the due date for filing the tax return or the date the tax is paid, whichever is later). Always contact an accountant before discarding records that may determine tax liability. Suggested retention periods are shown in Table 3–4.

A federal regulation mandates that assigned claims for Medicaid and Medicare be kept for 7 years; the physician is subject to auditing during that period.

Termination of a Case

A physician may wish to withdraw formally from further care of a patient because the patient discharged the physician, did not follow instructions, did not take the recommended medication, failed to return for an appointment, or discontinued payment on an overdue account. A physician may terminate a contract by:

▶ Sending a letter of withdrawal (Fig. 3–23) to the patient by registered or certified mail with return receipt (Fig. 3–24), so that proof of termination is in the patient's medical record.

▶ Sending a letter of confirmation of discharge when the patient states that he or she no longer desires care (Fig. 3–25). This should also be sent registered or certified mail with return receipt requested.

▶ Sending a letter confirming that the patient left the hospital against medical advice or the advice of the physician. If there is a signed statement in the patient's hospital records to this effect, it is not

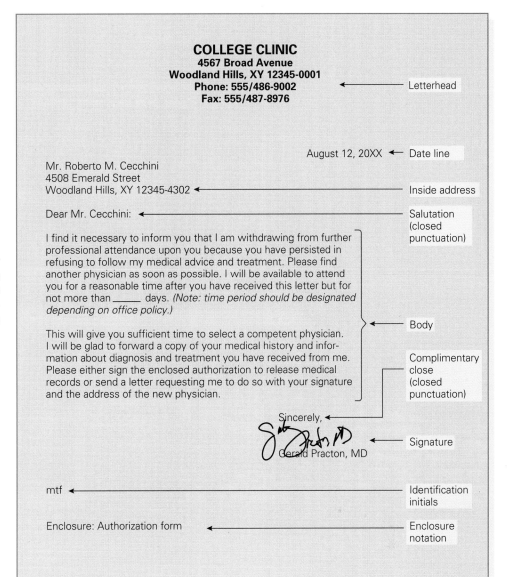

Figure 3–23. Example of letter of withdrawal from a case that is typed in modified-block style with closed punctuation and special notations (placement of parts of letter).

The letter content reads:

COLLEGE CLINIC
4567 Broad Avenue
Woodland Hills, XY 12345-0001
Phone: 555/486-9002
Fax: 555/487-8976 — Letterhead

August 12, 20XX — Date line

Mr. Roberto M. Cecchini
4508 Emerald Street
Woodland Hills, XY 12345-4302 — Inside address

Dear Mr. Cecchini: — Salutation (closed punctuation)

I find it necessary to inform you that I am withdrawing from further professional attendance upon you because you have persisted in refusing to follow my medical advice and treatment. Please find another physician as soon as possible. I will be available to attend you for a reasonable time after you have received this letter but for not more than _____ days. *(Note: time period should be designated depending on office policy.)*

This will give you sufficient time to select a competent physician. I will be glad to forward a copy of your medical history and information about diagnosis and treatment you have received from me. Please either sign the enclosed authorization to release medical records or send a letter requesting me to do so with your signature and the address of the new physician. — Body

Sincerely, — Complimentary close (closed punctuation)

Gerald Practon, MD — Signature

mtf — Identification initials

Enclosure: Authorization form — Enclosure notation

---

necessary to send a letter. If a letter is sent, a copy of the letter and return signature card from the post office must be filed with the patient's records.

Prevention of Legal Problems

After reading Chapters 1 through 3, you have discovered there are many instances in which an insurance biller must be careful in executing job duties to avoid the possibility of a lawsuit. A summary of guidelines for prevention of lawsuits is shown in Box 3–1.

RESOURCES ON THE INTERNET

A model compliance plan for small physician practices can be found at *http://oig.hhs.gov/authorities/docs/ physician.pdf*

A model compliance plan for Third Party Billing Companies can be found at *http://oig.hhs.gov/ fraud/docs/complianceguidance/thirdparty.pdf*

STUDENT ASSIGNMENT LIST

✔ Study Chapter 3.
✔ Answer the review questions in the *Workbook* to reinforce the theory learned in this chapter and help prepare you for a future test.
✔ Complete the assignments in the *Workbook* to give you experience in reviewing patients' medical reports and records.
✔ Turn to the Glossary at the end of this textbook for a further understanding of the Key Terms used in this chapter.

UNITED STATES POSTAL SERVICE

First-Class Mail
Postage & Fees Paid
USPS
Permit No. G-10

• Sender: Please print your name, address, and ZIP+4 in this box •

COLLEGE CLINIC
4567 BROAD AVENUE
WOODLAND HILLS, XY 12345 0001

A

Figure 3–24. A and **B** (front and back), A domestic return receipt Postal Service Form 3811 and, **C,** receipt for certified mail Postal Service Form 3800 (U.S. Government Printing Office) shown completed.

SENDER: *COMPLETE THIS SECTION*

■ Complete items 1, 2, and 3. Also complete item 4 if Restricted Delivery is desired.
■ Print your name and address on the reverse so that we can return the card to you.
■ Attach this card to the back of the mailpiece, or on the front if space permits.

1. Article Addressed to:

Mr. John Doe
2761 Fort Street
Woodland Hills, XY 12345

COMPLETE THIS SECTION ON DELIVERY

A. Received by (*Please Print Clearly*) | B. Date of Delivery

C. Signature

X

☐ Agent
☐ Addressee

D. Is delivery address different from item 1? ☐ Yes
   If YES, enter delivery address below: ☐ No

3. Service Type
   ☒ Certified Mail   ☐ Express Mail
   ☐ Registered   ☐ Return Receipt for Merchandise
   ☐ Insured Mail   ☐ C.O.D.

4. Restricted Delivery? (*Extra Fee*)   ☐ Yes

2. Article Number (*Copy from service label*)
   7000 0520 0020 3886 3129

PS Form 3811, July 1999   Domestic Return Receipt   102595-00-M-0952

B

PLACE STICKER AT TOP OF ENVELOPE
TO THE RIGHT OF RETURN ADDRESS.
FOLD AT DOTTED LINE

CERTIFIED MAIL

7000 0520 0020 3886 3129
7000 0520 0020 3886 3129

U.S. Postal Service
CERTIFIED MAIL RECEIPT
(Domestic Mail Only; No Insurance Coverage Provided)

Postage | $

Certified Fee

Return Receipt Fee
(Endorsement Required)

Restricted Delivery Fee
(Endorsement Required)

Total Postage & Fees | **$**

Postmark
Here

Recipient's Name *(Please Print Clearly) (To be completed by mailer)*
Mr. John Doe

Street, Apt. No.; or PO Box No.
2761 Fort Street

City, State, ZIP+4
Woodland Hills, XY 12345

PS Form 3800, February 2000   **See Reverse for Instructions**

C

COLLEGE CLINIC
4567 Broad Avenue
Woodland Hills, XY 12345-0001
Phone: 555/486-9002
Fax: 555/487-8976

September 3, 20XX

Mrs. Gregory Putnam
4309 North E Street
Woodland Hills, XY 12345-4398

Dear Mrs. Putnam

This will confirm our telephone conversation today during which you discharged me from attending you as your physician in your present illness. In my opinion, your medical condition requires continued treatment by a physician. If you have not already obtained the services of another physician, I suggest you do so without further delay.

You may be assured that, upon your written authorization, I will furnish your new physician with information regarding the diagnosis and treatment you have received from me.

Very truly yours

Gerald Procton, MD

mtf

Figure 3–25. Letter to confirm discharge by patient. Letter typed in modified block style (dateline, complimentary close, and signature indented) with open punctuation (no commas after salutation or complimentary close).

Prevention of Lawsuits—Guidelines for Insurance Billing Specialists

1. Keep information about patients strictly confidential.
2. Obtain proper instruction and carry out responsibilities according to the employer's guidelines.
3. Keep abreast of general insurance program guidelines, annual coding changes, and medical and scientific progress to help when handling insurance matters.
4. Secure proper written consent in all cases before releasing a patient's medical record.
5. Do not refer to consent or acknowledgment forms as "releases." Use the word "consent" or "authorization" forms, as required by law. This also produces a better understanding of the document to be signed.
6. Make sure documentation of patient care in the medical record corresponds with billing submitted on the insurance claim.
7. Exercise good judgment in what you write and how you word electronic mail because it does not give security against confidentiality.
8. Make every effort to reach an understanding with patients in the matter of fees by explaining what services will be received and what the "extras" may be. For hospital cases, it is advisable to explain that the fee the physician charges is for his or her services only and that charges for the bed or ward room, operating room, laboratory tests, and anesthesia will be billed separately in addition to the physician's charges.
9. Do not discuss other physicians with the patient. Patients sometimes invite criticism of the methods or results of former physicians. Remember that you are hearing only one side of the story.
10. Tell the physician immediately if you learn that a new patient is still under treatment by another physician and did not give this information to the physician during the initial interview.
11. Do not compare the respective merits of various forms of therapy and refrain from discussing patients' ailments with them. Patients come to talk to the physician about their symptoms, and you may give them incorrect information. Let the physician make the diagnosis. Otherwise, you may seriously embarrass the physician, yourself, or both of you.
12. Report a physician who is doing something illegal that you are aware of. You can be held responsible for being silent and failing to report an illegal action.
13. Say nothing to anyone except as required by the attorney of the physician or by the court if litigation is pending.
14. Be alert to hazards that may cause injury to anyone in the office and report such problems immediately.
15. Consult the physician before turning over a delinquent account to a collection agency.
16. Be courteous in dealing with patients and always act in a professional manner.

Diagnostic
Coding

- State the meaning of basic abbreviations and symbols in the code books.
- Define diagnostic code terminology.
- Perform diagnostic coding accurately after completing the problems in the *Workbook*.

OBJECTIVES*

After reading this chapter, you should be able to:

- State the history of diagnostic coding.
- Explain the purpose and importance of coding diagnoses.
- Use diagnostic code books properly and obtain accurate codes.

---

*Performance objectives and exercises for hands-on practical experience for this chapter appear in the *Workbook*.

The Diagnostic Coding System

This chapter deals with diagnostic coding for outpatient professional services, and the next chapter relates to coding of procedures. Proper coding can mean the financial success or failure of a medical practice. A working knowledge of medical terminology, including a basic course in anatomy and physiology, is essential to becoming a topnotch coder of diagnoses. The coding must be accurate because in many instances, such as with a patient under the Medicare program, payment for services may be based on the diagnosis. All diagnoses that affect the current status of the patient may be assigned a code. This includes conditions that exist at the time of the patient's initial contact with the physician as well as conditions that develop subsequently that affect the treatment received. Diagnoses that relate to a patient's previous medical problem that have no bearing on the patient's present condition are not coded. The American Health Information Management Association (AHIMA) diagnostic coding guidelines for outpatient services and diagnostic coding and reporting requirements for physician billing may be found by visiting the Web site listed in the Resources at the end of this chapter.

Types of Diagnostic Codes

Codes must be sequenced correctly on an insurance claim so that the chronology of patient care events and severity of disease can be understood. When submitting insurance claims for patients seen in a physician's office or an outpatient hospital setting, the **primary diagnosis,** which is the main reason for the encounter, must be listed first. In an office setting, this is commonly called the **chief complaint (CC).** The **secondary diagnosis,** listed subsequently, may contribute to the condition or define the need for a higher level of care but is not the underlying cause. The underlying cause of a disease is referred to as the **etiology** and is sequenced in the first position. The **principal diagnosis,** used in hospital coding, is the diagnosis obtained after study that prompted the hospitalization. It is possible that the primary and principal diagnosis codes may be the same. Note that the concept of a "principal diagnosis" is only applicable to inpatient hospital orders.

Reasons for the Development and Use of Diagnostic Codes

Diagnostic coding was developed for the following reasons:

1. Tracking of disease processes
2. Classification of causes of mortality
3. Medical research
4. Evaluation of hospital service utilization

Medical practices use diagnostic codes on insurance claims instead of writing out the diagnostic description. The consequences of not using ICD-9-CM codes are many. For example, the physician's level of reimbursement may be affected, claims can be denied, fines or penalties can be levied, and sanctions can be imposed. It is important to use diagnostic codes on all claims; payments are accurate and prompt if coding is correctly done. When records are comprehensive, statistics can be gathered to make future payments more realistic for the physicians in private practice.

Occasionally an insurance company replies to a claim with an explanation of benefits or remittance advice stating, "This procedure or item is not payable for the diagnosis as reported." For example, a patient has undergone magnetic resonance imaging (MRI) of the brain. Medicare will not reimburse for MRI for the diagnosis of transient ischemic attack or Alzheimer's disease but will pay for it with the diagnosis of cerebral insufficiency. The procedures that are diagnosis-related include most imaging services (radiography, computed tomography, and MRI), cardiovascular services (electrocardiograms, Holter monitors, echocardiography, Doppler and stress testing), neurologic services (electroencephalography and noninvasive ultrasonography), some laboratory services, and vitamin B_{12} injections. It is important to know the procedures that are diagnosis-related and exactly which diagnosis relates to the procedure being billed. A reference book may be helpful in this situation, such as *Ingenix's Medicare Correct Coding.*

Physician's Fee Profile

A **physician's fee profile** is a compilation of each physician's charges and the payments made to him or her over a given period of time for each specific professional service rendered to a patient. Each insurance company keeps a profile on every provider for services that are processed for statistical purposes. As charges are increased, so are payments, and the profile is then updated through the use of statistical computer data. There are two types of profiles: *individual customary profile* and *prevailing profile.* Inquire from each insurance carrier whether the carrier will update the physician's fee profile on an annual basis. If so, send in an annual updated fee profile to those third-party payers who implement this policy.

The use of nonspecific diagnostic codes may place the physician's practice at considerable risk concerning the development of his or her fee profile. Every claim form filed by a third-party payer is entered into permanent computerized records. The compiled data (fees charged, and procedure and diagnostic codes) may be used in the future as the basis for the physician's fee profile.

To ensure accuracy of future profiles, the insurance billing specialist should use specific diagnostic codes on a routine basis. The coding must be accurate and precise if profiles are to be established for realistic payments.

History of Coding Diseases

From the earliest days of medical treatment, people have tried to name and classify diseases. Although many attempts have been made to systematize and clarify disease terminology, no one method has ever been accepted by the entire medical community.

Around 1869, the American Medical Association prepared the *American Nomenclature of Diseases*. In 1903 the *Bellevue Hospital Nomenclature of Diseases* was published; it was subsequently replaced by the *Standard Nomenclature of Diseases and Operations*. In the 1960s the American Medical Association published *Current Medical Information and Terminology* (CMIT), which used a computer format to make frequent revisions easier. The medical terms were alphabetically arranged and included detailed descriptions of the diseases and two- and four-digit code numbers. Publication of the book ceased in 1991.

Institutions (within a facility), pathologists, and those involved with generating medical reports and billing for laboratory medicine procedures use a system for retrieving types of diagnoses. These codes are found in a book entitled *Systematized Nomenclature of Human and Veterinary Medicine (SNOMED International)*, Volumes I through IV.* In addition, this system is used for managing patient records, teaching medical information science (informatics), and indexing and managing research data.

International Classification of Diseases

History

The *International Classification of Diseases* (ICD) had its beginnings in England during the 17th century. The United States began using the ICD to report causes of death and prepare mortality statistics in the latter half of the 19th century. Hospitals began using the ICD in 1950 to classify and index diseases. The ninth revision of the *International Classification of Diseases* (ICD-9), published by the World Health Organization, is now being used by state health departments and the U.S. Public Health service for mortality reporting.

Organization and Format

In 1979 the ***International Classification of Diseases, Ninth Revision, Clinical Modification*** (ICD-9-CM) was published by the Department of Health Services in the United States. It is updated annually and has three volumes. Volume 1 is a Tabular List of Diseases, each having an assigned number. Volume 2 is an Alphabetic Index of Diseases. Volume 3 is a Tabular List and Alphabetic Index of Procedures used primarily in the hospital setting. The systematized arrangement in these books makes it possible to encode, computerize, store, and retrieve large volumes of information from the patient's medical record. ICD-9-CM is used by hospitals and other health care providers to code and report clinical information necessary for participation in various government programs, such as Medicare, Medicaid, and professional review organizations.

Volumes 1 and 2 are used in physicians' offices and other outpatient settings to complete insurance claims. These two volumes are almost completely compatible with the original international version (ICD-9). The code numbers have from three to five digits. Although abbreviated versions of the ICD-9-CM are available, it is preferable to obtain the complete ninth revision of Volumes 1 and 2.

The annual update of the ICD-9-CM occurs each October 1, and the changes are published in three publications—*Coding Clinic,* published by the American Hospital Association; the *American Health Information Management Association Journal,* published by the American Health Information Management Association; and the *Federal Register,* published by the U.S. Government Printing Office. Coding from an out-of-date manual can delay payment or cause costly mistakes that can lead to financial disaster. Many insurance carriers do not use the new codes until they have a chance to update their computer systems. Verify with each carrier exactly when it plans to begin using the new codes. Refer to Appendix A to learn the names and addresses of several companies that publish the ICD-9-CM.

Psychiatric disorders are coded using the *Diagnostic and Statistical Manual of Mental Disorders*, Fourth Edition (DSM-IV). This code system is not discussed in this text. Refer to Appendix B to find out where to obtain this code book.

Contents

Table 4–1 is an outline of Volumes 1 and 2 of the ICD-9-CM. Volume 1 lists chapter headings with associated codes. The Supplementary Classification

---

*Available from the College of American Pathologists, 325 Waukegan Road, Northfield, IL 60093-2750.

TABLE 4–1   **Outline of Volumes 1 and 2 of ICD-9-CM**

Volume I Chapter Headings	Codes
1 Infectious and Parasitic Diseases	001–139
2 Neoplasms	140–239
3 Endocrine, Nutritional, and Metabolic Diseases and Immunity Disorders	240–279
4 Diseases of the Blood and Blood-Forming Organs	280–289
5 Mental Disorders	290–319
6 Diseases of the Nervous System and Sense Organs	320–389
7 Diseases of the Circulatory System	390–459
8 Diseases of the Respiratory System	460–519
9 Diseases of the Digestive System	520–579
10 Diseases of the Genitourinary System	580–629
11 Complications of Pregnancy, Childbirth, and the Puerperium	630–676
12 Diseases of the Skin and Subcutaneous Tissue	680–709
13 Diseases of the Musculoskeletal System and Connective Tissue	710–739
14 Congenital Anomalies	740–759
15 Certain Conditions Originating in the Perinatal Period	760–779
16 Symptoms, Signs, and Ill-Defined Conditions	780–799
17 Injury and Poisoning	800–999
Supplementary Classification	
Classification of Factors Influencing Health Status and Contact with Health Service	V01–V82
Classification of External Causes of Injury and Poisoning	E800–E999
Appendices	
A Morphology of neoplasms	
B Glossary of mental disorders	
C Classification of drugs by American Hospital Formulary Service List Number and their ICD-9-CM equivalents	
D Classification of industrial accidents according to agency	
E List of three-digit categories	
Volume 2	
Section 1: Index to Diseases and Injuries, alphabetic	
Section 2: Table of Drugs and Chemicals	
Section 3: Index to External Causes of Injuries and Poisonings	

consists of V and E codes, which are discussed later in this chapter. Sections A, B, C, and D of the Appendices are not used in physician outpatient billing. Volume 2 contains three sections: an alphabetic index for diseases and injuries, a table of drugs and chemicals, and an alphabetic index to external causes of injuries and poisonings (E codes). An outline and information on how to find codes in Volume 3 are provided in Chapter 16. This reference is used primarily in the hospital setting.

How to Use the Diagnostic Code Books Properly

To become a proficient coder, it is important to develop an understanding of the conventions and terminology of ICD-9-CM. Read all of the information at the beginning of Volumes 1 and 2 before coding. Volume 1, the Tabular List for the disease classifications, makes use of certain abbreviations, punctuation, symbols, and other conventions, as shown in Box 4–1.

In Volume 2, the Alphabetic Index for the disease classification, the symbol of **slanted brackets** ([ ]) is used to indicate the need for another code. A code is given after a listing followed by slanted brackets enclosing an additional code. Record both of these codes in the same sequence as indicated in the index.

An **italicized code** in the Tabular List may never be sequenced as principal or primary diagnoses.

Coding Instructions

Code only the conditions or problems that the physician is actively managing at the time of the visit. However, some insurance carriers have restrictions on accepting codes and may allow only one or two codes per claim. In those situations, it may not be possible to code all active problems. Always use Volume 2, the Alphabetic Index, and Volume 1, the Tabular (numerical) List before assigning a code. Never use just one volume. Begin with the Alphabetic Index to locate the main term of the diagnosis. The main term is the condition. The primary arrangement of the Alphabetic Index, the disease index, is by *condition*. If you cannot find the condition listed, consider rearranging the word roots (e.g., crypt orchid/o or orchido crypt/o). Then substitute a similar suffix.

The use of a medical dictionary aids in accurate coding. Research any unfamiliar terminology; for example, amaurotic idiocy with severe mental retardation; impaludism.

Volume 2 elements are structured as follows:

▶ Main terms are classifications of diseases and injuries and appear as headings in **boldface** type.
▶ Subterms are listings under main terms and are indented two spaces to the right under main terms.
▶ Modifiers (often referred to as nonessential modifiers because their presence or absence does not affect the code assigned) provide additional description and are enclosed in parentheses.
▶ Carryover lines continue the text and are indented more than two spaces from the level of the preceding line.
▶ Subterms of subterms are additional listings and are indented two spaces to the right under the subterm (Box 4–2; see also Fig. 4–13).

Always code to the highest degree of specificity. The more digits a code has, the more specific the description. A three-digit code may be used only

---

BOX 4–1

ICD-9-CM Conventions

Abbreviations

NEC   **Not Elsewhere Classifiable** (in the coding books). The category number for the term including NEC is to be used with ill-defined terms and only when the coder lacks the information necessary to code the term in a more specific category.

Example: **Fibrosclerosis** Familial multifocal
NEC **710.8**

NOS   **Not Otherwise Specified** (by the physician). This abbreviation is the equivalent of "unspecified." It refers to a lack of sufficient detail in the diagnosis statement to be able to assign it to a more specific subdivision within the classification.

Example: 153.9 Colon, unspecified Large intestine NOS.

Punctuation

[ ]	Brackets are used to enclose synonyms, alternative wordings, or explanatory phrases.
[code]	Italicized (slanted) brackets enclosing a code, used in Volume 2, the Alphabetic Index, indicates the need for another code. Record both codes in the order as indicated in the index.
⊏	Large bracket may signal a new or revised code.
•	A bullet at a code or line of text indicates the entry is new.
( )	Parentheses are used to enclose supplementary words that may be present or absent in the statement of a disease or procedure without affecting the code number to which it is assigned.
▲	A Triangle in the Tabular list indicates the code title is revised. In the Alphabetical Index, the triangle indicates the code has changed.
:	Colons are used in the Tabular List after an incomplete term that needs one or more of the modifiers that follow to make it assignable to a given category.
►◄	When two triangle symbols meet at their points, they appear at the beginning and end of a section of new or revised text.
{ }	Braces are used to enclose a series of terms, each of which is modified by the statement appearing at the right of the brace.

Symbols

☐	The lozenge symbol printed in the left margin preceding the disease code indicates that the content of a four-digit category has been moved or modified.
DEF:	This symbol indicates a definition of disease or procedural term.
MSP:	This identifies specific trauma codes that alert the carrier that another carrier should be billed and Medicare billed second if payment from the first payer does not equal or exceed the amount Medicare would pay.
PDx:	This symbol identifies a V code that can only be used as a primary diagnosis.
SDx:	This symbol identifies a V code that can only be used as a secondary diagnosis. A V code without a symbol can be used as either a primary or secondary diagnosis.
♀♂	Age and Sex Symbols are used to detect inconsistencies between the patient's age and diagnosis. Examples are: Newborn Age: 0 Pediatric Age: 0–17 Maternity Age: 12–55 Adult Age: 15–124
§	The section mark symbol preceding a code denotes the placement of a footnote at the bottom of the page that is applicable to all subdivisions in that code.
④ ⑤ ✓4th ✓5th	Either of these symbols signals that a fourth or fifth digit is necessary for coding to indicate the highest level of specificity.

---

when the diagnostic statement cannot be further subdivided. When a three-digit code has subdivisions, the appropriate subdivision must be coded. Some insurance carrier computer systems kick out the lower-level codes (three-digit codes) and hold these claims for medical review, thereby delaying payment. *Do not* arbitrarily use a zero as a filler character when typing a diagnostic code number because this may be interpreted as indicating a different disease. The addition of a zero to a code number that does not require an additional digit also can cause a claim to be denied (Example 4–1).

Five-digit codes can appear:
1. At the beginning of a chapter
2. At the beginning of a section
3. At the beginning of a three-digit category
4. In a four-digit subcategory

The use of five digits is NOT optional; therefore select a code book that has the categories marked and color coded so it will not be easy to overlook fifth

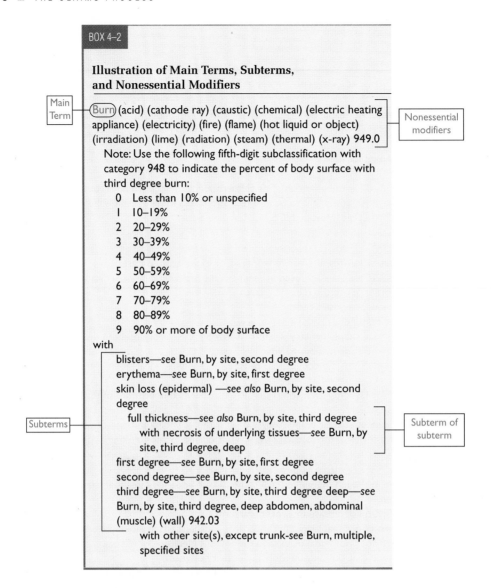

BOX 4–2

Illustration of Main Terms, Subterms, and Nonessential Modifiers

Main Term

Burn (acid) (cathode ray) (caustic) (chemical) (electric heating appliance) (electricity) (fire) (flame) (hot liquid or object) (irradiation) (lime) (radiation) (steam) (thermal) (x-ray) 949.0

Nonessential modifiers

Note: Use the following fifth-digit subclassification with category 948 to indicate the percent of body surface with third degree burn:

0   Less than 10% or unspecified
1   10–19%
2   20–29%
3   30–39%
4   40–49%
5   50–59%
6   60–69%
7   70–79%
8   80–89%
9   90% or more of body surface

with

blisters—*see* Burn, by site, second degree
erythema—*see* Burn, by site, first degree
skin loss (epidermal) —*see also* Burn, by site, second degree
   full thickness—*see also* Burn, by site, third degree
      with necrosis of underlying tissues—*see* Burn, by site, third degree, deep
first degree—*see* Burn, by site, first degree
second degree—*see* Burn, by site, second degree
third degree—*see* Burn, by site, third degree deep—*see* Burn, by site, third degree, deep abdomen, abdominal (muscle) (wall) 942.03
      with other site(s), except trunk-see Burn, multiple, specified sites

Subterms

Subterm of subterm

EXAMPLE 4–1

Invalid code caused by added zero	Valid code
373.20	373.2
496.0	496

digits. Near the end of this chapter (accompanying the section Rules for Coding, Diabetes Mellitus) is another example illustrating the use of five digits. Sometimes when the fourth or fifth digit is missing, the code is not complete and technically is not a code but rather a category (Example 4–2).

When you are billing Medicare, you will find that some diagnostic codes are designated as invalid from year to year. If you work in a medical practice that sees Medicare patients, it is essential to read the regional Medicare bulletins and attend Medicare seminars periodically to keep abreast of these changes.

PROCEDURE: Basic Steps in Coding

Use a standard method and establish a routine for locating a code. Follow these recommended steps for coding the first diagnosis. There are no shortcuts. For each subsequent diagnosis in a patient's medical record, repeat these steps. Refer to Figure 4–1 as you go through Step 1.

EXAMPLE 4–2

§645   Prolonged pregnancy
[0, 1, 3]   Postterm pregnancy
      Pregnancy that has advanced beyond 42 weeks of gestation

The section mark (§) requires a fifth digit; valid digits are in brackets [ ] under each code. Use 0 as the fourth digit for this category.

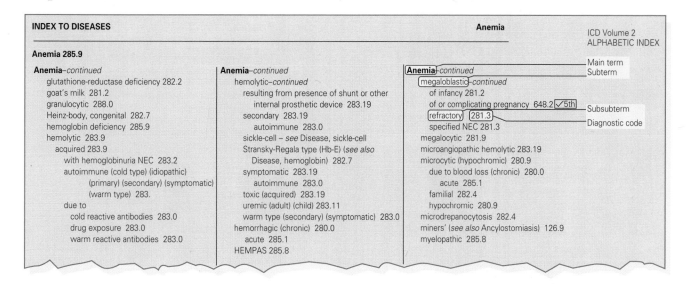

Figure 4–1. Excerpt from the Alphabetic Index of *International Classification of Diseases, 9th Revision, Clinical Modification* (ICD-9-CM), Volume 2.

1. **Locate the main term in the Alphabetic Index, Volume 2 (anemia).**

   ▶ Refer to any notes under the main term. (none shown)

   ▶ Read any terms enclosed in parentheses after the main term (nonessential modifiers). (none shown)

   ▶ Look for appropriate subterm. (megaloblastic) *Do not* skip over any subterms indented under the main term.

   ▶ Look for appropriate sub-subterm. (refractory)

   ▶ Follow any cross-reference instructions. (none given)

   ▶ Write down the code. (281.3)

2. **Verify the code number in the Tabular List, Volume 1 (Fig. 4–2).**

   ▶ Read and be guided by any instructional terms in the Tabular List. In this example, there are none given.

   ▶ Read complete description and assign the code to the highest specificity. (refractory megaloblastic anemia, 281.3)

   Now use a step-by-step approach to code chronic alcoholic liver disease and refer to each volume as shown in Example 4–3.

   Code initially from the Alphabetic Index, Volume 2. Then go to the Tabular List, Volume 1, to *verify* that

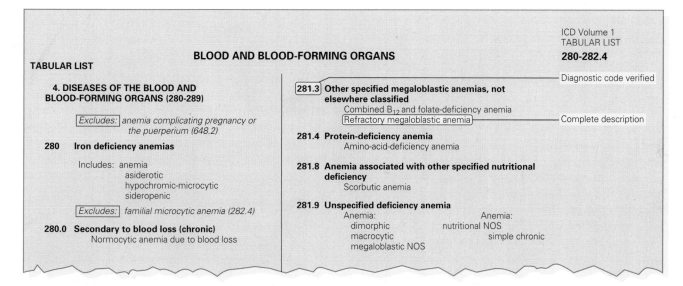

Figure 4–2. Excerpt from the Tabular List of *International Classification of Diseases, 9th Revision, Clinical Modification* (ICD-9-CM), Volume 1.

EXAMPLE 4–3

Coding Chronic Alcoholic Liver Disease

Step 1. Determine the diagnosis, *chronic alcoholic liver disease*, and identify the main term, *disease*.

Step 2. Look under main term, *disease* (the condition) in Volume 2.
  a. A note states "see also Syndrome" and would be followed if you cannot locate the code.
  b. There are no nonessential modifiers to read.
  c. Find the subterm *liver*.
  d. Locate the sub-subterm *chronic*.
  e. There are no cross-references listed.
  f. Write down the code number 571.3.

Step 3. Verify the code number—not the page number in Volume 1.
  a. Verify you are in the correct chapter, Diseases of the Digestive System.
  b. The three-digit code category is *Chronic liver disease and cirrhosis* (571).
  c. Note, there are no 5th-digit code requirements.
  d. The complete description reads "571.3 Alcoholic liver damage, unspecified." The code and its title refer to any liver damage caused by alcoholism, without specification as to the nature of the disorder. Because there are no exclusion notes, this is the correct code.

Step 4. Assign and record the correct code, 571.3.

The Patient's Diagnosis is Dyspepsia and Heartburn, Code Number 536.8.

Step 1. Look for the code number—not the page number—in Volume 1.
Step 2. Notice that there is an exclusion note for heartburn indicating the code number 787.1
Step 3. Be sure to check code number 787.1 in the Tabular Listing.

A

536.8 Dyspepsia and other specified disorders of function of stomach

Achylia gastrica	Hyperchlorhydria
Hourglass contraction of stomach	Hypochlorhydria
Hyperacidity	Indigestion

| *Excludes:* | achlorhydria (536.0) |
| | heartburn (787.1) |

B

Figure 4–3. A, Example of a disease to look up in the Tabular List and, **B,** illustration of coding showing an exclusion note from the Tabular List of *International Classification of Diseases, 9th Revision, Clinical Modification* (ICD-9-CM), Volume I.

the code number selected is in accord with the desired classification of the diagnosis. Look for important instructions that often appear. Check for exclusion notes, which refer to terms or conditions that are not included within the code. These may further direct the coder to the correct ICD-9-CM code assignment (Fig. 4–3).

An "excludes" box may appear listing diagnoses and additional codes to research to ensure that the correct code is assigned. As shown in Figure 4–3, *B*, this example appears on the insurance claim keyed without the decimal as: 5368.

Note: Heartburn is not coded because it is a symptom of dyspepsia and appears as an exclusion under dyspepsia in Volume 1.

Certain conditions are classified according to etiology (cause) of the disorder (Fig. 4–4). In these cases, you should follow the instructions "Code first underlying disease . . ." Code the etiology in the first position. Code the disorder in the second position. Words to look for in the diagnostic statement include "acquired," "congenital," "associated with," "obstetric," "nonobstetric," "transmissible," "not transmissible," "traumatic," and "nontraumatic."

When the patient's medical record states a "versus" diagnosis, such as "peptic ulcer versus gastroesophageal reflux," code the presenting symptoms. When a specific condition is stated in the

diagnosis as acute (or subacute) and chronic, and the Alphabetic Index provides separate codes at either the third-, fourth-, or fifth-digit level for acute and chronic, use both codes with the acute code given first (Example 4–4).

EXAMPLE 4–4

Acute and Chronic Pelvic Inflammatory Disease

Condition:	Disease
Subcategories:	Pelvis, Pelvic
Subsubcategory:	Inflammatory

	Acute	614.3
	Chronic	614.4

Four-digit subcategories .8 and .9 usually, but not always, are reserved for "other specified" and "unspecified" conditions, respectively. "Other specified" and "unspecified" subcategories are referred to as residual subcategories (Fig. 4–5). Residual subcategories are used for conditions that

---

713.1 Arthropathy associated with gastrointestinal conditions other than infections

Code first underlying disease as:
  regional enteritis (555.0–555.9)
  ulcerative colitis (556)

Figure 4–4. Coding by etiology.

Figure 4–5. Four-digit residual subcategories—specified, other specified, and unspecified disease conditions.

are specifically named in the medical record but not specifically listed under a code description. If there is a lack of details in the medical record and you cannot match to a specific subdivision, research the medical record for a qualifying statement in the physician's progress notes or history and physical examination report that will allow you to use a more specific diagnostic code (Fig. 4–6).

Diagnostic codes must match the age and gender of the patient. If an adult female patient with breast cancer is seen (excluding carcinoma in situ and skin cancer of breast), a code from 174.0 through 174.9 must be used. If a male with breast cancer is treated, a code from 175.0 through 175.9 must be chosen. Some codes apply only to newborns, such as code 775.10 for neonatal diabetes mellitus.

Special Points to Remember in Volume 1

▶ Use two or more codes if necessary to completely describe a given diagnosis. *Example:* Arteriosclerotic cardiovascular *disease* (429.2) with congestive heart *failure* (428.0).

▶ Search for one code when two diagnoses or a diagnosis with an associated secondary process (manifestation) or complication is present. There are instances when two diagnoses are classified with a single code number called a **combination code** (Fig. 4–7).

▶ Use category codes (three-digit codes) only if there are no subcategory codes (fourth-digit subdivisions) (Fig. 4–8).

Special Points to Remember in Volume 2

▶ Notice that appropriate sites or modifiers are listed in alphabetical order under the main terms, with further subterm listings as necessary.

▶ Examine all modifiers that appear in parentheses next to the main term.

▶ Check for nonessential modifiers that apply to any of the qualifying terms used in the statement of the diagnosis found in the patient's medical record (Fig. 4–9).

▶ Notice that eponyms appear as both main term entries and modifiers under main terms such as "disease" or "syndrome" and "operation." As mentioned in Chapter 3 and shown in Example 3–2, an *eponym* is the name of a disease, structure, operation, or procedure, usually derived from the name of a place or a person who discovered or described it first.

▶ Look for sublisted terms in parentheses that are associated with the eponym (Fig. 4–10).

▶ Locate closely related terms, code categories, and cross-referenced synonyms indicated by *see* and *see also* (Fig. 4–11).

Handy Hints in Diagnostic Coding

If your ICD-9-CM code books are not color-coded, mark manifestation (italicizzed) codes with a colored highlighter pen (e.g., 608.81 [italicized code]). This will remind you **to always code the underlying disease first.**

Many times you locate a diagnostic code in Volume 2 only to find that the cross-referenced code is the same when verified in Volume 1. Indicate these codes in Volume 2 with a colored highlighter pen to remind you that this code is correct as described in Volume 2, which saves the time you would spend checking Volume 1.

Figure 4–6. Insurance billing specialist looking up a patient's medical record file to verify documentation for a diagnostic code.

491.2 Obstructive chronic bronchitis

Bronchitis:
    emphysematous
    obstructive (chronic) (diffuse)
Bronchitis with:
    chronic airway obstruction
    emphysema

EXCLUDES *asthmatic bronchitis (acute) NOS (493.9)*
chronic obstructive asthma (493.2x)

491.20 Without mention of acute exacerbation

Emphysema with chronic bronchitis

491.21 With acute exacerbation

Combination code ──────→ Acute bronchitis with chronic obstructive
                           pulmonary disease [COPD]
Disease combinations ──→ Acute and chronic obstructive bronchitis
                        Acute exacerbation of chronic obstructive
                           pulmonary disease [COPD]
                        Emphysema with both acute and chronic bronchitis

Figure 4–7. Combination coding.

Keep a list of diagnostic and CPT procedure codes that go well together. Some insurance companies publish lists of codes specifying diagnostic codes that are acceptable for specific procedures. Reference books are available that show codes that link between diagnostic and procedure codes. The American Medical Association publishes a list of the most common diagnostic codes at the end of each of their minispecialty code books. See Appendix B for information on titles and how to obtain reference books that contain such data.

430 Subarachnoid hemorrhage

Meningeal hemorrhage
Ruptured:
    berry aneurysm
    (congenital) cerebral aneurysm NOS

| *Excludes:* | syphilitic ruptured cerebral aneurysm (094.87) |

Figure 4–8. Three-digit coding.

Eponym ──────→ **Cushing's**
                basophilism, disease, or syndrome
                    (iatrogenic) (idiopathic) (pituitary
                    basophilism) (pituitary dependent)
                    255.0

                Basophilism (corticoadrenal) (Cushing's)
                    (pituitary) (thymic) 255.0

Figure 4–10. Coding diagnoses associated with an eponym.

Obesity (constitutional) (exogenous) ◄─── Nonessential
    (familial) (nutritional) (simple) 278.0   modifiers
adrenal 255.8
due to hyperalimentation 278.00
endocrine NEC 259.9
endogenous 259.9
Fröhlich's (adiposogenital dystrophy) 253.8
glandular NEC 259.9
hypothyroid (*see also* Hypothyroidism) 244.9
morbid 278.01
of pregnancy 646.1
pituitary 253.8
thyroid (*see also* Hypothyroidism) 244.9

Figure 4–9. Coding with modifiers in parentheses.

Inflammation, inflamed, inflammatory
    (with exudation)-*continued*

spinal
    cord (*see also* Encephalitis) 323.9
        late effect—*see* category 326
        membrane—*see* Meningitis
        nerve—*see* Disorder, nerve

Figure 4–11. Cross-referencing synonyms, closely related terms, and code categories from the Alphabetic Index of the *International Classification of Diseases, 9th Revision, Clinical Modification* (ICD-9-CM), Volume 2.

V Codes

V codes are a supplementary classification of coding located in a separate section at the end of Volume 1, Tabular List. In Volume 2, the Alphabetic Index, the V codes are included in the major section Index of Diseases.

V codes are used when a person who is not currently sick encounters health services for some specific purpose, such as to act as a donor of an organ or tissue, receive a vaccination, discuss a problem that is not in itself a disease or injury, seek consultation about family planning, request sterilization, or to obtain supervision of a normal pregnancy (Example 4–5). These types of encounters are among the more common encounters for hospital outpatients and patients of private practitioners, health clinics, and others. In these situations, the V code appears as a primary code and is placed first.

EXAMPLE 4–5

Supervision of First Pregnancy, Normal

Step 1. Find the heading **pregnancy** in Volume 2.
Step 2. Look for the subheading **supervision.**
Step 3. Look for the second subheading **normal** and a further subheading **first,** which gives you the code V22.0.
Step 4. Find **V22.0** in Volume 1, Tabular List, and you will see "**Supervision of normal first pregnancy.**"

V codes also are used when some circumstance or problem is present that influences the person's health status but is not in itself a current illness or injury, such as when the person is known to have an allergy to a specific drug. In this instance, the V code cannot be used as a stand-alone code and should be used only as a supplementary code.

Additional code numbers are given for occupational health examinations and routine annual physical examinations; therefore select specific codes depending on the circumstances (Example 4–6).

Sometimes a patient receives a consultation for a preoperative medical evaluation as an inpatient or

EXAMPLE 4–6

Routine Annual Physical Examination

Step 1. Look up **examination,** and notice **annual** as a subterm and the code V70.0
Step 2. Find **V70** in Volume 1, Tabular List, and the wording "**Routine general medical examination at a health facility.**"

outpatient (Example 4–7), and the majority of the results are negative for chronic or current illness. A good-health diagnosis code will trigger a rejection by the insurance carrier. Use an admission (encounter) code from the V72.X code series for "other specified examinations" instead of a treatment code. The term "admission (encounter)" is equivalent to *encounter for* and does not refer to an admission to the hospital.

EXAMPLE 4–7

A patient to have surgery for gallstones is sent to a cardiologist for evaluation of suspected cardiovascular disease.
Step 1. In Volume 2, look up **admission** *(encounter)* **(for) examination, preoperative, cardiovascular V72.81.** Verify it in Volume 2.
Step 2. Code the reason for the surgery—574.xx, cholelithiasis.

When coding a healthy patient examination, V codes (V70.1 and V70.3 through V70.7) should be sequenced as primary diagnoses over all other diagnoses. Be cautious when using V codes as second or third diagnoses because Medicare will automatically reject the claim, and insurance companies that adopt Medicare policies may possibly do so, too.

E Codes

E codes are also a supplementary classification of coding in which you look for external causes of injury rather than disease. E codes are given in a separate section of Volume 1, Tabular List, after V codes. In Volume 2, the E codes are also in a separate section, Index to External Causes of Injury and Poisoning, which follows the regular alphabetical index. E codes are also used in coding adverse reactions to medications (Fig. 4–12).

The use of an E code after the primary or other acute secondary diagnosis explains the mechanism for the injury. Generally, E codes are not used for insurance claims submitted by physicians' offices, but some physicians may decide to use them for thoroughness when documenting a case. Instructions are included here for additional knowledge about the classification system.

The Table of Drugs and Chemicals found in Volume 2 (Table 4–2) contains a classification of drugs and other chemical substances for identifying poisoning states and external causes of adverse effects. Read the Foreword at the beginning of this table. Each of the substances listed in the table is assigned a code according to the poisoning classification (960 through 989). These codes are used when there is a state of poisoning, overdose, wrong substance given or taken, or intoxication.

INDEX TO EXTERNAL CAUSES

Heat (apoplexy) (collapse) (cramps) (effects of)
(excessive) (exhaustion) (fever)
(prostration) (stroke) E900.9
due to
man made conditions (as listed in E900.1,
except boat, ship, watercraft) E900.1
weather (conditions) E900.0
from
electric heating apparatus causing burning
E924.8
nuclear explosion
in
war operations E996
terrorism E979.5   ●
generated in, boiler, engine, evaporator, fire
room of boat, ship, watercraft E838 **✓4ᵗʰ**
inappropriate in local application or packing in
medical or surgical procedure E873.5
late effect of NEC E989

Figure 4–12. E coding.

Adverse effect is defined as an adverse or a pathologic reaction to a drug that occurs when appropriate doses are given to humans for prophylaxis (prevention of disease), diagnosis, and therapy (Example 4–8). When an adverse effect occurs (e.g., drug reaction, hypersensitivity, drug intolerance, idiosyncratic reaction), a code is assigned to the diagnosis that classifies the specific reaction or symptom (e.g., dermatitis, syncope, tachycardia, urticaria). The E code identifying the agent involved is taken solely from the Therapeutic Use column. An E code may never be sequenced in the first position.

Poisoning is defined as a condition resulting from an intentional overdose of drugs or chemical substances or from the wrong drug or agent given or taken in error (Example 4–9). Intoxication is defined as an adverse effect rather than a poisoning when drugs such as digitalis, steroid agents, and so on are involved. However, whenever the term *intoxication*

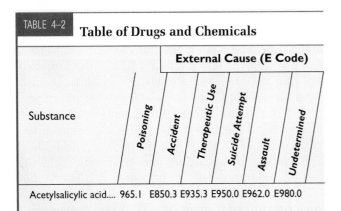

TABLE 4–2	**Table of Drugs and Chemicals**					
	External Cause (E Code)					
Substance	Poisoning	Accident	Therapeutic Use	Suicide Attempt	Assault	Undetermined
Acetylsalicylic acid.... 965.1	E850.3	E935.3		E950.0	E962.0	E980.0

EXAMPLE 4–8

Coding an Adverse Effect

The patient had an adverse effect (ventricular fibrillation) to the medication digoxin, which was prescribed by her physician and taken correctly.

Step 1. Refer to the Table of Drugs and Chemicals in volume 2 and look up **digoxin.**

Step 2. Because this medication was for *therapeutic use*, locate the correct E code number under that column.

Step 3. The correct number is *E942.1.*

Step 4. Locate the main term **fibrillation** in the Index to Diseases.

Step 5. Find the subterm **ventricular.**

Step 6. The correct code number is *427.41.*

Step 7. Verify the code number 427.41 in Volume I, *Tabular Listing.*

Sequencing: **427.41 Ventricular fibrillation (chief complaint)**
E942.1 Therapeutic use, Digoxin

Note: For outpatient billing, the E code would not be listed.

EXAMPLE 4–9

Poisoning Examples

- Taking the wrong medication
- Receiving the wrong medication
- Taking the wrong dose of the right medication
- Receiving the wrong dose of the right medication
- Ingesting a chemical substance not intended for human consumption
- Overdose of a chemical substance (drug)
- Prescription drug taken with alcohol
- Mixing prescription drugs and over-the-counter medications without the physician's advice or consent

Coding a Poisoning

Baby Kathy got into the kitchen cabinet and ingested liquid household ammonia.

Step 1. Refer to the Table of Drugs and Chemicals in Volume 2 and look up **ammonia.**

Step 2. Find the subterm **liquid (household)**

Step 3. Since this is a case of ingesting a chemical substance not intended for human use, locate the correct code number under the **Poisoning** column.

Step 4. Write down the code number **983.2.**

Step 5. Since this is an accident, locate the E code in the **Accident** column (**E861.4**).

Sequencing: 983.2 Poisoning, ammonia
E861.4 Poisoning, accidental, ammonia

Note: The manifestation (outcome of the poisoning, e.g., nausea and vomiting) would be coded in the first position if documented in the medical record. For outpatient billing, the E code would not be listed.

is used, the biller should clarify with the physician the circumstances surrounding the administration of the drug or chemical before assigning the appropriate code.

Rules for Coding

Signs, Symptoms, and Ill-Defined Conditions

Chapter 16 of the ICD-9-CM—Symptoms, Signs, and Ill-Defined Conditions (codes 780.0-799.9)—contains many but not all codes for symptoms. If the final diagnosis at the end of the encounter or at the time of discharge is qualified by any of the following terms ("suspected," "suspicion of," "questionable," "likely," "probable," or "rule out"), *do not code* these conditions as if they existed or were established. Instead, code the chief complaint, sign, or symptom. Do not type "ruled out" on the insurance claim. This condition was suspected at one time but was ruled out after study and is no longer an active diagnosis. *Example:* Diabetes mellitus, ruled out. The condition(s) should be documented to the highest degree of certainty for each encounter or visit (e.g., signs, symptoms, abnormal test results, or other reason for the visit).

This is contrary to coding practices used by hospital medical record departments for coding the diagnoses of hospital inpatients. If one were to follow hospital coding guidelines and the patient was suspected of having a heart attack, this would be interpreted as a confirmed case of a myocardial infarction. The same holds true for "possible epilepsy." If the patient had a convulsion and epilepsy was the probable cause but had not been proved, code the convulsion.

The following are instances in which sign and symptom codes can be used.

▶ No precise diagnosis can be made (Examples 4–10 and 4–11).
▶ Signs or symptoms are transient, and a specific diagnosis was not made (Example 4–12).

EXAMPLE 4–10

The patient has an enlarged liver, and further diagnostic studies may or may not be done. Use code 789.10 for hepatomegaly.

EXAMPLE 4–11

The patient complains of painful urination, and urinalysis is negative. Use code 788.1 for dysuria.

EXAMPLE 4–12

The patient complains of **chest pain on deep inspiration.** On examination, the physician finds nothing abnormal and tells the patient to return in 1 week. When the patient returns, the pain has ceased. **Use code 786.52 for painful respiration.**

EXAMPLE 4–13

On examination, the physician documents abnormal percussion of the chest. The patient is sent for a chest x-ray and asked to return for a recheck. The patient does not have the x-ray and fails to return. Use code **786.7 for abnormal chest sounds.**

EXAMPLE 4–14

A patient complains of nausea and vomiting and is referred to a gastroenterologist. Use code **787.01** for nausea with vomiting.

▶ Provisional diagnosis for a patient who does not return for further care (Example 4–13).
▶ A patient is referred for treatment before a definite diagnosis is made (Example 4–14).

Sterilization

The code V25.2 is used only when the sterilization is performed for the major purpose of contraception rather than being an incidental result of the treatment of a disease. If the sterilization is purely elective, code V25.2 suffices as a single code for the diagnosis. If the sterilization is performed for contraceptive purposes during a current admission for obstetric delivery, sequence code V25.2 in the second position. If the sterilization is the end result of a hysterectomy performed because of injury or damage to the uterus during delivery, do not use code V25.2 but instead code the condition or procedure.

Neoplasms

Neoplasms are new growths, and they may be benign or malignant tumors. A **benign tumor** is one that does not have the properties of invasion and metastasis (e.g., transfer of disease from one organ to another) and is usually surrounded by a fibrous capsule. Cysts and lesions are *not* neoplasms. A **malignant tumor** has the properties of invasion and metastasis. The term *carcinoma* refers to a cancerous

EXAMPLE 4–15

Primary cancerous tumor	189	**Malignant neoplasm of kidney and other and unspecified urinary organs.**

189.0 Kidney, except pelvis
Kidney NOS
Kidney parenchyma

Secondary cancerous tumor	198	**Secondary malignant neoplasm of other specified sites**

Excludes lymph node metastasis (196.0–196.9)
198.0 Kidney

or malignant tumor. Carcinoma **in situ** means cancer confined to the site of origin without invasion of neighboring tissues. A *primary* tumor means the original tumor site. A *secondary* tumor means a site of metastasis. If the diagnosis does not mention metastasis, then code the case as a primary tumor (Example 4–15). Lymphomas and leukemias are not classified using the primary and secondary terminology.

The diagnostic statement "metastatic from" indicates primary stage carcinoma, whereas "metastatic to" indicates secondary stage carcinoma. If the diagnostic statement is "malignant neoplasm spread to," then code the primary site spread to the secondary site. The phrase "recurrent malignancy" is a new primary neoplasm.

The main entry "Neoplasm" contains a table with the column headings Malignant, Benign, Uncertain Behavior, and Unspecified. The table is found in the alphabetic index under "Neoplasm" in Volume 2 (Table 4–3). Code numbers for neoplasms are given by anatomic site. For each site, there are six possible code numbers, indicating whether the neoplasm in question is malignant (primary, secondary, or

TABLE 4–3   Coding for Neoplasms

	Malignant				Uncertain	
	Primary	*Secondary*	*Ca in situ*	**Benign**	**Behavior**	**Unspecified**
Neoplasm, neoplastic	199.1	199.1	234.9	229.9	238.9	239.9

Notes: 1. The list provided gives the code numbers for neoplasms by anatomic site. For each site there are six possible code numbers according to whether the neoplasm in question is malignant, benign, in situ, of uncertain behavior, or of unspecified nature. The description of the neoplasm will often indicate which of the six columns is appropriate (e.g., malignant melanoma of skin, benign fibroadenoma of breast, carcinoma in situ of cervix uteri).

Where such descriptors are not present, the remainder of the Index should be consulted where guidance is given to the appropriate column for each morphologic (histologic) variety listed; e.g., Mesonephroma—see Neoplasm, malignant; Embryoma—see also Neoplasm, uncertain behavior; Disease, Bowen's—see Neoplasm, skin, in situ. However, the guidance in the Index can be overridden if one of the descriptors mentioned above is present (e.g., malignant adenoma of colon is coded to 153.9 and not to 211.3 because the adjective "malignant" overrides the Index entry "Adenoma—see also Neoplasm benign").

2. Sites marked with the sign * (e.g., face NEC*) should be classified to malignant neoplasm of skin of these sites if the variety of neoplasm is a squamous cell carcinoma or an epidermoid carcinoma and to benign neoplasm of skin of these sites if the variety of neoplasm is a papilloma (any type).

abdomen, abdominal	195.2	198.89	234.8	229.8	238.8	239.8
cavity	195.2	198.89	234.8	229.8	238.8	238.8
organ	195.2	198.89	234.8	229.8	238.8	238.8
viscera	195.2	198.89	234.8	229.8	238.8	239.8
wall	173.5	198.2	232.5	216.5	238.2	239.2
connective tissue	171.5	198.89	—	215.5	238.1	239.2
abdominopelvic	195.8	198.89	234.8	229.8	238.8	239.8
accessory sinus—see Neoplasm, sinus						
acoustic nerve	192.0	198.4	—	225.1	237.9	239.7
acromion (process)	170.4	198.5	—	213.4	238.0	239.2
adenoid (pharynx) (tissue)	147.1	198.89	230.0	210.7	235.1	239.0
adipose tissue (see also Neoplasm, connective tissue)	171.9	198.89	—	215.9	238.1	239.2
adnexa (uterine)	183.9	198.82	233.3	221.8	236.3	239.5
adrenal (cortex) (gland) (medulla)	194.0	198.7	234.8	227.0	237.2	239.7
ala nasi (external)	173.3	198.2	232.3	216.3	238.2	239.2
alimentary canal or tract NEC	159.9	197.8	230.9	211.9	235.5	239.0

> **EXAMPLE 4–16**
>
> ### Adenocarcinoma of the Breast with Metastases to the Pelvic Bone
>
> **Step 1.** Look up **adenocarcinoma** in Volume 2. Do not use the morphology code, M8140/3. Notice it states, "see also Neoplasm, by site, malignant."
>
> **Step 2.** Locate **neoplasm** in the table in Volume 2. At the top of the page notice the Malignant heading with the subheadings **Primary, Secondary,** and **Ca In Situ. Primary** means the first site of development of the malignancy. **Secondary** means metastasis from the primary site to a second site. **Ca In Situ** means cancer confined to the epithelium of the site of origin without invasion of the basement membrane tissue of the site.
>
> **Step 3.** Find the site of the adenocarcinoma (in this case the breast), and look under the Malignant and Primary headings. Note that the code given is **174.9.**
>
> **Step 4.** Next, find **bone** as a subterm in the Neoplasm Table and look for the subterm **pelvic.** Now look at the three columns under Malignant and, using the Secondary column, find the **correct code number 198.5.** In listing these diagnoses on the insurance claim, you give the following: **174.9 and 198.5.**

carcinoma in situ), benign, of uncertain behavior, or of unspecified nature. The description of the neoplasm often indicates which of the six code numbers is appropriate (e.g., malignant melanoma of skin, benign fibroadenoma of breast, carcinoma in situ of cervix uteri, and so on) (Example 4–16). For a tumor that has not been diagnosed as benign or malignant by the pathologist, use the codes in the column labeled "Uncertain Behavior." If a tumor is suspected and not confirmed, use "mass." For example, a breast mass would be coded 611.72. When coding a neoplasm, ask yourself the following questions:

◗ What is it now?
◗ Where did it start?
◗ What happened to it?

Anatomic sites marked with an asterisk (*) are always considered to be neoplasms of the skin.

In Appendix A of the Tabular List of Volume 2, there is a section entitled Morphology of Neoplasms, which gives M codes. These codes are not used for billing insurance claims by physicians' offices.

Circulatory System Conditions

Diseases of the circulatory system are difficult to code because of the variety and lack of specific terminology used by physicians in stating the diagnoses. Carefully read all inclusion, exclusion, and "use additional code" notations contained in the Tabular List of Volume 1.

Hypertension

The lay term "high blood pressure" is medically termed *hypertension*. Hypertension can *cause* various forms of heart and vascular disease, or it can *accompany* some heart conditions. In fact, there is a syndrome called *malignant hypertension* that has nothing to do with tumor formation. A *syndrome* is another name for a *symptom complex* (a set or complex of signs, symptoms, or other manifestations resulting from a common cause or appearing in combination, presenting a distinct clinical picture of a disease or inherited abnormality). Malignant hypertension is a symptom complex of markedly elevated blood pressure (diastolic pressure of more than 140 mm Hg) associated with papilledema. The term *malignant* here means "life threatening." *Benign hypertension* refers to high blood pressure that runs a relatively long and symptomless course.

When the diagnostic statement indicates a cause by stating "heart condition *due to* hypertension" or "hypertensive heart disease," use codes 402.0X through 402.9X. If the diagnostic statement reads "*with* hypertension" or "cardiomegaly *and* hypertension," you need two separate codes. Elevated blood pressure without mention of hypertension is coded 796.2. Secondary hypertension is coded 405.XX, and the cause of the hypertension should be coded when specified.

Myocardial Infarctions

A separate three-digit category (412) is provided for old myocardial infarction, healed myocardial infarction, or myocardial infarction diagnosed on electrocardiogram. Myocardial infarction of 8 weeks' duration or less is considered acute, if not specified otherwise. Symptoms of more than 8 weeks' duration are coded 414.8, Other Forms of Chronic Ischemic Heart Disease.

Chronic Rheumatic Heart Disease

The conditions presumed to be caused by rheumatic fever are as follows:

◗ Mitral valve of unspecified etiology 394
◗ Mitral valve insufficiency 394.1
◗ Mitral valve and aortic valve disorders of unspecified etiology 396
◗ Mitral stenosis 394.0

The following condition is *not* presumed to be caused by rheumatic fever:

◗ Aortic valve of unspecified etiology 424

Arteriosclerotic Cardiovascular Disease and Arteriosclerotic Heart Disease

Use code 429.2 for a patient who has a diagnosis of arteriosclerotic cardiovascular disease (ASCVD). Code 440.9 excludes ASCVD because it is in conflict with the note given for 429.2. Code 429.2 is primary when the additional code 440.9 is needed. However, a patient with arteriosclerotic heart disease (ASHD) is assigned code 414.0. At code 429.2 in your copy of Volume 1, write in "see code 440" after "use additional code to identify, if desired, the presence of arteriosclerosis." To distinguish between ASCVD and ASHD, cardiovascular means pertaining to heart and blood vessels throughout the body, whereas ASHD means acute or chronic heart disability resulting from an insufficient supply of oxygenated blood to the heart.

Diabetes Mellitus

The two types of diabetes are type I and type II. The following are the clinical features important in the classification of diabetes.

Type I Diabetes	Type II Diabetes
Insulin-dependent diabetes mellitus (IDDM)	Non–insulin-dependent diabetes mellitus (NIDDM)
Patients *must* be treated with insulin	Patients *may* be treated with insulin
Insulin levels are very low	Insulin levels may be high "normal," or low
Ketosis prone	Non–ketosis prone
Patients usually are lean	Patients usually are obese
Usually "juvenile onset" (peak onset at early puberty	Usually "adult onset," although occasionally seen in children
Often little family history of diabetes mellitus	Often strong family history of diabetes mellitus

In type I diabetes (IDDM), the patient's pancreas does not function and produce the necessary insulin. Thus this patient's body is dependent on insulin. In type II diabetes (NIDDM), the patient's pancreas produces some insulin, but the insulin is ineffective in doing its job, which is removing sugar from the bloodstream. This diabetic's problem may be controlled with diet, oral medication, or insulin.

Coding *always* requires five digits because of the types and complications that may accompany this disease. Here is the way this classification appears in ICD-9-CM, Volume 2:

Fifth-digit subclassification with code 250 is not based on severity or age grouping of the case (Fig. 4–13). It is a *type grouping;* use the following:

250.00 for non-insulin dependent diabetes (NIDDM)

Adult onset
Type two, Type II or unspecified
Stable or not stated as uncontrolled
Non-ketosis prone

250.01 for insulin-dependent diabetes (IDDM)

Juvenile onset
Type one, Type I
Stable or not stated as uncontrolled
Ketosis prone

250.02 for non-insulin-dependent diabetes (NIDDM)

Adult onset
Type two, Type II or unspecified
Uncontrolled

250.03 for insulin-dependent diabetes (IDDM)

Juvenile onset
Type one, Type I
Uncontrolled

Always ask the physician for further clarification when a medical record contains the statement "discharged on insulin" with no further explanation of the type of diabetes. Do not assume that a patient taking insulin has insulin-dependent diabetes.

Do not use code 250.0X if the diabetes is stated with delivery of a child or as a complication of pregnancy. Use code 648.01.

Pregnancy, Delivery, or Abortion

The following main sections are included:

630-633 Ectopic and Molar Pregnancy

634-639 Other Pregnancy with Abortive Outcome *(five-digit subclassifications must be used with categories 634-637)*

640-648 Complications Mainly Related to Pregnancy *(five-digit subclassifications must be used)*

650-659 Normal Delivery and Other Indications for Care in Pregnancy, Labor, and Delivery *(five-digit subclassifications must be used in categories 651-659)*

660-669 Complications Occurring Mainly in the Course of Labor and Delivery *(five-digit subclassifications must be used)*

670-677 Complications of the Puerperium *(five-digit subclassifications must be used for categories 670-676)*

The following guidelines are used:

1. Code 650 is used for a completely *normal* delivery. This means normal spontaneous delivery,

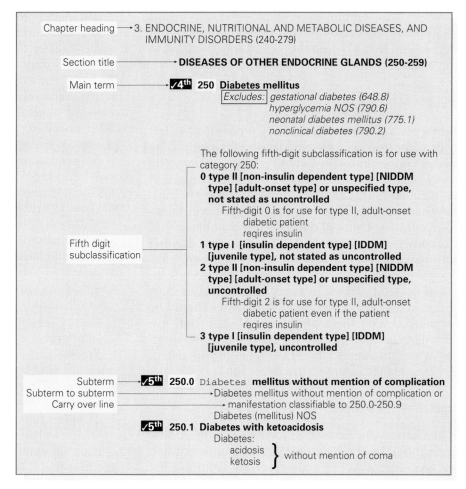

Chapter heading → 3. ENDOCRINE, NUTRITIONAL AND METABOLIC DISEASES, AND IMMUNITY DISORDERS (240-279)

Section title → **DISEASES OF OTHER ENDOCRINE GLANDS (250-259)**

Main term → **✓4th** **250** **Diabetes mellitus**
Excludes: gestational diabetes (648.8)
hyperglycemia NOS (790.6)
neonatal diabetes mellitus (775.1)
nonclinical diabetes (790.2)

The following fifth-digit subclassification is for use with category 250:
0 type II [non-insulin dependent type] [NIDDM type] [adult-onset type] or unspecified type, not stated as uncontrolled
Fifth-digit 0 is for use for type II, adult-onset diabetic patient reqires insulin

Fifth digit subclassification
1 type I [insulin dependent type] [IDDM] [juvenile type], not stated as uncontrolled
2 type II [non-insulin dependent type] [NIDDM type] [adult-onset type] or unspecified type, uncontrolled
Fifth-digit 2 is for use for type II, adult-onset diabetic patient even if the patient reqires insulin
3 type I [insulin dependent type] [IDDM] [juvenile type], uncontrolled

Subterm → **✓5th** **250.0** Diabetes **mellitus without mention of complication**
Subterm to subterm → Diabetes mellitus without mention of complication or
Carry over line → manifestation classifiable to 250.0-250.9
Diabetes (mellitus) NOS
✓5th **250.1 Diabetes with ketoacidosis**
Diabetes:
acidosis
ketosis } without mention of coma

Figure 4–13. Classification of diabetes mellitus showing fifth-digit subclassification from *International Classification of Diseases, 9th Revision, Clinical Modification* (ICD-9-CM), Volume 2.

cephalic (vertex) presentation of one live-born fetus, full-term gestation (with or without episiotomy), no manipulation necessary, and no laceration.

2. A code other than 650 should be used to provide greater detail about a **complication** of abortion, pregnancy, childbirth, or the puerperium when information is available, such as the presence of anemia, diabetes mellitus, or thyroid dysfunction (Example 4–17). Complication of the puerperium is a complication within 6 weeks after labor.

EXAMPLE 4–17		
648.01	250.00	Pregnancy (delivered) with diabetes mellitus
648.23	282.60	Pregnancy (antepartum) with sickle cell anemia

In most instances, an additional code is added to specify the patient's specific problem.

3. A multiple gestation (i.e., twins, triplets) is a complication of pregnancy and is considered high risk. When a patient delivers and experiences both antepartum and postpartum complications, different fifth digits may be applied on the codes to describe the episodes of care (Example 4–18).

EXAMPLE 4–18	
651.11	Triplet pregnancy (delivered)
675.02	Infection of nipple (postpartum)

Admitting Diagnoses

Some diagnosis codes are considered questionable when used as the first diagnosis on admittance of a patient to the hospital (e.g., 278.00 obesity, 401.1 benign hypertension). The inpatient admission diagnosis may be expressed as one of the following.

1. One or more significant findings (symptoms or signs) representing patient distress or abnormal findings on examination.
2. A diagnosis established on an ambulatory care basis or previous hospital admission.
3. An injury or poisoning.
4. A reason or condition not classifiable as an illness or injury, such as pregnancy in labor, follow-up inpatient diagnostic tests, and so on.

When your employer physician makes hospital visits, code the reason for the visit, which may *not* necessarily be the reason the patient was admitted to the hospital.

Burns

Burns always are coded using two codes. The first code is for the exact site and degree of the burn. The second code found in Category 948 describes the percentage of body surface area burned. A fifth digit is included in this category and is necessary to indicate how much of the total body surface had third-degree burns. Think of the body as a whole and not the body parts as a whole. The adult body is divided into regions: head, 9%; arms, 9% each; trunk, 18% front and 18% back; legs, 18% each; and perineum, 1% (Fig. 4–14). Children's and infants' bodies have different regional percentages. Burn codes should be sequenced with the highest-degree burn first, followed by the other burn codes. However, when a first- and a second-degree burn of the same site are listed, only the highest-degree burn of that site is coded.

Injuries and Late Effects

Diagnostic codes for injuries are listed in the Alphabetic Index by the type of injury and broken down by anatomic site. To code multiple injuries, list the diagnosis for the conditions treated in order of importance, with the diagnosis for the most severe problem listed first. If surgery is involved, the diagnostic code for the surgical problem should be listed first unless there is a severe injury of another part of the body. For example, in the case of an intracranial injury, managed medically, and a fractured phalanx, managed surgically, the intracranial injury is listed as the primary diagnosis and the diagnosis fractured phalanx is sequenced second. The most difficult part of assigning injury codes is knowing what words to look for in the Alphabetic Index. Codes 800 through 959 include fractures, dislocations, sprains, and other types of injury. Injuries are coded according to the general type of injury and broken down within each type by anatomic site. A list of common injury medical terms and the types of injuries included for each is shown in Table 4–4. An injury may have a late effect, which must be coded in a different fashion.

Use the following guides for coding injuries.

1. Decide whether a diagnosis represents a current injury or a late effect of an injury (Example 4–19).
2. Fractures are coded as closed if there is no indication of whether the fracture is open or closed.
3. The word "with" indicates involvement of both sites, and the word "and" indicates involvement of either one or two sites when multiple injury sites are given (Example 4–20).

Look up code 813 in your diagnostic code book and note that this code section relates to a fracture of the radius, ulna, or both.

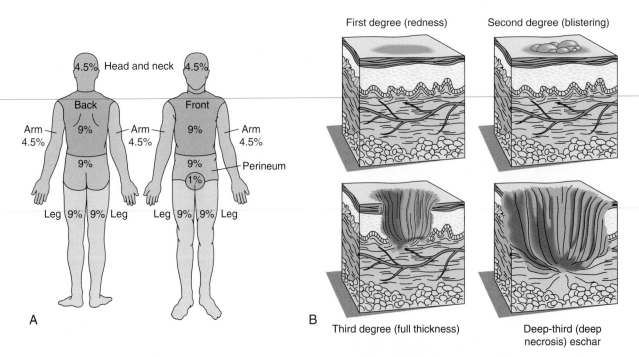

Figure 4–14. A, The rules of nines for burn injury to the body. **B,** The degrees of burn involving the layers of the skin, i.e., first-degree burns include the epidermis (redness), second-degree burns include the epidermis and dermis (blistering), third-degree burns include the first two layers and the subcutaneous tissues (full-thickness), and deep-third burns involve all layers of the skin with resulting eschar (deep necrosis).

TABLE 4–4	**Common Injury Medical Terms**
Contusion	Bruise and hematoma without a fracture or open wound
Crush	Crushing injury not complicated by concussion, fractures, injury to internal organs, or intracranial injury
Dislocation	Displacement and subluxation. Dislocation may be open or closed. Closed dislocation may be complete, partial, simple, or uncomplicated. Open dislocation may be either compound, infected, or with foreign body. A dislocation not indicated as closed or open is classified as closed.
Fracture	Fractures may be open or closed. A fracture not indicated as open or closed is classified as closed. An injury described as fracture dislocation is coded as a fracture. Open fractures may be described as compound, infected, missile, puncture, or with foreign body. Closed fractures may be described as comminuted, depressed, elevated, fissured, greenstick, impacted, linear, march, simple, slipped, epiphyseal, or spiral.
Injury, blood vessel	Described as either arterial hematoma, avulsion, laceration, rupture, traumatic aneurysm, or traumatic fistula
Injury, internal	Includes all injuries to internal organs such as the heart, lung, liver, kidney, and pelvic organs. Types of injuries to internal organs include laceration, tear, traumatic rupture, penetrating wounds, blunt trauma, crushing, blast injuries, or open wounds to internal organs with or without fracture in the same region.
Injury, intracranial	Includes concussion, cerebral laceration and contusion, or intracranial hemorrhage. These injuries may be open or closed. Intracranial injuries with skull fractures may be found under fracture.
Injury, superficial	Includes abrasion, insect bite (nonvenomous), blister, or scratch
Sprain/strain	Injury to the joint capsule, ligament, muscle, or tendon described by the following terms: avulsion, hemarthrosis, laceration (closed), rupture, or tear. Open laceration of these structures should be coded as open wounds.
Wound, open	Includes open wounds not involving internal organs. Wounds may be to skin, muscle, or tendon, described as animal bite, avulsion, cut, laceration, puncture wound, or traumatic amputation. Open wounds may be complicated or uncomplicated. Complicated includes injuries with mention of delayed healing, delayed treatment, foreign body, or major infection.

A **late effect** means "the residual effect (condition produced) after the acute phase of an illness or injury has terminated." An effect is considered to be late if the diagnosis reads "due to an old injury," "late," "due to" or "following" (previous illness or injury), or "due to an injury or illness that occurred 1 year or more before the current admission of encounter." If time has passed between the occurrence of the acute illness or injury and the development of the residual effect, such as scarring, late effects also may be coded.

Example 4–21 illustrates late effects. Residuals are shown in italics, and the causes are shown in bold print. Code both the residual effect and the cause. Use the following guides for coding late effects.

1. Refer to the main term "late" in ICD-9-CM Volume 2 when coding a case with late effects.

2. Use two codes when late effects are involved for both the present condition and the initial condition. The late effect code is usually a secondary diagnosis code, with the primary diagnosis code the current residual condition. In some cases, the late effect is the sole reason for the office visit; in such cases, the late effect code becomes the primary diagnosis.

Now that you have learned the basics of ICD-9-CM coding, the next step is to begin to learn the new system based on ICD-10.

ICD-10-CM Diagnosis and Procedure Codes

For the past 20 years the ICD-9-CM diagnosis system has been used. Although it has been updated, the system has outlived its usefulness because of advances in technology, discovery of new diseases, development of new procedures, and the need to report more details for statistical purposes. The time is fast approaching to adopt another system. Actually

EXAMPLE 4–19	
824.8	**Current injury:** Fracture, left ankle
	OR
733.81 and 905.4	Late effect: Malunion fracture left ankle

EXAMPLE 4–20	
806	Fracture of the vertebral column **with** spinal cord injury
813	Fracture of radius **and** ulna

EXAMPLE 4–21
Malunion **fracture,** right tibia
Traumatic *arthritis* following **fracture** of right knee *Hemiplegia* following **cerebrovascular thrombosis** 1 year previously
Scarring caused by third-degree **burn** of right arm
Contracture of right heel tendons caused by **poliomyelitis**

there are two systems, *International Classification of Diseases, 10th Revision, Clinical Modification* (ICD-10-CM—diagnostic codes) and *ICD-10 Procedure Coding System* (ICD-10-PCS—procedure codes). Both hospital and physician office insurance billers should be concerned with the new diagnosis codes, but only hospital billers need to concern themselves with the procedure codes.

ICD-10 Volume 1: Tabular List was published by the World Health Organization in 1992. It is being clinically modified (CM) by the National Center for Health Statistics (NCHS) before code adoption. The CM provides the specifics that the United States needs for collecting data on our health status. Reasons for clinical modification are the removal of procedural codes, unique mortality codes, and "multiple" codes. ICD-10-PCS was developed in the mid-1990s by 3M Health Information Systems under contract with the Centers for Medicaid and Medicare Services (CMS). This replaces Volume 3 of ICD-9-CM used in hospital billing but does not replace the *Current Procedural Terminology* (CPT) code book used in outpatient billing. Reasons for development of ICD-10-PCS are:

- ICD-10 did not have procedure classification.
- ICD-9-CM was not expandable, comprehensive, or multiaxial (broken down into many subdivisions).
- ICD-9-CM did not have standardized terminology and included diagnostic information.
- ICD-10-CM differs from ICD-9-CM in the following ways:

1. Major changes in code book organization exist.
2. Many new categories and chapters have been added.
3. There is a replacement of the traditional numeric coding system with a six-digit alphanumeric scheme for ICD-10-CM (Example 4–22).
4. Old injury (800-999) codes have been changed to S and T codes.
5. Explanatory notes and instructions for use have been greatly expanded.
6. The dagger-and-asterisk system of dual classification in ICD-10 has been considerably expanded for ICD-10-CM (Example 4–23).
7. The E and V codes in ICD-9-CM are now Chapters XX and XXI.
8. The coding system allows for assignment of unique codes as new procedures are developed.

The second part, section, or volume of the ICD-10-CM is an instruction manual that provides definitions, standards, and rules for the tabular list. The last part or volume is an alphabetical index. These systems allow more code choices and require greater documentation in the medical record. An experienced coder should develop a proactive, positive attitude toward accepting and learning the ICD-10-CM. A coder must have a higher level of clinical knowledge. It is wise to attend an anatomy and physiology course

EXAMPLE 4–22

ICD-9-CM

FRACTURE OF UPPER LIMB (810-819)

810   **Fracture of clavicle**
Includes: collar bone
interligamentous part of clavicle
The following fifth-digit subclassification is for use with category 810:
0   unspecified part
Clavicle NOS
1   sternal end of clavicle
2   shaft of clavicle
3   acromial end of clavicle

✓5th   **810.0**   Closed

ICD-10-CM

S42.00   Closed Fracture of Clavicle
  S42.001   Closed Fracture of *Right* Clavicle
  S42.002   Closed Fracture of *Left* Clavicle
  S42.009   Closed Fracture of Clavicle,
        Unspecified Side

a year before the new system is adopted if you have not already done so. There has been a monumental change from ICD-9-CM to ICD-10-CM. After coding guidelines have been developed, training workshops will be offered. To gain knowledge and proficiency, approximately 80 hours of instruction may be needed to learn the new system. Even after a person learns how to code, it takes a longer time to code under the new system, especially if ICD-10-PCS is used.

Publishers of ICD-10-CM may use different styles and format so it is important to study and compare the features of several books before making a decision to purchase. When choosing a book, the following questions should be asked: Is color coding being used for emphasis in locating items quickly? Are definitions or notes included to help one interpret and gain a better understanding of difficult medical

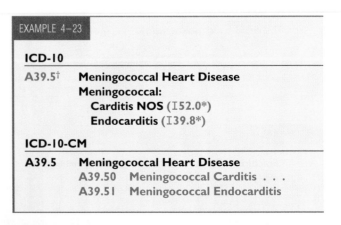

EXAMPLE 4–23

ICD-10

A39.5†   **Meningococcal Heart Disease**
    Meningococcal:
        Carditis NOS (I52.0*)
        Endocarditis (I39.8*)

ICD-10-CM

A39.5   **Meningococcal Heart Disease**
    A39.50   Meningococcal Carditis . . .
    A39.51   Meningococcal Endocarditis

terms and phrases? Are coding guidelines boxed for easy reference? All of these benefit the coder.

Possible errors may occur when using the Tabular List and when coding diseases or conditions that begin with categories "O" and "I." These can look like the numbers "zero" and "one" (e.g., I00 and O99 are correct and not 100 and 099). In these categories, special attention must be given.

As of the date of the printing of this textbook, guidelines have not been adopted, so training has not begun. The next edition of this textbook will feature how to code using ICD-10-CM.

RESOURCES ON THE INTERNET

 For AHIMA diagnostic code guidellines for outpatient services and diagnostic coding and reporting requirements for physician billing, visit the Web site: *http://www.ahima.org*

STUDENT ASSIGNMENT LIST

✔ Study Chapter 4.
✔ Answer the review questions in the *Workbook* to reinforce theory learned in this chapter and to help prepare you for a future test.
✔ Complete the assignments in the *Workbook* to gain hands-on experience in diagnostic coding.

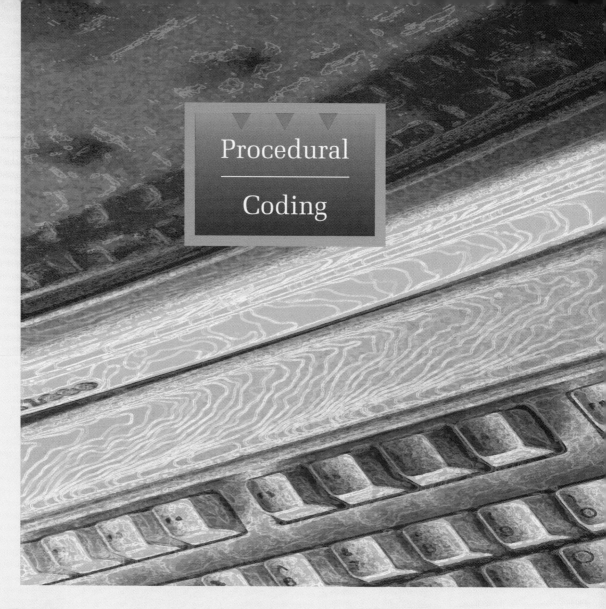

Procedural
Coding

5

- Code the *Workbook* problems using the CPT manual.
- Describe the differences between CPT and RVS coding systems.
- Describe various methods of payment by insurance companies and state and federal programs.

KEY TERMS

actual charge

bilateral

bundled codes

comprehensive code

conversion factor

Current Procedural Terminology (CPT)

customary fee

downcoding

fee schedule

global surgery policy

Healthcare Common Procedure Coding System (HCPCS)

modifier

prevailing charge

procedure code numbers

professional component (PC)

reasonable fee

relative value studies (RVS)

star symbol

surgical package

technical component (TC)

unbundling

upcoding

usual, customary, and reasonable (UCR)

OBJECTIVES*

After reading this chapter you should be able to:

- Explain the purpose of coding for professional services.
- Use procedure code books properly.
- Define procedure code terminology.
- Explain the importance and usage of modifiers in procedure coding.

---

*Performance objectives and exercises for hands-on practical experience for this chapter appear in the *Workbook*.

Understanding the Importance of Procedural Coding Skills

Now that you have learned some terminology and the basics of diagnostic coding, the next step is to learn how to code procedures.

Procedure coding is the transformation of written descriptions of procedures and professional services into numeric designations (code numbers). The physician rendering medical care either writes or dictates this information into the patient's medical record. Then the insurance billing specialist abstracts pertinent information and assigns procedure codes. Routine office visits and procedures usually are listed with codes and brief descriptions on the encounter form. These are circled or checked off by the physician when they are performed on the patient.

With the use of the computer to produce insurance claims and the use of telecommunications, magnetic tape billing, or optical scanning equipment to process payment of these claims, more emphasis is being placed on procedure coding. Coding must be correct if claims are to be paid promptly. Every procedure or service must be assigned correct and complete code numbers. Because of the complexity of procedural coding, a working knowledge of medical terminology, including anatomy and physiology, is essential.

Procedure codes are a standardized method used to precisely describe the services provided by physicians and allied health care professionals. They allow claim forms to be optically scanned by insurance companies. The general acceptance of the codes by insurance carriers and government agencies assures the physician who uses a standardized coding system that the services and procedures he or she performs can be objectively identified and priced. The American Health Information Management Association (AHIMA) diagnostic coding guidelines for outpatient services and procedure coding and reporting requirements for physician billing may be found by visiting the Web site in the Resources at the end of this chapter.

The primary coding system used in physicians' offices for professional services and procedures is *Current Procedural Terminology* (CPT), fourth edition,* published annually by the American Medical Association (AMA). Another rating scale, called relative value studies (RVS), is also used for services and procedures (see later in this chapter).

Some managed care plans develop a few "plan codes" for use by the plan only. Sometimes the codes are used for tracking; other times, they are used to provide reimbursement for a service not defined within CPT.

Various books are available for coding procedures for physicians. In some states medical societies and medical specialty associations publish books for this purpose.

HIPAA Compliance Alert

Coding Compliance Plan

Because the government is more involved in health care, each medical practice should establish and maintain a coding compliance program. This helps coders and physicians avoid fraud and abuse issues. A plan should include the medical practice's basic philosophy and policies, details of coding procedures, and a confidentiality statement. Billers and coders should sign a statement annually indicating that they have read, understood, and agree with the medical practice's standards of conduct (Chapter 1, Fig. 1–6). The plan should show how coders maintain correct coding and how medical records support the codes billed. An internal audit should be done periodically and action taken to correct the offense if noncompliance is discovered. Such plans must have a compliance officer or a committee that oversees the audits, monitors compliance issues, and trains employees in compliance issues.

Current Procedural Terminology

The first edition of *Physicians' Current Procedural Terminology* appeared in 1966, and the book was subsequently revised in 1970, 1973, and 1977. Since 1984, *Current Procedural Terminology* (CPT), fourth edition, has been updated and revised annually. Code numbers are added or deleted as new procedures are developed or existing procedures are modified. These changes are shown in each edition by the use of symbols, which are described and shown later in this chapter in Figure 5–2.

CPT uses a basic five-digit system for coding services rendered by physicians and two-digit add-on modifiers to indicate complications or special circumstances. **Procedure code numbers** represent diagnostic and therapeutic services on medical billing statements and insurance forms (see Example 5–1).†

---

*Available from Book and Pamphlet Fulfillment: OP-3416, American Medical Association, P.O. Box 10946, Chicago, IL 60610-0946 or visit CPT on the Web at *www.ama-assn.org/cpt*.

†Examples shown in this chapter reflect wording pertinent to coding a specific procedure and may be missing complete chart entries; therefore there may be a gap of information for the reader.

EXAMPLE 5–1

Current Procedural Terminology Procedure Code Numbers

A 45-year-old woman is seen for an initial office visit for evaluation of recurrent right shoulder pain. The examination required a detailed history and physical examination (D HX & PX) with low complexity medical decision making (LCMDM). Patient complains of pain radiating down right arm. Complete radiographs of the right shoulder were taken in the office and read by the physician. A corticosteroid solution was injected into the shoulder joint.

Current Procedural Terminology Code	Description of Services
99203	Office visit, new patient **(E/M service)**
73030	Radiologic examination, shoulder, two views **(Diagnostic service)**
20610	Arthrocentesis inj.; major joint, shoulder **(Therapeutic service)**

Almost all states use some method of procedural coding, and many states recommend CPT. CPT emerged as the procedural coding of choice when the federal government developed the Health Care Financing Administration (HCFA) Common Procedure Coding System (HCPCS) (pronounced "hick-picks") for the Medicare Program. Health Care Financing Administration changed its acronym to CMS (Centers for Medicare and Medicaid Services); therefore currently the HCPCS acronym is translated as **Healthcare Common Procedure Coding System.** The Medicare HCPCS consists of three levels of coding:

▶ Level I: the AMA CPT codes and modifiers (national codes).
▶ Level II: CMS–designated codes and alpha modifiers (national codes). Examples of this level may be found at the end of Appendix B of the *Workbook.*
▶ Level III: Codes specific to regional fiscal intermediary or individual insurance carrier (local codes) and not found in either levels I or II.

Level III, local codes, are used to identify new procedures or specific supplies for which there is no national code. These are five-digit alphanumeric codes and use the letters S and W through Z. You may discover that one case can be coded in two or even three coding levels. The CPT code should be used when both a CPT and level II code have the same description. The level II code should be used if the descriptions are not identical (e.g., if the CPT code narrative is generic and the HCPCS level II code is specific).

The formula for selecting a code that most accurately identifies the service reported is as follows:

Physician or provider service = CPT code
Supplies = HCPCS national code
Instructions to use from carrier = local code

Some private insurance companies have begun to accept level II HCPCS codes. It is always wise to check the carrier's provider manual or telephone the carrier before sending in claims for medications and durable medical equipment. The HCPCS is updated each spring. (See Chapter 11 for additional information on coding for Medicare cases.) In some states, the TRICARE and Medicaid programs accept HCPCS codes. In the majority of states, most private payers have adopted the HCPCS system.

Methods of Payment

Private insurance companies and federal and state programs adopt different methods for basing their payments on outpatient claims; they are (1) fee schedules; (2) usual, customary, and reasonable; and (3) relative value scales or schedules. Additional methods of payment for inpatient hospital claims are discussed in Chapter 16.

Fee Schedule

A **fee schedule** is simply a listing of accepted charges or established allowances for specific medical procedures. A medical practice can have more than one fee schedule unless specific state laws restrict this practice. The following situations can occur:

1. Providers *participating* in the Medicare program would typically have a fee schedule for Medicare patients and one for non–Medicare patients.
2. Providers *not participating* in the Medicare program typically have two fee schedules: one based on limiting charges for each service set by the Medicare program and one used for non–Medicare patients.
3. Providers having a contractual arrangement with a managed care plan (e.g., health maintenance organization, individual practice association, or preferred provider organization) probably use additional fee schedules.
4. Providers rendering services to those who have sustained industrial injuries use a separate workers' compensation fee schedule (Chapter 14).

Section 1128(b) of the Social Security Act says a physician may risk exclusion or suspension from the Medicare program if his or her Medicare charges are "substantially in excess of such individual's or entity's usual charges." Options are to lower private rates to the Medicare fee schedule amount or use a separate Medicare fee schedule. An exception is charges negotiated for managed care contracts that are not considered the physician's usual charges. In those cases, it is possible that Medicare patients may be charged more than managed care patients.

To prevent a possible violation of Section 1128(b) of the Social Security Act, it is suggested that the provider assign one set fee or amount for each procedure code when establishing a fee schedule. This is the fee billed to all carriers and to self-pay patients. Instead of different charges for different carriers, the provider can establish different reimbursement fees based on the amount that the carrier reimburses, which is based on the contract with the carrier. By establishing one fee instead of multiple fees for each procedure, the provider helps establish the usual and customary fee for his or her geographical area. It is also possible to observe when carriers raise their allowable rates, which cannot be done if sending a claim based on the carrier allowable. It is important as well to monitor carrier adjustments to determine how much revenue is lost because of poor contracts and to monitor employee theft.

The physician may want to evaluate one or all of the fee schedules in use to annually increase fees because of a rise in the cost of living. A process for accomplishing this is discussed and shown in the section of this chapter subtitled "Determining Relative Value Studies Conversion Factors."

Usual, Customary, and Reasonable

Usual, customary, and reasonable (UCR) is a complex system in which three fees are considered in calculating payment. UCR is used mostly in reference to fee-for-service reimbursement. Figure 5–1 illustrates how a surgeon's payment is determined under this method. The *usual fee* is the fee that a physician usually charges (submitted fee) for a given service to a private patient. A fee is **customary** if it is in the range of usual fees charged by providers of similar training and experience in a geographic area (e.g., the history of charges for a given service). The **reasonable fee** is the fee that meets the aforementioned criteria or is, in the opinion of the medical review committee, justifiable considering the special circumstances of the case. Reimbursement is based on the lower of the two fees (usual and customary) and determines the approved or allowed amount. In a UCR system, payment can be extremely low for a rarely performed but highly complex procedure because there may be no

Figure 5–1. Usual, customary, and reasonable calculation for four participating surgeons' cases.

PARTICIPATING SURGEON UCR CALCULATION

Four Example Cases

Surgeon's bill	Usual fee	compared to	Customary fee		Payment
1) $400	$350 ———————		$350 ———	▸declared reasonable (extenuating circumstances)	$400
2) $400	$350 ———————		$350 ———	▸declared customary (no unusual circumstances)	$350
3) $375	$350 ———————		$400 ———	▸declared customary (does not exceed customary level)	$375
4) $350	$350 ———————		$400 ———	▸declared customary (falls within customary range)	$350

Usual Fee– usual submitted fee for a given service to patient.

Customary Fee– in the range of usual fees charged by providers of similar training and experience in a geographical area (i.e., the history of charges for a given service).

Reasonable Fee– meets the aforementioned criteria or is, in the opinion of the medical review committee, justifiable considering the special circumstances of the case.

Payment– based on the lower of usual and customary fees.

history of billed charges from other physicians on which to base payment. Many rivate health insurance plans use this method and pay a physician's full charge if it does not exceed UCR charges. Depending on the insurance company policy, the UCR system is periodically updated. UCR is a method chosen by insurance carriers and not the provider. If the physician has a UCR that is significantly lower than those of other practices in his or her area, document this and ask the insurance carrier for a review and possible adjustment. Increasing numbers of plans are beginning to discontinue the UCR system and are adopting the Medicare Resource-Based Relative Value Scale (RBRVS) method for physician reimbursement. A description of this system is found under "Relative Value Studies," which follows, and additional information appears in Chapter 11.

Actual charge and prevailing charge are two other factors that Medicare takes into consideration while assigning UCR fees. The **actual charge** is the amount a physician actually bills a patient for a particular medical procedure or service. The **prevailing charge** is a charge that falls within the range of charges most frequently used in a locality for a particular medical service or procedure. Note that this is a general definition of UCR, and programs other than Medicare define it in a different way.

Relative Value Studies

In 1956 the California Medical Association Committee on Fees published the first edition of the *California Relative Value Studies (CRVS).*

It was subsequently revised and published in 1957, 1960, 1964, 1969, and 1974. **RVS** is referred to as either **relative value studies** or scale. It is a coded listing of procedures with *unit values* that indicate the relative value of the various services performed, taking into account the time, skill, and overhead cost necessary for each service (Example 5–2).

EXAMPLE 5–2

Relative Value Scale

Procedure Code	Description	Units
10060	Incision & Drainage of cyst	0.8

Using a hypothetical figure of **$153/unit,** this procedure is valued at $122.40.

Math: $153.00 × 0.8 = $122.40

The units in this scale are based on median charges of all physicians during the time period in which the RVS was published. A **conversion factor** is used to translate the abstract units in the scale to dollar fees for each service.

The RVS became a very sophisticated system for the coding and billing of professional services. After the successful use of the California RVS, many state and medical specialty associations adopted this method. In 1975 the Federal Trade Commission (FTC) challenged the legality of using the RVS as a fee schedule. Since that time, many medical societies and medical specialty associations have issued new publications that omit unit values for the procedures listed, retaining the procedure code portion of RVS.

Some states have passed legislation mandating the use of RVS codes for procedures and the unit values as the schedule of fees for workers' compensation claims. In these states the conversion factor to be used in applying the units is also stated in the law. The insurance carrier pays a specific dollar amount for each unit listed for each procedure in the RVS code book.

An insurer or other third party could devise an RVS based on its own data. This RVS would not be created by physicians desiring to regulate their own fees and therefore would be acceptable to the FTC. One such book available is *St. Anthony's Relative Values for Physicians (RVP)* (refer to Appendix B, Relative Value Studies, for information on where to obtain this book). A national RVS developed under a government contract may be acceptable and would not be in violation of antitrust laws.

The Resource-Based Relative Value Seale (RBRVS) is an RVS developed for the CMS by William Hsiao and associates of the Harvard School of Public Health. Centers for Medicaid and Medicare Services used it to devise the Medicare fee schedule that was phased in from 1992 through 1996. This approach to fees was developed to redistribute Medicare dollars more equitably among physicians. For further information, see Chapter 11, Medicare.

Determining Relative Value Studies Conversion Factors

A physician's fees can be adjusted if they are too high or low; but how to do this can present a problem. Determining the conversion factor can be of great assistance in realigning fees or setting a fee for a procedure for which the physician has not previously billed. Because there are six code sections in CPT, it is necessary to figure out the conversion factor for each section separately. Once the unit values and the RVS used by the insurance carriers being billed are known, the reimbursements can be monitored to ensure the payments are correct. It is legal to use an RVS guide for setting, realigning, or evaluating fees as long as the physician does not enter into any price-fixing agreements. To set fees based on an RVS, obtain an RVS and make up a set of separate conversion factors for the Evaluation and Management (E/M), Anesthesia, Surgery, Radiology, Pathology, and Medicine sections. The workers' compensation board or the insurance commissioner in your state can supply an RVS.

A radiology book is a valuable reference for physicians who take x-ray films in their offices and bill for them. See Appendix B for information on how to obtain the code books mentioned in this chapter.

Use the following steps to determine conversion factors.

PROCEDURE : Determining Conversion Factors

1. Choose 10 or more procedures in the same section (E/M, Anesthesia, Surgery, Radiology, Pathology, or Medicine) and put down the code numbers and fees you presently use.
2. Take each procedure and divide the fee you presently charge by the procedure's unit value. The unit value is listed next to the code number and procedure description in the RVS. Because some procedure descriptions change from year to year, be sure that the description of the service is the proper definition for the service you are giving for that particular fee.
3. Look at all the dollar figures in the section that you have determined. They should fall within the same general range. If they do not, then some of the fees that are too high or low may have to be reevaluated and readjusted, depending on the service descriptions and competition.
4. Add all the conversion factors in the E/M section. Divide the sum by the total number of services in that sampling. Use this as the conversion factor for the Medicine section. Remember this is only a guideline, and the physician may elect to use the highest, lowest, or median figure depending on his or her own judgment and circumstances.

Repeat these steps with each of the sections to obtain at least five conversion factors. Once you have determined the conversion factors for each section, you can determine a dollar figure for a new procedure within the same general grouping by multiplying the unit value by the dollar conversion factor. This will give an approximate cost of each procedure's relative worth. After determining how to obtain a conversion factor, you may wish to evaluate the fee schedules annually to decide whether fees should be raised for certain procedures or services.

How To Use the CPT Code Book

The following are guidelines for the 2003 edition of the CPT. This code book is a systematic listing of five-digit code numbers with no decimals. It is divided into seven code sections with categories and subcategories. The main code sections and appendices are as follows:

Evaluation and Management (E/M)	99201 to 99499
Anesthesia	00100 to 01999
Surgery	10040 to 69990
Radiology, Nuclear Medicine, and Diagnostic Ultrasound	70010 to 79999
Pathology and Laboratory	80048 to 89399
Medicine	90281 to 99569
Category II Codes	0001T to 0026T
Appendix A	Modifiers
Appendix B	Summary of Additions, Deletions, and Revisions
Appendix C	Update to Short Descriptors
Appendix D	Clinical Examples
Appendix E	Summary of CPT Add-on Codes
Appendix F	Summary of Codes Exempt from Modifier -51

Within each of the main sections are categories and subcategories divided according to anatomic body systems, procedure, condition, description, and specialties.

Read through the clinical examples presented in Appendix D. These will help familiarize you with some of the case scenarios that commonly occur for the codes that appear in the E/M section of the CPT.

When on the job, you might want to make your CPT into a reference manual by customizing it. This would help you find codes, modifiers, and rules, making your job easier. Break apart the manual into as many sections as necessary by the specialty where you work. Three-hole punch it, and place it into a binder. Add indexes with tabs to the frequently used sections. You can add coding edits, Medicare updates, and notes at any place in the binder. Color code any codes you usually have to add modifiers to or that should not be used until you have reviewed certain data. For example, use red to highlight codes, descriptions, or entire sections, to alert you or anyone using the reference to codes often denied. Use yellow highlight to indicate a code that needs to be checked before using it in combination with other codes. Use a symbol (e.g., * or ?) to identify services not covered under certain conditions. Because Appendix A is a comprehensive list of the modifiers, add any insurance plan bulletins pertinent to modifiers that affect the specialty you bill for in this section of the binder. Customizing the CPT with a reference like this can save you time and reduce errors made in coding claims.

Category I, II, and III Codes

To improve the existing CPT code system, a CPT-5 Project was implemented, which includes two new code sets: category II codes, intended for performance measurement; and category III codes, intended for new and emerging technology. Existing CPT codes are considered category I.

Category II codes are being tested and as the publication date, have not been released for use. They will be assigned an alphanumeric identifier with a letter in the last field (e.g., 1234F) to distinguish them from category I CPT codes. Use of these codes is optional and not necessary for correct coding.

Category III codes are a temporary set of tracking codes used for new emerging technologies. They are intended to expedite data collection and assessment of new services and procedures to substantiate widespread use and clinical effectiveness. Category III codes can take the place of temporary local codes (HCPCS Level III) that are being phased out and eliminated under the Health Insurance Portability and Accountability Act (HIPAA). These codes appear in CPT 2003 in a separate section after the Medicine section. They also have an alphanumeric identifier with a letter in the last field (e.g., 0025T, determination of corneal thickness with interpretation and report, bilateral) to distinguish them from category I codes.

Code Book Symbols

With each new issuance of CPT, new codes and description changes are added. Become familiar with the new codes and any description changes for the specialized areas that will be used. Figure 5–2 shows

Figure 5–2. Symbols that appear in *Current Procedural Terminology* (CPT) code book.

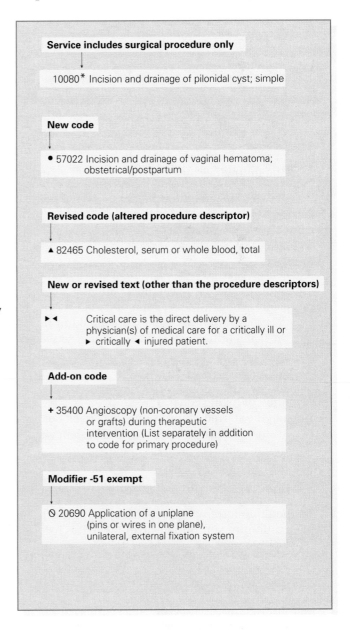

Service includes surgical procedure only

10080* Incision and drainage of pilonidal cyst; simple

New code

● 57022 Incision and drainage of vaginal hematoma; obstetrical/postpartum

Revised code (altered procedure descriptor)

▲ 82465 Cholesterol, serum or whole blood, total

New or revised text (other than the procedure descriptors)

►◄ Critical care is the direct delivery by a physician(s) of medical care for a critically ill or ► critically ◄ injured patient.

Add-on code

+ 35400 Angioscopy (non-coronary vessels or grafts) during therapeutic intervention (List separately in addition to code for primary procedure)

Modifier -51 exempt

⊘ 20690 Application of a uniplane (pins or wires in one plane), unilateral, external fixation system you how to identify new codes and description changes by following the symbols that are used.

When using a new code, marked with a bullet (•), remember that it may take as long as 6 months before an insurance carrier has a mandatory value assignment; therefore reimbursements are received in varying amounts during that time. For revised codes or revised text, marked with a triangle (▲) or (▶ ◀), highlight what is new or deleted. This will save time in trying to figure out what was changed and will prevent using these codes incorrectly. Appendices B and C in the code book provide a summary of the additions, deletions, and revisions. Add-on codes, shown with a plus sign (+), and modifier-51 exempt, shown with a symbol (O), are explained at the end of this chapter.

In the Surgery section, a **star symbol** (*)[1] next to a procedure number means that certain relatively small surgical services involve a readily identifiable surgical procedure but include variable preoperative and postoperative services (e.g., incision and drainage of an abscess, injection of a tendon sheath, manipulation of a joint under anesthesia, or dilation of the urethra). Because of the indefinite preoperative and postoperative services the usual "package" concept for surgical services (see the preceding) cannot be applied. Such procedures are identified by a star (*) following the procedure code number.

When a star (*) follows a surgical procedure code number, the following rules apply:

1. The service as listed includes the surgical procedure only. Associated preoperative and postoperative services are not included in the service as listed.
2. Preoperative services are considered one of the following:
   a. When the starred (*) procedure is carried out at the time of an initial visit (new patient) and this procedure constitutes the major service at that visit, procedure number 99025 is listed in lieu of the usual initial visit as an additional service. Many carriers do not recognize 99025, therefore to be paid for the visit, use the appropriate evaluation and management code. See correct method of listing codes in Example 5–3.
   b. When the starred (*) procedure is carried out at the time of an initial or established patient visit involving significant identifiable services, the appropriate visit is listed with the modifier "-25" appended in addition to the starred (*) procedure and its follow-up care.
   c. When the starred (*) procedure requires hospitalization, an appropriate hospital visit is listed in addition to the starred (*) procedure and its follow-up care.

EXAMPLE 5–3

Medicine Section Code 99025 and Star Procedure

A new patient (NP) presents in the physician's office complaining of a skin abscess. The physician takes a problem-focused history, performs a problem-focused physical examination (PF HX PX), and decides to make an incision and drain the abscess; straightforward decision making (SF MDM).

99025[2]   Initial new patient visit (used in lieu of E/M code)
10060*   Incision and drainage of abscess (star procedure)

This scenario indicates that the starred surgical procedure, performed on a new patient, constitutes the major service. All three requirements have been met to use code 99025.

---

3. All postoperative care is added on a service-by-service basis (e.g., office or hospital visit, or cast change).
4. Complications are added on a service-by-service basis (as with all surgical procedures).

Evaluation and Management Section

The insurance billing specialist must become familiar with the terminology in the procedure code book to use it efficiently. Basic procedural code terminology was reviewed in Chapter 3 to give you a good foundation to begin coding. By now you should know the differences between a new and an established patient, a consultation and a referral, and concurrent care versus continuity of care. This section familiarizes you with specific coding policies in relation to some of the terminology you have learned thus far.

Consultation

Some insurance policies pay for only one consultation per patient per year and often require a written report to be generated.

A consulting physician must submit a written report to the requesting physician. Codes for consultations are as follows:

▶ Office or other outpatient consultations (new or established patient): 99241 through 99245
▶ Initial inpatient consultations (new or established patient): 99251 through 99255
▶ Follow-up inpatient consultations (established patient): 99261 through 99263
▶ Confirmatory consultations (new or established patient): 99271 through 99275. This type of

---

[1]As of the publication of this textbook, it is projected that CPT 2004 may eliminate the asterisk or "star" symbol from CPT surgical codes so refer to CPT for current guidelines.
[2]As of the publication of this textbook, it is projected that CPT 2004 may eliminate the 99025 code so refer to CPT for current guidelines.

consultation calls for an opinion only. Modifier -32 (mandated services) is added if a second opinion is necessary by the insurance company.

Do not use the follow-up consultation codes if the consulting physician assumes responsibility for management of a portion or all of the patient's conditions (after a consultation is completed). In the office setting, use the appropriate initial consultation code for the initial encounter and then the appropriate established patient code. In a hospital setting, use the appropriate inpatient hospital consultation code and then subsequent hospital care codes.

Critical Care

According to CPT guidelines, critical care is the direct delivery by a physician(s) of medical care for a critically ill or injured patient. A critical illness or injury acutely impairs one or more vital organ systems that makes imminent or life-threatening deterioration in the patient's condition highly probable. Critical care involves high complexity decision making to assess, manipulate, and support vital system function(s) to treat single or multiple vital organ system failure or prevent further life-threatening deterioration of the patient's condition. Examples of vital organ system failure include, but are not limited to: central nervous system failure; circulatory failure; and shock, renal, hepatic, metabolic, or respiratory failure.

Although critical care typically requires interpretation of multiple physiologic parameters or application of advanced technology(s), critical care may be provided in life-threatening situations when these elements are not present. Critical care may be provided on multiple days, even if no changes are made in the treatment rendered to the patient, provided that the patient's condition continues to require the level of physician attention described in the preceding.

Providing medical care to a critically ill, injured, or postoperative patient qualifies as a critical care service only if both the illness or injury and the treatment being provided meet the preceding requirements. Critical care is usually, but not always, given in a critical care area, such as the coronary care unit, intensive care unit, pediatric intensive care unit, respiratory care unit, or the emergency care facility.

Critical care services provided to infants 31 days through 24 months of age are reported with pediatric critical care codes 99293 and 99294. The pediatric critical care codes are reported as long as the infant or young child qualifies for critical care services during the hospital stay. Critical care services provided to neonates (30 days of age or less) are reported with the neonatal critical care codes 99295 and 99296. The neonatal critical care codes are reported as long as the neonate qualifies for critical care

services through the thirtieth postnatal day. The reporting of the pediatric and neonatal critical care services is not based on time or the type of unit (e.g., pediatric or neonatal critical care unit) and it is not dependent on the type of provider delivering the care. For additional instructions on reporting these services, see the Neonatal and Pediatric Critical Care section and codes 99293 through 99296.

Services for a patient who is not critically ill but happens to be in a critical care unit are reported by use of other appropriate E/M codes.

Critical care and other E/M services may be provided to the same patient on the same date by the same physician.

The following services are included in reporting critical care when performed during the critical period by the physician(s) providing critical care: the interpretation of cardiac output measurements (93561, 93562); chest radiographs (71010, 71015, 71020); pulse oximetry (94760, 94761, 94762); blood gases, and information data stored in computers (e.g., electrocardiograms, blood pressures, hematologic data [99090]); gastric intubation (43752, 91105); temporary transcutaneous pacing (92953); ventilator management (94656, 94657, 94660, 94662); and vascular access procedures (36000, 36410, 36415, 36540, 36600).

Any services performed that are not listed in the preceding should be reported separately. Many carriers attempt to downcode your claim by stating the procedure is included with Critical Care. You should appeal these denials by attaching supporting documentation, such as a copy of the critical care guidelines. At first the carrier may tell you the codes are inclusive. Then they may tell you the codes are not a covered benefit. Continue to dispute the denials until you get paid.

Codes 99291 through 99292 should be reported for the physician's attendance during the transport of critically ill or injured patients more than 24 months of age to or from a facility or hospital. For physician transport services of critically ill or injured pediatric patients 24 months of age or less see 99289 and 99290.

The critical care codes 99291 and 99292 are used to report the total duration of time spent by a physician providing critical care services to a critically ill or injured patient, even if the time spent by the physician on that date is not continuous. For any given period of time spent providing critical care services, the physician must devote his or her full attention to the patient, and therefore cannot provide services to any other patient during the same period of time.

Time spent with the individual patient should be recorded in the patient's record. The time that can be reported as critical care is the time spent engaged in work directly related to the individual patient's care, whether that time was spent at the immediate bedside or elsewhere on the floor or unit. For example, time spent on the unit or at the nursing station on the floor reviewing test results or imaging studies, discussing the critically ill patient's care with other medical staff, or documenting critical care services in the medical record is reported as critical care, even though it does not occur at the bedside. Also, when the patient is unable or clinically incompetent to participate in discussions, time spent on the floor or unit with family members or surrogate decision makers obtaining a medical history, reviewing the patient's condition or prognosis, or discussing treatment or limitation(s) of treatment may be reported as critical care, provided that the conversation bears directly on the management of the patient.

Time spent in activities that occur outside of the unit or off the floor (e.g., telephone calls, whether taken at home, in the office, or elsewhere in the hospital) may not be reported as critical care because the physician is not immediately available to the patient.

Time spent in activities that do not directly contribute to the treatment of the patient may not be reported as critical care, even if they are performed in the critical care unit (e.g., participation in administrative meetings or telephone calls to discuss other patients). Time spent performing separately reportable procedures or services should not be included in the time reported as critical care time.

Code 99291 is used to report the first 30 to 74 minutes of critical care on a given date. It should be used only once per date even if the time spent by the physician is not continuous on that date. Critical care of less than 30 minutes total duration on a given date should be reported with the appropriate E/M code.

Code 99292 is used to report additional block(s) of time, of up to 30 minutes each, beyond the first 74 minutes.

Neonatal and Pediatric Critical Care

According to CPT guidelines, the following codes (99293 through 99296) are used to report services provided by a physician directing the care of a critically ill neonate or infant. The same definitions for critical care services apply for the adult, child, and neonate.

The initial day neonatal critical care code (99295) can be used in addition to codes 99360, 99436, or 99440 as appropriate, when the physician is present for the delivery and newborn resuscitation is necessary. Other procedures performed as a necessary part of the resuscitation (e.g., endotracheal intubation) are also reported separately.

Codes 99295 and 99296 are used to report services provided by a physician directing the care of a critically ill neonate through the first 30 days of life. They represent care starting with the date of admission

(99295) and subsequent day(s) (99296) and may be reported only once per day per patient. Once the neonate is no longer considered critically ill, the Intensive Low Birth Weight Services codes for those with present body weight of less than 2500 grams (99298 and 99299) or the codes for Subsequent Hospital Care (99231 through 99233) for those with present body weight more than 2500 grams should be used.

Codes 99293 and 99294 are used to report services provided by a physician directing the care of a critically ill infant or young child from 31 days of postnatal age up through 24 months of age. They represent care starting with the date of admission (99293) and subsequent day(s) (99294) and may be reported by a single physician only once per day, per patient in a given setting. The critically ill or injured child older than 2 years when admitted to an intensive care unit is reported with hourly critical care service codes (99291 and 99292). Once an infant is no longer considered to be critically ill but continues to require intensive care, the Intensive Low Birth Weight Services codes (99298 and 99299) should be used to report services for infants with present body weight of less than 2500 grams. When the present body weight of those infants exceeds 2500 grams, the Subsequent Hospital Care (99231 through 99233) codes should be used.

Care rendered under 99293 through 99296 includes management, monitoring, and treatment of the patient, including: respiratory and pharmacologic control of the circulatory system, enteral and parenteral nutrition, metabolic and hematologic maintenance, parent and family counseling, case management services, and personal direct supervision of the health care team in the performance of cognitive and procedural activities.

The pediatric and neonatal critical care codes include those procedures previously listed for the hourly critical care codes (99291 and 99292). In addition, the following procedures also are included in the bundled (global) pediatric and neonatal critical care service codes (99293 to 99296): umbilical venous (36510) and umbilical arterial (36660) catheters, central (36488 and 36490) or peripheral vessel catheterization (36000), other arterial catheters (36140 and 36620), oral or nasogastric tube placement (43752), endotracheal intubation (31500), lumbar puncture (62270), suprapubic bladder aspiration (51000), bladder catheterization (53670), initiation and management of mechanical ventilation (94656, 94657) or continuous positive airway pressure (94660), surfactant administration, intravascular fluid administration (90780 and 90781), transfusion of blood components (36430 and 36440), vascular punctures (36420 and 36600), invasive or noninvasive electronic monitoring of vital signs, bedside pulmonary function testing (94375), or monitoring or interpretation of blood gases or oxygen saturation (94760 through 94762). Any services performed that are not listed in the preceding should be reported separately.

Emergency Care

Codes 99281 through 99285 describe various levels of emergency care that is provided in an emergency department. An emergency department is defined as an organized hospital-based facility for the provision of unscheduled episodic services to patients who present for immediate medical attention. Code 99288 is used when advanced life support is necessary during emergency care. If office services are provided on an emergency basis, code 99058 (found in the Medicine Section) may be used when billing private insurance cases. CPT codes 99281 through 99285 are not to be used to report emergency care provided in an office setting. Medicare does not pay when code 99058 is used, and other carriers also may deny this code. When a physician spends several hours attending to a patient, coding for prolonged services (modifier -21), in addition to an office visit, might be indicated. See the section on modifiers for further explanation.

If a patient comes into the office requiring emergency care for a wound trauma, and you bill for the office visit, suturing of the laceration, and the surgical tray, most insurance carriers will pay only for the suturing. The carrier will state that the office visit is included or bundled (codes grouped together that are related to a procedure) with the surgical procedure. The carrier will also state that the surgical tray is included or bundled with the surgical procedure. If you view the CMS Correct Coding Initiative (CCI) edits, you can see which codes are inclusive with another. If the CCI edits do not show the codes as being inclusive, you should appeal the carrier's decision or bill the patient if allowed by state law. This topic is explained later in this chapter under "Coding Guidelines for Code Edits." However, if you code the claim for office services provided on an emergency basis, most carriers will reimburse for the office visit (see Example 5–4). Remember that starred surgical procedures should be billed with an E/M code. Non-starred surgical procedures can stand alone and be billed without an E/M code. The exception is when the patient presents with other reasons for the visit; for example, if the patient has an extensive open wound of the arm only, a bill may be submitted only for the wound repair. If the patient has an extensive wound of the arm with abrasions of the shoulder, contusions of the ribs, and a sprained finger, then a bill should be submitted for the wound repair and an E/M code. The wound diagnosis can support the wound repair, and the other injuries support the E/M. Make sure the appropriate modifiers are used

EXAMPLE 5–4	**Office Emergency**
Incorrect Coding	
99212	Office visit, level 2, established patient
12005	Simple repair of scalp laceration, 12.6 cm
99070	Surgical tray (itemized)
Correct Coding	
99212	Office visit, level 2, established patient
99058	*Office services provided on an emergency basis*
12005	Simple repair of scalp laceration, 12.6 cm

with your claim. For example, modifier -25 is used to report a significant and separate procedure that was performed in addition to an E/M.

Miscellaneous service codes 99050 through 99054 can be used depending on the hour at which the patient is seen as an emergency in the physician's office. Many carriers, including Medicare, do not pay for these codes. Some carriers might pay for these codes and require documentation from the provider to support the code. Other codes under Miscellaneous Services in the Medicine Section may be applicable for a patient receiving emergency care, so these should be scrutinized carefully. New codes have been added to the prolonged services section and case management section in the 2003 CPT manual as follows:

▪ 99358 Prolonged evaluation and management service before or after direct (face-to-face) patient care (e.g., review of extensive records and tests, or communication with other professionals or the patient and family); first hour (list separately in addition to code[s] for other physician service[s] or inpatient or outpatient E/M service)

▪ 99359 Prolonged evaluation and management service before or after direct (face-to-face) patient care (e.g., review of extensive records and tests, or communication with other professionals or the patient and family); each additional 30 minutes (list separately in addition to code for prolonged physician service)

▪ 99360 Physician standby service, requiring prolonged physician attendance, each 30 minutes (e.g., operative standby, standby for frozen section, cesarean and high-risk delivery, electroencephalogram [EEG] monitoring)

▪ 99361 Medical conference by a physician with interdisciplinary team of health professionals or representatives of community agencies to coordinate activities of patient care (patient not present); approximately 30 minutes

▪ 99362 Medical conference by a physician with interdisciplinary team of health professionals or representatives of community agencies to coordinate activities of patient care (patient not present); approximately 60 minutes

▶ 99371 Telephone call by a physician to patient or for consultation or medical management or for coordinating medical management with other health care professionals (e.g., nurses, therapists, social workers, nutritionists, physicians, or pharmacists); simple or brief (e.g., to report on tests or laboratory results, clarify or alter previous instructions, integrate new information from other health professionals into the medical treatment plan, or adjust therapy)

▶ 99372 Telephone call by a physician to patient or for consultation or medical management or for coordinating medical management with other health care professionals (e.g., nurses, therapists, social workers, nutritionists, physicians, or pharmacists); intermediate (e.g., to provide advice to an established patient on a new problem, initiate therapy that can be handled by telephone, discuss test results in detail, coordinate medical management of a new problem in an established patient, discuss and evaluate new information and details, or initiate new plan of care)

▶ 99373 Telephone call by a physician to patient or for consultation or medical management or for coordinating medical management with other health care professionals (e.g., nurses, therapists, social workers, nutritionists, physicians, or pharmacists); complex or lengthy (e.g., lengthy counseling session with anxious or distraught patient, detailed or prolonged discussion with family members about seriously ill patient, or lengthy communication necessary to coordinate complex services of several different health professionals working on different aspects of the total patient care plan)

Counseling

Codes 99381 through 99397 include counseling that is provided at the time of the initial or periodic comprehensive preventive medicine examination. Codes 99401 through 99412 should be used for reporting counseling given at an encounter separate from the preventive medicine examination.

Categories and Subcategories

The E/M section of CPT has categories and subcategories that have from three to five levels for reporting purposes. These levels are based on key components, contributory factors, and face-to-face time with the patient or family. To begin the coding process, the insurance billing specialist must identify the category (e.g., office, hospital inpatient or outpatient, or consultation) and then select the subcategory (e.g., new patient or established patient). The description should be read thoroughly to note the *key components* (e.g., history, examination, or medical decision making) and the *contributory factors* (e.g., counseling, coordination of care, or nature of the presenting problem), the face-to-face time of the service should be noted. Review the sample in Figure 5–3 illustrating an E/M code for a new patient

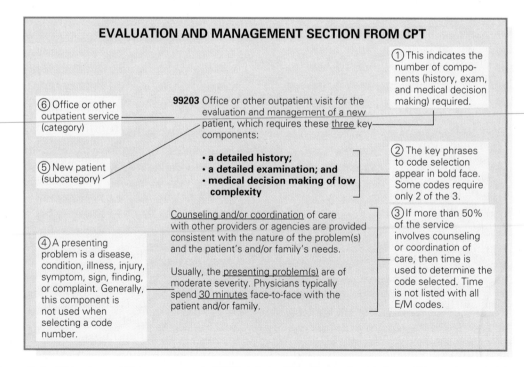

Figure 5–3. Evaluation and Management code 99203 defining the main words and phrases. This code is used for a new patient seen in the office or in an outpatient or ambulatory setting.

seen in the office or in an outpatient or ambulatory setting.

Because key components are clinical in nature, the physician must give these factors and document them in the patient's record to assist in coding each case. In a case in which counseling and coordination of care dominate (more than 50%) the face-to-face physician–patient encounter, then *time* is considered the key component to qualify for a particular level of E/M services. Tables 5–1 and 5–2 give a concise view of the components for each code number.

Many physicians began ranking the E/M codes on a scale of from 1 to 5, with 5 the highest, most complex level and 1 the lowest, least complex level. These levels coincide with the last digit of the CPT code. It is common to hear a physician say, "Ted Brown was seen for a level 4 today." This terminology may appear on encounter forms with five-digit CPT code numbers and be referred to as levels 1 through 5 (Example 5–5).

EXAMPLE 5–5

Current Procedural Terminology Code Digit Analysis

Code book
Section   Type Level

| 9 | 9 | 2 | 0 | 2 |

E/M Section   New
                 Patient   II

Alternatively, this terminology may be seen abbreviated as L-1, L-2, and so on, but this usage is not preferred because it can be confused with the nomenclature for the sections of the lumbar vertebrae. The level also may be written out as level one, level two, and so on, depending on the complexity of the case. A breakdown of the E/M levels with code numbers is shown in Table 5–3.

In some billing cases, it is necessary to use a two-digit modifier to give a more accurate description of the services rendered. This is used in addition to the procedure code. Refer to the comprehensive list of modifiers at the end of this chapter for more information.

Surgery Section

Coding from an Operative Report

Obtain a copy of the patient's operative report from the hospital when coding surgery. Make a photocopy that you can write on as you make notes. When scanning the report, use a ruler or highlighter pen. Use the ruler to read the report line by line. Highlight words that may indicate that the procedure performed may be altered by specific circumstances and when billing can remind you that a code modifier may be needed. Look up any unfamiliar terms and write the definition in the margin.

When coding a complex surgical procedure, either include an operative report or give a brief explanation in the proper block of the insurance claim form so that the claims adjuster clearly understands the case and maximum payment is generated.

Use of code numbers that describe a part of the body treated may increase reimbursement (e.g., suturing of a facial laceration pays a higher rate than suturing of an arm laceration).

Code only the operations that actually were documented in the report. Do not code using only the name of the procedure given in the heading of the operative report. Read the report thoroughly before coding to see whether additional procedures were performed and whether they were part of the main procedure, performed independently, or unrelated. Information on how to code multiple procedures that are not inherent in a major procedure may be found at the end of this chapter under modifier -51.

Reread the report to make certain that all procedural and diagnostic codes have been identified. Compare the content with the codes you are using. You cannot code circumstances the physician relays to you verbally. Be sure the words "extensive complications" are in the report if there are such complications.

Surgical code descriptions may define a correct coding relationship where one code is part of another based on the language used in the description (Example 5–6).

Confirm that the report findings agree with the procedure codes on the claim.

Surgical Package

Surgical package is a phrase commonly encountered when billing. Procedures not followed by a star (*) include the "package" concept. Generally, a surgical procedure includes:

▶ The operation
▶ Local infiltration; topical anesthesia or metacarpal, metatarsal, or digital block

| TABLE 5–1 | | **Selection of Evaluation and Management Codes** | | | | |

Code	History	Examination	Medical Decision Making	Problem Severity	Coordination of Care and Counseling	Time Spent (avg)
Office or Other Outpatient Services (Includes Hospital Observation Area)						
New Patient*						
99201	Problem focused	Problem focused	Straightforward	Minor or self-limited	Consistent with problem(s) and patient's needs	10 min face to face
99202	Expanded problem focused	Expanded problem focused	Straightforward	Low to moderate	Consistent with problem(s) and patient's needs	20 min face to face
99203	Detailed	Detailed	Low complexity	Moderate	Consistent with problem(s) and patient's needs	30 min face to face
99204	Comprehensive	Comprehensive	Moderate complexity	Moderate to high	Consistent with problem(s) and patient's needs	45 min face to face
99205	Comprehensive	Comprehensive	High complexity	Moderate to high	Consistent with problem(s) and patient's needs	60 min face to face
Established Patient*†						
99211	—	—	Physician supervision, but presence not required	Minimal	Consistent with problem(s) and patient's needs	5 min face to face
99212	Problem focused	Problem focused	Straightforward	Minor or self-limited	Consistent with problem(s) and patient's needs	10 min face to face
99213	Expanded problem focused	Expanded problem focused	Low complexity	Low to moderate	Consistent with problem(s) and patient's needs	15 min face to face
99214	Detailed	Detailed	Moderate complexity	Moderate to high	Consistent with problem(s) and patient's needs	25 min face to face
99215	Comprehensive	Comprehensive	High complexity	Moderate to high	Consistent with problem(s) and patient's needs	40 min face to face
Hospital Observation Services						
99217	—	—	—	—	—	—
99218	Detailed or comprehensive	Detailed or comprehensive	Straightforward or low complexity	Low	Consistent with problem(s) and patient's needs	—
99219	Comprehensive	Comprehensive	Moderate complexity	Moderate	Consistent with problem(s) and patient's needs	—
99220	Comprehensive	Comprehensive	High complexity	High	Consistent with problem(s) and patient's needs	—

Selection of Evaluation and Management Codes—cont'd

Code	History	Examination	Medical Decision Making	Problem Severity	Coordination of Care and Counseling	Time Spent (avg)
			Hospital Inpatient Services			
			Initial Care‡			
99221	Detailed or comprehensive	Detailed or comprehensive	Straightforward or low complexity	Low	Consistent with problem(s) and patient's needs	30 min unit/ floor
99222	Comprehensive	Comprehensive	Moderate complexity	Moderate	Consistent with problem(s) and patient's needs	50 min unit/ floor
99223	Comprehensive	Comprehensive	High complexity	High	Consistent with problem(s) and patient's needs	70 min unit/ floor
			Hospital Inpatient Services			
			Subsequent Care‡§			
99231	Problem focused interval	Problem focused	Straightforward or low complexity	Stable, recovering or improving	Consistent with problem(s) and patient's needs	15 min unit/ floor
99232	Expanded problem focused interval	Expanded problem focused	Moderate complexity	Inadequate response to treatment; minor complication	Consistent with problem(s) and patient's needs	25 min unit/ floor
99233	Detailed interval	Detailed	High complexity	Unstable; significant new problem(s) or complication(s)	Consistent with problem(s) and patient's needs	35 min unit/ floor
99238	Hospital discharge day management					

*Key component: For new patients for initial office and other outpatient services, all three components (history, physical examination, and medical decision making) are essential in selecting the correct code. For established patients, at least two of these three components are required.
†Includes follow-up, periodic reevaluation, and management of new problems.
‡Key components: For initial care, all three components (history, physical examination, and medical decision making) are essential in selecting the correct code. For subsequent care, at least two of these three components are required.
§All subsequent levels of service include a review of the medical record, diagnostic studies, and changes in the patient's status, such as history, physical condition, and response to treatment since the last assessment.

▶ Subsequent to the decision for surgery, one related E/M encounter on the date immediately before or on the date of procedure (including history and physical)
▶ Immediate postoperative care, including dictating operative notes and talking with the family and other physicians
▶ Writing orders
▶ Evaluating the patient in the postanesthesia recovery area
▶ Typical postoperative follow-up care (hospital visits, discharge, or follow-up office visits)

This is referred to as a "package" for surgical procedures, and one fee covers the whole package (Fig. 5–4, *A*). The majority of surgical procedures, including fracture care, are handled in this manner.

Preoperative services such as consultations, office visits, and initial hospital care often are billed separately. An appropriate five-digit E/M code should be selected. Payment of these services depends on third-party payment policy.

There are variations among insurance policies and managed care plans about what is included in the package fee. Some follow Medicare guidelines; some

| TABLE 5–2 | **Code Selection Criteria for Consultations** |

E/M Code	History*	Examination	Medical Decision Making*	Problem Severity	Coordination of Care; Counseling	Time (avg)
Office and Other Outpatient						
99241	Problem focused	Problem focused	Straightforward	Minor or self-limited	Consistent with problem(s) and patient's needs	15 min face to face
99242	Expanded problem focused	Expanded problem focused	Straightforward	Low	Consistent with problem(s) and patient's needs	30 min face to face
99243	Detailed	Detailed	Low complexity	Moderate	Consistent with problem(s) and patient's needs	40 min face to face
99244	Comprehensive	Comprehensive	Moderate complexity	Moderate to high	Consistent with problem(s) and patient's needs	60 min face to face
99245	Comprehensive	Comprehensive	High complexity	Moderate to high	Consistent with problem(s) and patient's needs	80 min face to face
Initial Inpatient†						
99251	Problem focused	Problem focused	Straightforward	Minor or self-limited	Consistent with problem(s) and patient's needs	20 min unit/ floor
99252	Expanded problem focused	Expanded problem focused	Straightforward	Low	Consistent with problem(s) and patient's needs	40 min unit/ floor
99253	Detailed	Detailed	Low complexity	Moderate	Consistent with problem(s) and patient's needs	55 min unit/ floor
99254	Comprehensive	Comprehensive	Moderate complexity	Moderate to high	Consistent with problem(s) and patient's needs	80 min unit/ floor
99255	Comprehensive	Comprehensive	High complexity	Moderate to high	Consistent with problem(s) and patient's needs	110 min unit/ floor
Follow-Up Inpatient†						
99261	Problem focused	Problem focused	Straightforward or low complexity	Stable, recovering or improving	Consistent with problem(s) and patient's needs	10 min unit/ floor
99262	Expanded problem focused interval	Expanded problem focused	Moderate complexity	Inadequate response to treatment; minor complication	Consistent with problem(s) and patient's needs	20 min unit/ floor
99263	Detailed interval	Detailed	High complexity	Unstable; significant new problem(s) or complication	Consistent with problem(s) and patient's needs	30 min unit/ floor
Confirmatory						
99271	Problem focused	Problem focused	Straightforward	Minor or self-limited	Consistent with problem(s) and patient's needs	—

TABLE 5–2	Code Selection Criterial for Consultations—cont'd					
E/M Code	History*	Examination	Medical Decision Making*	Problem Severity	Coordination of Care; Counseling	Time (avg)
99272	Expanded problem focused	Expanded problem focused	Straightforward	Low	Consistent with problem(s) and patient's needs	—
99273	Detailed	Detailed	Low complexity	Moderate	Consistent with problem(s) and patient's needs	—
99274	Comprehensive	Comprehensive	Moderate	Moderate to high	Consistent with problem(s) and patient's needs	—
99275	Comprehensive	Comprehensive	High	Moderate to high	Consistent with problem(s) and patient's needs	—

*Key component: For office and initial inpatient consultations, all three components (history, physical examination, and medical decision making) are crucial for selecting the correct code. Two of these three components are required for follow-up consultations.

†These codes also are used for residents of nursing facilities.

do not. Plans may include all visits several weeks before surgery, or they may include only visits that occur 1 day before the surgery. When a decision is made for surgery, a common question asked is whether a charge may be made for the consultation or office visit and admission if done on the same day. In most cases, the admission should be charged listing initial hospital care codes 99221 through 99223. However, the guidelines are different for surgeons. For example, surgical package rules apply if a surgeon sees a patient in consultation and recommends that the patient receive immediate transfer of care to the surgeon and admission for surgery. The consultation that resulted in the decision for surgery may be billed by adding modifier -57 (decision for surgery) to the consultation procedure code number. The surgeon may not charge for an admission because all E/M services provided within 24 hours of surgery are bundled into the surgical fee.

> Remember the rule: Not documented, not done.

Medicare Global Package

Medicare has a **global surgery policy** for major operations that is similar to the surgical package concept. The Medicare global fee is a single fee for all necessary services normally furnished by the surgeon before, during, and after the procedure. This became

TABLE 5–3	Levels with Code Numbers			
	Office Visits		Consultations	
	New	Established	Office	Hospital
Level 1	99201	99211	99241	99251
Level 2	99202	99212	99242	99252
Level 3	99203	99213	99243	99253
Level 4	99204	99214	99244	99254
Level 5	99205	99215	99245	99255

EXAMPLE 5–6

Integral Code Descriptions

Partial and complete, which means the partial procedure is included in the complete procedure.
56620   Vulvectomy simple; partial
56625   Complete

Partial and total, which means the partial procedure is included in the total procedure.
58940   Oophorectomy, partial or total, unilateral or bilateral

Unilateral and bilateral, which means the unilateral procedure is included in the bilateral procedure.
58900   Biopsy of ovary, unilateral or bilateral

Single and multiple, which means the single procedure is included in the multiple procedure.
49321   Laparoscopy, surgical; with biopsy (*single* or *multiple*)

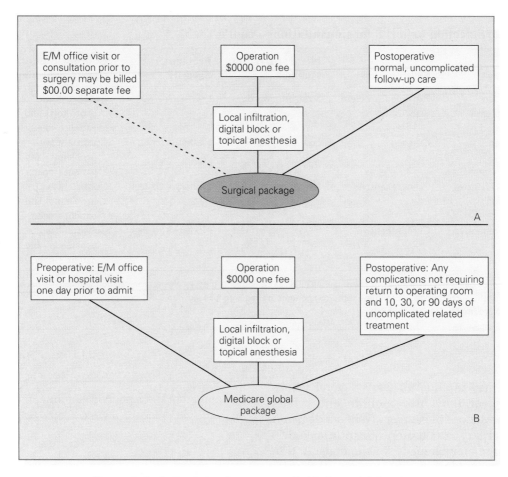

Figure 5–4. A, Surgical package concept. **B,** Medicare global package.

effective January 1, 1992 (Fig. 5–4, *B*). Included in the package are:

▶ Preoperative visits (1 day before or day of surgery)
▶ Intraoperative services that are a usual and necessary part of the surgical procedure
▶ Complications after surgery that do not require additional trips to the operating room (medical and surgical services)
▶ Postoperative visits including hospital visits, discharge, and office visits for variable postoperative periods: 0, 10, or 90 days

In addition, procedures in the global period column of the *Federal Register* may show one of the following:

MMM This is a service furnished in uncomplicated maternity cases, which includes prenatal care, delivery, and postnatal care.
XXX No global period. Visits, procedures, and follow-up services may be charged separately.

YYY The global period will be determined by the local Medicare carrier because the code is for an unlisted procedure.
ZZZ The code is part of another service and falls within that service's global period.

Services provided for a Medicare patient *not included* in the global surgery package are the following:

▶ Initial consultation or evaluation (regardless of when it occurs)
▶ Postoperative visits unrelated to the diagnosis for which the surgical procedure was performed (modifier -24 applies)
▶ Treatment necessary to stabilize a seriously ill patient before surgery
▶ Diagnostic tests and procedures
▶ Related procedure for postoperative complications that requires a return trip to the operating room (modifier -78 applies)
▶ Immunosuppressive therapy after transplant surgery

If a Medicare patient is discharged from one hospital facility and admitted to a different hospital or facility on the same day, a provider may get paid for both, depending on the circumstances of the case. A low-level admission code (e.g., 99221) is used for the second hospital admit. A higher-level admission code may be used when the patient goes from a regular room to a specialized hospital of some type. Two separate claim forms, one for the discharge and another for the admission, must be used.

Follow-up Days

The number of follow-up days that are allowed after surgery at no additional charge varies. The CPT code book does not specify how many days should be given, so an additional reference manual is needed. Most states use an RVS for workers' compensation cases, which lists the follow-up days allowed for most surgical procedures. Another source that lists surgical follow-up days for Medicare services is published in the *Federal Register* at the end of each year. Locate Appendix B (the Medicare Fee Schedule) and follow-up days are listed as a global fee period in the ninth column. Obtain the RVS used in your state or a copy of the *Federal Register* for this information.

Medicare lists a 90-day global period for all major procedures. A number of commercial insurance carriers have a 45-day global period for all or some major procedures. Some commercial carriers treat major procedures like minor procedures in the surgical package. To obtain specific carrier information, send the insurance company a list of the most common surgical procedures and ask for the surgical package rules and the number of global days that apply to each code. If this information is not available, it is wise to bill the private carrier for the preoperative and all postoperative visits. When this information is received, a table should be created that shows global days on a payer-by-payer and procedure-by-procedure basis. On the chart of each patient scheduled for surgery, the type of surrgery and how many days the insurance policy allows should be indicated. A bill should be submitted for all visits after the surgical package period expires.

For office visits by the physician during the postoperative period, use CPT code number 99024 to indicate "No Charge." This code is located in the Medicine Section under Special Services and Reports; Miscellaneous Services. It has no value, is unbundled with other codes, and is used for tracking purposes. Always use 99024 for postoperative visits on itemized billing statements, because this lets the patient know how many office visits after surgery are being billed at no charge. There is no Medicare guideline for this code. Generally it is not necessary to list this code when completing an insurance claim unless the insurance carrier has specific instructions requesting that it be shown. If the patient has to be seen beyond the normal postoperative period, the reason should be documented in the patient's medical record and an applicable procedure code and fee for this service should be indicated on the claim form. A bill may be submitted for the office visit if the patient returns to the provider during the postoperative (global) period and the reason for the visit is not related to wound repair or infection. The diagnosis codes will support the visit. If the provider did not perform the surgery but is performing the postoperative care, the provider can charge for the visits.

Repair of Lacerations

If multiple lacerations are repaired with the same technique and are in the same anatomic category, the insurance billing specialist should add up the total length of all the lacerations and report one code to obtain maximum reimbursement. Anatomic categories are the scalp, neck, axillae, external genitalia, trunk, extremities (hands or feet), face, ears, eyelids, nose, lips, or mucous membranes. If the patient had three repairs and each was listed with a different code, the second and third codes are downcoded so a smaller payment is generated. If a patient has lacerations on both sides of the face, the lengths of all the lacerations should be combined because the anatomic region is the same, and a claim should be submitted for the total length. No modifier is used, and the right and left side of the face are not billed separately (Example 5–7).

EXAMPLE 5–7   **Repair of Multiple Lacerations**

Three lacerations of the face totaling 8.2 cm

Incorrect Coding

12011	Repair 2.5-cm laceration of face
12013	Repair 2.7-cm laceration of face
12013	Repair 3-cm laceration of face

Correct Coding

12015	Repair 8.2-cm laceration of face.

Multiple Lesions

The descriptions for the surgical codes that relate to accessory structures and lesions found in the integumentary system can cause confusion. Code descriptions, including indentations, should be read completely with attention paid to terms such as complex, complicated, extensive, and multiple (lesions). Lesion excision code selection is not based on lesion diameter but on excised diameter. Excised diameter is the greatest clinical diameter of the apparent lesion plus the narrowest margin necessary for complete excision. See Example 5–8 as a guide to obtain maximum reimbursement for paring of seven corns.

EXAMPLE 5–8	**Paring of Seven Corns**
Incorrect Coding	
11055	Paring; single lesion
11056-51	Two to four lesions
11057-51	More than four lesions
or	
11055 × 7	Paring; single lesion (× seven corns)
Correct Coding	
11057	Paring; more than four lesions (seven corns)

Delay submission of the insurance claim for removal of a lesion or lesions until the pathology report is received. Usually, a malignant lesion is reimbursed at a higher rate because of the more detailed nature of the procedure.

Supplies

When billing for office surgery and supplies used, checklists for the items used on the sterile tray (Fig. 5–5, *A*) and for determining complete and incomplete records (Fig. 5–5, *B*) should be used. These items can only be charged for if the surgery required the use of *additional* items not normally used for this type of surgery.

Prolonged Services, Detention, or Standby

Code numbers 99354 through 99359 should be used to indicate prolonged services with direct face-to-face patient contact; for example, the physician has spent time beyond the usual amount allotted the service (e.g., 30 to 60 minutes). There are specific codes for face-to-face contact and without direct face-to-face contact. Prolonged service that is less than 30 minutes should not be billed using these codes because the time is included in the total work of the E/M codes. Time should be documented in the medical record to justify use of these codes. Reimbursement for prolonged detention in the hospital is higher than payment for many other types of care, and reimbursement for critical care is even higher.

Physician standby services are billed using code 99360. Some insurance programs or plans (e.g., Medicare) do not pay for operative standby, so be sure to check before billing to see whether the commercial carrier will pay. The charge is based on what the physician feels is the value of an hour of her or his time. An example is when a pediatrician is on standby during a high-risk cesarean section on a pregnant woman.

A   MINOR OPERATING ROOM INSTRUMENT TRAY SUPPLY CHECKLIST

1 Adson Brown tissue forceps   _____
1 Adson tissue forceps with teeth   _____
1 long tissue forceps   _____
2 mosquito clamps   _____
1 Peck Joseph dissecting scissors   _____
1 Kahn dissecting scissors   _____
1 Reynolds dissecting scissors   _____
1 Stratte needle holder   _____
1 Webster needle holder   _____
4 small piercing towel clips   _____
2 double-skin hooks   _____
2 single-skin hooks   _____
1 knife handle   _____
1 #15 blade   _____
10 4 x 4s   _____
2 cotton-tipped applicators   _____
1 small basin   _____
3 sterile towels (drapes)   _____
1 Bovie pencil   _____
Sutures:_____ _____ _____
Dressings:½ inch Steri-strips   _____

B   OFFICE SURGERY MEDICAL RECORD CHECKLIST

Patient information sheet   _____
H and P or progress note   _____
Consent form   _____
Diagnostic studies   _____
Pathology report(s)   _____
Anesthesia record   _____
Circulating nurse's note   _____
Doctor's orders   _____
Discharge note   _____
Operative report   _____
Signature/operative report   _____

Figure 5–5. A, Checklist to document supplies used when billing for office surgery. This list can be kept with the patient's medical record. **B,** Checklist for identifying complete and incomplete medical records used for a patient receiving office surgery. As each item or document is completed, it is checked off so that the person reviewing the chart can see at a glance what needs to be finalized.

PROCEDURE: How to Code Effectively

To code effectively, follow these steps.

1. Always read the *Introduction* section at the beginning of the code book, which changes annually with each edition.
2. Read the *Guidelines* at the beginning of each of the six sections of the book. These define commonly used terms, explain classifications within each section, and give instructions specific to each section.

3. Read the *notes* and special subsection information throughout the Surgery, Radiology, Pathology, and Medicine sections. This information is listed throughout each section.
4. Use the index at the back of the book to locate a specific item by generalized code numbers, NOT by page numbers. Listings are given in four primary classes of main entries:
    a. Procedure or service
       Example: Anastomosis; Endoscopy; Splint
    b. Organ or other anatomic site
       Example: Salivary Gland; Tibia; Colon
    c. Condition
       Example: Abscess; Entropion; Tetralogy of Fallot
    d. Synonyms, eponyms, and abbreviations
       Example: EEG; Bricker operation; Clagett procedure

If the procedure performed is not listed, check for the organ involved. If the procedure or organ is difficult to find, look up the condition. Key words, such as synonyms or eponyms, and abbreviations will help you find the appropriate code.

5. Locate the code number in the code section and read through the narrative description to locate the most appropriate number to apply to the patient's procedure. Always start with the main term when reading the description. A semicolon (;) separates common portions from subordinate

11040	Debridement; skin, partial thickness
11041	skin, full thickness
11042	skin, and subcutaneous tissue
11043	skin, subcutaneous tissue, and muscle
11044	skin, subcutaneous tissue, muscle, and bone

Figure 5–6. Use of a semicolon.

designations; subterms are indented (Fig. 5–6). Any terminology after the semicolon has a dependent status, as do the subsequent indented entries. In Figure 5–6 you see that procedure code number 11044 should read as follows: Debridement; skin, subcutaneous tissue, muscle, and bone. Figure 5–7 shows an insurance claim for a patient who has had six corns pared.

6. When trying to locate an E/M code, identify the place or type of service rendered. Then identify whether the patient is new or established and locate the category or subcategory. Review any guidelines or instructions pertaining to the category or subcategory. Read the descriptors of the levels of E/M service. Identify the requirements necessary for code assignment. Make sure the components necessary were performed by the physician and documented in the chart, and then assign the E/M code.

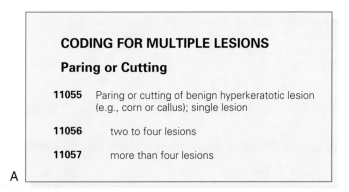

Figure 5–7. A, Procedure codes from the Surgery Section of *Current Procedural Terminology.* **B,** Blocks 24A through 24K of the CMS-1500 insurance claim form showing placement of the code on Line 2.

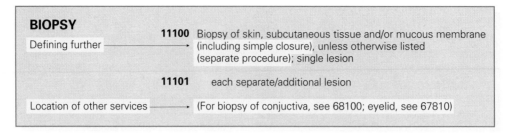

Figure 5–8. Use of parentheses in the Surgery Section of *Current Procedural Terminology.*

7. Transfer the five-digit code number to the claim form exactly as given for each procedure. Be careful not to transpose code numbers. Also note the following:

   ▶ Parentheses ( ) further define the code and tell where other services are located (Fig. 5–8).

   ▶ Measurements throughout the code book are based on the metric system (Fig. 5–9).

   ▶ All anesthesia services are reported by use of the five-digit anesthesia code plus a physical status modifier. The use of other modifiers to explain a procedure further is optional. *Example:* Patient is a healthy 23-year-old Caucasian woman. Anesthesia given for a vaginal delivery. The procedure code is 00946-P1.

▶ The Surgery section is the largest segment of the code book. It has many subsections and subheadings. You must be able to break down a procedure and identify various terms that will direct you to the correct code. Blocks 24A through 24K of the CMS-1500 insurance claim form show placement of the code on Line 2 (Example 5–9, bottom).

Unlisted Procedures

When a service is rendered, the unlisted code with a description stating "unlisted" (Example 5–10) should be used rather than than a "guessed" or incorrect code, and a cover letter should be sent explaining the

---

EXAMPLE 5–9   **Blocks 24A through 24K of the CMS-1500 Claim Form**

Closed manipulative treatment of a clavicular fracture.
Section: Surgery, Musculoskeletal System
Anatomic subheading: Shoulder
Condition: Fracture or Dislocation
Code: 23505

Thus when completing an insurance claim form for closed manipulative tx, clavicular fracture, the billing portion appears as follows:

24. A DATE(S) OF SERVICE From MM DD YYYY	To MM DD YYYY	B Place of Service	C Type of Service	D PROCEDURES, SERVICES, OR SUPPLIES (Explain Unusual Circumstances) CPT/HCPCS ⎸ MODIFIER	E DIAGNOSIS CODE	F $ CHARGES	G DAYS OR UNITS	H EPSDT Family Plan	I EMG	J COB	K RESERVED FOR LOCAL USE
010720XX		11		99203	1	00 00	1			46	27889700
010720XX		11		23505	1	00 00	1			46	27889700

Figure 5–9. Metric measurements from the Surgery Section of *Current Procedural Terminology.*

13150	Repair, complex, eyelids, nose, ears and/or lips; 1.0 cm or less (See also 40650–40654, 67961–67975)
13151	1.1 cm to 2.5 cm
13152	2.6 cm to 7.5 cm

Unlisted Procedure Code

99429   Unlisted preventive medicine service.

service. Unlisted codes end in -99 and are found at the end of each section or subsection. A comprehensive listing of unlisted codes is found at the beginning of each section. Some Medicare fiscal agents do not pay for any of the special-99 adjunct codes.

Follow these guidelines when submitting a claim with an unlisted code to obtain maximum payment:

▶ Always send supporting documentation with the claim that clearly identifies the procedure performed and the medical necessity for it. If detailed documentation cannot be electronically submitted or faxed to the carrier, send a paper claim with supporting documentation in a large envelope so it is not folded. Do not use paper clips, staples, or tape to affix the attachments to the claim. Mark each attachment with the patient's name, insurance identification number, date of service, page number of the attachment, and total number of pages submitted (e.g., page 2 of 3). This helps the claim's processor match the documentation to the claim in the event they become separated.

▶ When unlisted procedures are performed frequently, ask the insurance carrier to assign a temporary a local code so that it is not necessary to submit supporting documentation each time. This avoids manual processing and delays.

▶ File claims with unlisted procedure codes in a separate "tickler" file. Follow up the status of the claim if there is no response within 1 month.

Coding Guidelines for Code Edits

In 1996 the Medicare program implemented a Correct Coding Initiative (CCI). This initiative involves a code edit system consistent with Medicare policies to eliminate inappropriate reporting of CPT codes. *Code edit* is a function of computer software that performs online checking of codes on an insurance claim to detect unbundling, splitting of codes, and other types of improper code submissions. Such software is used by private payers, other federal programs, and state Medicaid programs also. Some code pairs in the CCI edits are followed by a 0 and others by a 1. If the superscript 0 appears with a code pair, it means Medicare never allows a modifier to be used, so the pair could be reported together. The superscript 1 means that you may use a modifier

under certain circumstances to get both codes reimbursed.

Because every medical practice has billing problems and questions unique to its specialty that arise because of denial or reduction in payment of claims, the billing specialist must become a detective and discover how to obtain maximum reimbursements in the appropriate specialty. The best way is to experiment by trying new coding options and noting improvements in reimbursement. Coding takes expertise. It is an art, not an exact science. The following explanations of various ways of coding claims assist in obtaining maximum reimbursement for each service rendered and avoiding denials, lowered reimbursement, and possible audit.

Comprehensive and Component Edits

A **comprehensive code** means a single code that describes or covers two or more component codes that are bundled together as one unit. Each component code represents a portion of the service described in the comprehensive code and should be used only if a portion of the comprehensive service was performed (Example 5–11).

Comprehensive and Component Codes

Comprehensive code	**93015** Cardiovascular stress test	
Component codes	**93016, 93017, 93018**	
93015	Cardiovascular stress test using maximal or submaximal treadmill or bicycle exercise, continuous electrocardiographic monitoring, or pharmacological stress; with physician supervision, with interpretation and report	
93016	Physician supervision only, without interpretation and report	
93017	Tracing only, without interpretation and report	
93018	Interpretation and report only	

Under the Medicare program, *component edits* are made involving procedures that meet any of the following criteria:

1. Code combinations that are specified as "separate procedures" by the CPT
2. Codes that are included as part of a more extensive procedure
3. Code combinations that are restricted by the guidelines outlined in the CPT

Separate Procedure

Separate procedure example: Inguinal hernia repair with lesion excised from spermatic cord

Comprehensive code: 49505 Repair initial hernia age 5 years or older; reducible

Component code: 55520 Excision of lesion of spermatic cord (**separate procedure**)

---

4. Component codes that are used incorrectly with the comprehensive code

If any one of these restricted code combinations is billed, Medicare allows payment for the procedure with the higher relative value (Example 5–12).

When performing an inguinal hernia repair, the surgeon makes an incision in the groin and dissects tissue to expose the hernia sac, internal oblique muscle, and spermatic cord. If a lesion is excised from the spermatic cord, it is considered a component of the comprehensive hernia repair procedure and not separately billable. Medicare will deny code 55520 as a component of procedure code 49505 when performed at the same operative session.

Mutually Exclusive Code Denials

Mutually exclusive edits relate to procedures that meet any of the following criteria:

1. Code combinations that are restricted by the guidelines outlined in the CPT
2. Procedures that represent two methods of performing the same service
3. Procedures that cannot reasonably be done during the same session
4. Procedures that represent medically impossible or improbable code combinations (see Example 5–13)

Mutually Exclusive Code

| 47605 | **Excision,** Cholecystectomy; with cholangiography |
| 47563 | **Laparoscopy,** surgical; cholecystectomy with cholangiography |

Note: Different methods of accomplishing same procedure.

Because both of these procedures are different methods of accomplishing removal of the gallbladder with cholangiography and represent duplication of efforts and overlapping of services, Medicare would deny code 47563 as mutually exclusive to code 47605.

Bundled Codes

When related to insurance claims, the phrase **bundled codes** means to group codes together that are related to a procedure. To completely understand bundled codes, one must have a thorough knowledge of the service or procedure that is being provided or use an unbundling book as a reference guide.

Example 5–14 illustrates one type of bundling found in the CPT code book. Because code 19271 does not include mediastinal lymphadenectomy and code 19272 does include it, reporting both codes together would be a contradiction in the actual performance of the services at the same session. Hence, when mediastinal lymphadenectomy is part of the procedure, submit code 19272 because code 19271 is bundled with it.

Bundled Code

| Component code | 19271 | Excision of chest wall tumor involving ribs, with plastic reconstruction; without mediastinal lymphadenectomy |
| Comprehensive code | 19272 | with mediastinal lymphadenectomy |

In the Medicare program, a number of services may be affected because CMS considers the services bundled. Because many commercial carriers may follow Medicare guidelines, an understanding of this bundling concept is necessary. When dealing with private insurance, an Explanation of Benefits document may print out with a statement "Benefits have been combined," which means the same thing as bundling.

For example, when listing a sterile tray for an in-office surgical procedure, the tray is bundled with the procedure unless additional supplies are needed more than and above those usually used. CPT code 99070 (supplies and materials) is not recognized by Medicare for any supplies; however, level 2 alphanumeric codes may be used in such cases. The costs of some services and most supplies are bundled into E/M codes (e.g., telephone services and reading of test results). However, Medicare pays for slings, splints, rib belts, cast supplies, Hexcelite and light casts, pneumatic ankle-control splints, and prosthetics, but a supplier number is needed to bill for take-home surgical supplies and durable medical equipment (DME). Claims for supplies and DME go to one of four regional DME carriers whose addresses are listed in Appendix A. A reference book published by St. Anthony Publishing has comprehensive lists of the codes that CMS considers bundled

---

for the Medicare program. (See Appendix B for further information.)

When appealing a claim, a great deal of time may be spent on paperwork only to discover that the code is bundled and denial is imminent. Whenever in doubt about whether services are combined or not, contact the insurance carrier and ask.

Unbundling

Unbundling is coding and billing numerous CPT codes to identify procedures that usually are described by a single code. It is also known as *exploding* or *à la carte* medicine.

Some practices do this unwittingly, but it is considered fraud if it is done intentionally to gain increased reimbursement. Unbundling can lead to downward payment adjustments and possible audit of claims.

Types of unbundling are shown in Examples 5–15 through 5–18.

- ▶ Fragmenting one service into component parts and coding each component part as if it were a separate service (Example 5–15)
- ▶ Reporting separate codes for related services when one comprehensive code includes all related services (Example 5–16)
- ▶ Coding **bilateral** (both sides of the body) procedures as two codes when one code is proper (Example 5–17)
- ▶ Separating a surgical approach from a major surgical service that includes the same approach (Example 5–18)

EXAMPLE 5–17

Unbundling (Bilateral)

Incorrect Coding

76090-RT	Right mammography
76090-LT	Left mammography

Correct Coding

76091	Mammography; bilateral

EXAMPLE 5–18

Unbundling (Surgical Approach)

Incorrect Coding

49000	Exploratory laparotomy
44150	Colectomy, total, abdominal

Correct Coding

44150	Colectomy, total, abdominal (correct since it *includes* exploration of the surgical field)

EXAMPLE 5–15

Unbundled Code

Incorrect Coding

43235	Upper gastrointestinal (GI) endoscopy
43600	Biopsy of stomach

Correct Coding

43239	Upper GI endoscopy with biopsy of stomach

EXAMPLE 5–16

Unbundling (Comprehensive Code)

Unbundled Claim		**Claim Coded Correctly**	
58150	Total abdominal hysterectomy (corpus and cervix) with removal of tubes and with removal of ovary ($1200)	**58150**	Comprehensive code for all three services ($1200)
58700	Salpingectomy ($650)		
58940	Oophorectomy ($685)		
Total charge: $2535		Total charge: $1200	

Insurers use special software that detects unbundling. To avoid this problem, always use up-to-date CPT and RVS code books. The use of outdated codes often inadvertently results in unbundling. Find out from insurers what edition they are using and always use the same edition as the insurer, especially during a transition period at the first of the year. A new technology or technique may have its own code when it is developed, but may be bundled with another code as it becomes commonplace. If the practice uses a billing service, request in writing that its computer system include no unbundling programming.

Downcoding

Approximately 35 different procedural coding systems are used in various regions across the United States. Generally, only three to five procedural coding systems are in use in any one given region at the same time. CPT and relative value study codes are emphasized in this chapter because they are the most commonly accepted, depending on what type of case you are billing—private, federal, state, or industrial. **Downcoding** occurs when the coding system used on a claim submitted to an insurance carrier does not match the coding system used by the company receiving the claim. The computer system converts the code submitted to the closest code in use, which is usually down one level from the submitted code. The payment that is generated is usually less than if the claim was not downcoded. In many states, it is illegal for an insurance company to downcode a claim. Insurance Commissioners have published bulletins warning carriers to cease this practice of claims adjudication. When a carrier receives a claim, the carrier is allowed to pay or deny the claim. If additional information is needed to adjudicate the claim, it is requested from the patient or provider. The carrier is limited to the number of days it has to review the claim. On completion of the review, the carrier must pay or deny the claim. Make sure that the documentation from the provider supports the code that is being submitted to prevent downcoding. Use current CPT manuals. Review all Medicare updates for changes to HCPCS codes. Always monitor reimbursements and monitor downcodes to become knowledgeable about which codes are affected. Call the insurance carrier and find out which code system is in use and obtain a reference list so you can code using the appropriate system (Example 5–19). However, many carriers do not release any information about their coding system and state it is proprietary to them.

document. If the two do not match, the carrier will reimburse according to the lowest paying code that fits the description given (Example 5–20). See Chapter 8 for additional information and solutions to downcoding.

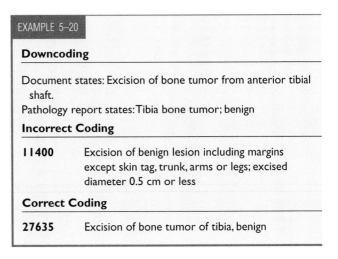

EXAMPLE 5–20

Downcoding

Document states: Excision of bone tumor from anterior tibial shaft.
Pathology report states: Tibia bone tumor; benign

Incorrect Coding

11400	Excision of benign lesion including margins except skin tag, trunk, arms or legs; excised diameter 0.5 cm or less

Correct Coding

27635	Excision of bone tumor of tibia, benign

Upcoding

The term **upcoding** is used to describe deliberate manipulation of CPT codes for increased payment. This practice can be spotted by Medicare fiscal intermediaries and insurance carriers using prepayment and postpayment screens or "stop alerts," which are built into most coding computer software programs. An example of intentional upcoding is when a physician selects one level of service code for all visits with the theory that the costs even out. This opens the door to audits and in the end may cost the practice money. Upcoding may occur unintentionally if the coder is ill informed or does not keep current. Join a free list service (listserv) to keep current, make national coding contacts, and post questions to someone who may know the answer to a current coding or billing dilemma; for example, go to the Web site *www.partbnews.com/enroll,* fill out the enrollment form, and click "Done."

EXAMPLE 5–19　　**Downcoding**

Incorrect Coding

20010	Incision of abscess with suction irrigation

(Note: 20010 has been deleted from CPT and would result in downcoding.)

Correct Coding

20005	Incision of abscess, deep or complicated

Code Monitoring

Monitoring of CPT codes is done to maximize reimbursement from all insurance carriers. First determine which codes are used most often in the physician's practice. Many computer programs can generate a list of codes, ranking them according to frequency of use. If the practice does not have a computer, take a sampling of the charge slips to find out the prevalent codes. Once the high volume codes are known, focus on coding strategies for maximum reimbursement (Fig. 5–10).

Downcoding also occurs when the claims examiner converts the CPT code submitted to a code in the RVS being used by the carrier. When there is a choice between two or three somewhat similar codes, the claims examiner chooses the lowest paying code. Any time the code that was submitted is changed, appeal the change immediately.

Downcoding also may occur when a claims examiner compares the code used with the written description of the procedure included in an attached

CODE/PAYMENT TRACKING LOG					Date: 1-XX
CPT CODE	Practice fee	Medicare date and amount paid	Medicaid date and amount paid	TRICARE date and amount paid	Blue Shield date and amount paid
99201	$00.00	11-XX $00.00	8-XX $00.00	7-XX $00.00	4-XX $00.00
99202	$00.00	12-XX $00.00	9-XX $00.00	10-XX $00.00	6-XX $00.00
99211	$00.00	12-XX $00.00			11-XX $00.00
99212	$00.00				12-XX $00.00
99221	$00.00				
99231	$00.00				
99232	$00.00				
99241	$00.00				

Figure 5–10. Example of a code/payment tracking log.

Monitor every RA/EOB that comes in directly or via patients. Every private, Medicare, Medicaid, and TRICARE payment received should be checked for accuracy to see whether it is consistently the same or downcoding has occurred. Incorrect payments should be investigated and possibly appealed. Examine all payments made for codes that do not match those submitted. Be sure to appeal every payment that is less than half of what the physician bills. An example of a code and payment tracking log to help monitor payments received is shown in Figure 5–10.

Helpful Hints in Coding

Office Visits

When an established patient is seen for an office visit and the medical assistant incidentally takes the patient's blood pressure per the physician's order, the physician includes that service with the appropriate level of E/M code number (e.g., 99213 or 99214). If the medical assistant takes the blood pressure and the patient is not seen by the physician but the physician reviews the results, the appropriate code number is 99211 (presence of physician not necessary). If more than one office visit is necessary per day, the requirements for use of modifiers -25 and -59 should be read before submitting a claim to determine if one of them may be applicable.

Some insurance policies allow only two moderate- or high-complexity office visits per patient per year. Therefore contact the insurance company to learn about any limitations. A physician's practice should have a system in place to track this.

Drugs and Injections

If the insurance claim has a description section (Block 19 on the CMS-1500 claim form), give the name, amount, and strength of the medication as well as how it was administered. This information must be documented in the patient's medical record also. If a drug is experimental or expensive, it is good practice to include a copy of the invoice when sending in the insurance claim. Codes for injections are 90471, 90472, and 90780 through 90799. Separate codes are used to identify the product being administered (see codes 90281 through 90399 and 90476 through 90749). Separate codes are available for combination vaccines. See codes 95004 through 95199 for allergy testing and immunotherapy. If an anesthetic agent is being used, determine whether it is diagnostic, therapeutic, or prophylactic for pain. Medicare bills for immunosuppressive therapy are submitted to durable medical equipment carriers.

Adjunct Codes

Adjunct codes are referred to in the Medicine Section of the CPT as Special Services and Reports and fall under the category of Miscellaneous Services. They are important to consider when billing because these codes provide the reporting physician with a means of identifying special services and reports that are an adjunct to the basic services provided. The circumstances that are covered under these codes (99000 through 99090) include handling of laboratory specimens, telephone calls, seeing patients at odd hours, office emergency services, supplies and materials, special reports, travel, and educational services rendered to patients. Explain the circumstances or include a report to justify the use of these codes if there is room on the insurance claim. Some insurance companies pay, but others do not.

Basic Life or Disability Evaluation Services

Use code 99450 when reporting examinations done on patients for the purpose of trying to obtain life or disability insurance. Codes 99455 and 99456 may be used for work-related or medical disability examinations. Additional information about life or health insurance examinations is given in Chapter 6.

Code Modifiers

The use of a CPT code's two-digit add-on **modifier** permits the physician to indicate circumstances in which a procedure as performed differs in some way from that described by its usual five-digit code (Example 5–21). A modifier can indicate:

EXAMPLE 5–21

Code Modifier

2-digit 27590-**80** Amputation, thigh; **Assistant surgeon**

▶ A service or procedure has either a professional or technical component.
▶ A service or procedure was performed by more than one physician or in more than one location.
▶ A service or procedure has been increased or reduced.
▶ A service or procedure was provided more than once.
▶ Only part of a service was performed.
▶ An adjunctive service was performed.
▶ A bilateral procedure was performed.
▶ Unusual events occurred.

Modifiers should be considered an exception when coding services or procedures. The majority of professional services or procedures rendered are performed exactly as described by the CPT codes. Modifiers do not change the definition of a code but are used to describe modifying circumstances. It may be necessary when using a modifier to include an operative, pathology, x-ray, or special report to justify its use when submitting an insurance claim. A statement as to when a report is appropriate to include is noted for each modifier listed in Table 5–4.

Correct Use of Common CPT Modifiers

A choice of any modifier that fits the situation that is being coded may be used except when the modifier definition restricts the use of specific codes; for example, -51 Multiple procedures: "When multiple

procedures, *other than Evaluation and Management Services . . .*" Some of the most commonly used modifiers are discussed in detail here.

-21 Prolonged Evaluation and Management Services

This modifier is used to report a service longer than or greater than that described in the highest level evaluation and management service code (e.g., 99205, 99215, or 99223). In addition, there are some five-digit codes for prolonged services involving *direct* (face-to-face) patient contact in either the inpatient or outpatient setting (99354 through 99357) and *without direct* (face-to-face) contact (99358 and 99359). Prolonged service of less than 30 minutes is not reported separately so these codes are used to report for time beyond that. Refer to the CPT for an illustration of correct reporting for these codes. Example 5–22 shows use of this modifier.

EXAMPLE 5–22

Prolonged E/M Service

An 80-year-old diabetic woman is seen in a skilled nursing facility (SNF) by her internist for stage II decubitus ulcer with cellulitis. A revision in the treatment plan is indicated because of her condition. The physician performs a detailed interval history and a comprehensive physical examination, and the medical decision making is of moderate complexity. The physician meets with the patient's family to discuss treatment plans and future care (55 minutes).

99313-**21** Subsequent nursing facility care-prolonged E/M service

---

-22 Unusual Procedural Service

Modifier -22 is used when the service(s) provided is greater than that usually necessary for the listed procedure. If you add the modifier -22 for unusual service, then the operative report must state that unusual service was performed within the context of the normal procedure. Encourage your physician to use appropriate descriptions in the report, and call these words to his or her attention. Three guidelines are: (1) the complications cannot be indicated by a separate code; (2) the procedure is lengthy and unusual; and (3) the services provided by the physician are increased because of unusual circumstances or complexities. This modifier may not be used with

TABLE 5–4	CPT Modifier Codes

Modifier Code	Explanation
-21	**Prolonged Evaluation and Management Services:** When the face-to-face or floor/unit service(s) provided is prolonged or otherwise greater than that usually required for the highest level of evaluation and management service within a given category, it may be identified by adding modifier -21 to the evaluation and management code number. A report also may be appropriate.* **Example:** A physician spends an hour with a spouse and hospital inpatient, then an additional hour reviewing laboratory studies and x-ray films and reports, setting up a treatment plan with nurses, and coordinating care by two other specialists. **Medicare Payment Rule:** No effect on payment.
-22	**Unusual Procedural Services:** When the services provided are greater than that usually required for the listed procedure, they may be identified by adding modifier -22 to the usual procedure number. A report may also be appropriate.† **Example:** Removal of foreign body from stomach, which usually takes about 45 minutes, takes 2 hours on a particular patient; use modifier -22. A discharge summary or specially dictated statement should be attached to the claim form. This modifier increases the payment. **Medicare Payment Rule:** May result in increased payment based on supporting documentation of the unusual circumstances and complexity of the procedure performed.
-23	**Unusual Anesthesia:** Occasionally, a procedure that usually requires either no anesthesia or local anesthesia must be done under general anesthesia because of unusual circumstances. This circumstance may be reported by adding the modifier -23 to the procedure code of the basic service.† **Examples:** A proctoscopy might require no anesthesia. A skin biopsy or excision of a subcutaneous tumor might require local anesthesia. If general anesthesia is needed, append the procedure code with -23.
-24	**Unrelated Evaluation and Management Service by the Same Physician During a Postoperative Period:** The physician may need to indicate that an evaluation and management service was performed during a postoperative period for a reason(s) unrelated to the original procedure. This circumstance may be reported by adding the modifier -24 to the appropriate level of E/M service.† **Example:** A patient seen for a postoperative visit after an appendectomy complains of a lump on the leg. The physician takes a history and examines the site, and a biopsy is scheduled. The E/M code 99024 is used for the postsurgery examination, and the modifier -24 is added for unrelated service rendered during a postoperative period. **Medicare Payment Rule:** No effect on payment: however, failure to use this modifier when appropriate may result in denial of the E/M service.
-25	**Significant, Separately Identifiable Evaluation and Management Service by the Same Physician on the Day of a Procedure or Other Service:** The physician may need to indicate that on the day a procedure or service identified by a CPT code was performed, the patient's condition required a significant, separately identifiable E/M service above and beyond the other service provided or beyond the usual preoperative and postoperative care associated with the procedure that was performed. The E/M service may be prompted by the symptom or condition for which the procedure or service was provided. As such, different diagnoses are not required for reporting the E/M service on the same date. **Example:** A patient is seen for a diabetic follow-up and the physician discovers a suspicious mole on the patient's neck (0.4 cm), which is removed. The physician makes a minor adjustment of the oral diabetes medication. This case illustrates a significant E/M service provided on the same day as a procedure, so -25 is added to the E/M code. Code 11420 is used for removal of the benign lesion. **Note:** This modifier is not used to report an E/M service that resulted in a decision to perform surgery. See modifier -57.† **Medicare Payment Rule:** No effect on payment; however, failure to use this modifier when appropriate may result in denial of the E/M service.
-26	**Professional Component:** Certain procedures are a combination of a professional physician component and a technical component. When the professional (physician) component is reported separately, the service may be identified by adding the modifier -26 to the usual procedure number.* **Note:** The **professional component** comprises only the professional services performed by the physician during x-ray, laboratory, and other diagnostic procedures. These services include a portion of a test or procedure that the physician does, such as interpretation of the results. The **technical component** includes personnel, materials, including usual contrast media and drugs, film or xerograph, space, equipment, and other facilities but excludes the cost of radioisotopes. When billing for the technical component, use the usual five-digit procedure number with modifier -TC. **Example:** 70450-26 Computed axial tomography, head or brain; without contrast material. The modifier -26 indicates the physician interpreted this test only. 70450-TC Computed axial tomography, head or brain; without contrast material. The modifier indicates the facility is billing only for the use of the equipment.

Continued.

TABLE 5–4	**CPT Modifier Codes—cont'd**

Modifier Code | **Explanation**

-27 **Multiple Outpatient Hospital E/M Encounters on the Same Date:** For hospital outpatient reporting purposes, utilization of hospital resources related to separate and distinct E/M encounters performed in multiple outpatient hospital settings on the same date may be reported by adding the modifier -27 to each appropriate level outpatient or emergency department E/M code(s). This modifier provides a means of reporting circumstances involving E/M services provided by physician(s) in more than one (multiple) outpatient hospital setting(s) (e.g., hospital emergency department, clinic). Do not use this modifier for physician reporting of multiple E/M services performed by the same physician on the same date. See E/M, emergency department, or preventive medicine services codes.

Example: Patient is seen in a hospital outpatient clinic. The patient falls in the treatment room and receives a cut on the right arm. The patient is taken to the emergency department for two stitches and a dressing.

Medicare Payment Rule: Do not use modifier -27 for Medicare outpatients. Continue to use the -G0 (G-zero) modifier that HCFA established to cover multiple procedures, same patient, same day.

-32 **Mandated Services:** Services related to mandated consultation or related services (e.g., PRO, third-party payer, governmental, legislative or regulatory requirement), may be identified by adding the modifier -32 to the basic procedure.‡

Example: A patient is referred to the physician by an insurance company for an unbiased opinion regarding permanent disability after a year of treatment following an accident. Add modifier -32 to the E/M code because the second opinion is mandated by the insurance company.

Medicare Payment Rule: No effect on payment.

-47 **Anesthesia by Surgeon:** Regional or general anesthesia provided by the surgeon may be reported by adding the modifier -47 to the basic service (this does not include local anesthesia).†

Note: Modifier -47 is not used for anesthesia procedures 00100 through 01999.

Example: A gastroenterologist performs an endoscopy for removal of esophageal polyps using the snare technique. The physician sedates the patient with Versed to perform the procedure.

43217 Esophagoscopy with removal of polyps by snare technique

43217-47 Administered Versed

Medicare Payment Rule: Medicare will not reimburse the surgeon to administer anesthesia (any type).

-50 **Bilateral Procedure:** Unless otherwise identified in the listings, bilateral procedures requiring a separate incision performed during the same operative session should be identified by the appropriate five-digit code describing the first procedure. The second (bilateral) procedure is identified by adding modifier -50 to the procedure number.

Note: It is important to read each surgical description carefully to look for the word "bilateral."

Example A:

71060 Bronchography, bilateral (would be listed with no modifier)

Example B:

19200 Mastectomy, radical

19200-50 Mastectomy, radical; bilateral

Medicare Payment Rule: Payment is based on 150% (200% for radiographs) of the fee schedule amount.

-51 **Multiple Procedures:** When multiple procedures, other than E/M services, are performed at the same session by the same provider, the primary procedure or service may be reported as listed. The additional procedure(s) or service(s) may be identified by adding the modifier -51 to the additional procedure or service code(s).

Note: This modifier should not be appended to designated "add-on" codes (see Appendix E of CPT). Always list the procedure of highest dollar value first.

Example: Patient had herniated disk in lower back with stabilization of the area where the disk was removed.

63030 Lumbar laminectomy with disk removal

22612-51 Arthrodesis

(modifier used after the lesser of the two procedures)

Medicare Payment Rules: Standard multiple surgery policy—100% of the fee schedule amount is allowed for the highest valued procedure, 50% for the second through fifth procedures, and "by report" for subsequent procedures.

-52 **Reduced Services:** Under certain circumstances a service or procedure is partially reduced or eliminated at the physician's election. Under these circumstances the service provided can be identified by its usual procedure number and the addition of the modifier -52, signifying that the service is reduced. This provides a means of reporting reduced services without disturbing the identification of the basic service.

Note: This means there will be no effect on the physician's fee profile in the computer data. It is not necessary to attach a report to the claim when using this modifier, because it indicates a reduced fee. When a physician performs a procedure but does not charge for the service, such as a postoperative follow-up visit that is included in a global service, remember to use code 99024. Some physicians prefer to bill the insurance carrier the full amount and accept

TABLE 5–4	CPT Modifier Codes—cont'd

Modifier Code	Explanation
	what the carrier pays as payment in full. In such cases, a modifier is not used. If only part of a procedure is performed and the physician feels a reduction in the service is warranted, to develop a reduced fee try calculating the reduced service by time. Calculate the amount (cost) per minute of the complete procedure by dividing the amount (cost) by the usual time it takes to complete the procedure. To determine how long the reduced procedure took, multiply the amount (cost) per minute by the time it took to do the reduced procedure. **Example:** A patient is not able to participate or cooperate in a minimal psychiatric interview (90801) and the physician decides to attempt this at a later date. Modify the code with -52. **Medicare Payment Rule:** Payment is based on the extent of the procedure or service performed. Submit documentation with the claim.
-53	**Discontinued Procedure:** Under certain circumstances, the physician may elect to terminate a surgical or diagnostic procedure. Because of extenuating circumstances or those that threaten the well-being of the patient, it may be necessary to indicate that a surgical or diagnostic procedure was started but discontinued. This circumstance may be reported by adding the modifier -53 to the code for the discontinued procedure. **Note:** This modifier is not used to report the elective cancellation of a procedure before the patient's anesthesia induction or surgical preparation in the operating suite. For outpatient hospital or ambulatory surgery center (ACS), see modifiers -73 and -74. **Example:** The physician is beginning a cholecystectomy on a patient. An earthquake of great magnitude occurs and the electricity is shut off. The backup generator comes on and electricity is restored; however, because of the disarray in the operative suite, the physician decides to discontinue the surgery. Code 47562 is used with -53 appended to it. **Medicare Payment Rule:** The carrier will determine the amount of payment "by report." Submit documentation with the claim identifying the extent of the procedure performed and the extenuating circumstances.
-54	**Surgical Care Only:** When one physician performs a surgical procedure and another provides preoperative or postoperative management, surgical services may be identified by adding the modifier -54 to the usual procedure number.* **Note:** Because many surgical procedures encompass a "package" concept that includes normal uncomplicated follow-up care, the surgeon is paid a reduced fee when using this modifier. **Example:** A patient presents in the emergency department with severe abdominal pain. Dr. A, the on-call surgeon, examines the patient and performs an emergency appendectomy. Dr. A is leaving on vacation the next morning so he calls his friend and colleague Dr. B. He asks him to visit the patient in the hospital the following day and take over the postoperative care. Dr. A bills using the appendectomy procedure code 44950 and modifies it with -54. **Medicare Payment Rule:** Payment is limited to the amount allotted for intraoperative services only.
-55	**Postoperative Management Only:** When one physician performs the postoperative management and another physician performs the surgical procedure, the postoperative component may be identified by adding the modifier -55 to the usual procedure number. **Note:** The fee to list would be approximately 30% of the surgeon's fee. **Example:** The Dunmires are relocating to Memphis, Tennessee, when she discovers a lump on her arm. She visits her family physician, Dr. A, who tells her it needs to be excised. She wants her physician (Dr. A) to do the surgery and Dr. A agrees if she promises to arrange for a physician in Memphis to follow her postoperatively. She makes arrangements with Dr. B in Memphis. Dr. B bills using the correct excision code that he obtained from Dr. A and modifies it with -55. **Medicare Payment Rule:** Payment is limited to the amount allotted for postoperative services only. Payment to more than one physician for split surgical care of a patient may not exceed the amount paid for the total global surgical package.
-56	**Preoperative Management Only:** When one physician performs the preoperative care and evaluation and another physician performs the surgical procedure, the preoperative component may be identified by adding the modifier -56 to the usual procedure number.† **Example:** Dr. A sees Mrs. Jones and determines she needs to have a lung biopsy. He admits her to the hospital and Dr. A becomes ill. Dr. B is called in and performs the surgery. Dr. A bills for the preoperative care using the surgical code he obtained from Dr. B and modifies it with -56. **Medicare Payment Rule:** Payment for this component is included in the allowable for the surgery. If another physician performed the surgery, use an appropriate E/M code to bill for the preoperative service.
-57	**Decision for Surgery:** An evaluation and management service that resulted in the initial decision to perform the surgery may be identified by adding the modifier -57 to the appropriate level of E/M service.‡ **Example:** A patient is referred to a surgeon for a consultation to determine whether surgery is necessary. The patient consents to surgery. The surgeon bills the E/M consultation code and adds the -57 modifier. By adding this modifier, the third-party payer is informed that the consultation is not part of the global surgical procedure. Medicare will pay if it is

Continued.

TABLE 5–4	CPT Modifier Codes—cont'd

Modifier Code	Explanation
	for major surgery that requires a 90-day postoperative follow-up but not for a minor surgical procedure (0- to 10-day postoperative follow-up).
	Medicare Payment Rule: Payment is made for the E/M service in addition to the global surgery payment.
-58	**Staged or Related Procedure or Service by the Same Physician During the Postoperative Period:** The physician may need to indicate that the performance of a procedure or service during the postoperative period was (a) planned prospectively at the time of the original procedure (staged); (b) more extensive than the original procedure; or (c) for therapy after a diagnostic surgical procedure. This circumstance may be reported by adding the modifier -58 to the staged or related procedure.‡
	Note: This modifier is not used to report the treatment of a problem that requires a return to the operating room. See modifier -78.
	Example: A patient has breast cancer, and a surgeon performs a mastectomy. During the postoperative global period, the surgeon inserts a permanent prosthesis. The -58 modifier is added to the code for inserting the prosthesis, indicating that this service was planned at the time of the initial operation. If the modifier is not used, the insurance carrier may reject the claim because surgery occurred during the surgery's global period.
-59	**Distinct Procedural Service:** Under certain circumstances, the physician may need to indicate that a procedure or service was distinct or independent from other services performed on the same day. Modifier -59 is used to identify procedures and services that are not normally reported together but are appropriate under the circumstances. This may represent a different session or patient encounter, different procedure or surgery, different site or organ system, separate incision or excision, separate lesion, or separate injury (or area of injury in extensive injuries) not ordinarily encountered or performed on the same day by the same physician. However, when another already established modifier is appropriate, it should be used rather than modifier -59. Only if no more descriptive modifier is available, and the use of modifier -59 best explains the circumstances, should modifier -59 be used.
	Example: The patient is scheduled for a hysterectomy. She asks the physician if he will remove a lipoma (2.2 cm) from the right upper thigh area while she is under anesthesia. The surgeon bills for the hysterectomy, and bills for the lipoma removal (11403), modifying it with -59.
	Medicare Payment Rule: No effect on payment amount; however, failure to use modifier when appropriate may result in denial of payment for the services.
-62	**Two Surgeons:** When two surgeons work together as primary surgeons performing distinct parts of a single reportable procedure, each surgeon should report his or her distinct operative work using the same procedure code and adding the modifier -62. If additional procedures (including add-on procedures) are performed during the same surgical session, separate codes may be reported without the modifier -62.
	Note: If the co-surgeon acts as an assist in the performance of additional procedure(s) during the same surgical session, those services may be reported using separate procedure code(s) with modifier -80 or -81.
	Example: A procedure for scoliosis is performed by a thoracic surgeon who does the anterior approach and an orthopedic surgeon who does the posterior approach and repair.
	Medicare Payment Rule: Medicare allows 125% of the approved fee schedule amount for the -62 modifier if reported by both surgeons. That total fee is divided in half and dispersed to each surgeon at 62.5% of the approved amount.
-63	**Procedure Performed on Infants less than 4 kg:** Procedures performed on neonates and infants up to a present body weight of 4 kg may involve significantly increased complexity and physician work commonly associated with these patients. This circumstance may be reported by adding the modifier -63 to the procedure number.
	Note: Unless otherwise designated, this modifier may be appended only to procedures or services listed in the 20000 through 69999 code series. Modifier -63 should not be appended to any codes listed in the Evaluation and Management Services, Anesthesia, Radiology, Pathology or Laboratory, or Medicine sections.
-66	**Surgical Team:** Under some circumstances, highly complex procedures (requiring the concomitant services of several physicians, often of different specialties, plus other highly skilled, specially trained personnel and various types of complex equipment) are carried out under the "surgical team" concept. Such circumstances may be identified by each participating physician with the addition of the modifier -66 to the basic procedure number used for reporting services.*
	Example: A kidney transplant, requiring use of a vascular surgeon, urologist, and nephrologist, with the assistance of an anesthesiologist and pathologist, or open heart surgery using perfusion personnel, three cardiologists, and an anesthesiologist.
	Medicare Payment Rule: Carrier medical staff determines the payment amounts for team surgeries on a report basis. Submit supporting documentation with the claim.
-73	**Discontinued Outpatient Hospital or ASC Procedure Prior to the Administration of Anesthesia:** Because of extenuating circumstances or those that threaten the well-being of the patient, the physician may cancel a surgical or

| TABLE 5–4 | **CPT Modifier Codes—cont'd** |

Modifier Code | **Explanation**

diagnostic procedure subsequent to the patient's surgical preparation (including sedation when provided, and being taken to the room where the procedure is to be performed), but prior to the administration of anesthesia (local, regional block[s] or general). Under these circumstances, the intended service that is prepared for but canceled can be reported by its usual procedure number and the addition of modifier -73.

Note: The elective cancellation of a service prior to the administration of anesthesia or surgical preparation of the patient should not be reported. For physician reporting of a discontinued procedure, see modifier -53.

-74 **Discontinued Outpatient Hospital or ASC Procedure After Administration of Anesthesia:** Because of extenuating circumstances or those that threaten the well-being of the patient, the physician may terminate a surgical or diagnostic procedure after the administration of anesthesia (local, regional block[s] or general) or after the procedure was started (incision made, intubation started, scope inserted). Under these circumstances, the procedure started but terminated can be reported by its usual procedure number and the addition of modifier -74.

Note: The elective cancellation of a service prior to the administration of anesthesia or surgical preparation of the patient should not be reported. For physician reporting of a discontinued procedure, see modifier -53.

-76 **Repeat Procedure by Same Physician:** The physician may need to indicate that a procedure or service was repeated subsequent to the original service. This circumstance may be reported by adding modifier -76 to the repeated service.[†]

Example: A femoral-popliteal bypass graft (35556) is performed, the graft clots later that day, and the entire procedure is repeated. The original procedure is reported and the repeat procedure is reported using modifier -76. A report should be attached to the insurance claim when using this modifier.

Medicare Payment Rule: Failure to use this modifier when appropriate (and to submit supporting documentation) may result in denial of the subsequent surgery.

-77 **Repeat Procedure by Another Physician:** The physician may need to indicate that a basic procedure performed by another physician had to be repeated. This situation may be reported by adding modifier -77 to the repeated service.[†]

Example: A femoral-popliteal bypass graft (35556) is performed in the morning and in the afternoon it becomes clotted. The original surgeon is not available and a different surgeon performs the repeat operation later in the day. The original surgeon reports 35556. The second surgeon reports 35556-77.

Medicare Payment Rule: Failure to use this modifier when appropriate (and to submit supporting documentation) may result in denial of the subsequent surgery.

-78 **Return to the Operating Room for a Related Procedure During the Postoperative Period:** The physician may need to indicate that another procedure was performed during the postoperative period of the initial procedure. When this subsequent procedure is related to the first, and requires the use of the operating room, it may be reported by adding the modifier -78 to the related procedure. (For repeat procedures on the same day, see -76.)[†]

Example: A patient has an open reduction with fixation of a fracture of the elbow. While still hospitalized, the patient develops an infection and is returned to surgery for removal of the pin because it appears to be the cause of an allergic reaction. The original procedure is billed for the open treatment of the fracture. The pin removal is billed with modifier -78 because it is a related procedure.

Medicare Payment Rule: Medicare will pay the full value of the intraoperative portion of a given procedure. Documentation should be submitted with the claim to describe the clinical circumstances.

-79 **Unrelated Procedure or Service by the Same Physician During the Postoperative Period:** The physician may need to indicate that the performance of a procedure or service during the postoperative period was unrelated to the original procedure. This circumstance may be reported by using the modifier -79. (For repeat procedures on the same day, see -76).[†]

Example: A patient in the hospital has colon resection surgery and is discharged home. After 7 days, the patient develops acute renal failure, is hospitalized, does not recover renal function, and hemodialysis is ordered. A nephrologist inserts a cannula for the dialysis. When billing for the nephrologist, the code for hemodialysis is shown with a -79 modifier, indicating that this is unrelated to the initial surgery. If modifier -79 is not used, the insurance carrier may not realize the service is not related to the initial surgery and may reject the claim.

Medicare Payment Rule: No effect on payment; however, failure to use this modifier when appropriate may result in denial of the subsequent surgery. Specific diagnostic codes substantiate the medical necessity of the unrelated procedure. Documentation may be required to describe the clinical circumstances. A new global period begins for any procedure modified by -79.

-80 **Assistant Surgeon:** Surgical assistant services may be identified by adding the modifier -80 to the usual procedure number(s).*

Note: Some insurance policies do not include payment for assistant surgeons, such as for 1-day surgery, but do pay for major or complex surgical assistance. In some instances, prior approval may be indicated because of the patient's physiologic condition. Medicare will not pay assistant surgeons for operations that are not life threatening. Therefore,

Continued.

TABLE 5–4	**CPT Modifier Codes—cont'd**

Modifier Code	Explanation
	Medigap insurance will not pay on this service because the service is nonallowable. Assisting surgeons usually charge 16% to 30% of the primary surgeon's fee.
	Example: The primary surgeon performs a right ureterectomy submitting code 50650-RT. The assistant surgeon bills using the primary surgeon's code with modifier -80 (50650-80).
	Medicare Payment Rule: Payment is based on the billed amount or 16% of the global surgical fee, whichever is lower, for procedures approved for assistant-at-surgery. Medicare will deny payment for an assistant-at-surgery for surgical procedures in which a physician is used as an assistant in less than 5% of the cases nationally.
-81	**Minimum Assistant Surgeon:** Minimum surgical assistant services are identified by adding the modifier -81 to the usual procedure number.
	Note: Payment is made to physicians but not registered nurses or technicians who assist during surgery.*
	Example: A primary surgeon plans to perform a surgical procedure but during the operation circumstances arise that require the services of an assistant surgeon for a relatively short period of time. In this scenario, the second surgeon provides minimal assistance and may report using the procedure code with the -81 modifier appended.
-82	**Assistant Surgeon:** (When qualified resident surgeon is not available.) The unavailability of a qualified resident surgeon is a prerequisite for use of modifier -82 appended to the usual procedure code number(s).*
	Note: This modifier usually is used for services rendered at a teaching hospital.
	Example: A resident surgeon is scheduled to assist with an anorectal myomectomy (45108). Surgery is delayed because of the previous surgery, the shift rotation changes, and the resident is not available. A nonresident assists with the surgery and reports the procedure appending it with modifier -82 (45108-82).
-90	**-90 Reference (Outside) Laboratory:** When laboratory procedures are performed by a party other than the treating or reporting physician, the procedure may be identified by adding the modifier -90 to the usual procedure number.†
	Note: Use this modifier when the physician bills the patient for the laboratory work and the laboratory is not doing its own billing.
	Example: Dr. Input examines the patient, performs venipuncture, and sends the specimen to an outside laboratory for a liver panel. The physician has an arrangement with the laboratory to bill for the test, and, in turn, he bills the patient. Dr. Input bills for the examination (E/M code), venipuncture (36415 or for Medicare 0001), and liver panel (80058), using modifier -90 (80058-90) to append to the liver panel code.
-91	**Repeat Clinical Diagnostic Laboratory Test:** In the course of treatment of the patient, it may be necessary to repeat the same laboratory test on the same day to obtain subsequent (multiple) test results. Under these circumstances, the laboratory test performed can be identified by its usual procedure number and the addition of modifier -91.
	Note: This modifier may not be used when tests are rerun to confirm initial results; because of testing problems with specimens or equipment; or for any other reason when a normal, one-time, reportable result is all that is required. This modifier may not be used when other code(s) describe a series of test results (e.g., glucose tolerance tests, evocative or suppression testing). This modifier may only be used for laboratory test(s) performed more than once on the same day on the same patient.
	Example: A patient is scheduled for a nonobstetrical dilation and curettage for dysfunctional uterine bleeding. When the patient arrives at the office, a routine hematocrit is obtained. During the procedure, the patient bleeds excessively. After the procedure, the physician orders a second hematocrit to check the patient for anemia caused by blood loss. The first hematocrit is billed using CPT code 85013. The second hematocrit is billed using the same code appended with modifier -91 (85013-91).
-99	**Multiple Modifiers:** Under certain circumstances, two or more modifiers may be necessary to delineate a service completely. In such situations modifier -99 should be added to the basic procedure, and other applicable modifiers may be listed as part of the description of the service.‡
	Example: An assistant surgeon helps repair an enterocele where unusual circumstances appear because of extensive hemorrhaging.
	57270-99 Repair of enterocele
	-22 Extensive hemorrhaging (unusual service)
	-80 Assistant surgeon
	Medicare Payment Rule: No effect on payment; however, the individual modifier payment policies apply, including any inherent effect they may have on payment.

Modified from the American Medical Association, Chicago, IL.
*This modifier may have an effect on reimbursement.
†This modifier may affect reimbursement, depending on the payer.
‡Modifier is informational in nature. Do not ask for an adjustment in reimbursement. Monitor reimbursement when using this modifier.
§This modifier affects reimbursement but not the physician's fee profile.

E/M services. Most insurance carriers send an insurance claim to medical review before payment is made if modifier -22, indicating unusual services, appears on the claim. Because payments may be delayed, be cautious when using this modifier. Comprehensive documentation obtains 20% to 30% more reimbursement for the basic procedure. An operative report should be submitted with the claim. However, some Medicare carriers routinely deny any claim with modifier -22. An appeal for review can be made in such denials. See Chapter 8 for details on the Medicare review and appeal process.

-25 Significant, Separately Identifiable Evaluation and Management Service by the Same Physician on the Same Day of the Procedure or Other Service

For information on this modifier, see the explanation of modifier -57.

-26 Professional Component

Certain procedures are a combination of a **professional component (PC)** and a **technical component (TC).** Usually these are seen in the radiology and pathology sections of CPT. The professional (physician) component refers to a portion of a test or procedure that the physician does, such as interpreting an electrocardiogram (ECG), reading an x-ray film, or making an observation and determination using a microscope. The technical component refers to the use of the equipment and the operator who performs the test or procedure, such as ECG machine and technician, radiography machine and technician, and microscope and technician. Do not modify procedures that are either 100% technical or 100% professional or when the physician performs both the professional and technical components. Modifier -26 represents the professional component only. Use of this modifier alerts the insurance company to expect a separate claim from another provider or facility for the technical component.

In Example 5–23, the physician is performing only one of two services—he or she is interpreting the results of bilateral hip x-ray films.

The facility where the patient had the x-ray bills only for the technical component by modifying the same code with a -TC (73520-TC). If the physician owns the equipment and reads the x-ray film, there is no need to modify the x-ray code (73520).

-51 Multiple Procedures

There are many occasions when multiple procedures are performed at the same session by the same provider. In such cases, report the primary service or

---

EXAMPLE 5–23

Professional/Technical Components

73520-**26**	Professional component only for a radiograph of both hips. *Use to bill physician's fee for interpretation and of X-ray film.*	$
73520-**TC**	Technical component only for a radiograph of both hips. *Use to bill facility fee that owns equipment and employs technician.*	$
		=
73520	Radiologic examination, hips, bilateral. Minimum of two views of each hip. *Use to bill complete fee when physician owns equipment, employs technician, and interprets x-ray film.*	$$

---

procedure, which can be determined easily by highest dollar value, as listed. Identify all additional services or procedures by appending code(s) with modifier -51 (Example 5–24).

EXAMPLE 5–24

Multiple Procedure Modifier -51

Excision of 2.0-cm benign lesion on the nose and at the same session a biopsy of the skin and subcutaneous tissue of the forearm.

Code	Fee	Description of Services
11442	$$	Excision, other benign lesion including margins, face, ears, eyelids, nose, lips, mucous membrane; excised diameter 1.1 to 2.0 cm
11100-**51**	$	Biopsy of skin, subcutaneous tissue or mucous membrane (including simple closure), unless otherwise listed; single lesion (**second; multiple procedure**)

The operative report should clearly state which procedures were done through separate incisions and which were done through the same incision. There are many circumstances when multiple procedures are performed. Modifier -51 may be used to identiy the following:

▶ Multiple medical procedures performed at the same session by the same provider
▶ Multiple, related surgical procedures performed at the same session by the same provider

▶ Surgical procedures performed in combination at the same session, whether through the same or another incision or involving the same or different anatomy

▶ A combination of medical and surgical procedures performed at the same session by the same provider

Usually payment for the primary code is 100% of the allowable charge, second code 50%, third code 25%, fourth and remaining codes 10%. However, Medicare pays 50% of the allowable for two to five secondary procedures and does not require the assignment of modifier -51. The computer system can determine code order and automatically make the code adjustment. Always bill the full amount and let the insurance carrier make the payment adjustments for percentage considerations. For all insurance carriers, it is recommended to monitor the Remittance Advice/Explanation of Benefits to ensure correct payment. A decision flow chart is provided for reference to simplify applying modifiers to multiple surgical procedures. As you read through the remainder of this chapter, follow the steps by answering the questions in Figure 5–11, *A* as they apply to your billing scenario and refer to Figure 5–11, *B* for key information and descriptions.

Do not use this modifier with Evaluation and Management services, add-on codes designated with a "+" (see Appendix E in CPT), or codes listed as exempt to modifier -51 (see Appendix F in CPT). Add-on codes are codes that cannot stand alone. When billing with add-on codes, you *always* have to list another code referred to as the "parent code" to give full description for service billed (Example 5–25).

When making a decision about when to use an add-on code, look for a clue phrase that indicates additional procedures, such as "each additional," "list in addition to," and "second lesion."

It is wise to provide an explanation of why the service was reduced. A cover letter or a copy of the operative report should not accompany these claims because usually they are not sent to medical review and such documents may impede processing. Never use this modifier if the fee is reduced because of a patient's inability to pay.

-57 Decision for Surgery

This modifier is used strictly to report an E/M service that resulted in the initial decision to perform a major surgical procedure within 24 hours of the office visit (e.g., those with a 90-day follow-up period); see Examples 5–26 and 5–27. A -57 modifier may be used for inpatient or outpatient consultations, inpatient hospital visits, and new or established patient visits that occur the day of or the day before surgery. Do not attach modifier -57 to a hospital visit code for the day before surgery or the day of surgery when a decision for a major surgical procedure was made a week before surgery. Think of -57 as telling the insurance company that the office visit *is not* part of the global fee.

EXAMPLE 5–26

Decision for Surgery

A new patient is seen in the office complaining of a great deal of pain. Cholangiography is done and reveals blocked bile ducts. The patient is scheduled for surgery the next day.

8-1-20xx	99204-**57**	New patient office visit	$00.00
8-2-20xx	47600	Cholecystectomy	$000.00

EXAMPLE 5–25

Add-On Code

Parent code	11000	Biopsy of skin . . . single lesion
Add-on code	+11101	each separate/additional lesion (list separately in addition to code for primary procedure)

-52 Reduced Services

Use of this modifier indicates that under certain circumstances a service or procedure is partially reduced or eliminated at the physician's discretion.

-25 Significantly Separately Identifiable E/M Service

In some cases, you may be confused whether to assign modifier -25 or -57. Modifier -25 is defined as "Significant, separately identifiable evaluation and management service by same physician on the same day of the procedure or other service." The industry standard is to use -25 when a diagnostic procedure or minor *nonstarred procedure* is involved (e.g., those with a 0- to 10-day follow-up period). Typically, E/M services that are modified with -25 are office visits performed on the day of a minor (nonstarred) procedure for an established patient. However, the confusion results because the CPT code book states, "This modifier is not used to report an E/M service that resulted in a decision to perform surgery. See modifier -57."

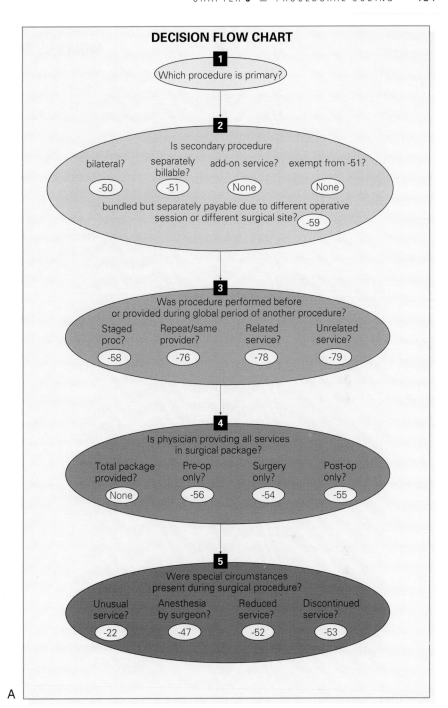

Figure 5–11. A, Decision flow chart for surgical procedures.   *Continued.*

Another consideration when a decision to perform surgery takes place on the same day as the procedure is code 99025 from the Medicine Section of CPT, Special Services and Reports, Miscellaneous Services. However, code 99025 can only be used in lieu of an E/M code for an initial (new patient) visit, when a starred (*) surgical procedure constitutes major services at that visit (Example 5–3).

Consult Figure 5–12 when making the decision about which code or modifier to use for a surgical procedure that is performed within 24 hours of an office visit.

In Medicare cases, the CMS has published in the *Correct Coding Initiative* the specific codes for modifier -25 use after October 2000. Refer to the bulletin or newsletter pertinent to this update.

MULTIPLE SURGICAL PROCEDURES

Multiple services must be related to:
- Same patient
- Same provider
- Same date of service

- List all procedures in order of reimbursement, highest to lowest
- Most comprehensive service brings greatest reimbursement and is considered primary
- Check all procedures to make sure there is no unbundling, i.e., using two codes when one code describes procedure
- Decision making expands at this point. Follow numbered question to determine correct modifier usage

-50 bilateral procedure, not described by code
-51 not bundled, separately billable
-59 ordinarily bundled, separately payable due to special circumstance

- The term "primary procedure" can also refer to the first procedure initiating a global surgical period
-58 Current service was planned prospectively at time of first service
-76 Physician repeats procedure subsequent to original procedure
-78 Return to operating room for subsequent procedure, complication relating to original procedure
-79 Unrelated procedure performed during global period of previous surgery

4

- Surgical package means one fee covers the whole package, surgical procedure and postoperative care

5

-22 An extremely difficult procedure due to altered anatomy or unusual circumstances (add 10% to 30% reimbursement)
-47 When the surgeon administers regional or general anesthesia
-52 Procedure/service reduced or eliminated at the discretion of the physician
-53 Procedure is discontinued due to extenuating circumstances or because of threat to the patient

B

Figure 5–11, cont'd. B, Guidelines and description of modifiers for multiple surgical procedures flow chart.

-58 Staged or Related Procedure

This modifier is used to indicate that the performance of a procedure or service during the postoperative period was
▶ Planned (staged) at the time of the original procedure.
▶ More extensive than the original procedure.
▶ For therapy after a diagnostic surgical procedure.

Such circumstances should be reported by adding modifier -58 to the staged or related procedure. The use of this modifier requires accurate documentation of events leading up to surgeries and any subsequent surgeries. It is only possible to modify procedures if the coder has all of the relevant facts and circumstances. In Example 5–27, the fracture is considered

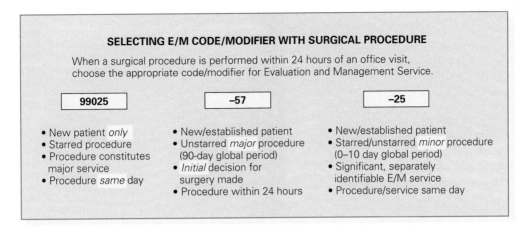

Figure 5–12. Three selections, with criteria to evaluate, when choosing the appropriate code or modifier for evaluation and management services when a surgical procedure is performed within 24 hours of an office visit.

EXAMPLE 5–27

Decision for Surgery

A new patient comes to the office after sustaining a fall while in-line skating. She is in distress, complaining of right wrist pain and swelling of the joint. The injury is evaluated **(1)** with an x-ray film **(2)**. It is determined that the patient has a Smith fracture and manipulation is performed. A long-arm cast is applied **(3)** using fiberglass (Hexcelite) material **(4)**.

(1)   99203-57   Initial office evaluation (detailed)
                  with decision for surgery

(2)   73100-RT   Radiologic examination, right wrist, AP and lat views

(3)   25605   Closed treatment of distal radial fracture (e.g., Colles or Smith type), with manipulation

(4)   99070   Supplies: Casting material (private carrier) Medicine Section code

          or

                  Supplies: Hexcelite material (Medicare carrier)

      A4590   HCPCS Level II code

The patient returns in 4 weeks for follow-up care **(1)**. The wrist is radiographed again **(2)**, the long-arm cast is removed **(3)**, and a short-arm cast is applied **(4)** using plaster material **(5)**.

(1)   No code   Follow-up care included in global fee

(2)   73100-RT   Radiologic examination, right wrist, AP and lat views

(3)   No code   Cast removal included in original fracture care (25605)

(4)   29075-58   Application, plaster, elbow to finger (short arm) **staged procedure**

(5)   99070   Supplies: Casting material (private carrier) Medicine Section code

          or

                  Supplies: Plaster material (Medicare carrier)

      A4580   HCPCS Level II code

---

surgery because it is in the surgery section of the CPT book. All fracture codes have 90-day postoperative periods.

-62, -66, -80, -81, -82 More than One Surgeon

If more than one surgeon is involved, clarify for whom you are billing by using two-digit modifiers (-62, co-surgeon; -66, team surgery; -80, assistant at surgery; -81, minimum assistant surgeon, or -82, assistant surgeon when a qualified resident surgeon is not available) (Examples 5–21 and 5–28).

Modifier -80 (assistant at surgery) is commonly used when billing for a physician who assists another (primary) physician in performing a surgical procedure (Example 5–28).

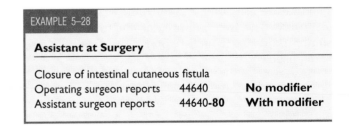

EXAMPLE 5–28

Assistant at Surgery

Closure of intestinal cutaneous fistula
Operating surgeon reports   44640   **No modifier**
Assistant surgeon reports   44640-80   **With modifier**

The assisting doctor is usually paid a fee of 16% to 30% of the allowed fee the primary surgeon receives for performing the surgery. The assisting physician uses the same surgical code as the primary surgeon and adds the -80 modifier to it. The fee indicating a reduced percentage typically is listed as the fee on the claim form. However, some insurance carriers may prefer having the full fee listed and making the reduction on their end. Under Medicare guidelines,

HCPCS LEVEL II ALPHANUMERIC MODIFIERS

26596-F3 Excision of Constricting Ring on Ring Finger of Left Hand

Figure 5–13. HCPCS level II alpha modifiers (LT and RT used to identify right and left hands) and alphanumeric modifiers (FA through F9) used to identify digits (fingers) of right and left hands.

there may be some surgical procedures that restrict payment for an assistant surgeon, so refer to the provider manual or contact the fiscal intermediary for information.

-99 Multiple Modifiers

If a procedure requires more than one modifier code, use the two-digit modifier -99 after the usual five-digit code number, all typed on one line; then each modifier is typed on a separate line (Example 5–29). Some insurance companies require -99 with a separate note in Block 19 of the CMS-1500 claim form or in the freeform area of electronic submissions, indicating which two or more modifiers are being used.

HCPCS

Besides CPT and RVS modifiers, HCPCS level II and III modifiers are used by Medicare and level II may be used by some commercial carriers. Healthcare Common Procedure Coding System level II modifiers may be two alpha digits (Example 5–30), two alphanumeric characters (Fig. 5–13), or a single alpha digit used for reporting ambulance services or results of positron emission tomography scans. A brief list of these modifiers may be found in Appendix A of the CPT code book. A comprehensive list may be found in an HCPCS national level II code book. Healthcare Common Procedure Coding System reference books may be obtained from resources listed in Appendix B.

EXAMPLE 5–29

Multiple Modifiers

A physician sees a patient who is grossly obese. The operative report documents that a bilateral sliding-type inguinal herniorrhaphy was performed, and the procedure took 2 hours 15 minutes.

49525-99	Bilateral repair sliding inguinal hernia requiring 2 hours 15 minutes
-50	
-22	

EXAMPLE 5–30

HCPCS Modifiers

When taking x-ray films of both feet, the billing portion of the insurance claim appears as follows:

05/06/XX 73620 **RT** Radiologic examination, foot—right
05/06/XX 73620 **LT** Radiologic examination, foot—left

Use the two-digit HCPCS modifiers whenever they are necessary. Healthcare Common Procedure Coding System modifiers further describe the services provided and can *increase* or *decrease* the physician's fee. If not used properly, they can drastically affect the physician's fee profile by reducing future payments to the physician.

Comprehensive List of Modifier Codes

Now that you have learned about some basic modifiers, read through the comprehensive list shown in Table 5–4 to gain information on additional modifiers and their use illustrated by clinical examples.

RESOURCES ON THE INTERNET

 For AHIMA diagnostic code guidelines for outpatient services and diagnostic coding and reporting requirements for physician billing, visit the Web site: *http://www. ahima.org.*

STUDENT ASSIGNMENT LIST

✔ Study Chapter 5.
✔ Answer the review questions in the *Workbook* to reinforce the theory learned in this chapter and help prepare you for a future test.
✔ Complete the assignments in the *Workbook* to assist you in hands-on practical experience in procedural coding as well as learning medical abbreviations.
✔ Turn to the Glossary at the end of this textbook for a further understanding of the Key Terms used in this chapter.

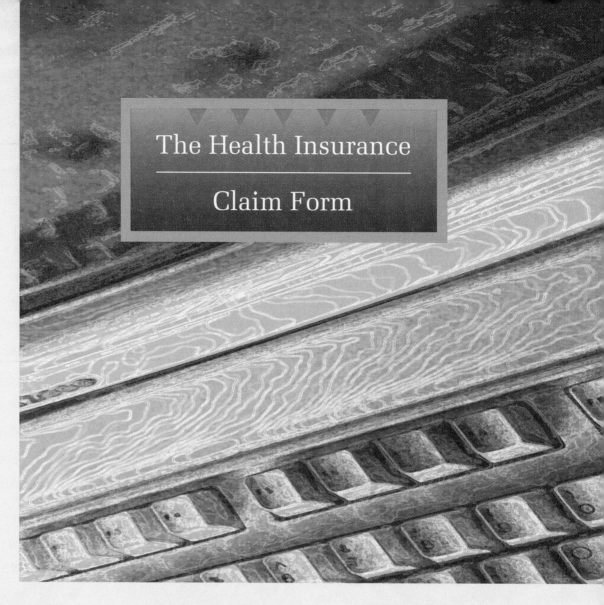

The Health Insurance
Claim Form

6

- Explain the difference between clean, pending, rejected, incomplete, and invalid claims.
- Abstract from the patient record relevant information for completing the CMS-1500 insurance claim form.
- Describe reasons why claims are rejected.
- Minimize the number of insurance forms returned because of improper completion.
- Identify techniques required for optically scanned insurance claims.
- Execute general guidelines for completing the CMS-1500 claim form for federal, state, and private payer insurance contracts.

OBJECTIVES*

After reading this chapter, you should be able to:

- Give the history of the Health Insurance Claim Form (CMS-1500).
- State when the CMS-1500 claim form may or may not be used.
- Expedite the handling and processing of the CMS-1500 insurance claim form.
- Define two types of claims submission.

KEY TERMS

clean claim

digital fax claim

dingy claim

dirty claim

durable medical equipment (DME) number

electronic claim

employer identification number (EIN)

facility provider number

group provider number

Health Insurance Claim Form (CMS-1500)

incomplete claim

intelligent character recognition (ICR)

invalid claim

national provider identifier (NPI)

optical character recognition (OCR)

"other" claims

paper claim

pending claim

performing provider identification number (PPIN)

physically clean claim

provider identification number (PIN)

rejected claim

Social Security number (SSN)

state license number

unique provider identification number (UPIN)

---

*Performance objectives and exercises for hands-on practical experience for this chapter appear in the *Workbook*.

History

In 1958 the Health Insurance Association of America (HIAA) and the American Medical Association (AMA) attempted to standardize the insurance claim form by jointly developing the Standard Form. It was not universally accepted by all third-party payers, and as the types of coverage became more variable, new claim forms were instituted that required more information than the original Standard Form. The form eventually became known as COMB-1, or Attending Physician's Statement. In 1968 the HIAA decided to revamp the form so that it would be more adaptable to electronic data processing.

In April 1975 the AMA approved a "universal claim form," called the **Health Insurance Claim Form (HCFA-1500)** and currently referred to as **CMS-1500,** which could be used for both group and individual claims. The CMS-1500 claim form answered the needs of many health insurers processing claims manually. The National Association of Blue Shield Plans Board of Directors adopted a motion supporting the concept of a uniform national claim form.

In 1990 the CMS-1500 was revised and printed in red ink, which allowed claims to be optically scanned by the insurance carriers. Beginning on May 1, 1992, all services for Medicare patients from physicians and suppliers except for ambulance services had to be billed on the scannable CMS-1500 form.

The revised form was adopted by TRICARE Management Activity (TMA), formerly known as the Office of Civilian Health and Medical Programs of the Uniformed Services (OCHAMPUS). It also received the approval of the AMA Council on Medical Services. The HIAA endorses and recommends that their members, which are private insurance companies, accept the form. In some states, the Medicaid program, as well as industrial (workers' compensation) cases, use this form to process claims.

Widespread use of this form will save time and simplify processing of claims for both physicians and carriers because it eliminates the need to complete the many various insurance forms brought into the office by patients. Another way of billing that may be accepted by insurance companies is to complete the CMS-1500 and attach it to the patient's form. The patient's and employer's portions of the private insurance form should be complete and accurate, and the patient should sign the release of information box and the assignment of benefits, if applicable. Both forms are sent directly to the insurance carrier. If the patient is insured with two companies, release of information and assignment for both insurance carriers should be obtained. The primary carrier should be determined and the claim submitted to that carrier first. After the primary insurance carrier has paid, a claim should be submitted to the secondary carrier.

Insurance carriers with various computer programs and equipment that optically scan claims may have instructions on completion of the form that vary from locality to locality and program to program. Local representatives of insurance carriers should always be contacted to find out whether the form is acceptable before any claims are submitted. A photocopy is not acceptable if the form is processed by the insurance carrier through scanning equipment. Quantities of the CMS-1500 can be purchased from many medical office supply companies as well as from the American Medical Association, 515 North State Street, Chicago, IL 60610.

In this chapter, instructions for completing a claim using optical character recognition format is emphasized. However, the federal government prefers electronic claims submission to reduce costs and expedite reimbursement. Chapter 7 explains the intricacies of transmitting electronic claims as well as the do's and don'ts of transmitting a digital fax claim.

HIPAA Compliance Alert

Compliance Issues Related to Insurance Claim Forms

With the advent of the Health Insurance Portability and Accountability Act (HIPAA) of 1996, a number of federal laws affect insurance claim submission. The patient must sign either Block 12 authorizing release of information, or a consent document with similar wording to be retained in the office files. The provider rendering the service or procedure must be properly identified with the correct provider number. Claims must only show services rendered that have been properly documented and are medically necessary without evidence of fraud or abuse issues. If and when a National Provider Identifier (NPI) system for health care providers is used, the NPI must be used in connection with the electronic transactions identified in HIPAA.

Types of Claims

Claims are paper or electronic and can be designated as clean or pending (in suspense). The term "encounter record" is a buzz term for a claim.

A **paper claim** is one that is submitted on paper, including optically scanned claims that are converted to electronic form by insurance companies. Paper claims may be typed or generated via computer.

An **electronic claim** is one that is submitted to the insurance carrier via a central processing unit (CPU), tape diskette, direct data entry, direct wire, dial-in telephone, or personal computer via modem. Electronic claims are never printed on paper.

A **digital fax claim** is sent to the insurance carrier as a paper claim via fax but never printed to paper at the receiving end. The fax is encoded by an optical code reader and is transmitted into the claims processing system. It is not considered an electronic claim.

Claim Status

A **clean claim** means that the claim was submitted within the program or policy time limit and contains all necessary information so it can be processed and paid promptly. A **physically clean claim** is one that has no staples or highlighted areas and on which the bar code area has not been deformed.

A **pending claim** is an insurance claim that is held in suspense because of review or other reason. These claims may be cleared for payment or denied.

Medicare Claim Status

In the Medicare program, besides the phrase "clean claims," specific terms, such as *incomplete, rejected, invalid, dirty,* and *dingy,* are used to describe various claim processing situations. These terms may or may not be used by other insurance programs.

A *clean claim* means the following:

1. The claim has no deficiencies and passes all electronic edits.
2. The carrier does not need to investigate outside of the carrier's operation before paying the claim.
3. The claim is investigated on a postpayment basis, meaning a claim is not delayed before payment and may be paid.
4. The claim is subject to medical review with attached information or forwarded simultaneously with electronic medical claim (EMC) records.

Medicare claims not considered "clean" claims, which require investigation or development on a prepayment basis (developed for Medicare Secondary Payer information), are known as **"other" claims.**

Participating provider electronic submissions are processed within approximately 14 days of receipt. Participating provider paper submissions and nonparticipating provider claims are not processed until at least 27 days after receipt.

An **incomplete claim** is any Medicare claim missing required information. It is identified to the provider so it can be resubmitted.

A **rejected claim** is one that requires investigation and needs further clarification and possibly answers to some questions. Such a claim should be resubmitted.

An **invalid claim** is any Medicare claim that contains complete, necessary information but is illogical or incorrect (e.g., listing an incorrect provider number for a referring physician). An invalid claim is identified to the provider and may be resubmitted.

A **dirty claim** is a claim submitted with errors, one requiring manual processing for resolving problems, or one rejected for payment. Pending or suspense claims are placed in this category because something is holding the claim back from payment, perhaps review or some other problem.

A **dingy claim** happens when the Medicare contractor cannot process a claim for a particular service or bill type. These claims are held until the necessary systems changes are implemented to pay the claim correctly.

Abstracting from Medical Records

Abstraction of technical information from patient records may be requested for three situations: (1) to complete insurance claim forms; (2) when sending a letter to justify a health insurance claim after professional services are rendered; or (3) when a patient applies for life, mortgage, or health insurance. Abstracting to complete insurance claims is discussed later in this chapter.

Cover Letter Accompanying Insurance Claims

A letter accompanying insurance claims should include the patient's name; subscriber identification number; date and type of service; a short history; and a clear but concise explanation of the medical necessity, difficulty or complexity, or unusual circumstance (e.g., emergency). The letter and insurance claim should be sent to the attention of the claims supervisor so it may be directed to the appropriate person for processing.

Life or Health Insurance Applications

When a patient applies for insurance, the insurance company may request information from the patient's private physician, require a physical examination, or both.

On some application forms (Fig. 6–1), the release of medical information signed by the patient may appear as a separate sheet or as a perforated attachment to a multiple-paged form. In the latter, page 1 is completed by the insurance agent when interviewing the client, page 2 is filled in by the prospective insured, and page 3 is completed by the physician at the time of the physical examination of the prospective insured. Sometimes a form is sent to the client's attending physician along with a check requesting medical information (Fig. 6–2). The amount of the check may vary, depending on how much information is requested. If the check is not included, the physician should request a fee based on the length of the report before sending in the completed report form. The fee is required before completion of the form or payment may not be received.

Be extremely accurate when abstracting medical information from the patient's record. Figure 6–3 is a

PART II of Application to the MASSACHUSETTS INDEMNITY AND LIFE INSURANCE COMPANY

PROPOSED INSURED OR ANNUITANT: _Jason F. Reed_

Date of Birth _March 10, 1972_
Mo.   Day   Year

1. a. Name and address of your personal physician? _Gerald Practon, MD 4567 Broad Ave.,_
(If none, so state)
   b. Date and reason last consulted? _November 4, 1999   Woodland Hills, XY 12345_
   c. What treatment was given or medication prescribed? _Rx Humadine_

	Yes	No
2. Have you ever been treated for or ever had any known indication of:		
a. Disorder of eyes, ears, nose, or throat?	☐	☑
b. Dizziness, fainting, convulsions, recurrent headache, speech defect, paralysis or stroke, mental or nervous disorder?	☐	☑
c. Shortness of breath, persistent hoarseness or cough, blood spitting, bronchitis, pleurisy, asthma, emphysema, tuberculosis or chronic respiratory disorder?	☐	☑
d. Chest pain, palpitation, high blood pressure, rheumatic fever, heart murmur, heart attack or other disorder of the heart or blood vessels?	☐	☑
e. Jaundice, intestinal bleeding, ulcer, hernia, appendicitis, colitis, diverticulitis, hemorrhoids, recurrent indigestion, or other disorder of the stomach, intestines, liver or gallbladder?	☐	☑
f. Sugar, albumin, blood or pus in urine, venereal disease, stone or other disorder of kidney, bladder, prostate or reproductive organs?	☐	☑
g. Diabetes, thyroid or other endocrine disorders?	☐	☑
h. Neuritis, sciatica, rheumatism, arthritis, gout or disorder of the muscles or bones, including the spine, back, or joints?	☐	☑
i. Deformity, lameness or amputation?	☐	☑
j. Disorder of skin, lymph glands, cyst, tumor or cancer?	☐	☑
k. Allergies, anemia or other disorder of the blood?	☐	☑
l. Excessive use of alcohol, tobacco, sedatives, or any habit-forming drugs?	☐	☑
3. Are you now under observation or taking treatment?	☐	☑
4. Have you had any change in weight in the past year?	☐	☑
5. Other than above, have you within the past 5 years:	☐	☑
a. Had any mental or physical disorder not listed above?	☑	☐
b. Had a (checkup) consultation, illness, injury, surgery?		
c. Been a patient in a hospital, clinic, sanatorium, or other medical facility?	☐	☑
d. Had electrocardiogram, X-ray, blood sugar, basal metabolism, other (diagnostic test?)	☑	☐
e. Been advised to have any diagnostic test, hospitalization, or surgery which was not completed?	☐	☑
6. Have you ever had military service deferment, rejection or discharge because of a physical or mental condition?	☐	☑
7. Have you ever requested or received a pension, benefits, or payment because of an injury, sickness or disability?	☐	☑
8. Family History: Tuberculosis, (diabetes) cancer, high blood pressure, heart or kidney disease, mental illness or suicide?	☑	☐

DETAILS of "Yes" answers. (IDENTIFY QUESTION NUMBER, CIRCLE APPLICABLE ITEMS: Include diagnoses, dates, duration and names and addresses of all attending physicians and medical facilities.)

5b. Last checkup 1997
(G. Procton MD)

5d. Blood serology

8. Father is diabetic

	Age if Living	Cause of Death?	Age at Death?
Father	55		
Mother	54		
Brothers and Sisters	2		
No. Living			
No. Dead			

(For non-medical cases only)
Height _____ Weight _____

9. Females only:		Yes	No
a. Have you ever had any disorder of menstruation, pregnancy or of the female organs or breasts?		☐	☐
b. To the best of your knowledge and belief are you now pregnant?		☐	☐

I HEREBY DECLARE that, to the best of my knowledge and belief, the statements and answers in Part II of this Application are full, complete, and true. These statements and answers are to be considered as the basis for any insurance written hereon.

Signed at: (City & State) _Woodland Hills, XY_   Dated: _January 25, 20XX_

x _Jason F. Reed_

Signature of witness   Signature of PROPOSED INSURED

Form MD (70)a

Figure 6–1. The prospective insured completes this side of the insurance application form.

PART III—PHYSICIAN'S EXAMINATION REPORT

Acct. No. _145_ District or Agency_____ Name of Agent _James Santor_

Date _Jan. 25, 20xx_ Name of Insuring Company _Hartman Insurance Company_

PROPOSED INSURED: _Reed_ (Last Name) _Jason_ (First Name) _F._ (Middle Initial) Date of Birth _3_ Mo. _10_ Day _1972_ Year

10a.

Height (In Shoes)	Weight (Clothed)	Chest (Full Inspiration)	Chest (Forced Expiration)	Abdomen, at Umbilicus
5 ft. 11 in.	180 lbs.	43 in.	42 in.	38 in.

Details of "Yes" answers. (Identify item.)

b. Did you weigh?...... ☒ Yes ☐ No Did you measure?.................. ☒ Yes ☐ No

c. Is appearance unhealthy or older than stated age?................ ☐ Yes ☒ No

11. Blood Pressure (Record ALL readings)

Systolic	120	
Diastolic { 4th phase	80	
5th phase		

12. Pulse:

	At Rest	After Exercise	3 minutes later
Rate	60	86	66
Irregularities per min.			

13. Heart: Is there any:

Enlargement............... ☐ Yes ☒ No Dyspnea............. ☐ Yes ☒ No

Murmur(s)................. ☐ Yes ☒ No Edema............. ☐ Yes ☒ No

(describe below—if more than one, describe separately)

MCL

Location		

Indicate:

			Apex by X
Constant	☐	☐	Murmur area by ↻
Inconstant	☐	☐	
Transmitted	☐	☐	Point of greatest intensity by O
Localized	☐	☐	
Systolic	☐	☐	Transmission by ►
Presystolic	☐	☐	
Diastolic	☐	☐	
Soft (Gr. 1–2)	☐	☐	For comments and your impression?
Mod. (Gr. 3–4)	☐	☐	
Loud (Gr. 5–6)	☐	☐	
After Exercise:			
Increased	☐	☐	
Absent	☐	☐	
Unchanged	☐	☐	
Decreased	☐	☐	

14. Is there on examination any abnormality of the following: (Circle applicable items and give details.)

	Yes	No
(a) Eyes, ears, nose, mouth, pharynx? _____	☐	☒
(If vision or hearing markedly impaired, indicate degree and correction)		
(b) Skin (incl. scars); lymph nodes; varicose veins or peripheral arteries?....................	☐	☒
(c) Nervous system (include reflexes, gait, paralysis)?.........	☐	☒
(d) Respiratory system?	☐	☒
(e) Abdomen (include scars)?	☐	☒
(f) Genitourinary system (include prostate)?..............	☐	☒
(g) Endocrine system (include thyroid and breasts)?	☐	☒

	Yes	No
(h) Musculoskeletal system (include spine, joints, amputations, deformities)?....................	☐	☒
(A confidential report may be sent to the Medical Director)		
15. (a) Are there any hernias?	☐	☒
(b) Any hemorrhoids?	☐	☒
16. Are you aware of any additional medical history?..............	☐	☒
17. Was the examination conducted in the English language?....	☒	☐
If No, complete the following:		
a. Was an interpreter used?..................	☐	☒

b. What language was used? _____

c. Relationship of interpreter to proposed insured?_____

Urinalysis: Specific Gravity

Albumin	Sugar
0	trace

Is specimen being sent?_____ ☒ Yes ☐ No
If Yes, where?_____ _ABC laboratory_

Send Specimen: (Details according to Company) _____

Date: _1-25-20xx_ Time: _10_ (A.M. / P.M.) City: _Woodland Hills_ State: _XY_

Signature of Medical Examiner: _Gerald Practon_ M.D. Physical Measurements Information_____

PMI-188R—1-88

Figure 6–2. Sample of a life insurance application form with the check to the physician omitted. The physician completes this side of the form at the time of the examination of the patient, the prospective insured.

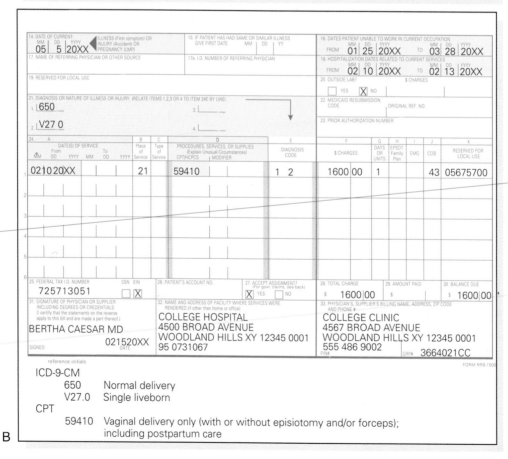

Figure 6–3. A, Example of a chart note illustrating important information to read through and abstract for insurance claim completion. **B,** The location of the abstracted information placed in the blocks on a CMS-1500 insurance claim form in OCR format.

chart note identifying important abstracting components. Abbreviations on the chart must be understood, and only requested information is provided. If the form has questions about high blood pressure, kidney infection, or heart problems, the patient could be prohibited from obtaining life, health, or mortgage insurance if the answers are derogatory. If the urine sample shows albumin or sugar, a person also could be denied insurance. If a patient has had a chronic illness, the physician should be asked if a euphemism can be substituted. A *euphemism* is a word or phrase substituted for one considered offensively explicit, such as "remains" for "corpse."

If a patient tests positive for human immunodeficiency virus (HIV), legal counsel may be necessary because some state laws allow information on HIV infection and acquired immunodeficiency syndrome (AIDS) to be given only to the patient or to the patient's spouse. In some states, it is illegal to require a blood test for HIV antibodies, a urinalysis for HIV, or an HIV antigen test as a condition of coverage. It also may be illegal to question applicants about HIV status or prior symptoms of and treatment for AIDS or other forms of immune deficiency. Sometime, private group plans allow medical coverage for people testing positive for HIV or an AIDS-related illness through a state major risk medical insurance program. However, the waiting period may exceed 1 year if the maximum enrollment number has been reached.

Sometime a narrative report dictated by the physician is preferable to filling in the form, especially if there are long columns to check and no space for comments. It even may be necessary to attach a copy of an operative, pathology, laboratory, or radiology report and an electrocardiogram (ECG) tracing. Electrocardiogram tracings mounted upside-down have resulted in rejections of insurance applications.

A "Please Read" note should be placed on the insurance questionnaire to have the physician check it over thoroughly before signing it and to make sure that the information is accurate and properly stated.

An insurance company may ask a copy service to come to your office to photocopy the patient's record. Usually this is done at the office's convenience, and an appointment should be made. The insurance company should be reminded that an authorization form signed by the patient is necessary to release medical information. An appropriate fee for this service is charged and quoted at the time of the telephone request. The physician should review the records in advance to see that they are in proper order.

Health Insurance Claim Form (CMS-1500)

Basic Guidelines for Submitting a Claim

The CMS-1500 insurance claim form should be used as often as possible. It is accepted by nearly all private insurance carriers as well as Medicaid, Medicare, TRICARE, and workers' compensation.

A claim form should be completed and submitted whenever a patient asks, even if it is suspected that the patient has no coverage, unless the patient accepts the tactful suggestion that he or she is not covered. If in question, the insurance carrier should be contacted about eligibility status. An official rejection from the insurance company is the best answer to present to the patient in this situation. The patient may be unaware of major medical credits accrued because of nonpayment of benefits from a basic plan. It is feasible to bill and get paid for services rendered even though the patient may not think that he or she is covered.

Individual Insurance

When a patient brings in a form from a private insurance plan that is not like the CMS-1500 claim form, he or she should sign it. In addition, the patient should sign the CMS-1500 claim form in two places (the Assignment of Benefits and Release of Information, Blocks 12 and 13). The patient's portion of the private insurance form should be checked to ensure that it is complete and accurate. The forms should then be mailed together to the insurance carrier. Some companies allow staples and some do not. It is not recommended to let patients direct their own forms to insurance companies or employers. Patients have been known to lose forms or alter data on documents before mailing, forget to send them, or mail them to an incorrect address.

Group Insurance

When a patient has group insurance through an employer, the employer's section of the private insurance should be completed. If it is not completed, the form should be sent to the employer before the physician's section of the CMS-1500 claim form is completed. If the employer's section is complete, both forms should be sent directly to the insurance carrier after the physician's portion is completed.

Secondary Insurance

When two insurance policies are involved (sometimes called dual coverage), one is considered primary and the other secondary (Example 6–1). The

---

EXAMPLE 6–1   Primary/Secondary Insurance Plans

A husband and wife have insurance through their employers and each has added the spouse to their plans for secondary coverage. If the wife is seen for treatment, then the insurance plan sponsored by her employer is primary and her husband's plan is secondary.

24. A						B	C	D		E	F	G	H	I	J	K
DATE(S) OF SERVICE						Place	Type	PROCEDURES, SERVICES, OR SUPPLIES		DIAGNOSIS	$ CHARGES	DAYS	EPSDT	EMG	COB	RESERVED FOR
From			To			of	of	(Explain Unusual Circumstances)		CODE		OR	Family			LOCAL USE
MM	DD	YY	MM	DD	YY	Service	Service	CPT/HCPCS	MODIFIER			UNITS	Plan			
1 10 04 20XX			10 08 20XX			21		99232		1	55	56	5		32	783127XX
2																

primary policy is the policy held by the patient when the patient and his or her spouse are both insured. The patient's signature should always be acquired for release of information and assignment of benefits for both insurance companies.

After payment is made by the primary plan, a claim is submitted with a copy of the explanation of benefits from the primary carrier to the secondary carrier.

Completion of Insurance Claim Forms

Private insurance carriers should be contacted to see if they optically scan insurance claim forms. If a claim is optically scanned by the insurance company, *no* comments should be put in blocks that are unanswerable or do not apply. They should be left blank. The computer scanner will kick out the claim if any marks are entered into nonapplicable blocks. If a form is not optically scanned by the insurance carrier, it may be a good idea to answer all questions on the form. If any are unanswerable, DNA (Does Not Apply), NA, or N/A (Not Applicable) should be typed or a dashed line inserted.

Diagnosis

In Block 21, diagnosis field, all accurate diagnostic codes that affect the patient's condition should be inserted, with the primary diagnosis code listed first followed by any secondary diagnosis codes. A diagnosis should never be submitted without supporting documentation in the medical record. The diagnosis must agree with the treatment. If there is no formal diagnosis at the conclusion of an encounter, the code(s) for the patient's symptom(s) should be submitted.

To avoid confusion, it is best to list only one illness or injury and its treatment per form, unless there are concurrent conditions.

Service Dates

Ditto dates for services performed should not be used. Charges for services rendered in different years on the same claim form should not be submitted. Sometimes such practices can be affected by deductible and eligibility factors, thereby delaying reimbursement.

Consecutive Dates

Some carriers allow hospital or office visits to be grouped if each visit is consecutive, occurs in the

same month, uses the same procedure code, and results in the same fee. The fee for a single procedure should be listed in Block 24F, and the number of times the procedure was performed should be listed in Block 24G as illustrated in the graphic at the top of this page. However, private insurance carriers should be contacted because some carriers require a total fee listed in Block 24F rather than the fee for a single procedure. If there is a difference in the procedure code or fee for several visits listed on the claim, each hospital or office visit must be itemized and each procedure code and charge entered on a separate line.

No Charge

No claim should be submitted for services that have no charge unless the patient requests that it be sent in. These services should appear documented in the patient's medical and financial records.

Physicians' Identification Numbers

Insurance companies and federal and state programs require certain identification numbers on claim forms submitted from individuals and facilities who provide and bill for services to patients. This can be confusing to the beginner, as well as someone experienced in insurance billing procedures, because there are so many different numbers; therefore an explanation is given.

▶ **State License Number:** To practice within a state, each physician must obtain a physician's **state license number.** Sometimes this number is requested on forms and used as a provider number.

E	F	G	H	I	J	K
DIAGNOSIS CODE	$ CHARGES	DAYS OR UNITS	EPSDT Family Plan	EMG	COB	RESERVED FOR LOCAL USE
						C16021

▶ **Employer Identification Number:** In a medical group or solo practice, each physician must have his or her own federal tax identification number, known as an **employer identification number (EIN).** This is issued by the Internal Revenue Service for income tax purposes.

25. FEDERAL TAX I.D. NUMBER	SSN EIN
74 10640XX	☐ ☒

▶ **Social Security Number:** In addition, each physician has a **Social Security number (SSN)** for other personal use and may have one or more *tax identification numbers (TIN)* for financial reasons. These are not typically used on the claim form unless the provider does not have an EIN.

> 25. FEDERAL TAX I.D. NUMBER   SSN EIN
> 082 XX 1707   ☒ ☐

Provider Numbers

Claims may require three provider identification numbers: one for the referring physician, one for the ordering physician, and one for the performing physician (billing entity). It is possible that the ordering physician and the performing physician are the same. On rare occasions, the number may be the same for all three, but more frequently three different numbers are required, depending on the circumstances of the case. For placement of the provider number on the CMS-1500 claim form, refer to the block-by-block instructions for Blocks 17a and 24J-K. Keep in mind what role the physician(s) and their numbers represent in relationship to the provider listed in Block 33. The following examples of blocks from the CMS-1500 insurance claim form show where these numbers are commonly placed.

To assist with claims completion, a reference list of provider numbers should be compiled for all ordering physicians and physicians who frequently refer patients. Physicians' provider numbers can be obtained by calling their offices or through the Medicare carrier. Refer to Appendix A for all physician provider numbers when completing Workbook assignments.

▶ **Provider Identification Number:** Every physician who renders services to patients may be issued a carrier-assigned **provider identification number (PIN)** by the insurance company.

> 33. PHYSICIAN'S, SUPPLIER'S BILLING NAME, ADDRESS, ZIP CODE
> & PHONE #
> JOHN DOE MD 555 486 9001
> 123 ANY STREET
> ANYTOWN XY 12345
> PIN# 70 98765XX   GRP#

▶ **Unique Provider Identification Number:** The Medicare program issues each physician a **unique provider identification number (UPIN).**

> 17a. I.D. NUMBER OF REFERRING PHYSICIAN
> 46278897XX

▶ **Performing Provider Identification Number:** Each physician has a separate **performing provider identification number (PPIN)** for each group

office or clinic in which he or she practices. If a doctor practices in two of the group's four offices, he or she has two PPINs. In the Medicare program, each member of a group is issued an eight-character PPIN, which correlates to that particular group's location in addition to a group number (Example 6–2).

EXAMPLE 6–2 **Performing Provider Identification Number**

College Clinic
4567 Broad Avenue
Woodland Hills, XY
12345-0001   **Group PIN: 3664021CC**
Cosmo Graff, MD   **PPIN: WA 24516B**
College Clinic
20 South Main Street
Louisville, XY 12670-0341   **Group PIN: 3664021CC**
Cosmo Graff, MD   **PPIN: WA 01021A**

▶ **Group Provider Number:** The **group provider number** is used instead of the individual PIN for the performing provider who is a member of a group practice that submits claims to insurance companies under the group name.

> 33. PHYSICIAN'S, SUPPLIER'S BILLING NAME, ADDRESS, ZIP CODE
> & PHONE #
> COLLEGE CLINIC 555 486 9002
> 4567 BROAD AVENUE
> WOODLAND HILLS XY 12345 0001
> PIN#   GRP# 3664021CC

▶ **National Provider Identifier:** In 1997 the Centers for Medicare and Medicaid Services (CMS) began issuing each provider a Medicare lifetime 10-digit **NPI,** but an implementation date has not been released as of this printing. When adopted, it will be recognized by Medicaid, Medicare, TRICARE, and CHAMPVA programs and eventually may be used by private insurance carriers. It may replace some of the existing identification numbers.

F	G	H	I	J	K
$ CHARGES	DAYS OR UNITS	EPSDT Family Plan	EMG	COB	RESERVED FOR LOCAL USE
					46 278897XX

NPI root
check digit
locator code

▶ **Durable Medical Equipment Number:** Medicare providers who charge patients a fee for supplies and equipment, such as crutches, urinary catheters, ostomy supplies, surgical dressings, and so forth must bill Medicare using a **durable medical equipment (DME) number.**

```
33. PHYSICIAN'S, SUPPLIER'S BILLING NAME, ADDRESS, ZIP CODE
    & PHONE #
    COLLEGE CLINIC  555 486 9002
    4567 BROAD AVENUE
    WOODLAND HILLS XY 12345   0001
PIN#  34007600XX    GRP#
```

DME #

▶ **Facility Provider Number:** Each facility (e.g., hospital, laboratory, radiology office, skilled nursing facility) is issued a **facility provider number** to be used by the performing physician to report services done at the location.

```
32. NAME AND ADDRESS OF FACILITY WHERE SERVICES WERE
    RENDERED (if other than home or office)
    COLLEGE HOSPITAL
    4500 BROAD AVENUE
    WOODLAND HILLS XY 12345
    95  07310XX
```

A FINAL NOTE: A PIN Number Pays!

Physician's Signature

The physician should sign the insurance claim form above or under the typed or preprinted physician's name. A stamped signature is allowed in some instances and discussed later in this chapter. A removable indicator "Sign Here" tag may be used to help the physician locate where to sign the claim.

Insurance Biller's Initials

The insurance billing specialist should place his or her initials in the bottom left or top right corner of the claim form. Placement of this reference should be consistent. There are three good reasons to adopt this habit:

▶ To identify who in the office is responsible for the insurance form
▶ To decrease errors
▶ To avoid being accused of someone else's error, especially if the previous biller submitted a fraudulent claim

Proofread

Every claim should be proofread for transposition of numbers (group, policy, physician's ID, procedure and diagnostic codes), misspelled name, missing date of birth, blanks, and attachments. Larger, more complex claims require special attention because they involve greater sums of money and may be more difficult to complete.

Supporting Documentation

Occasionally claims need supporting documents to further explain services billed and obtain maximum reimbursement.

On any submitted report, the patient's name, subscriber's name (if different from that of the patient), and insurance identification number should be included in case the document becomes separated from the claim during processing.

If a medication is expensive or experimental, a copy of the invoice received from the supply house or pharmacy should be sent.

When a procedure is complicated, a copy of all pertinent reports (operative, radiology, laboratory, pathology, and discharge summary) should be included.

For a treatment not listed in the procedure code book, a detailed report should be sent that gives the nature, extent, and need for the services. If the claim is submitted electronically, this description should be typed in the narrative field. The correct code number should be used for unlisted services or procedures, which usually end in "99" (Example 6–3).

EXAMPLE 6–3   **Unlisted Procedure**

Unlisted Allergy Testing Procedure 95199

Office Pending File

As mentioned in Chapter 2, the office copy of the insurance form should be filed in a separate alpha (tickler) file for insurance claim copies (preferred) or in the back of the patient's medical chart.

Common Reasons Why Claim Forms Are Delayed or Rejected

It is wise to be aware of common billing errors and how to correct them for quicker claim settlements and to reduce the number of appeals. This may help avoid additional administrative burdens, such as telephone calls, resubmission of claims, appeal letters, and so on. Also see Chapter 8 for information on solutions to denied or delayed claims as well as prevention measures. The following is a list of some reasons why claims are rejected or delayed and suggested solutions when completing the CMS-1500 insurance claim form blocks.

Problem: **Block 1.** Claim submitted to the secondary insurer instead of the primary insurer.

Solution: Obtain data from the patient during the first office visit as to which company is the primary insurer, depending on illness, injury, or accident. Submit the claim to the primary carrier and then send in a claim with the explanation of benefits (EOB) to the secondary carrier.

Problem: Blocks 1 to 13. Information missing on patient portion of the claim form.

Solution: Obtain a complete patient registration form from which information can be extracted. Educate patients on data requirements at the time of the first visit to the physician's office if patients are filling out their portion.

Problem: Block 1a. Patient's insurance number is incorrect or transposed (especially in Medicare and Medicaid cases).

Solution: Proofread numbers carefully from source documents. Always photocopy front and back sides of insurance identification cards.

Problem: Block 2. Patient's name and insured's name are entered as the same when the patient is a dependent.

Solution: Verify the insured party and check for Sr., Jr., and correct birth date.

Problem: Block 3. Incorrect gender identification, resulting in a diagnosis or procedure code that is inconsistent with patient's gender.

Solution: Proofread claim before mailing and review patient's medical record to locate gender, especially if the patient's first name could be male or female.

Problem: Blocks 9a to d. Incomplete entry for other insurance coverage.

Solution: Accurately abstract data from the patient's registration form. Telephone the patient if information is incomplete.

Problem: Block 10. Failure to indicate whether patient's condition is related to employment or an "other" type of accident.

Solution: Review patient's medical history to find out details of injury or illness and proofread claim before mailing. Telephone the employer to see if permission was given to treat the patient as a workers' compensation case.

Problem: Blocks 12 and 13. Patient's signature is missing.

Solution: Always check the form after the patient signs this block or check the patient's medical record to see if the patient's signature is on file.

Problem: Block 14. Date of injury is missing, date of last menstrual period (LMP), or dates of onset of illness are omitted. This information is important for determining whether accident benefits apply, patient is eligible for maternity benefits, or there was a preexisting condition.

Solution: Do not list unless dates are clearly documented in the patient's medical record. Read the patient's medical history and call the patient to obtain the date of accident or LMP. Compose an addendum to the record, if necessary. Always proofread the claim before mailing so no data are missing.

Problem: Blocks 17 to 17a. Incorrect or missing name or UPIN/NPI of referring physician on claim for consultation or other services requiring this information.

Solution: Check the patient registration form and the chart note for reference to the referring physician. Obtain a list of UPIN/NPI numbers for all physicians in the area.

Problem: Block 19. Attachments (e.g., prescription, operative report, manufacturer's invoice) or Medicaid verification (e.g., labels, identification numbers) is missing.

Solution: Submit all information required for pricing or coverage on 8.5- × 11-inch paper with the patient's name, subscriber name (if other than patient), and insurance identification number on each attachment (enclosure). Type the word "ATTACHMENT" in Block 19 or 10d. Never staple or clip documentation to a claim.

Problem: Block 21. The diagnostic code is missing, incomplete, invalid, not in standard nomenclature (e.g., missing fourth or fifth digit), includes a written description, or does not correspond to the treatment (procedure code) rendered by the physician.

Solution: Update encounter forms annually. Verify and submit correct diagnostic codes by referring to an updated diagnostic code book and reviewing the patient record. Check with the physician if the diagnosis code listed does not go with the procedure code shown.

Problem: Block 24A. Omitted, incorrect, overlapping, or duplicate dates of service.

Solution: Verify against the encounter form or medical record that all dates of service are listed and accurate and appear on individual lines. Date spans for multiple services must be adequate for the number and types of services provided. Each month should be on a separate line and each year should be on a separate claim.

Problem: **Block 24B.** Missing or incorrect place of service code.

Solution: Verify the place of service from the encounter form or medical record and list the correct code for place of service and submitted procedure.

Problem: **Block 24C.** Missing or incorrect type of service code for Medicaid, TRICARE, or workers' compensation claims.

Solution: Verify and list the type of service code and confirm that it is correct for the submitted procedure code(s).

Problem: **Block 24D.** Procedure codes are incorrect, invalid, or missing.

Solution: Verify the coding system used by the insurance company and submit correct procedure code(s) by referring to a current procedure code book. For Medicare patients and certain private insurance plans, check the HCPCS manual for CMS national and local procedure codes.

Problem: **Block 24D.** Incorrect or missing modifier(s).

Solution: Verify usage of modifiers by referring to a current procedure code book and HCPCS manual. Submit valid modifiers with the correct procedure codes (Chapter 5).

Problem: **Block 24F.** Omitted or incorrect amount billed.

Solution: Be certain the fee column is filled in. Check the amounts charged with the appropriate fee schedule.

Problem: **Block 24G.** Reasons for multiple visits made in 1 day are not stated on an attachment sheet.

Solution: Depending on insurance guidelines, submit documentation explaining reason for multiple visits. Use appropriate modifiers or upcode evaluation and management services to include all visits.

Problem: **Block 24G.** Incorrect quantity billed.

Solution: Verify charge amounts. Make sure that the number of units listed is equal to the date span when more than one date of service is billed (e.g., hospital visits).

Problem: **Blocks 24J-K.** Provider's identification number is missing.

Solution: Verify and insert the required provider's number in these blocks.

Problem: **Blocks 24A to K, Line 6.** Squeeze in more than six lines per claim form.

Solution: Insert service date and corresponding procedure on lines one to six only. Complete an additional claim form if more services should be billed.

Problem: **Block 28.** Total amounts do not equal itemized charges.

Solution: Total charges for each claim and verify amounts with patient account. If number of units listed in 24G is more than 1, multiply the units by the fee listed in 24F and add to all other charges listed.

Problem: **Block 31.** Physician's signature is missing.

Solution: Have the physician or physician's representative sign the claim using a removable indicator "Sign Here" tag to indicate the correct location.

Problem: **Block 32.** Information is not centered in block as required.

Solution: Enter data centered in block.

Problem: **Block 33.** Provider's address, PIN, or group number is missing.

Solution: Obtain provider's data from a list that contains all physicians' professional information.

Additional Reasons Why Claim Forms Are Delayed

Problem: No record of the claim at the insurance company.

Solution: Always keep copies of paper claims or electronic transmission receipts. Send claims with large dollar amounts by certified mail, return receipt requested.

Problem: Claim form submitted is illegible.

Solution: Never hand write a claim form. Check printer ink, toner, or typewriter ribbon and replace when necessary.

Problem: Untimely or lack of response to claim development letters.

Solution: Pay close attention to the due date shown in the letter, and reply to development letters (insurance company's request for additional information) as soon as possible. Send a copy of the claim with the letter and appropriate medical documentation listing the claim control number, if assigned.

Optical Scanning Format Guidelines

Optical Character Recognition

Optical character recognition (OCR) or **intelligent character recognition (ICR)** devices (scanners) are being used more frequently across the nation in processing insurance claims because of their speed and efficiency. A scanner can transfer printed or typed text and bar codes to the insurance company's computer memory. Scanners read at such a fast speed that they reduce data entry cost and decrease processing time.

More control is gained over data input by using OCR. It improves accuracy, thus reducing coding errors because the claim is entered exactly as coded by the insurance biller.

Do's and Don'ts for Optical Character Recognition

The CMS-1500 form was developed so insurance carriers could process claims efficiently by OCR or ICR. Typing or keying a form for OCR scanning requires different techniques than preparing one for standard claims submission. Because the majority of insurance carriers accept the OCR format, it is suggested that it be routinely used. Basic do's and don'ts for completing claims using OCR format are given.

Do: use original claim forms printed in red ink; photocopies cannot be scanned.

Don't: hand write information on the document. Handwriting is only accepted for signatures. Handwritten claims require manual processing.

2 nd request

Do: align the typewriter or printer correctly so characters appear in the proper fields. Enter all information within designated fields.

Don't: allow characters to touch lines.

Correct

Incorrect

Don't: use script, slant, minifont, or italicized fonts or expanded, compressed, bold, or proportional print. If typing on a typewriter, use an OCR or Manifold typing element in pica Courier 10 or 12 fonts so that shifting for capitals is unnecessary. Use fonts that have the same width for each character.

Do: use black typewriter ink, high carbon content one-time Mylar or OCR printer ribbons. Change ribbons or cartridges frequently for clear print quality.

Do: enter all information in upper case (CAPITAL) letters. Keep characters within the borders of each field.

Correct

Incorrect

Don't: strike over any errors when correcting or crowd preprinted numbers; OCR equipment does not read corrected characters on top of correction tape or correction fluid.

Correct

Incorrect

Do: indicate a deletion for a delete field and go to the next line to insert the data if an optically scanned form has a delete field. Lines, marks, or characters entered in a delete field cause deletion of the entire line.

Do: complete a new form for additional services if the case has more than six lines of service.

Correct

6	04 07 20XX		11	99214

24.	A				B	C	D
	DATE(S) OF SERVICE				Place	Type	PROCEDURES, SERVIC
	From		To		of	of	(Explain Unusual Ci
MM	DD	YY	MM	DD	YY	Service	Service	CPT/HCPCS	MODI
1	04 10 20XX				21		30520

Incorrect

6	04 07 20XX		11	99214
	04 10 20XX		21	30520

Don't: use highlighter pens or colored ink on claims because OCR equipment will not pick these up.

Do: use alpha or numeric symbols.

Don't: use symbols (#, -, /), periods (.), ditto marks, parentheses, or commas (,).

Correct

25. FEDERAL TAX I.D. NUMBER   SSN EIN
123 XX 6789   [X] [ ]

Incorrect

25. FEDERAL TAX I.D. NUMBER   SSN EIN
123-XX-6789   [ ] [ ]

Don't: use decimals in Block 21 or dollar ($) signs in the money column.

Correct

F
$ CHARGES
10000

Incorrect

F
$ CHARGES
$10000

Don't: use narrative descriptions of procedures, modifiers, or diagnoses; code numbers are sufficient.

Correct

D		
PROCEDURES, SERVICES, OR SUPPLIES		
(Explain Unusual Circumstances)		
CPT/HCPCS	MODIFIER	
42820		

Incorrect

D		
PROCEDURES, SERVICES, OR SUPPLIES		
(Explain Unusual Circumstances)		
CPT/HCPCS	MODIFIER	
42820	tonsill-ectomy	

Don't: use N/A or DNA when information is not applicable. Leave the space blank.

Correct

17. NAME OF REFERRING PHYSICIAN OR OTHER SOURCE

Incorrect

17. NAME OF REFERRING PHYSICIAN OR OTHER SOURCE
DNA

Do: enter comments in Block 19 (e.g., ATTACH-MENT) for primary EOB submitted with claim to secondary insurance company.

Correct

19. RESERVED FOR LOCAL USE
ATTACHMENT

Incorrect

PRIMARY EOB ATTACHED

1. MEDICARE	MEDICAID	CHAMPUS	CHAMPVA
[ ] (Medicare #)	[ ] (Medicaid #)	[ ] (Sponsor's SSN)	[ ] (VA File #)

2. PATIENT'S NAME (Last Name, First Name, Middle Initial)
FOREHAND HARRY N

5. PATIENT'S ADDRESS
1456 MAIN STREET

CITY	STATE
WOODLAND HILLS	XY

ZIP CODE	TELEPHONE (Include Area Code)
12345 0000	(555) 555 9876

Don't: use paper clips, cellophane tape, or staples.

Don't: staple over the bar code area of the claim form.

Do: enter eight-digit date formats: 06012000 or 06 01 2000, depending on the block instructions.

Correct

Incorrect

Do: keep signature within signature block. Rubber stamps may be used if they are accepted by insurance carrier and produce complete, clean images, without smudges or missing letters.

Correct

Incorrect

Don't: overtrim or undertrim forms when bursting. Use care in separating forms and discard any form with tears or holes.

Don't: fold or spindle forms when mailing because they will not feed into OCR equipment properly if creased or torn.

Do: enter information via machine printing (e.g., typewriter, word processor, or computer keyboard). Use clean equipment and quality ink jet, laser, or letter-quality matrix printers, if possible, not dot matrix. Clean line printers frequently. Adjust hammer density to prevent shadows and satellites. Monitor phase adjustment to ensure character clarity side to side and top to bottom.

PROCEDURE : Instructions for the Health Insurance Claim Form (CMS-1500)

The Health Insurance Claim Form is divided into two major sections: patient information and physician information. The Patient and Insured (Subscriber) Information section is the upper portion of the claim form and contains 13 blocks numbered 1 through 13 (11 data elements and two signature blocks). The Physician or Supplier Information section is the lower portion of the claim form and consists of 20 blocks numbered 14 through 33 (19 data elements and 1 signature block). Some of the blocks are subdivided with subdivisions labeled a, b, c, d, and so forth. There are a total of more than 100 places to enter specific information.

The instructions are straightforward and contain all pertinent information needed to complete a claim (see Figs. 6–6 through 6–15). Much information on specific coverage guidelines, program policies, and practice specialties could not be included here.

A brief description of each block and of its applicability to the requirements of private insurance payers, Medicaid, Medicare, TRICARE, CHAMPVA, and workers' compensation is presented. Because guidelines vary at the state and local levels for completing the CMS-1500 claim form for the aforementioned insurance plans, consult your local intermediary or private carriers. For completing MediCal claims in California, refer to Appendix C.

When generating paper claims via computer, many software programs insert the insurance carrier's name and address in the top right corner of the CMS-1500 claim form. When typing a claim form, it is suggested that this same procedure be followed.

Block numbers match those on the Health Insurance Claim Form. Italicized sections refer students to guidelines in completing the *Workbook* assignments when there are optional ways of completing a block. Icon meanings are as follows:

 All Payers: All payer guidelines, including all private insurance companies and all federal and state programs.

All private payers: All private insurance companies.

 Medicaid: State Medicaid programs.

 Medicare: Federal Medicare programs, Medicare/Medicaid, Medicare/Medigap, and Medicare Secondary Payer (MSP).

 TRICARE: TRICARE Standard (formerly CHAMPUS), TRICARE Prime, TRICARE Extra.

 CHAMPVA: Civilian Health and Medical Program of the Department of Veterans' Affairs.

 Workers' Compensation: State workers' compensation programs.

Top of Form

Enter name and address of insurance company in the top right corner of the insurance form using all capital letters and no punctuation.

PLEASE
DO NOT
STAPLE
IN THIS
AREA

PRUDENTIAL INSURANCE COMPANY
5450 WILSHIRE BOULEVARD
WOODLAND HILLS XY 12345 0000

HEALTH INSURANCE CLAIM FORM

MEDICARE	MEDICAID	CHAMPUS	CHAMPVA	GROUP HEALTH PLAN	FECA BLK LUNG	OTHER	1a. INSURED'S I.D. NUMBER	(FOR PROGRAM IN ITEM 1)
(Medicare #)	(Medicaid #)	(Sponsor's SSN)	(VA File #)	X (SSN or ID)	(SSN)	(ID)	111704521	A482

2. PATIENT'S NAME (Last Name, First Name, Middle Initial)
FOREHAND HARRY N

3. PATIENT'S BIRTH DATE 01 | 06 | 1946 SEX M[X] F[ ]

4. INSURED'S NAME (Last Name, First Name, Middle Initial)
SAME

Block 1

PLEASE
DO NOT
STAPLE
IN THIS
AREA

PRUDENTIAL INSURANCE COMPANY
5450 WILSHIRE BOULEVARD
WOODLAND HILLS XY 12345 0000

| | PICA | | | | | | | HEALTH INSURANCE CLAIM FORM | | PICA | | |

1. MEDICARE	MEDICAID	CHAMPUS	CHAMPVA	GROUP HEALTH PLAN	FECA BLK LUNG	OTHER	1a. INSURED'S I.D. NUMBER	(FOR PROGRAM IN ITEM 1)
☐ (Medicare #)	☐ (Medicaid #)	☐ (Sponsor's SSN)	☐ (VA File #)	☒ (SSN or ID)	☐ (SSN)	☐ (ID)	111704521	A482

2. PATIENT'S NAME (Last Name, First Name, Middle Initial)	3. PATIENT'S BIRTH DATE	SEX	4. INSURED'S NAME (Last Name, First Name, Middle Initial)
FOREHAND HARRY N	MM 01 DD 06 YY 1946	M ☒ F ☐	SAME

All private payers: Individual Health Plan: Check "Other" for an individual who is covered under an individual policy. **Group Health Plan:** Check this box for those covered under any group contract insurance (e.g., insurance obtained through employment); also for patients who receive services paid by managed care programs (e.g., HMOs, PPOs, IPAs).
▶ *When completing the* Workbook *assignments, if the insured is employed, assume the insurance is through the employer and is "group" insurance; otherwise assume it is an individual policy and enter "other."*

Medicaid: Check for person receiving Medicaid benefits.

Medicare: Check for patient who receives Medicare benefits.
   Medicare/Medicaid: Check "Medicare" and "Medicaid" if the patient is covered under Medicare and Medicaid programs.
Medicare/Medigap: Check "Medicare" and, if the patient has group or individual or Medigap coverage, check "Group" or "Other," depending on health plan.
▶ *When completing the* Workbook *assignments, if the insured is employed, assume the insurance is through the employer and is "group" insurance; otherwise assume it is an individual policy and enter "other."*
MSP: Check "Group" or "Other" (depending on health plan) and "Medicare" when a Medicare patient has insurance primary to Medicare coverage.

TRICARE: Check "CHAMPUS" for individual receiving TRICARE benefits.

CHAMPVA: Check "CHAMPVA" for individual receiving CHAMPVA benefits.

Workers' Compensation: Check "Other" for all workers' compensation claims except FECA Black Lung. Check "FECA Black Lung" for patients who receive black lung benefits under the Federal Employee Compensation Act.

Block 1a

PLEASE
DO NOT
STAPLE
IN THIS
AREA

PRUDENTIAL INSURANCE COMPANY
5450 WILSHIRE BOULEVARD
WOODLAND HILLS XY 12345 0000

HEALTH INSURANCE CLAIM FORM

								1a. INSURED'S I.D. NUMBER	(FOR PROGRAM IN ITEM 1)
PICA									PICA
1. MEDICARE	MEDICAID	CHAMPUS	CHAMPVA	GROUP HEALTH PLAN	FECA BLK LUNG	OTHER		111704521	A482
(Medicare #)	(Medicaid #)	(Sponsor's SSN)	(VA File #)	[X] (SSN or ID)	(SSN)	(ID)			

2. PATIENT'S NAME (Last Name, First Name, Middle Initial)	3. PATIENT'S BIRTH DATE MM DD YY	SEX	4. INSURED'S NAME (Last Name, First Name, Middle Initial)
FOREHAND HARRY N	01 06 1946	M [X] F ☐	SAME

 All private payers: Enter the patient's policy (identification or certificate) number in the left portion of the block and the group number, if applicable, in the right portion of the block as it appears on the insurance card, without punctuation.

 Medicaid: Enter the Medicaid number in the left portion of the block. Do not enter dashes or other special characters in this block.

Medicare: Enter the patient's Medicare Health Insurance Claim (HIC) number from the patient's Medicare card in the left portion of this block, regardless of whether Medicare is the primary or secondary payer.
Medicare/Medicaid: Enter the patient's Medicare number in the left portion of this block.
Medicare/Medigap: Enter the patient's Medicare number in the left portion of this block.
MSP: Enter the patient's Medicare number in the left portion of this block. Refer to Block 11 for primary insurance.

TRICARE: First enter sponsor's Social Security number (SSN) in the left portion of this block. Then, if the patient is a NATO beneficiary, add "NATO" or, if sponsor is a security agent, add "SECURITY." Do not provide the patient's SSN unless the patient and sponsor are the same.

CHAMPVA: Enter the Veterans Affairs file number (omit prefix or suffix) or sponsor's Social Security number in the left portion of this block. Do not use any other former service numbers.

 Workers' Compensation: Enter the claim number. If none is assigned, enter the employer's policy number or patient's Social Security number.

Block 2

PLEASE
DO NOT
STAPLE
IN THIS
AREA

PRUDENTIAL INSURANCE COMPANY
5450 WILSHIRE BOULEVARD
WOODLAND HILLS XY 12345 0000

	PICA							HEALTH INSURANCE CLAIM FORM		PICA		
1. MEDICARE	MEDICAID	CHAMPUS	CHAMPVA	GROUP HEALTH PLAN	FECA BLK LUNG	OTHER	1a. INSURED'S I.D. NUMBER		(FOR PROGRAM IN ITEM 1)			
(Medicare #)	*(Medicaid #)*	*(Sponsor's SSN)*	*(VA File #)*	X *(SSN or ID)*	*(SSN)*	*(ID)*	111704521		A482			
2. PATIENT'S NAME (Last Name, First Name, Middle Initial)				3. PATIENT'S BIRTH DATE MM DD YY		SEX	4. INSURED'S NAME (Last Name, First Name, Middle Initial)					
FOREHAND HARRY N				01 | 06 | 1946	M X	F	SAME					

All Payers: Enter the last name, first name, and middle initial of the patient—in that order—as shown on the patient's identification card, even if it is misspelled. Do not use nicknames or abbreviations. Do not use commas. A hyphen may be used if a name is hyphenated (Example 6–4).

EXAMPLE 6–4

Hyphenated name: Smith-White = SMITH-WHITE
Prefixed name: MacIverson = MACIVERSON
Seniority name with numeric suffix: John R. Ellis, III = ELLIS III JOHN R

Block 3

PLEASE
DO NOT
STAPLE
IN THIS
AREA

PRUDENTIAL INSURANCE COMPANY
5450 WILSHIRE BOULEVARD
WOODLAND HILLS XY 12345 0000

	PICA							HEALTH INSURANCE CLAIM FORM		PICA		
1. MEDICARE	MEDICAID	CHAMPUS	CHAMPVA	GROUP HEALTH PLAN	FECA BLK LUNG	OTHER	1a. INSURED'S I.D. NUMBER		(FOR PROGRAM IN ITEM 1)			
(Medicare #)	*(Medicaid #)*	*(Sponsor's SSN)*	*(VA File #)*	X *(SSN or ID)*	*(SSN)*	*(ID)*	111704521		A482			
2. PATIENT'S NAME (Last Name, First Name, Middle Initial)				3. PATIENT'S BIRTH DATE MM DD YY		SEX	4. INSURED'S NAME (Last Name, First Name, Middle Initial)					
FOREHAND HARRY N				01 | 06 | 1946	M X	F	SAME					

All Payers: Enter the patient's birth date using eight digits (01272000). The patient's age must be as follows to correlate with the diagnosis in Block 21:
▶ Birth: Newborn diagnosis
▶ Birth to 17 years: Pediatric diagnosis
▶ 12 to 55 years: Maternity diagnosis
▶ 15 to 124 years: Adult diagnosis
Check the appropriate box for the patient's sex. If left blank, gender block defaults to "female."

Block 4

PLEASE
DO NOT
STAPLE
IN THIS
AREA

PRUDENTIAL INSURANCE COMPANY
5450 WILSHIRE BOULEVARD
WOODLAND HILLS XY 12345 0000

HEALTH INSURANCE CLAIM FORM

	PICA								1a. INSURED'S I.D. NUMBER	(FOR PROGRAM IN ITEM 1)	PICA	
1. MEDICARE	MEDICAID	CHAMPUS	CHAMPVA	GROUP HEALTH PLAN	FECA BLK LUNG	OTHER						
(Medicare #)	(Medicaid #)	(Sponsor's SSN)	(VA File #)	X (SSN or ID)	(SSN)	(ID)		111704521	A482			

2. PATIENT'S NAME (Last Name, First Name, Middle Initial)

FOREHAND HARRY N

3. PATIENT'S BIRTH DATE
MM | DD | YY
01 | 06 | 1946   SEX   M [X]   F [ ]

4. INSURED'S NAME (Last Name, First Name, Middle Initial)

SAME

All private payers: Enter "SAME" when the insured is also the patient. If the insured is not the patient, enter the name of the insured (last name first).

Medicaid: Refer to Medicare guidelines.

Medicare: Leave blank if the insured is also the patient. Enter the insured's name if different from the patient's.
Medicare/Medicaid: Refer to Medicare guidelines.
Medicare/Medigap: Refer to Medicare guidelines.
MSP: Enter the name of the insured (last name first).

TRICARE: Enter the sponsor's last name, first name, and middle initial, not a nickname or abbreviation. Do not complete if "self" is checked in Block 6.

CHAMPVA: Enter the veteran's name, last name first.

Workers' Compensation: Enter the employer's name. If the employer is a large corporation, enter the name of the insured corporation in Block 4 and the local employer in Block 11b (e.g., Elsevier is the insured corporation [4] and Saunders is the employer and is typed in Block 11b).

Block 5

5. PATIENT'S ADDRESS			6. PATIENT RELATIONSHIP TO INSURED		7. INSURED'S ADDRESS (No., Street)	
1456 MAIN STREET			Self [X] Spouse [ ] Child [ ] Other [ ]			
CITY		STATE	8. PATIENT STATUS		CITY	STATE
WOODLAND HILLS		XY	Single [ ] Married [X] Other [ ]			
ZIP CODE	TELEPHONE (Include Area Code)		Employed [X] Full-Time Student [ ] Part-Time Student [ ]		ZIP CODE TELEPHONE (Include Area Code)	
12345 0000	(555) 490 9876				( )	

 All private payers: Enter the patient's mailing address and residential telephone number.

 Medicaid: Enter the patient's mailing address and residential telephone number.

Medicare: Enter the patient's mailing address and residential telephone number. On the first line, enter the street address; on the second line, the city and two-character state code (e.g., AZ = Arizona); on the third line, the ZIP code and residential telephone number. Punctuation is not necessary (e.g., ST Louis, no period after ST).
Medicare/Medicaid: Enter the patient's mailing address and residential telephone number.
Medicare/Medigap: Enter the patient's mailing address and residential telephone number.
MSP: Enter the patient's mailing address and residential telephone number.

TRICARE: Enter the patient's mailing address and residential telephone number. Do not enter a post office box number; provide the actual place of residence. If a rural address, the address must contain the route and box number. An APO/FPO address should not be used unless that person is residing overseas.

CHAMPVA: Enter the patient's mailing address and residential telephone number. Do not enter a post office box number; provide the actual place of residence. If a rural address, the address must contain the route and box number. An APO/FPO address should not be used unless that person is residing overseas.

 Workers' Compensation: Enter the patient's mailing address and residential telephone number.

Block 6

5. PATIENT'S ADDRESS			6. PATIENT RELATIONSHIP TO INSURED	7. INSURED'S ADDRESS (No., Street)	
1456 MAIN STREET			Self [X] Spouse [ ] Child [ ] Other [ ]		
CITY		STATE	8. PATIENT STATUS	CITY	STATE
WOODLAND HILLS		XY	Single [ ] Married [X] Other [ ]		
ZIP CODE	TELEPHONE (Include Area Code)		Employed [X] Full-Time Student [ ] Part-Time Student [ ]	ZIP CODE	TELEPHONE (Include Area Code)
12345 0000	(555) 490 9876				( )

All private payers: Check the patient's relationship to the insured. If the patient is an unmarried "domestic partner," check "Other."

Medicaid: Leave blank. Check appropriate box only if there is third-party coverage.

Medicare: Indicate relationship to insured when Block 4 is completed; otherwise leave blank.
Medicare/Medicaid: Refer to Medicare guidelines.
Medicare/Medigap: Refer to Medicare guidelines.
MSP: Indicate relationship to insured.

TRICARE: Check the patient's relationship to the sponsor. If the patient is the sponsor, check "self" (e.g., retiree). If the patient is a child or stepchild, check the box for child. If "other" is checked, indicate how the patient is related to the sponsor in Block 19 or on an attachment (e.g., former spouse).

CHAMPVA: Indicate the patient's relationship to the sponsor. If the patient is the sponsor, check "self." If the patient is a child or stepchild, check the box for child. If "other" is checked, indicate how the patient is related to the sponsor (e.g., former spouse) in Block 19 or on an attachment.

Workers' Compensation: Check "Other."

Block 7

5. PATIENT'S ADDRESS 1456 MAIN STREET		6. PATIENT RELATIONSHIP TO INSURED Self [X] Spouse [ ] Child [ ] Other [ ]	7. INSURED'S ADDRESS (No., Street)	
CITY WOODLAND HILLS	STATE XY	8. PATIENT STATUS Single [ ] Married [X] Other [ ]	CITY	STATE
ZIP CODE 12345 0000	TELEPHONE (Include Area Code) (555) 490 9876	Employed [X] Full-Time Student [ ] Part-Time Student [ ]	ZIP CODE	TELEPHONE (Include Area Code) ( )

All private payers: Leave blank if Block 4 indicates "same." Enter "SAME" if Block 4 is completed and the address is identical to that listed in Block 5. Enter address if different from that listed in Block 5.

Medicaid: Refer to Medicare guidelines.

Medicare: Leave blank if Block 4 is blank. Enter "SAME" if Block 4 is completed and the address is identical to that listed in Block 5. Enter address if different from that listed in Block 5.
Medicare/Medicaid: Refer to Medicare guidelines.
Medicare/Medigap: Refer to Medicare guidelines.
MSP: Complete only when Block 4 is completed. If insured is other than the patient, list insured's address and if the address is the same as in Block 5, enter "SAME."

TRICARE: Enter "SAME" if address is the same as that of the patient listed in Block 5. Enter the sponsor's address (e.g., an APO/FPO address or active duty sponsor's duty station or the retiree's mailing address) if different from the patient's address.

CHAMPVA: Enter "SAME" if address is the same as that of the patient. Enter the sponsor's address if different from the patient's address.

Workers' Compensation: Enter the employer's address.

Block 8

5. PATIENT'S ADDRESS		6. PATIENT RELATIONSHIP TO INSURED		7. INSURED'S ADDRESS (No., Street)		
1456 MAIN STREET		Self ☒ Spouse ☐ Child ☐ Other ☐				
CITY	STATE	8. PATIENT STATUS		CITY		STATE
WOODLAND HILLS	XY	Single ☐ Married ☒ Other ☐				
ZIP CODE	TELEPHONE (Include Area Code)	Employed ☒ Full-Time Student ☐ Part-Time Student ☐		ZIP CODE	TELEPHONE (Include Area Code)	
12345 0000	(555) 490 9876				( )	

All private payers: Check the appropriate box for the patient's marital status and whether employed or a student. The "other" box should be checked when a patient is covered under his or her children's health insurance plan or for a domestic partner. For individuals between the ages of 19 and 23, some insurance carriers require documentation from the school verifying full-time student status. This may be obtained as a signed letter from the school or by using a special form supplied by the insurance company.

Medicaid: Leave blank.

Medicare: Check the appropriate box or boxes for the patient's marital status and whether employed or a student (e.g., a beneficiary may be employed, a student, and married). Check "single" if widowed or divorced. In some locales, this block is not required by Medicare.
Medicare/Medicaid: Check appropriate box for the patient's marital status and whether employed or a student. Check "single" if widowed or divorced.
Medicare/Medigap: Check appropriate box for the patient's marital status and whether employed or a student. Check "single" if widowed or divorced.
MSP: Check appropriate box for the patient's marital status and whether employed or a student. Check "single" if widowed or divorced.

TRICARE: Check the appropriate box for the patient's marital status and whether employed or a student.

CHAMPVA: Check the appropriate box for the patient's marital status and whether employed or a student.

Workers' Compensation: Check "Employed." Some workers' compensation carriers may have requirements for marital status; otherwise leave blank.
▶ *When completing the* Workbook *assignments, leave marital status blank.*

Block 9

9. OTHER INSURED'S NAME (Last Name, First Name, Middle Initial)	10. IS PATIENT'S CONDITION RELATED TO:	11. INSURED'S POLICY GROUP OR FECA NUMBER
a. OTHER INSURED'S POLICY OR GROUP NUMBER	a. EMPLOYMENT? (CURRENT OR PREVIOUS) ☐ YES ☒ NO	a. INSURED'S DATE OF BIRTH MM ┆ DD ┆ YY SEX M ☐ F ☐
b. OTHER INSURED'S DATE OF BIRTH MM ┆ DD ┆ YY M ☐ SEX F ☐	b. AUTO ACCIDENT? PLACE (State) ☐ YES ☒ NO	b. EMPLOYER'S NAME OR SCHOOL NAME
c. EMPLOYER'S NAME OR SCHOOL NAME	c. OTHER ACCIDENT? ☐ YES ☒ NO	c. INSURANCE PLAN NAME OR PROGRAM NAME
d. INSURANCE PLAN NAME OR PROGRAM NAME	10d. RESERVED FOR LOCAL USE	d. IS THERE ANOTHER HEALTH BENEFIT PLAN? ☐ YES ☒ NO *If yes,* return to and complete item 9 a-d.

All private payers: For submission to primary insurance, leave blank. If patient has secondary insurance, enter patient's full name in last name, first name, and middle initial order.

Medicaid: For primary insurance, leave blank. For secondary insurance, enter patient's full name in last name, first name, and middle initial order.

Medicare: For primary insurance, leave blank. Do not list Medicare supplemental coverage (private, not Medigap) on the primary Medicare claim. Beneficiaries are responsible for filing a supplemental claim if the private insurer does not contract with Medicare to send claim electronically.
Medicare/Medicaid: Enter Medicaid patient's full name in last name, first name, and middle initial order.
Medicare/Medigap: Enter the last name, first name, and middle initial of the Medigap enrollee if it differs from that in Block 2; otherwise enter "SAME." Only Medicare participating physicians and suppliers should complete Block 9 and its subdivisions, and only when the beneficiary wishes to assign his or her benefits under a Medigap policy to the participating physician or supplier. If no Medigap benefits are assigned, leave blank.
MSP: Leave blank.

TRICARE: For primary insurance, leave blank. For secondary insurance held by someone other than the patient, enter the name of the insured. Blocks 11a to d should be used to report *other health insurance held by the patient.*

CHAMPVA: For primary insurance, leave blank. For secondary insurance held by someone other than the patient, enter the name of the insured. Blocks 11a to d should be used to report *other health insurance held by the patient.*

Workers' Compensation: Leave blank. If case is pending and not yet declared workers' compensation, insert other insurance.

Block 9a

All private payers: Enter the policy or group number of the other (secondary) insured's insurance coverage.

Medicaid: Leave blank.

Medicare: Refer to appropriate secondary coverage guidelines.

Medicare/Medicaid: Enter Medicaid policy number here or in Block 10d. However, some states may have different guidelines; so check with your local fiscal intermediary if in doubt.

▶ *When completing the* Workbook *assignments, enter the Medicaid policy number in Block 10d.*

Medicare/Medigap: Enter the policy or group number of the Medigap enrollee preceded by the word "MEDIGAP," "MG," or "MGAP." In addition to Medicare/Medigap, if a patient has a third insurance (e.g., employer-supplemental), all information for the third insurance should be submitted on an attachment.

▶ *When completing the* Workbook *assignments, enter the word "MEDIGAP."*

MSP: Leave blank.

TRICARE: Enter the policy or group number of the other (secondary) insured's insurance policy.

CHAMPVA: Enter the policy or group number of the other (secondary) insured's insurance policy.

Workers' Compensation: Leave blank.

Block 9b

All private payers: Enter the other insured's date of birth and gender.

Medicaid: Leave blank.

Medicare: Refer to appropriate secondary coverage guidelines.
Medicare/Medicaid: Enter the Medicaid enrollee's birth date, using eight digits (e.g., 03062000), and gender. If same as patient's, leave blank.
Medicare/Medigap: Enter the Medigap enrollee's birth date, using eight digits (e.g., 03062000), and gender. If same as patient's, leave blank.
MSP: Leave blank.

 TRICARE: For secondary coverage held by someone other than the patient, enter the other insured's date of birth and check the appropriate box for gender.

 CHAMPVA: For secondary coverage held by someone other than the patient, enter the other insured's date of birth and check the appropriate box for gender.

 Workers' Compensation: Leave blank.

Block 9c

 All private payers: For secondary coverage, enter employer's name, if applicable.

 Medicaid: Leave blank.

 Medicare: Refer to appropriate secondary coverage guidelines.
Medicare/Medicaid: Leave blank.
Medicare/Medigap: Enter the Medigap insurer's claims processing address. Ignore "employer's name or school name." Abbreviate the street address to fit in this block by deleting the city and using the two-letter state postal code and ZIP code. For example, 1234 Wren Drive, Any City, Pennsylvania 19106 would be typed "1234 WREN DR PA 19106." **Note:** *If a carrier-assigned unique identifier (sometimes called "Other Carrier Name and Address," or OCNA) for a Medigap insurer appears in Block 9d, then Block 9c may be left blank.*
MSP: Leave blank.

TRICARE: For secondary coverage held by someone other than the patient, enter the name of the other insured's employer or name of school.

 CHAMPVA: For secondary coverage held by someone other than the patient, enter the name of the other insured's employer or name of school.

 Workers' Compensation: Leave blank.

Block 9d

 All private payers: Enter name of secondary insurance plan or program.

 Medicaid: Leave blank.

 Medicare: Refer to appropriate secondary coverage guidelines.
Medicare/Medicaid: Leave blank.
Medicare/Medigap: Enter the Medigap insurer's nine-digit alphanumeric PAYERID number if known (often called the OCNA key), and Block 9c may be left blank. If not known, enter the name of the Medigap enrollee's insurance company. If you are a participating provider, all of the information in Blocks 9 through 9d must be complete and correct or the Medicare carrier cannot electronically forward the claim information to the Medigap insurer. For multiple insurance information, enter "ATTACHMENT" in Block 10d and provide information on an attached sheet.
MSP: Leave blank.

 TRICARE: For secondary coverage held by someone other than the patient, insert name of insured's other health insurance program. On an attached sheet, provide a complete mailing address for all other insurance information and enter the word "ATTACHMENT" in Block 10d. If the patient is covered by a Health Maintenance Organization, attach a copy of the brochure showing that the service is not covered by the HMO.

 CHAMPVA: For secondary coverage held by someone other than the patient, insert name of insured's other health insurance program. On an attached sheet, provide a complete mailing address for all other insurance information and enter the word "ATTACHMENT" in Block 10d. If the patient is covered by a Health Maintenance Organization, attach a copy of the brochure showing that the service is not covered by the HMO.

Workers' Compensation: Leave blank.

Block 10a

9. OTHER INSURED'S NAME (Last Name, First Name, Middle Initial)	10. IS PATIENT'S CONDITION RELATED TO:	11. INSURED'S POLICY GROUP OR FECA NUMBER
a. OTHER INSURED'S POLICY OR GROUP NUMBER	a. EMPLOYMENT? (CURRENT OR PREVIOUS) ☐ YES ☒ NO	a. INSURED'S DATE OF BIRTH MM DD YY SEX M ☐ F ☐
b. OTHER INSURED'S DATE OF BIRTH MM DD YY SEX M ☐ F ☐	b. AUTO ACCIDENT? PLACE (State) ☐ YES ☒ NO	b. EMPLOYER'S NAME OR SCHOOL NAME
c. EMPLOYER'S NAME OR SCHOOL NAME	c. OTHER ACCIDENT? ☐ YES ☒ NO	c. INSURANCE PLAN NAME OR PROGRAM NAME
d. INSURANCE PLAN NAME OR PROGRAM NAME	10d. RESERVED FOR LOCAL USE	d. IS THERE ANOTHER HEALTH BENEFIT PLAN? ☐ YES ☒ NO *If yes*, return to and complete item 9 a-d.

 All Payers: Check "yes" or "no" to indicate whether patient's diagnosis described in Block 21 is the result of an accident or injury that occurred on the job or an industrial illness.

Block 10b

 All private payers: A "yes" checked in Block 10b indicates a third-party liability case; file the claim with the other liability insurance or automobile insurance company. List the abbreviation of the state in which the accident took place (e.g., CA for California).

 Medicaid: Check appropriate box.

Medicare: Check "no." If "yes," bill the liability insurance as primary insurance and Medicare as secondary insurance.
Medicare/Medicaid: Refer to Medicare guidelines.
Medicare/Medigap: Refer to Medicare guidelines.
MSP: Refer to Medicare guidelines.

TRICARE: Check "yes" or "no" to indicate whether automobile liability applies to one or more of the services described in Block 24. If "yes," provide information concerning potential third-party liability. If a third party is involved in the accident, the beneficiary must complete Form DD 2527 (Statement of Personal Injury—Possible Third-Party Liability) and attach it to the claim.

CHAMPVA: Check "yes" or "no" to indicate whether automobile liability applies to one or more of the services described in Block 24. If "yes," provide information concerning potential third-party liability.

 Workers' Compensation: Check "yes" to indicate an automobile accident that occurred while the patient was on the job.

Block 10c

 All private payers: Check "yes" or "no" to indicate whether the patient's condition is related to an accident other than automobile or employment. Verify primary insurance.

 Medicaid: Check if applicable.

Medicare: Check "yes" or "no" to indicate whether the patient's condition is related to an accident other than automobile or employment. Verify primary insurance.
Medicare/Medicaid: Refer to Medicare guidelines.
Medicare/Medigap: Refer to Medicare guidelines.
MSP: Refer to Medicare guidelines.

TRICARE: Check "yes" or "no" to indicate whether another accident (not work related or automobile) applies to one or more of the services described in Block 24. If so, provide information concerning potential third-party liability. If third party is involved in the accident, the beneficiary must complete Form DD 2527 (Statement of Personal Injury—Possible Third-Party Liability) and attach it to the claim.

 CHAMPVA: Refer to TRICARE guidelines.

 Workers' Compensation: Check "no."

Block 10d

 All private payers: Leave blank.

 Medicaid: Generally this block is used exclusively for Medicaid as a secondary payer. Enter the patient's Medicaid (MCD) number preceded by "MCD." Note, however, that this guideline is under discussion, so carriers may not yet notify providers of a usage change for this block. Some carriers state that if more than one type of other insurance applies to the claim, the identifiers for each type should be shown, for example:
Medicare/Medigap and Medicaid coverage = MG/MCD
Medicare/Medigap and Employer—Supplemental coverage = MG/SP
Medicaid and Employer—Supplemental coverage = MCD/SP
Primary (MSP) and Medicaid Secondary coverage = MSP/MCD
Two primary insurance plans = 2MSP
▶ *When completing the* Workbook *assignments, enter the patient's Medicaid number preceded by "MCD."*

Medicare: Leave blank.
Medicare/Medicaid: Enter the patient's Medicaid (MCD) number preceded by "MCD."
Medicare/Medigap: Leave blank.
MSP: Leave blank.

TRICARE: Generally leave blank unless regional fiscal intermediary gives special guidelines. However, if Block 11d is checked "yes," the mailing address of the insurance carrier must be attached to the claim form, and in this block enter "ATTACHMENT."
▶ *When completing the* Workbook *assignments, leave blank.*

CHAMPVA: Generally leave blank unless regional fiscal intermediary gives special guidelines. If Block 11d is checked "yes," the mailing address of the insurance carrier must be attached to the claim form, and in this block enter "ATTACHMENT."
▶ *When completing the* Workbook *assignments, leave blank.*

Workers' Compensation: Leave blank.

Block 11

9. OTHER INSURED'S NAME (Last Name, First Name, Middle Initial)	10. IS PATIENT'S CONDITION RELATED TO:	11. INSURED'S POLICY GROUP OR FECA NUMBER
a. OTHER INSURED'S POLICY OR GROUP NUMBER	a. EMPLOYMENT? (CURRENT OR PREVIOUS) ☐ YES ☒ NO	a. INSURED'S DATE OF BIRTH MM DD YY SEX M ☐ F ☐
b. OTHER INSURED'S DATE OF BIRTH MM DD YY SEX M ☐ F ☐	b. AUTO ACCIDENT? PLACE (State) ☐ YES ☒ NO	b. EMPLOYER'S NAME OR SCHOOL NAME
c. EMPLOYER'S NAME OR SCHOOL NAME	c. OTHER ACCIDENT? ☐ YES ☒ NO	c. INSURANCE PLAN NAME OR PROGRAM NAME
d. INSURANCE PLAN NAME OR PROGRAM NAME	10d. RESERVED FOR LOCAL USE	d. IS THERE ANOTHER HEALTH BENEFIT PLAN? ☐ YES ☒ NO *If yes*, return to and complete item 9 a-d.

All private payers: Leave Blocks 11 through 11c blank if no private secondary coverage. If (private) secondary insurance, see Blocks 9 to 9d.

Medicaid: Generally leave blank. Enter a rejection code if the patient has other third-party insurance coverage and the claim was rejected.

Medicare: If other insurance is not primary to Medicare, enter "NONE" and go to Block 12. Block 11 must be completed. By completing this block, the physician, supplier, or both acknowledge having made a good faith effort to determine whether Medicare is the primary or secondary payer.

Medicare/Medicaid: Refer to Medicare guidelines.

Medicare/Medigap: Refer to Medicare guidelines.

MSP: When insurance is primary to Medicare, enter the insured's policy or group number, or both, and complete Blocks 11a through 11c.

TRICARE: Leave blank.

CHAMPVA: Enter the three-digit number of the VA station that issued the identification card.

Workers' Compensation: Leave blank.

Block 11a

 All private payers: Leave blank.

 Medicaid: Leave blank.

 Medicare: Leave blank.
Medicare/Medicaid: Leave blank.
Medicare/Medigap: Leave blank.
MSP: Enter the insured's eight-digit date of birth (06122000) and gender if different from that listed in Block 3.

 TRICARE: Enter sponsor's date of birth and gender, if different from that listed in Block 3.

 CHAMPVA: Enter sponsor's date of birth and gender, if different from that listed in Block 3.

 Workers' Compensation: Leave blank.

Block 11b

 All private payers: When submitting to secondary insurance, enter the name of the employer, school, or organization if primary policy is a group plan; otherwise leave blank.

 Medicaid: Leave blank.

Medicare: Leave blank.
Medicare/Medicaid: Leave blank.
Medicare/Medigap: Leave blank.
MSP: Enter the employer's name of primary insurance. Also use this block to indicate a change in the insured's insurance status (e.g., "RETIRED" and the eight-digit retirement date). Submit paper claims with a copy of the primary payer's Remittance Advice (RA) document to be considered for Medicare Secondary Payer benefits. Instances when Medicare may be secondary include the following:

1. Group health plan coverage
   a. Working aged
   b. Disability (large group health plan)
   c. End-stage renal disease
2. No fault, other liability, or both
   a. Automobile
   b. Homeowner
   c. Commercial
3. Work-related illness, injury, or both
   a. Workers' compensation
   b. Black lung
   c. Veterans' benefits

 TRICARE: Indicate sponsor's branch of service, using abbreviations (e.g., United States Navy = USN).

 CHAMPVA: Indicate sponsor's branch of service, using abbreviations (e.g., United States Army = USA).

 Workers' Compensation: If a large corporation's name is listed in Block 4, enter the name of the patient's local employer; otherwise leave this block blank.

Block 11c

 All private payers: When submitting to secondary insurance, enter the name of the primary insurance plan; otherwise leave this block blank.

 Medicaid: Leave blank.

Medicare: Leave blank.
Medicare/Medicaid: Leave blank.
Medicare/Medigap: Leave blank.
MSP: Enter the complete name of the insurance plan or program that is primary to Medicare. Include the primary payer's claim processing address directly on the EOB.

TRICARE: Leave blank.

CHAMPVA: Indicate name of the secondary coverage held by the patient, if applicable; otherwise leave this block blank.

Workers' Compensation: Leave blank.

Block 11d

All private payers: Check "yes" or "no" to indicate if there is another health plan. If "yes," Blocks 9a through 9d must be completed.

Medicaid: Leave blank.

Medicare: Generally leave blank; some regions require "yes" or "no" checked, so verify this requirement with your local fiscal intermediary.
▶ *When completing the* Workbook *assignments, leave blank.*
Medicare/Medicaid: Refer to Medicare guidelines.
Medicare/Medigap Refer to Medicare guidelines.
MSP: Leave blank.

TRICARE: Check "yes" or "no" to indicate if there is another health plan. If "yes," Blocks 9a through 9d must be completed.

CHAMPVA: Check "yes" or "no" to indicate if there is another health plan. If "yes," Blocks 9a through 9d must be completed.

 Workers' Compensation: Leave blank.

Block 12

READ BACK OF FORM BEFORE COMPLETING & SIGNING THIS FORM.	13. INSURED'S OR AUTHORIZED PERSON'S SIGNATURE I authorize
12. PATIENT'S OR AUTHORIZED PERSON'S SIGNATURE I authorize the release of any medical or other information necessary to process this claim. I also request payment of government benefits either to myself or to the party who accepts assignment below.	payment of medical benefits to the undersigned physician or supplier for services described below.
SIGNED *Harry N. Forehand* DATE *March 3, 20XX*	SIGNED *Harry N. Forehand*

or

READ BACK OF FORM BEFORE COMPLETING & SIGNING THIS FORM.	13. INSURED'S OR AUTHORIZED PERSON'S SIGNATURE I authorize
12. PATIENT'S OR AUTHORIZED PERSON'S SIGNATURE I authorize the release of any medical or other information necessary to process this claim. I also request payment of government benefits either to myself or to the party who accepts assignment below.	payment of medical benefits to the undersigned physician or supplier for services described below.
SIGNED SOF DATE	SIGNED SOF

 All private payers: A signature here authorizes the release of medical information for claims processing. Have the patient or authorized representative sign and date this block. If the patient has signed a consent form, "Signature on File" or "SOF" can be entered here. The consent form must current, may be lifetime, and must be in the physician's file. When the patient's representative signs, that person's relationship to the patient **must** be indicated. If the signature is indicated by a mark (X), a witness must sign his or her name and enter the address next to the mark.
▶ *When completing the* Workbook *assignments, enter "SOF" in this block.*

 Medicaid: Leave blank.

Medicare: A signature here authorizes payment of benefits to the physician (if the physician accepts assignment) *and* release of medical information for claims processing. Have the patient or authorized representative sign and date this block. If the patient has signed a consent form, "Signature on File" or "SOF" can be typed here. Be sure the form includes both authorizations just mentioned. The form must be current, may be lifetime, and must be in the physician's file. When the patient's representative signs, that person's relationship to the patient **must** be indicated. If the signature is by mark (X), a witness must sign his or her name and enter the address next to the mark.
▶ *When completing the* Workbook *assignments, enter "SOF" in this block.*
Medicare/Medicaid: Refer to Medicare guidelines.
Medicare/Medigap: Refer to Medicare guidelines.
MSP: Guidelines for this block are the same as for Medicare.

TRICARE: A signature here authorizes payment of benefits to the physician (if the physician accepts assignment) and release of medical information for claims processing. Have the patient or the authorized representative sign and date this block. If the patient has signed a consent form, "Signature on File" or "SOF" can be typed here. Be sure the form includes both authorizations just mentioned. The form must be current, may be lifetime, and must be in the physician's file. When the patient's representative signs, that person's relationship to the patient **must** be indicated. If the signature is by mark (X), a witness must sign his or her name and enter the address next to the mark.

▶ *When completing the* Workbook *assignments, enter "SOF" in this block.*

 CHAMPVA: Refer to TRICARE guidelines.

Workers' Compensation: No signature is necessary.

Block 13

READ BACK OF FORM BEFORE COMPLETING & SIGNING THIS FORM.	13. INSURED'S OR AUTHORIZED PERSON'S SIGNATURE I authorize
12. PATIENT'S OR AUTHORIZED PERSON'S SIGNATURE I authorize the release of any medical or other information necessary to process this claim. I also request payment of government benefits either to myself or to the party who accepts assignment below.	payment of medical benefits to the undersigned physician or supplier for services described below.
SIGNED *Harry N. Forehand* DATE *March 3, 20XX*	SIGNED *Harry N. Forehand*

or

READ BACK OF FORM BEFORE COMPLETING & SIGNING THIS FORM.	13. INSURED'S OR AUTHORIZED PERSON'S SIGNATURE I authorize
12. PATIENT'S OR AUTHORIZED PERSON'S SIGNATURE I authorize the release of any medical or other information necessary to process this claim. I also request payment of government benefits either to myself or to the party who accepts assignment below.	payment of medical benefits to the undersigned physician or supplier for services described below.
SIGNED SOF DATE	SIGNED SOF

All private payers: Patient's signature is necessary when benefits are assigned. "SOF" may be listed if the patient's signature is on file.

▶ *When completing the* Workbook *assignments, enter "SOF" in this block.*

 Medicaid: Leave blank.

Medicare: Leave blank.

Medicare/Medicaid: Leave blank.

Medicare/Medigap: For participating provider, a signature here authorizes payment of "mandated"-Medigap benefits when required Medigap information is included in Blocks 9 through 9d. List the signature of the patient or authorized representative, or list "SOF" if the signature is on file as a separate Medigap authorization.

▶ *When completing the* Workbook *assignments, enter "SOF" in this block.*

MSP: The signature of the patient or authorized representative should appear in this block, or list "SOF" if the signature is on file for benefits assigned from the primary carrier.

▶ *When completing the* Workbook *assignments, enter "SOF" in this block.*

TRICARE: Leave blank.

CHAMPVA: Leave blank.

Workers' Compensation: Leave blank. All payment goes directly to the physician.

Block 14

14. DATE OF CURRENT: MM | DD | YY ILLNESS (First symptom) OR INJURY (Accident) OR PREGNANCY (LMP)	15. IF PATIENT HAS HAD SAME OR SIMILAR ILLNESS. GIVE FIRST DATE MM | DD | YY	16. DATES PATIENT UNABLE TO WORK IN CURRENT OCCUPATION MM | DD | YY MM | DD | YY
03 | 01 | 20XX		FROM TO
17. NAME OF REFERRING PHYSICIAN OR OTHER SOURCE PERRY CARDI MD	17a. I.D. NUMBER OF REFERRING PHYSICIAN 67805027XX	18. HOSPITALIZATION DATES RELATED TO CURRENT SERVICES MM | DD | YY MM | DD | YY FROM TO
19. RESERVED FOR LOCAL USE		20. OUTSIDE LAB? $ CHARGES ☐ YES ☒ NO

All private payers: Enter the eight-digit date the patient's first symptoms occurred from the current illness, if stated in the medical record; date of injury or accident; or for pregnancy, first day of last menstrual period. For chiropractic treatment, enter the eight-digit date that treatment began.

Medicaid: Leave blank.

Medicare: Enter the eight-digit date the patient's first symptoms occurred from the current illness, if stated in the medical record; date of injury or accident; or for pregnancy, first day of last menstrual period. For chiropractic treatment, enter the eight-digit date that treatment began.
Medicare/Medicaid: Refer to Medicare guidelines.
Medicare/Medigap: Refer to Medicare guidelines.
MSP: Refer to Medicare guidelines.

 TRICARE: Enter the eight-digit date the patient's first symptoms occurred from the current illness, if stated in the medical record; date of injury or accident; or for pregnancy, first day of last menstrual period. For chiropractic treatment, enter the eight-digit date that treatment began.

 CHAMPVA: Refer to TRICARE guidelines.

 Workers' Compensation: Enter first date of injury, accident, or industrial illness; it should coincide with the date specified in the Doctor's First Report of Injury.

Block 15

14. DATE OF CURRENT: ILLNESS (First symptom) OR INJURY (Accident) OR PREGNANCY (LMP) MM DD YY 03 01 20XX	15. IF PATIENT HAS HAD SAME OR SIMILAR ILLNESS. GIVE FIRST DATE MM DD YY	16. DATES PATIENT UNABLE TO WORK IN CURRENT OCCUPATION MM DD YY MM DD YY FROM TO
17. NAME OF REFERRING PHYSICIAN OR OTHER SOURCE PERRY CARDI MD	17a. I.D. NUMBER OF REFERRING PHYSICIAN 67805027XX	18. HOSPITALIZATION DATES RELATED TO CURRENT SERVICES MM DD YY MM DD YY FROM TO
19. RESERVED FOR LOCAL USE		20. OUTSIDE LAB? $ CHARGES ☐ YES ☒ NO

 All private payers: Enter date when patient had same or similar illness, if applicable, and documented in the medical record.

 Medicaid: Leave blank.

 Medicare: Leave blank.
Medicare/Medicaid: Leave blank.
Medicare/Medigap: Leave blank.
MSP: Leave blank.

TRICARE: Enter date when patient had same or similar illness, if applicable, and documented in the medical record.

 CHAMPVA: Refer to TRICARE guidelines.

 Workers' Compensation: Enter date if appropriate and documented in the medical record.

Block 16

14. DATE OF CURRENT: MM DD YY	ILLNESS (First symptom) OR INJURY (Accident) OR PREGNANCY (LMP)	15. IF PATIENT HAS HAD SAME OR SIMILAR ILLNESS. GIVE FIRST DATE MM DD YY	16. DATES PATIENT UNABLE TO WORK IN CURRENT OCCUPATION MM DD YY MM DD YY FROM TO
03 01 20XX			
17. NAME OF REFERRING PHYSICIAN OR OTHER SOURCE PERRY CARDI MD		17a. I.D. NUMBER OF REFERRING PHYSICIAN 67805027XX	18. HOSPITALIZATION DATES RELATED TO CURRENT SERVICES MM DD YY MM DD YY FROM TO
19. RESERVED FOR LOCAL USE			20. OUTSIDE LAB? $ CHARGES ☐ YES ☒ NO

 All private payers: Enter dates patient is employed but cannot work in current occupation. *From:* Enter first *full* day patient was unable to perform job duties. *To:* Enter last day patient was disabled before returning to work.

 Medicaid: Leave blank.

 Medicare: Enter eight-digit dates patient is employed but cannot work in current occupation. *From:* Enter first *full* day patient was unable to perform job duties. *To:* Enter last day patient was disabled before returning to work.
Medicare/Medicaid: Refer to Medicare guidelines.
Medicare/Medigap: Refer to Medicare guidelines.
MSP: Refer to Medicare guidelines.

 TRICARE: Refer to Medicare guidelines.

 CHAMPVA: Refer to Medicare guidelines.

Workers' Compensation: May be completed but is not mandatory and must be verified with documentation in Doctor's First Report of Injury. *From:* Enter first *full* day patient was unable to perform job duties. *To:* Enter last day patient was disabled before returning to work.

▶ *When completing the* Workbook *assignments, enter information when documented in the medical record.*

Block 17

14. DATE OF CURRENT: MM DD YY ◀ ILLNESS (First symptom) OR INJURY (Accident) OR PREGNANCY (LMP)	15. IF PATIENT HAS HAD SAME OR SIMILAR ILLNESS. GIVE FIRST DATE MM DD YY	16. DATES PATIENT UNABLE TO WORK IN CURRENT OCCUPATION MM DD YY MM DD YY FROM TO
03 01 20XX		
17. NAME OF REFERRING PHYSICIAN OR OTHER SOURCE PERRY CARDI MD	17a. I.D. NUMBER OF REFERRING PHYSICIAN 67805027XX	18. HOSPITALIZATION DATES RELATED TO CURRENT SERVICES MM DD YY MM DD YY FROM TO
19. RESERVED FOR LOCAL USE		20. OUTSIDE LAB? ☐ YES ☒ NO $ CHARGES

All private payers: Enter complete name and degree of referring physician, when applicable. Do not list other referrals (e.g., family or friends).

Medicaid: Enter complete name and degree of referring physician, when applicable. Do not list other referrals (e.g., family or friends).

Medicare: Enter the name and degree of the referring or ordering physician on all claims for Medicare-covered services and items resulting from a physician's order or referral. Use a separate claim form for each referring or ordering physician.

Surgeon: A surgeon must complete this block. When the patient has not been referred, enter the surgeon's name. On an assistant surgeon's claim, enter the primary surgeon's name.

Referring physician: A physician who requests a service for the beneficiary for which payment may be made under the Medicare program. When a physician extender (e.g., nurse practitioner) refers a patient for a consultative service, enter the name of the physician supervising the physician extender.

Ordering physician: A physician who orders nonphysician services for the patient, such as diagnostic radiology, laboratory, or pathology tests; pharmaceutical services; durable medical equipment (DME); parenteral and enteral nutrition; or immunosuppressive drugs, and consultations.

When the ordering physician is also the performing physician (e.g., the physician who actually performs the in-office laboratory tests), the performing physician's name and assigned UPIN/NPI number must appear in Blocks 17 and 17a.

When a patient is referred to a physician who also orders and performs a diagnostic service, *a separate claim form* is necessary for the diagnostic service.

▶ Enter the original referring physician's name and NPI in Blocks 17 and 17a of the first claim form.

▶ Enter the ordering (performing) physician's name and NPI in Blocks 17 and 17a of the second claim form.

Medicare/Medicaid: Refer to Medicare guidelines.

Medicare/Medigap: Refer to Medicare guidelines.

MSP: Refer to Medicare guidelines.

TRICARE: Enter name, degree, and address of referring provider. This is necessary for all consultation claims. If the patient was referred from a Military Treatment Facility (MTF), enter the name of the MTF and attach DD Form 2161 or SF 513, "Referral for Civilian Medical Care."

CHAMPVA: Refer to TRICARE guidelines.

Workers' Compensation: Indicate name and degree of referring provider.

Block 17a

14. DATE OF CURRENT: MM | DD | YY 03 | 01 | 20XX	ILLNESS (First symptom) OR INJURY (Accident) OR PREGNANCY (LMP)	15. IF PATIENT HAS HAD SAME OR SIMILAR ILLNESS. GIVE FIRST DATE MM | DD | YY	16. DATES PATIENT UNABLE TO WORK IN CURRENT OCCUPATION MM | DD | YY MM | DD | YY FROM TO
17. NAME OF REFERRING PHYSICIAN OR OTHER SOURCE PERRY CARDI MD		17a. I.D. NUMBER OF REFERRING PHYSICIAN 67805027XX	18. HOSPITALIZATION DATES RELATED TO CURRENT SERVICES MM | DD | YY MM | DD | YY FROM TO
19. RESERVED FOR LOCAL USE			20. OUTSIDE LAB? $ CHARGES ☐ YES ☒ NO

All private payers: Enter the referring physician's UPIN/NPI number.

Medicaid: Enter the referring physician's UPIN/NPI number.

Medicare: Enter the CMS-assigned UPIN/NPI of the referring or ordering physician (or the supervising physician for a physician extender) as detailed in Medicare Block 17. Temporary "surrogate" NPIs are issued until permanent ones are assigned for physicians in the following categories: residents and interns, retired physicians, nonphysicians (nurse practitioners, clinical nurse specialists, and other state licensed nonphysicians), Veterans Affairs/US Armed Services, Public Health/Indian Health Services, and any physician not meeting the described criteria for a surrogate who has not been issued an NPI.

Medicare/Medicaid: Refer to Medicare guidelines.

Medicare/Medigap: Refer to Medicare guidelines.

MSP: Refer to Medicare guidelines.

TRICARE: Enter the referring physician's state license number. If the patient is referred from a Military Treatment Facility, leave blank.

CHAMPVA: Refer to TRICARE guidelines.

 Workers' Compensation: Leave blank.

Block 18

14. DATE OF CURRENT: ILLNESS (First symptom) OR INJURY (Accident) OR PREGNANCY (LMP)			15. IF PATIENT HAS HAD SAME OR SIMILAR ILLNESS. GIVE FIRST DATE MM DD YY	16. DATES PATIENT UNABLE TO WORK IN CURRENT OCCUPATION
MM 03	DD 01	YY 20XX		MM DD YY FROM TO MM DD YY
17. NAME OF REFERRING PHYSICIAN OR OTHER SOURCE PERRY CARDI MD			17a. I.D. NUMBER OF REFERRING PHYSICIAN 67805027XX	18. HOSPITALIZATION DATES RELATED TO CURRENT SERVICES MM DD YY FROM TO MM DD YY
19. RESERVED FOR LOCAL USE				20. OUTSIDE LAB? ☐ YES ☒ NO $ CHARGES

 All Payers: Complete this block when a medical service is furnished as a result of, or subsequent to, a related (inpatient) hospitalization, skilled nursing facility, or nursing home visit. Do not complete for outpatient hospital services, ambulatory surgery, or emergency department services. Enter eight-digit admitting and discharge dates. If the patient is still hospitalized at the time of the billing, enter eight zeros in the "TO" field.

Block 19

14. DATE OF CURRENT: ILLNESS (First symptom) OR INJURY (Accident) OR PREGNANCY (LMP)			15. IF PATIENT HAS HAD SAME OR SIMILAR ILLNESS. GIVE FIRST DATE MM DD YY	16. DATES PATIENT UNABLE TO WORK IN CURRENT OCCUPATION
MM 03	DD 01	YY 20XX		MM DD YY FROM TO MM DD YY
17. NAME OF REFERRING PHYSICIAN OR OTHER SOURCE PERRY CARDI MD			17a. I.D. NUMBER OF REFERRING PHYSICIAN 67805027XX	18. HOSPITALIZATION DATES RELATED TO CURRENT SERVICES MM DD YY FROM TO MM DD YY
19. RESERVED FOR LOCAL USE				20. OUTSIDE LAB? ☐ YES ☒ NO $ CHARGES

All private payers: This block may be completed in a number of different ways depending on commercial carrier guidelines. Some common uses are:

▶ Enter the word "ATTACHMENT" when an operative report, discharge summary, invoice, or other attachment is included.

▶ Enter an explanation about unusual services or unlisted services.

▶ Enter all applicable modifiers when modifier -99 is used in Block 24D (e.g., 99-80 51). If -99 appears with more than one procedure code, list the line number (24-1, -2, -3, and so on) for each -99 listed (Example 6–5).

EXAMPLE 6–5

2-80 51   3-80 51

▶ Enter the drug name and dosage when submitting a claim for Not Otherwise Classified (NOC) drugs. Enter the word "ATTACHMENT" and attach the invoice.

▶ Describe the supply when the code 99070 is used.

▶ Enter the x-ray date for chiropractic treatment.

Medicaid: Check with the regional fiscal intermediary who may have special guidelines for entries in this block.

▶ *When completing the* Workbook *assignments, refer to private payer guidelines.*

 Medicare: Although the block is labeled "Reserved for Local Use," CMS guidelines state it may be completed in a number of different ways depending on the circumstances of the services provided to the patient. This block can only contain up to three conditions per claim. Some common uses are:

▶ Enter the attending physician's NPI and the eight-digit date of the patient's latest visit for claims submitted by a physical or occupational therapist, psychotherapist, chiropractor, or podiatrist.
▶ Enter the drug's name and dosage when submitting a claim for Not Otherwise Classified (NOC) drugs. Enter the word "ATTACHMENT" and include a copy of the invoice.
▶ Describe the procedure for *unlisted procedures.* If there is not sufficient room in this block, send an attachment.
▶ Enter all applicable modifiers when modifier -99 is used in Block 24D (e.g., 99-80 51). If -99 appears with more than one procedure code, list the line number (24–1, –2, –3, and so on) for each -99 listed (Example 6–5).
▶ Enter "Homebound" when an independent laboratory renders an electrocardiogram or collects a specimen from a patient who is homebound or institutionalized.
▶ Enter the statement "Patient refuses to assign benefits" when a Medicare beneficiary refuses to assign benefits to a participating provider. No payment to the physician will be made on the claim in this case.
▶ Enter "Testing for hearing aid" when submitting a claim to obtain an intentional denial from Medicare as the primary payer for hearing aid testing and a secondary payer is involved.
▶ Enter the specific dental surgery for which a dental examination is being performed.
▶ Enter the name and dosage when billing for low osmolar contrast material for which there is no level II HCPCS code.
▶ Enter the eight-digit assumed and relinquished dates of care for each provider when providers share postoperative care for global surgery claims.
▶ Enter the statement "Attending physician, not hospice employee" when a physician gives service to a hospice patient but the hospice in which the patient resides does not employ the physician.

Medicare/Medicaid: Refer to Medicare guidelines.
Medicare/Medigap: Refer to Medicare guidelines.
MSP: Refer to Medicare guidelines.

 TRICARE: Generally this block is reserved for local use (e.g., to indicate referral number or enter x-ray date for chiropractic treatment).

 CHAMPVA: Refer to TRICARE guidelines.

Workers' Compensation: Leave blank.

Block 20

14. DATE OF CURRENT: ILLNESS (First symptom) OR INJURY (Accident) OR PREGNANCY (LMP)	15. IF PATIENT HAS HAD SAME OR SIMILAR ILLNESS. GIVE FIRST DATE MM DD YY	16. DATES PATIENT UNABLE TO WORK IN CURRENT OCCUPATION MM DD YY MM DD YY
MM DD YY 03 01 20XX		FROM TO
17. NAME OF REFERRING PHYSICIAN OR OTHER SOURCE PERRY CARDI MD	17a. I.D. NUMBER OF REFERRING PHYSICIAN 67805027XX	18. HOSPITALIZATION DATES RELATED TO CURRENT SERVICES MM DD YY MM DD YY FROM TO
19. RESERVED FOR LOCAL USE		20. OUTSIDE LAB? $ CHARGES ☐ YES ☒ NO

 All private payers: Enter "yes" or "no" when billing diagnostic laboratory tests. *NO* means the tests were performed by the billing physician or laboratory. *YES* means that the laboratory test was performed *outside* of the physician's office and that the physician is billing for the laboratory services. If "yes," enter purchase price of the test in the Charges portion of this block and complete Block 32.

 Medicaid: Check "no"; outside laboratories must bill directly.

 Medicare: Enter "yes" or "no" when billing diagnostic laboratory tests. *NO* means the tests were performed by the billing physician or laboratory. *YES* means that the laboratory test was performed *outside* of the physician's office and that the physician is billing for the laboratory services. If "yes," enter purchase price of the test in the Charges portion of this block and complete Block 32. *Clinical laboratory services must be billed to Medicare on an assigned basis.*
Medicare/Medicaid: Refer to Medicare guidelines.
Medicare/Medigap: Refer to Medicare guidelines.
MSP: Refer to Medicare guidelines.

TRICARE: Refer to Medicare guidelines.

CHAMPVA: Refer to TRICARE guidelines.

 Workers' Compensation: Refer to Medicare guidelines.

Block 21

21. DIAGNOSIS OR NATURE OF ILLNESS OR INJURY. (RELATE ITEMS 1,2,3 OR 4 TO ITEM 24E BY LINE)		22. MEDICAID RESUBMISSION CODE _____ ORIGINAL REF. NO.
1. 382 00 3.		
		23. PRIOR AUTHORIZATION NUMBER
2.	4.		

24. A DATE(S) OF SERVICE						B Place of Service	C Type of Service	D PROCEDURES, SERVICES, OR SUPPLIES (Explain Unusual Circumstances) CPT/HCPCS | MODIFIER	E DIAGNOSIS CODE	F $ CHARGES	G DAYS OR UNITS	H EPSDT Family Plan	I EMG	J COB	K RESERVED FOR LOCAL USE
From			To												
MM	DD	YY	MM	DD	YY										
1															

All payers: Enter up to four diagnostic codes in priority order, with the primary diagnosis in the first position. Codes must be carried out to their highest degree of specificity. Do not use decimal points or add any code narratives unless required in your locale. Code only the conditions or problems that the physician is actively treating and that relate directly to the services billed.

Block 22

21. DIAGNOSIS OR NATURE OF ILLNESS OR INJURY. (RELATE ITEMS 1,2,3 OR 4 TO ITEM 24E BY LINE)		22. MEDICAID RESUBMISSION CODE _____ ORIGINAL REF. NO.
1. 382 00 3.		
		23. PRIOR AUTHORIZATION NUMBER
2.	4.		

24. A DATE(S) OF SERVICE						B Place of Service	C Type of Service	D PROCEDURES, SERVICES, OR SUPPLIES (Explain Unusual Circumstances) CPT/HCPCS | MODIFIER	E DIAGNOSIS CODE	F $ CHARGES	G DAYS OR UNITS	H EPSDT Family Plan	I EMG	J COB	K RESERVED FOR LOCAL USE
From			To												
MM	DD	YY	MM	DD	YY										
1									1						

All private payers: Leave blank.

Medicaid: Complete for resubmission.

Medicare: Leave blank.
Medicare/Medicaid: Refer to Medicaid guidelines.
Medicare/Medigap: Leave blank.
MSP: Leave blank.

TRICARE: Leave blank.

CHAMPVA: Leave blank.

 Workers' Compensation: Leave blank.

Block 23

21. DIAGNOSIS OR NATURE OF ILLNESS OR INJURY. (RELATE ITEMS 1,2,3 OR 4 TO ITEM 24E BY LINE)					22. MEDICAID RESUBMISSION CODE		ORIGINAL REF. NO.
1. 382 00			3.		23. PRIOR AUTHORIZATION NUMBER		
2.			4.				

24. A DATE(S) OF SERVICE						B Place of Service	C Type of Service	D PROCEDURES, SERVICES, OR SUPPLIES (Explain Unusual Circumstances)		E DIAGNOSIS CODE	F $ CHARGES	G DAYS OR UNITS	H EPSDT Family Plan	I EMG	J COB	K RESERVED FOR LOCAL USE
From MM	DD	YY	To MM	DD	YY			CPT/HCPCS	MODIFIER							
1										1						

 All private payers: Enter the professional or peer review organization (PRO) 10-digit prior authorization number.

Medicaid: Enter the PRO 10-digit prior authorization or precertification number for procedures requiring PRO prior approval. If billing for an investigational device, enter the Investigational Device Exemption (IDE) number.

Medicare: Although this block is labeled "Prior Authorization Number," CMS guidelines state it may be completed in a number of different ways depending on the circumstances of the services provided to the patient. Some common uses are:

▶ Enter the Professional (Peer) Review Organization (PRO) 10-digit prior authorization or precertification number for procedures requiring PRO prior approval.
▶ Enter the Investigational Device Exemption (IDE) number if billing for an investigational device.
▶ Enter the 10-digit Clinical Laboratory Improvement Amendments (CLIA) federal certification number when billing for laboratory services billed by a physician office laboratory.
▶ Enter the six-digit Medicare provider number of the hospice or home health agency (HHA) when billing for care plan oversight services.

Medicare/Medicaid: Refer to Medicare guidelines.
Medicare/Medigap: Refer to Medicare guidelines.
MSP: Refer to Medicare guidelines.

TRICARE: Enter the PRO 10-digit prior authorization or precertification number for procedures requiring PRO prior approval. If billing for an investigational device, enter the IDE number. Attach a copy of the authorization.

CHAMPVA: Refer to TRICARE guidelines.

 Workers' Compensation: Leave blank.

Blocks 24A through 24K may not contain more than six detail lines. If the case requires more than six detail lines, put the additional information on a separate claim form, treat it as an independent claim, and total all charges on each claim. Claims cannot be "continued" from one to another. Do not list a procedure on the claim form for which there is no charge.

Block 24A

24. A DATE(S) OF SERVICE		B Place of Service	C Type of Service	D PROCEDURES, SERVICES, OR SUPPLIES (Explain Unusual Circumstances) CPT/HCPCS | MODIFIER	E DIAGNOSIS CODE	F $ CHARGES	G DAYS OR UNITS	H EPSDT Family Plan	I EMG	J COB	K RESERVED FOR LOCAL USE
From MM DD YY	To MM DD YY										
030320XX		11		99203	1	70 92	1			12	458977XX

25. FEDERAL TAX I.D. NUMBER SSN EIN	26. PATIENT'S ACCOUNT NO.	27. ACCEPT ASSIGNMENT? (For govt. claims, see back)	28. TOTAL CHARGE	29. AMOUNT PAID	30. BALANCE DUE
74 10640XX ☐ ☒	010	☒ YES ☐ NO	$ 70 92	$	$ 70 92

24. A DATE(S) OF SERVICE		B Place of Service	C Type of Service	D PROCEDURES, SERVICES, OR SUPPLIES (Explain Unusual Circumstances) CPT/HCPCS | MODIFIER	E DIAGNOSIS CODE	F $ CHARGES	G DAYS OR UNITS	H EPSDT Family Plan	I Initials	Date
From MM DD YY	To MM DD YY								EMG COB	RESERVED FOR LOCAL USE
113020XX		21		99231	1	37 74	1		32	783127XX
120120XX	120320XX	21		99231	1	37 74	3		32	783127XX

25. FEDERAL TAX I.D. NUMBER SSN EIN	26. PATIENT'S ACCOUNT NO.	27. ACCEPT ASSIGNMENT? (For govt. claims, see back)	28. TOTAL CHARGE	29. AMOUNT PAID	30. BALANCE DUE
75 67210XX ☐ ☒	102	☒ YES ☐ NO	$ 150 96	$	$ 150 96

 All private payers: Enter the month, day, and year (eight digits with no spaces) for each procedure, service, or supply reported in Block 24D. Make sure the dates shown are no earlier than the date of the current illness if listed in Block 14. If the "from" and "to" dates are the same, enter only the "from" date. Enter the "to" date when reporting a consecutive range of dates for the same procedure code. Use a separate line for each month. Some third-party payers may use different date formats (e.g., December 4, 20XX = 20001204).

Medicaid: Enter an eight-digit "from" date (month, day, and year with no spaces) for each service or supply. Leave "to" date blank. No date ranging is allowed for consecutive dates.

Medicare: Enter the month, day, and year (eight digits with no spaces) for each procedure, service, or supply reported in Block 24D. Make sure the dates shown are no earlier than the date of the current illness if listed in Block 14. If the "from" and "to" dates are the same, enter only the "from" date. Enter the "to" date when reporting a consecutive range of dates for the same procedure code. Use a separate line for each month except when reporting weekly radiation therapy, durable medical equipment, or oxygen rental.
Medicare/Medicaid: Refer to Medicare guidelines.
Medicare/Medigap: Refer to Medicare guidelines.
MSP: Refer to Medicare guidelines.

TRICARE: Enter the month, day, and year (eight digits with no spaces) for each procedure, service, or supply reported in Block 24D. Make sure the dates shown are no earlier than the date of the current illness if listed in Block 14. If the "from" and "to" dates are the same, enter only the "from" date. Enter the "to" date when reporting a consecutive range of dates for the same procedure code. Use a separate line for each month.

CHAMPVA: Refer to TRICARE guidelines.

 Workers' Compensation: Enter the month, day, and year (eight digits with no spaces) for each procedure, service, or supply reported in Block 24D. Date ranging is not the preferred format for consecutive dates.

Block 24B

24. A DATE(S) OF SERVICE From MM DD YY To MM DD YY	B Place of Service	C Type of Service	D PROCEDURES, SERVICES, OR SUPPLIES (Explain Unusual Circumstances) CPT/HCPCS | MODIFIER	E DIAGNOSIS CODE	F $ CHARGES	G DAYS OR UNITS	H EPSDT Family Plan	I EMG	J COB	K RESERVED FOR LOCAL USE
1 030320XX	11		99203	1	70 92	1			12	458977XX
2										
3										
4										
5										
6										

25. FEDERAL TAX I.D. NUMBER	SSN EIN	26. PATIENT'S ACCOUNT NO.	27. ACCEPT ASSIGNMENT? (For govt. claims, see back)	28. TOTAL CHARGE	29. AMOUNT PAID	30. BALANCE DUE
74 10640XX	☐ ☒	010	☒ YES ☐ NO	$ 70 92	$	$ 70 92

All Payers: Enter the appropriate "Place of Service" code shown in Figure 6–4. Identify by location where the service was performed or an item was used. Use the inpatient hospital code only when a service is provided to a patient admitted to the hospital for an overnight stay. Enter the name, address, and provider number of the hospital in Block 32.

BLOCK 24B
PLACE OF SERVICE CODES

01-02	Unassigned
03	School
04	Homeless shelter
05	Indian health service free-standing facility
06	Indian health service provider-based facility
07	Tribal 638 free-standing facility
08	Tribal 638 provider-based facility
09-10	Unassigned
11	Doctor's office
12	Patient's home
13-14	Unassigned
15	Mobile unit
16-19	Unassigned
20	Urgent care facility
21	Inpatient hospital
22	Outpatient hospital
23	Emergency department—hospital
24	Ambulatory surgical center
25	Birthing center
26	Military treatment facility/uniformed service treatment facility
27-30	Unassigned
31	Skilled nursing facility (swing bed visits)
32	Nursing facility (intermediate/long-term care facilities)
33	Custodial care facility (domiciliary or rest home services)
34	Hospice (domiciliary or rest home services)
35-40	Unassigned
41	Ambulance—land
42	Ambulance—air or water
43-49	Unassigned
50	Federally qualified health center
51	Inpatient psychiatric facility
52	Psychiatric facility—partial hospitalization
53	Community mental health care (outpatient, twenty-four-hours-a-day services, admission screening, consultation, and educational services)
54	Intermediate care facility/mentally retarded
55	Residential substance abuse treatment facility
56	Psychiatric residential treatment center
57-59	Unassigned
60	Mass immunization center
61	Comprehensive inpatient rehabilitation facility
62	Comprehensive outpatient rehabilitation facility
63-64	Unassigned
65	End-stage renal disease treatment facility
66-70	Unassigned
71	State or local public health clinic
72	Rural health clinic
73-80	Unassigned
81	Independent laboratory
82-98	Unassigned
99	Other place of service

Figure 6–4.

Block 24C

24.	A DATE(S) OF SERVICE						B Place of Service	C Type of Service	D PROCEDURES, SERVICES, OR SUPPLIES (Explain Unusual Circumstances) CPT/HCPCS | MODIFIER		E DIAGNOSIS CODE	F $ CHARGES		G DAYS OR UNITS	H EPSDT Family Plan	I EMG	J COB	K RESERVED FOR LOCAL USE
	From MM	DD	YY	To MM	DD	YY												
1	03	03	20XX				11		99203		1	70	92	1			12	458977XX
2																		
3																		
4																		
5																		
6																		

25. FEDERAL TAX I.D. NUMBER	SSN	EIN	26. PATIENT'S ACCOUNT NO.	27. ACCEPT ASSIGNMENT? (For govt. claims, see back)		28. TOTAL CHARGE		29. AMOUNT PAID	30. BALANCE DUE
74 10640XX	☐	X	010	X YES	☐ NO	$ 70	92	$	$ 70 92

All private payers: Leave blank.

Medicaid: Enter the appropriate "Type of Service" code from Figure 6–5.

BLOCK 24C
TYPE OF SERVICE CODES FOR MEDICAID,
TRICARE, AND WORKERS' COMPENSATION

These codes should be selected depending on the procedure code used on each line. Codes may vary according to regions and claim administrators.

1 Medical care (e.g., evaluation and management services)
2 Surgery
3 Consultation
4 Diagnostic x-ray (e.g., ultrasound and nuclear testing)
5 Diagnostic laboratory
6 Radiation therapy
7 Anesthesia
8 Assistant at surgery
9 Other medical service (e.g., laboratory, venipuncture, handling of specimen)
0 Blood or packed red cells
A DME rental/purchase
B Drugs
C Ambulatory surgery
D Hospice
E Second opinion on elective surgery
F Maternity
G Dental
H Mental health care
I Ambulance
J Program for persons with disabilities
L Renal supply in home
M Alternate payment for maintenance
N Kidney donor
V Pneumococcal vaccine
Z Third opinion on elective surgery

Figure 6–5.

Medicare: Leave blank. "Type of Service" codes are used on Medicare Remittance Advice (RA) documents and electronic claims.

Medicare/Medicaid: Refer to Medicare guidelines.

Medicare/Medigap: Refer to Medicare guidelines.

MSP: Refer to Medicare guidelines.

TRICARE: Enter the appropriate "Type of Service" code from Figure 6–5. Codes may vary according to regions and claim administrators.

▶ *When completing the* Workbook *assignments, use the codes shown in Figure 6–5.*

CHAMPVA: Refer to TRICARE guidelines.

Workers' Compensation: Enter the appropriate "Type of Service" code shown in Figure 6–5. These codes may not be used or may vary according to regions and claim administrators.

▶ *When completing the* Workbook *assignments, use the codes shown in Figure 6–5.*

Block 24D

24.	A DATE(S) OF SERVICE			B Place of Service	C Type of Service	D PROCEDURES, SERVICES, OR SUPPLIES (Explain Unusual Circumstances) CPT/HCPCS | MODIFIER	E DIAGNOSIS CODE	F $ CHARGES	G DAYS OR UNITS	H EPSDT Family Plan	I EMG	J COB	K RESERVED FOR LOCAL USE
	From MM DD YY	To MM DD YY											
1	030320XX			11		99203	1	70 92	1			12	458977XX
2													
3													
4													
5													
6													

25. FEDERAL TAX I.D. NUMBER	SSN EIN	26. PATIENT'S ACCOUNT NO.	27. ACCEPT ASSIGNMENT? (For govt. claims, see back)	28. TOTAL CHARGE	29. AMOUNT PAID	30. BALANCE DUE
74 10640XX	☐ ☒	010	☒ YES ☐ NO	$ 70 92	$	$ 70 92

CPT   99203   Office visit, new patient

All private payers: Enter the appropriate CPT/HCPCS code for each procedure, service, or supply and applicable modifier without a hyphen. If it is necessary to use more than two modifiers with a procedure code, enter modifier -99 in Block 24D and list applicable modifiers in Block 19.

Medicaid: Enter the appropriate CPT/HCPCS code for each procedure, service, or supply and applicable modifier without a hyphen.

Medicare: Enter CPT/HCPCS code and applicable modifiers without a hyphen for procedures, services, and supplies without a narrative description. When procedure codes do not require modifiers, leave modifier area blank—do not enter 00 or any other combination. For multiple surgical procedures, list the procedure with the highest fee first. For unlisted procedure codes, include a narrative description in Block 19 (e.g., 99499, "Unlisted Evaluation and Management Service"). If information does not fit in Block 19, include an attachment. When entering an unlisted surgery code, submit the operative notes with the claim as an attachment.
Medicare/Medicaid: Refer to Medicare guidelines.
Medicare/Medigap: Refer to Medicare guidelines.
MSP: Refer to Medicare guidelines.

TRICARE: Enter the appropriate CPT/HCPCS code for each procedure, service, or supply and applicable modifier without a hyphen. If it is necessary to use more than two modifiers with a procedure code, enter modifier -99 in Block 24D and list applicable modifiers in Block 19. When Not Otherwise Classified (NOC) codes are submitted (e.g., supplies and injections), provide a narrative of the service in Block 19 or on an attachment.

CHAMPVA: Refer to TRICARE guidelines.

 Workers' Compensation: Enter appropriate RVS codes and applicable modifiers (without a hyphen) used in your state or region.
► *When completing the* Workbook *assignments, use appropriate CPT codes.*

Block 24E

21. DIAGNOSIS OR NATURE OF ILLNESS OR INJURY (RELATE ITEMS 1,2,3 OR 4 TO ITEM 24E BY LINE)		22. MEDICAID RESUBMISSION CODE	ORIGINAL REF. NO.
1. 382 00	3.		
2.	4.	23. PRIOR AUTHORIZATION NUMBER	

24. A DATE(S) OF SERVICE				B Place of Service	C Type of Service	D PROCEDURES, SERVICES, OR SUPPLIES (Explain Unusual Circumstances) CPT/HCPCS | MODIFIER	E DIAGNOSIS CODE	F $ CHARGES	G DAYS OR UNITS	H EPSDT Family Plan	I EMG	J COB	K RESERVED FOR LOCAL USE
From MM DD YY		To MM DD YY											
1	030320XX			11		99203	1	70 92	1			12	458977XX
2													
3													
4													
5													
6													

25. FEDERAL TAX I.D. NUMBER	SSN EIN	26. PATIENT'S ACCOUNT NO.	27. ACCEPT ASSIGNMENT? (For govt. claims, see back)	28. TOTAL CHARGE	29. AMOUNT PAID	30. BALANCE DUE
74 10640XX	☐ ☒	010	☒ YES ☐ NO	$ 70 92	$	$ 70 92

All private payers: Enter only one diagnosis code reference "pointer" number per line item (unless you have verified that independent carriers allow more than one) linking the diagnostic code listed in Block 21. When multiple services are performed, enter the corresponding diagnostic reference number for each service (e.g., 1, 2, 3, or 4). DO NOT USE ACTUAL ICD-9-CM CODES IN THIS BLOCK.

▶ *When completing* Workbook *assignments, more than one diagnosis reference "pointer" number per line item is allowed.*

 Medicaid: Refer to Medicare guidelines. In some states, completion may not be required.

Medicare: Enter only one diagnosis code reference "pointer" number per line item linking the diagnostic codes listed in Block 21. When multiple services are performed, enter the corresponding diagnostic reference number for each service (e.g., 1, 2, 3, or 4). DO NOT USE ACTUAL ICD-9-CM CODES IN THIS BLOCK.

Medicare/Medicaid: Refer to Medicare guidelines.
Medicare/Medigap: Refer to Medicare guidelines.
MSP: Refer to Medicare guidelines.

TRICARE: Enter the diagnosis reference number (e.g., indicating up to four ICD-9-CM codes) as shown in Block 21 to relate the date of service and the procedures performed to the appropriate diagnosis. If multiple procedures are performed, enter the diagnosis code reference number for each service.

 CHAMPVA: Refer to TRICARE guidelines.

Workers' Compensation: Enter all appropriate diagnosis code reference "pointer" numbers from Block 21 to relate appropriate diagnosis to date of service and procedures performed. A maximum of four diagnosis pointers may be referenced. Place commas between multiple diagnosis reference pointers on the same line.

Block 24F

24. A DATE(S) OF SERVICE From MM DD YY	To MM DD YY	B Place of Service	C Type of Service	D PROCEDURES, SERVICES, OR SUPPLIES (Explain Unusual Circumstances) CPT/HCPCS | MODIFIER	E DIAGNOSIS CODE	F $ CHARGES	G DAYS OR UNITS	H EPSDT Family Plan	I EMG	J COB	K RESERVED FOR LOCAL USE
1	030320XX		11		99203		1	70 92	1			12	458977XX
2												
3												
4												
5												
6												

25. FEDERAL TAX I.D. NUMBER	SSN EIN	26. PATIENT'S ACCOUNT NO.	27. ACCEPT ASSIGNMENT? (For govt. claims, see back)	28. TOTAL CHARGE	29. AMOUNT PAID	30. BALANCE DUE
74 10640XX	☐ ☒	010	☒ YES ☐ NO	$ 70 92	$	$ 70 92

All private payers: Enter the fee for each listed service from the appropriate fee schedule. DO NOT ENTER DOLLAR SIGNS OR DECIMAL POINTS. ALWAYS INCLUDE CENTS. If the same service is performed on consecutive days, list the fee for one service in this block and the number of units (times it was performed) in Block 24G. The total for consecutive services should be computed and added into the claim total shown in Block 28.

▶ *When completing the* Workbook *assignments for private, Medicaid, TRICARE, and workers' compensation cases, use the Mock Fee. For Medicare participating provider cases, use the Participating Provider Fee. For nonparticipating provider cases, use the Limiting Charge.*

Block 24G

24. A DATE(S) OF SERVICE						B Place of Service	C Type of Service	D PROCEDURES, SERVICES, OR SUPPLIES (Explain Unusual Circumstances)		E DIAGNOSIS CODE	F $ CHARGES		G DAYS OR UNITS	H EPSDT Family Plan	I EMG	J COB	K RESERVED FOR LOCAL USE
From			To					CPT/HCPCS	MODIFIER								
MM	DD	YY	MM	DD	YY												
03	03	20XX				11		99203		1	70	92	1			12	458977XX

25. FEDERAL TAX I.D. NUMBER	SSN	EIN	26. PATIENT'S ACCOUNT NO.	27. ACCEPT ASSIGNMENT? (For govt. claims, see back)	28. TOTAL CHARGE	29. AMOUNT PAID	30. BALANCE DUE
74 10640XX	☐	☒	010	☒ YES ☐ NO	$ 70 92	$	$ 70 92

All private payers: Enter the number of days or units that apply to each line of service. This block is important for calculating multiple visits, anesthesia minutes, or oxygen volume.

Medicaid: Each service must be listed on separate lines (no date ranging). Indicate that each service was performed one time by listing "1" in this block. List number of visits in 1 day.

Medicare: Enter the number of days or units that apply to each line of service. This block is important for calculating multiple visits, number of miles, units of supplies including drugs, anesthesia minutes, or oxygen volume. See the Medicare Manual for reporting anesthesia time or units and for rounding out figures when billing gas and liquid oxygen units.
Medicare/Medicaid: Refer to Medicare guidelines.
Medicare/Medigap: Refer to Medicare guidelines.
MSP: Refer to Medicare guidelines.

TRICARE: Refer to Medicare guidelines.

CHAMPVA: Refer to Medicare guidelines.

Workers' Compensation: Refer to Medicare guidelines.

Block 24H

24. A DATE(S) OF SERVICE						B Place of Service	C Type of Service	D PROCEDURES, SERVICES, OR SUPPLIES (Explain Unusual Circumstances) CPT/HCPCS MODIFIER			E DIAGNOSIS CODE	F $ CHARGES		G DAYS OR UNITS	H EPSDT Family Plan	I EMG	J COB	K RESERVED FOR LOCAL USE
From MM	DD	YY	To MM	DD	YY													
1	03	03	20XX				11		99203			1	70	92	1			12	458977XX
2																		
3																		
4																		
5																		
6																		

25. FEDERAL TAX I.D. NUMBER	SSN EIN	26. PATIENT'S ACCOUNT NO.	27. ACCEPT ASSIGNMENT? (For govt. claims, see back)	28. TOTAL CHARGE	29. AMOUNT PAID	30. BALANCE DUE
74 10640XX	☐ ☒	010	☒ YES ☐ NO	$ 70 92	$	$ 70 92

 All private payers: Leave blank.

 Medicaid: EPSDT means early, periodic, screening, diagnosis, and treatment, and this refers to a Medicaid service program for children 12 years of age or younger. Enter "E" for EPSDT services or "F" for family planning services, if applicable.

 Medicare: Leave blank.
Medicare/Medicaid: Leave blank.
Medicare/Medigap: Leave blank.
MSP: Leave blank.

 TRICARE: Leave blank.

 CHAMPVA: Leave blank.

Workers' Compensation: Leave blank.

Block 24I

24. A DATE(S) OF SERVICE		B Place of Service	C Type of Service	D PROCEDURES, SERVICES, OR SUPPLIES (Explain Unusual Circumstances) CPT/HCPCS | MODIFIER	E DIAGNOSIS CODE	F $ CHARGES	G DAYS OR UNITS	H EPSDT Family Plan	I EMG	J COB	K RESERVED FOR LOCAL USE
From MM DD YY	To MM DD YY										
030320XX		11		99203	1	70 92	1			12	458977XX

25. FEDERAL TAX I.D. NUMBER	SSN EIN	26. PATIENT'S ACCOUNT NO.	27. ACCEPT ASSIGNMENT? (For govt. claims, see back)	28. TOTAL CHARGE	29. AMOUNT PAID	30. BALANCE DUE
74 10640XX	☐ ☒	010	☒ YES ☐ NO	$ 70 92	$	$ 70 92

All private payers: Leave blank.

Medicaid: EMG stands for the word "emergency" and means that the service was rendered in *hospital* emergency department. Enter "X" if emergency care is provided in an emergency department.

Medicare: Leave blank.
Medicare/Medicaid: Leave blank.
Medicare/Medigap: Leave blank.
MSP: Leave blank.

TRICARE: Enter "X" in this block to indicate that the service was provided in a hospital emergency department.

CHAMPVA: Enter "X" in this block to indicate that the service was provided in a hospital emergency department.

Workers' Compensation: Leave blank.

Block 24J

24. A DATE(S) OF SERVICE						B Place of Service	C Type of Service	D PROCEDURES, SERVICES, OR SUPPLIES (Explain Unusual Circumstances) CPT/HCPCS | MODIFIER	E DIAGNOSIS CODE	F $ CHARGES	G DAYS OR UNITS	H EPSDT Family Plan	I EMG	J COB	K RESERVED FOR LOCAL USE
From MM	DD	YY	To MM	DD	YY										
1 03	03	20XX				11		99203		1	70 | 92	1			12 458977XX
2															
3															
4															
5															
6															

25. FEDERAL TAX I.D. NUMBER	SSN EIN	26. PATIENT'S ACCOUNT NO.	27. ACCEPT ASSIGNMENT? (For govt. claims, see back)	28. TOTAL CHARGE	29. AMOUNT PAID	30. BALANCE DUE
74 10640XX	☐ ☒	010	☒ YES ☐ NO	$ 70 | 92	$	$ 70 | 92

 All private payers: Refer to the note for Block 24K.

 Medicaid: COB means coordination of benefits. Check, if applicable, when the patient has other insurance.

 Medicare: Refer to the note for Block 24K.
Medicare/Medicaid: Refer to the note for Block 24K.
Medicare/Medigap: Refer to the note for Block 24K.
MSP: Refer to the note for Block 24K.

 TRICARE: Leave blank.

 CHAMPVA: Leave blank.

Workers' Compensation: Leave blank.

Block 24K

24. A DATE(S) OF SERVICE From MM DD YY	To MM DD YY	B Place of Service	C Type of Service	D PROCEDURES, SERVICES, OR SUPPLIES (Explain Unusual Circumstances) CPT/HCPCS | MODIFIER	E DIAGNOSIS CODE	F $ CHARGES	G DAYS OR UNITS	H EPSDT Family Plan	I EMG	J COB	K RESERVED FOR LOCAL USE
1 030320XX		11		99203 |	1	70 92	1			12	458977XX
2				|							
3				|							
4				|							
5				|							
6				|							

25. FEDERAL TAX I.D. NUMBER	SSN EIN	26. PATIENT'S ACCOUNT NO.	27. ACCEPT ASSIGNMENT? (For govt. claims, see back)	28. TOTAL CHARGE	29. AMOUNT PAID	30. BALANCE DUE
74 10640XX	☐ ☒	010	☒ YES ☐ NO	$ 70 92	$	$ 70 92

All private payers: Enter the CMS-assigned Provider Identification Number (PIN) or National Provider Identifier (NPI) for each line of service when the performing physician or supplier is in a *group practice* and billing under a group ID number. An individual physician's PIN/NPI is not required if he or she is in solo practice or when billing under his or her individual ID number. **Note:** *Enter the first two digits of the NPI in Block 24J. Enter the remaining eight digits of the NPI in Block 24K, including the two-digit location identifier.*

Medicaid: Leave blank.

Medicare: Enter the CMS-assigned Provider Identification Number (PIN) or National Provider Identifier (NPI) for each line of service when the performing physician or supplier is in a *group practice* and billing under a group ID number. An individual physician's PIN/NPI is not required if he or she is in solo practice or when billing under his or her individual ID number. **Note:** *Enter the first two digits of the NPI in Block 24J. Enter the remaining eight digits of the NPI in Block 24K, including the two-digit location identifier.*
Medicare/Medicaid: Refer to Medicare guidelines.
Medicare/Medigap: Refer to Medicare guidelines.
MSP: Refer to Medicare guidelines.

TRICARE: Enter the physician's state license number when billing for a group practice using one group ID number. The state license number is an alpha character followed by six numeric digits. If there are not six digits, enter appropriate number of zero(s) after the alpha character (e.g., A1234 would be A001234).

CHAMPVA: Refer to TRICARE guidelines.

Workers' Compensation: Leave blank.

Block 25

25. FEDERAL TAX I.D. NUMBER	SSN EIN	26. PATIENT'S ACCOUNT NO.	27. ACCEPT ASSIGNMENT? (For govt. claims, see back)	28. TOTAL CHARGE	29. AMOUNT PAID	30. BALANCE DUE
74 10640XX	☐ ☒	010	☒ YES ☐ NO	$ 70 | 92	$	$ 70 | 92

31. SIGNATURE OF PHYSICIAN OR SUPPLIER INCLUDING DEGREES OR CREDENTIALS (I certify that the statements on the reverse apply to this bill and are made a part thereof.)	32. NAME AND ADDRESS OF FACILITY WHERE SERVICES WERE RENDERED (If other than home or office)	33. PHYSICIAN'S, SUPPLIER'S BILLING NAME, ADDRESS, ZIP CODE & PHONE #
CONCHA ANTRUM MD 030320XX SIGNED *Concha Antrum MD* DATE	SAME	COLLEGE CLINIC 4567 BROAD AVENUE WOODLAND HILLS XY 12345 0001 555 486 9002 PIN# GRP# 3664021CC

reference initials

 All Payers: Enter the physician or supplier's federal tax ID. This number may be the Employer Identification Number (EIN) or Social Security Number (SSN). Check the corresponding box.
▶ A Medicaid case may or may not require a physician's tax ID number, depending on individual state guidelines.
▶ In a Medicare/Medigap case, the physician's federal tax ID number is necessary for Medigap transfer.
▶ *When completing the* Workbook *assignments, enter the physician's EIN number and check the appropriate box.*

Block 26

25. FEDERAL TAX I.D. NUMBER	SSN EIN	26. PATIENT'S ACCOUNT NO.	27. ACCEPT ASSIGNMENT? (For govt. claims, see back)	28. TOTAL CHARGE	29. AMOUNT PAID	30. BALANCE DUE
74 10640XX	☐ ☒	010	☒ YES ☐ NO	$ 70 | 92	$	$ 70 | 92

31. SIGNATURE OF PHYSICIAN OR SUPPLIER INCLUDING DEGREES OR CREDENTIALS (I certify that the statements on the reverse apply to this bill and are made a part thereof.)	32. NAME AND ADDRESS OF FACILITY WHERE SERVICES WERE RENDERED (If other than home or office)	33. PHYSICIAN'S, SUPPLIER'S BILLING NAME, ADDRESS, ZIP CODE & PHONE #
CONCHA ANTRUM MD 030320XX SIGNED *Concha Antrum MD* DATE	SAME	COLLEGE CLINIC 4567 BROAD AVENUE WOODLAND HILLS XY 12345 0001 555 486 9002 PIN# GRP# 3664021CC

reference initials

 All Payers: Enter the patient's account number assigned by the physician's accounting system Do not use dashes or slashes. When Medicare is billed electronically, this block *must be completed.*
▶ *When completing the* Workbook *assignments, list the patient account number when provided.*

Block 27

25. FEDERAL TAX I.D. NUMBER	SSN EIN	26. PATIENT'S ACCOUNT NO.	27. ACCEPT ASSIGNMENT? (For govt. claims, see back)	28. TOTAL CHARGE	29. AMOUNT PAID	30. BALANCE DUE
74 10640XX	☐ ☒	010	☒ YES ☐ NO	$ 70 | 92	$	$ 70 | 92

31. SIGNATURE OF PHYSICIAN OR SUPPLIER INCLUDING DEGREES OR CREDENTIALS (I certify that the statements on the reverse apply to this bill and are made a part thereof.)	32. NAME AND ADDRESS OF FACILITY WHERE SERVICES WERE RENDERED (If other than home or office)	33. PHYSICIAN'S, SUPPLIER'S BILLING NAME, ADDRESS, ZIP CODE & PHONE #
CONCHA ANTRUM MD 030320XX SIGNED *Concha Antrum MD* DATE	SAME	COLLEGE CLINIC 4567 BROAD AVENUE WOODLAND HILLS XY 12345 0001 555 486 9002 PIN# GRP# 3664021CC

reference initials

All private payers: Check "yes" or "no" to indicate whether the physician accepts assignment of benefits. If yes, then the physician agrees to accept the allowed amount paid by the third party plus any copayment or deductible as payment in full.
▶ *When completing the* Workbook *assignments, check "yes."*

 Medicaid: Check "Yes."

Medicare: Check "yes" or "no" to indicate whether the physician accepts assignment of benefits. If yes, then the physician agrees to accept the allowed amount paid by the third party plus any copayment or deductible as payment in full. If this field is left blank, "no" is assumed, and a participating physician's claim will be denied. The following provider or supplier must file claims on an assignment basis:

▶ Clinical diagnostic laboratory services performed in physician's office.
▶ Physicians wishing to accept assignment on clinical laboratory services but not other services should submit two separate claims, one "assigned" for laboratory and one "nonassigned" for other services. Submit all charges on a nonassigned claim, as indicated in Block 27, and write "I accept assignment for the clinical laboratory tests" at the bottom of Block 24.
▶ Participating physician or supplier services.
▶ Physician's services to Medicare/Medicaid patients.
▶ Services of: physician assistants, nurse practitioners, clinical nurse specialists, nurse midwives, certified registered nurse anesthetists, clinical psychologists, and clinical social workers.
▶ Ambulatory surgical center services.
▶ Home dialysis supplies and equipment paid under Method II (monthly capitation payment).
▶ *When completing the* Workbook *assignments, check "yes."*

Medicare/Medicaid: Check "yes."
Medicare/Medigap: Check "yes."
MSP: Check "yes" or "no" to indicate whether the physician accepts assignment of benefits for primary insurance and Medicare.
▶ *When completing the* Workbook *assignments, check "yes."*

TRICARE: Refer to Medicare guidelines. However, participation in TRICARE may be made on a case-by-case basis.

CHAMPVA: Refer to Medicare guidelines.

Workers' Compensation: Leave blank.

Block 28

25. FEDERAL TAX I.D. NUMBER	SSN	EIN	26. PATIENT'S ACCOUNT NO.	27. ACCEPT ASSIGNMENT? (For govt. claims, see back)	28. TOTAL CHARGE	29. AMOUNT PAID	30. BALANCE DUE
74 10640XX		X	010	X YES ☐ NO	$ 70 92	$	$ 70 92

31. SIGNATURE OF PHYSICIAN OR SUPPLIER INCLUDING DEGREES OR CREDENTIALS (I certify that the statements on the reverse apply to this bill and are made a part thereof.)	32. NAME AND ADDRESS OF FACILITY WHERE SERVICES WERE RENDERED (If other than home or office)	33. PHYSICIAN'S, SUPPLIER'S BILLING NAME, ADDRESS, ZIP CODE & PHONE #
CONCHA ANTRUM MD 030320XX	SAME	COLLEGE CLINIC 4567 BROAD AVENUE WOODLAND HILLS XY 12345 0001 555 486 9002
SIGNED *Concha Antrum MD* DATE		PIN# GRP# 3664021CC

reference initials

All Payers: Enter total charges for services listed in Block 24F. If more than one unit is listed in Block 24G, multiply the number of units by the charge and add the amount into the total charge. Do not enter dollar signs or decimal points. Always include cents.

Block 29

25. FEDERAL TAX I.D. NUMBER SSN EIN	26. PATIENT'S ACCOUNT NO.	27. ACCEPT ASSIGNMENT? (For govt. claims, see back)	28. TOTAL CHARGE	29. AMOUNT PAID	30. BALANCE DUE
74 10640XX ☐ ☒	010	☒ YES ☐ NO	$ 70 | 92	$	$ 70 | 92

31. SIGNATURE OF PHYSICIAN OR SUPPLIER INCLUDING DEGREES OR CREDENTIALS (I certify that the statements on the reverse apply to this bill and are made a part thereof.)	32. NAME AND ADDRESS OF FACILITY WHERE SERVICES WERE RENDERED (If other than home or office)	33. PHYSICIAN'S, SUPPLIER'S BILLING NAME, ADDRESS, ZIP CODE & PHONE #
CONCHA ANTRUM MD 030320XX	SAME	COLLEGE CLINIC 4567 BROAD AVENUE WOODLAND HILLS XY 12345 0001
SIGNED *Concha Antrum MD* DATE		PIN# 555 486 9002 GRP# 3664021CC

reference initials

 All private payers: Enter only the amount paid for the charges listed on the claim.

 Medicaid: Enter only the payment on claim by a third-party payer, excluding Medicare.

 Medicare: Enter only the amount paid for the charges listed on the claim.
Medicare/Medicaid: Refer to Medicare guidelines.
Medicare/Medigap: Enter only the amount paid for the charges listed on the claim.
MSP: Enter only the amount paid for the charges listed on the claim. It is mandatory to enter amount paid by primary carrier and attach an explanation of benefits document when billing Medicare.

 TRICARE: Enter only amount paid by *other carrier* for the charges listed on the claim. If the amount includes payment by any other health insurance, the other health insurance explanation of benefits, work sheet, or denial showing the amounts paid must be attached to the claim. Payment from the beneficiary should not be included.

 CHAMPVA: Refer to TRICARE guidelines.

Workers' Compensation: Leave blank.

Block 30

25. FEDERAL TAX I.D. NUMBER	SSN EIN	26. PATIENT'S ACCOUNT NO.	27. ACCEPT ASSIGNMENT? (For govt. claims, see back)	28. TOTAL CHARGE	29. AMOUNT PAID	30. BALANCE DUE
74 10640XX	☐ ☒	010	☒ YES ☐ NO	$ 70|92	$	$ 70|92

31. SIGNATURE OF PHYSICIAN OR SUPPLIER INCLUDING DEGREES OR CREDENTIALS (I certify that the statements on the reverse apply to this bill and are made a part thereof.)	32. NAME AND ADDRESS OF FACILITY WHERE SERVICES WERE RENDERED (If other than home or office)	33. PHYSICIAN'S, SUPPLIER'S BILLING NAME, ADDRESS, ZIP CODE & PHONE #
CONCHA ANTRUM MD 030320XX SIGNED *Concha Antrum MD* DATE	SAME	COLLEGE CLINIC 4567 BROAD AVENUE WOODLAND HILLS XY 12345 0001 555 486 9002 PIN# GRP# 3664021CC

reference initials

 All private payers: Enter balance due on claim (Block 28 less Block 29).

 Medicaid: Leave blank or enter balance due on claim depending on individual state guidelines. ▶ *When completing the* Workbook *assignments, enter the balance due.*

 Medicare: Leave blank.
Medicare/Medicaid: Leave blank.
Medicare/Medigap: Leave blank.
MSP: Leave blank.

 TRICARE: Enter balance due on claim (Block 28 less Block 29).

 CHAMPVA: Enter balance due on claim (Block 28 less Block 29).

 Workers' Compensation: Enter balance due on claim (Block 28 less Block 29).

Block 31

25. FEDERAL TAX I.D. NUMBER	SSN EIN	26. PATIENT'S ACCOUNT NO.	27. ACCEPT ASSIGNMENT? (For govt. claims, see back)	28. TOTAL CHARGE	29. AMOUNT PAID	30. BALANCE DUE
74 10640XX	☐ ☒	010	☒ YES ☐ NO	$ 70|92	$	$ 70|92

31. SIGNATURE OF PHYSICIAN OR SUPPLIER INCLUDING DEGREES OR CREDENTIALS (I certify that the statements on the reverse apply to this bill and are made a part thereof.)	32. NAME AND ADDRESS OF FACILITY WHERE SERVICES WERE RENDERED (If other than home or office)	33. PHYSICIAN'S, SUPPLIER'S BILLING NAME, ADDRESS, ZIP CODE & PHONE #
CONCHA ANTRUM MD 030320XX SIGNED *Concha Antrum MD* DATE	SAME	COLLEGE CLINIC 4567 BROAD AVENUE WOODLAND HILLS XY 12345 0001 555 486 9002 PIN# GRP# 3664021CC

reference initials

All Payers: Type the provider's name and show the signature of the physician or the physician's representative above or below the name. Enter the eight-digit date the form was prepared. Most insurance carriers will accept a stamped signature, but the stamp must be completely inside the block. *Do not* type the name of the association or corporation.

Block 32

25. FEDERAL TAX I.D. NUMBER	SSN EIN	26. PATIENT'S ACCOUNT NO.	27. ACCEPT ASSIGNMENT? (For govt. claims, see back)	28. TOTAL CHARGE	29. AMOUNT PAID	30. BALANCE DUE
74 10640XX	☐ ☒	010	☒ YES ☐ NO	$ 70 | 92	$	$ 70 | 92

31. SIGNATURE OF PHYSICIAN OR SUPPLIER INCLUDING DEGREES OR CREDENTIALS (I certify that the statements on the reverse apply to this bill and are made a part thereof.)	32. NAME AND ADDRESS OF FACILITY WHERE SERVICES WERE RENDERED (If other than home or office)	33. PHYSICIAN'S, SUPPLIER'S BILLING NAME, ADDRESS, ZIP CODE & PHONE #
CONCHA ANTRUM MD 030320XX	SAME	COLLEGE CLINIC 4567 BROAD AVENUE WOODLAND HILLS XY 12345 0001 555 486 9002
SIGNED *Concha Antrum MD* DATE		PIN# GRP# 3664021CC

reference initials

 All private payers: Enter the word "SAME" in the center of the block if the facility furnishing services is the same as that of the biller listed in Block 33. *If other* than home, office, nursing facility, or community mental health center, enter the name, address, and provider number of the facility (e.g., hospital name for physician's hospital services). For durable medical equipment, enter the *location* where the *order is taken.* If a test is performed by a mammography screening center, enter the six-digit certification number approved by the Food and Drug Administration (FDA). When billing for purchased diagnostic tests performed outside the physician's office but billed by the physician, enter the facility's name, address, and CMS-assigned NPI where the test was performed.

 Medicaid: Refer to Medicare guidelines when completing this block; however, use Medicaid facility provider number.

 Medicare: Enter "SAME" in the center of the block if the facility furnishing services is the same as that of the biller listed in Block 33. *If other* than home, office, nursing facility, or community mental health center, enter the name, address, and provider number of the facility (e.g., hospital name for physician's hospital services). For hospital services performed by a physician, the Medicare provider number must be preceded by "HSP." For durable medical equipment, enter the *location* where the *order is taken.* If the test is performed by a mammography screening center, enter the six-digit FDA-approved certification number. When billing for purchased diagnostic tests performed outside the physician's office but billed by the physician, enter the facility's name, address, and CMS-assigned NPI where the test was performed.

Medicare/Medicaid: Refer to Medicare guidelines.

Medicare/Medigap: Refer to Medicare guidelines.

MSP: Refer to Medicare guidelines.

 TRICARE: Refer to private payer guidelines. For partnership providers, indicate the name of the Military Treatment Facility.

CHAMPVA: Refer to private payer guidelines.

Workers' Compensation: Refer to private payer guidelines.

Block 33

25. FEDERAL TAX I.D. NUMBER	SSN EIN	26. PATIENT'S ACCOUNT NO.	27. ACCEPT ASSIGNMENT? (For govt. claims, see back)	28. TOTAL CHARGE	29. AMOUNT PAID	30. BALANCE DUE
74 10640XX	☐ ☒	010	☒ YES ☐ NO	$ 70 | 92	$	$ 70 | 92

31. SIGNATURE OF PHYSICIAN OR SUPPLIER INCLUDING DEGREES OR CREDENTIALS (I certify that the statements on the reverse apply to this bill and are made a part thereof.)	32. NAME AND ADDRESS OF FACILITY WHERE SERVICES WERE RENDERED (If other than home or office)	33. PHYSICIAN'S, SUPPLIER'S BILLING NAME, ADDRESS, ZIP CODE & PHONE #
CONCHA ANTRUM MD 030320XX	SAME	COLLEGE CLINIC 4567 BROAD AVENUE WOODLAND HILLS XY 12345 0001 555 486 9002
SIGNED *Concha Antrum MD* DATE		PIN# GRP# 3664021CC

reference initials

 All private payers: Refer to Medicare guidelines.

 Medicaid: Refer to Medicare guidelines, except use Medicaid's facility provider number.

Medicare: Enter the name, address, and telephone number for the physician, clinic, or supplier billing for services. Either enter the PIN/NPI for a performing physician or supplier who is *not* a member of a group practice in the lower left section of the block or enter the *group number* for a performing physician or supplier who belongs to a group practice and is billing under the group ID number in the right lower section of the block.
Medicare/Medicaid: Refer to Medicare guidelines.
Medicare/Medigap: Refer to Medicare guidelines.
MSP: Refer to Medicare guidelines.

TRICARE: Enter the name, address, and telephone number for the physician, clinic, or supplier billing for services. Radiologists, pathologists, and anesthesiologists may use their billing address if they have no *physical address.* Enter the physician's Tax Identification Number (TIN) in the lower left section of the block; *the group number is not required.*
▶ *When completing the Workbook assignments, enter the performing physician's NPI in the lower left section of the block.*

CHAMPVA: Refer to TRICARE guidelines.

 Workers' Compensation: Enter the name, address, and telephone number of the physician. Individual or group provider numbers or state license number generally are required depending on the insurance carrier's requirements.
▶ *When completing Workbook assignments, follow Medicare guidelines.*

BOTTOM OF FORM

Enter insurance billing specialist's initials in lower left corner of the insurance claim form.

Insurance Program Templates

The following pages show completed CMS-1500 insurance claim forms and templates for the most common insurance programs encountered in a medical practice. Screened areas on each form do not apply to the insurance program example shown and should be left blank. Add a tab at the page margin for ease in flipping to this reference section when completing *Workbook* assignments. Examples illustrating entries for basic cases are:

Figure 6–6   Private payer

Figure 6–7   Back of CMS-1500 insurance claim form

Figure 6–8   Medicaid

Figure 6–9   Medicare

Figure 6–10   Medicare/Medicaid—a crossover claim

Figure 6–11   Medicare/Medigap—a crossover claim

Figure 6–12   MSP—other insurance primary and Medicare secondary

Figure 6–13   TRICARE—Standard

Figure 6–14   CHAMPVA

Figure 6–15   Workers' Compensation

RESOURCES ON THE INTERNET

For a reference list of audio tapes, books, newsletters, periodicals, software, and videotapes, see Appendix B.
HIPAA regulations (information)
Web site: *http://www.hhs.gov*
Standard Code Set (rules and information for electronic claim submission)
Web site: *http://www.aspe.hhs.gov/*
UPIN access: Click "Professionals," click "UPIN Search," scroll down the list of states, enter the physician's name, and submit
Web site: *http://www.hgsa.com*

STUDENT ASSIGNMENT LIST

✔ Study Chapter 6.
✔ Answer the review questions in the *Workbook* to reinforce the theory learned in this chapter and to help prepare you for a future test.
✔ Complete the assignments in the *Workbook* to give you hands-on experience in abstracting information from case histories and financial accounting record cards as well as completing insurance claim forms.
✔ Study the claim sample in the *Workbook* and try to locate as many errors as possible based on the instructions you have been given in this chapter.
✔ Turn to the Glossary at the end of this textbook for a further understanding of the Key Terms used in this chapter.

COMPUTER ASSIGNMENT

Do the exercises for Cases 1 through 6 on the computer disk to review concepts you have learned for this chapter. Follow private insurance OCR guidelines and refer to Block Help when needed. These cases increase in difficulty. The first five cases use an encounter form and Case 6 uses a medical record from which you are required to abstract information and code diagnoses and procedures.

PRIVATE PAYER
No secondary coverage

PRIVATE INSURANCE COMPANY NAME
MAILING ADDRESS
CITY STATE ZIP CODE

1. MEDICARE	MEDICAID	CHAMPUS	CHAMPVA	GROUP HEALTH PLAN	FECA BLK LUNG	OTHER	1a. INSURED'S I.D. NUMBER	(FOR PROGRAM IN ITEM 1)
☐ (Medicare #)	☐ (Medicaid #)	☐ (Sponsor's SSN)	☐ (VA File #)	☒ (SSN or ID)	☐ (SSN)	☐ (ID)	111704521	A482

2. PATIENT'S NAME (Last Name, First Name, Middle Initial)
FOREHAND   HARRY   N

3. PATIENT'S BIRTH DATE
MM 01 | DD 06 | YYYY 1946   M ☒   SEX   F ☐

4. INSURED'S NAME (Last Name, First Name, Middle Initial)
SAME

5. PATIENT'S ADDRESS (No., Street)
1456 MAIN STREET

6. PATIENT RELATIONSHIP TO INSURED
Self ☒ Spouse ☐ Child ☐ Other ☐

7. INSURED'S ADDRESS (No., Street)

CITY
WOODLAND HILLS   STATE XY

8. PATIENT STATUS
Single ☐   Married ☒   Other ☐

CITY   STATE

ZIP CODE
12345 0000   TELEPHONE (include Area Code) (555) 490 9876

Employed ☒   Full-Time Student ☐   Part-Time Student ☐

ZIP CODE   TELEPHONE (include Area Code) (   )

9. OTHER INSURED'S NAME (Last Name, First Name, Middle Initial)

10. IS PATIENT'S CONDITION RELATED TO:

11. INSURED'S POLICY GROUP OR FECA NUMBER

a. OTHER INSURED'S POLICY OR GROUP NUMBER

a. EMPLOYMENT? (CURRENT OR PREVIOUS)
☐ YES   ☒ NO

a. INSURED'S DATE OF BIRTH
MM | DD | YYYY   M ☐   SEX   F ☐

b. OTHER INSURED'S DATE OF BIRTH
MM | DD | YYYY   M ☐   SEX   F ☐

b. AUTO ACCIDENT?   PLACE (State)
☐ YES   ☒ NO

b. EMPLOYER'S NAME OR SCHOOL NAME

c. EMPLOYER'S NAME OR SCHOOL NAME

c. OTHER ACCIDENT?
☐ YES   ☒ NO

c. INSURANCE PLAN NAME OR PROGRAM NAME

d. INSURANCE PLAN NAME OR PROGRAM NAME

10d. RESERVED FOR LOCAL USE

d. IS THERE ANOTHER HEALTH BENEFIT PLAN?
☐ YES   ☒ NO   If yes, return to and complete item 9 a-d.

READ BACK OF FORM BEFORE COMPLETING AND SIGNING THIS FORM.
12. PATIENT'S OR AUTHORIZED PERSON'S SIGNATURE I authorize the release of any medical or other information necessary to process this claim. I also request payment of government benefits either to myself or to the party who accepts assignment below.

SIGNED *Harry N. Forehand*   DATE *March 3, 20XX*

13. INSURED'S OR AUTHORIZED PERSON'S SIGNATURE I authorize payment of medical benefits to the undersigned physician or supplier for services described below.

SIGNED *Harry N. Forehand*

14. DATE OF CURRENT:
MM 03 | DD 01 | YYYY 20XX
ILLNESS (First symptom) OR INJURY (Accident) OR PREGNANCY (LMP)

15. IF PATIENT HAS HAD SAME OR SIMILAR ILLNESS GIVE FIRST DATE   MM | DD | YYYY

16. DATES PATIENT UNABLE TO WORK IN CURRENT OCCUPATION
MM | DD | YYYY   FROM   TO   MM | DD | YYYY

17. NAME OF REFERRING PHYSICIAN OR OTHER SOURCE
PERRY CARDI MD

17a. I.D. NUMBER OF REFERRING PHYSICIAN
67805027XX

18. HOSPITALIZATION DATES RELATED TO CURRENT SERVICES
MM | DD | YYYY   FROM   TO   MM | DD | YYYY

19. RESERVED FOR LOCAL USE

20. OUTSIDE LAB? $ CHARGES
☐ YES   ☒ NO

21. DIAGNOSIS OR NATURE OF ILLNESS OR INJURY (RELATE ITEMS 1,2,3 OR 4 TO ITEM 24E BY LINE)
1. 38200   3.
2.   4.

22. MEDICAID RESUBMISSION CODE   ORIGINAL REF. NO.

23. PRIOR AUTHORIZATION NUMBER

24. A. DATE(S) OF SERVICE						B. Place of Service	C. Type of Service	D. PROCEDURES, SERVICES, OR SUPPLIES (Explain Unusual Circumstances) CPT/HCPCS | MODIFIER	E. DIAGNOSIS CODE	F. $ CHARGES	G. DAYS OR UNITS	H. EPSDT Family Plan	I. EMG	J. COB	K. RESERVED FOR LOCAL USE
From MM 03	DD 03	YYYY 20XX	To MM	DD	YYYY	11		99203	1	70 92	1			12	45897700

25. FEDERAL TAX I.D. NUMBER   SSN EIN
74 1064090   ☐ ☒

26. PATIENT'S ACCOUNT NO.
010

27. ACCEPT ASSIGNMENT? (For govt. claims, see back)
☒ YES ☐ NO

28. TOTAL CHARGE
$ 70 92

29. AMOUNT PAID
$

30. BALANCE DUE
$ 70 92

31. SIGNATURE OF PHYSICIAN OR SUPPLIER INCLUDING DEGREES OR CREDENTIALS (I certify that the statements on the reverse apply to this bill and are made a part thereof.)
CONCHA ANTRUM MD 030320XX

SIGNED *Concha Antrum MD* DATE

32. NAME AND ADDRESS OF FACILITY WHERE SERVICES WERE RENDERED (if other than home or office)

SAME

33. PHYSICIAN'S, SUPPLIER'S BILLING NAME, ADDRESS, ZIP CODE AND PHONE #
COLLEGE CLINIC
4567 BROAD AVENUE
WOODLAND HILLS XY 12345 0001
555 486 9002
PIN#   GRP# 3664021CC

reference initials

Figure 6–6. Front side of the scannable (red ink) Health Insurance Claim Form approved by the American Medical Association's Council on Medical Service. This form is also known as the CMS-1500 and is shown illustrating completion to a private insurance company with no secondary coverage. Third-party payer, state, and local guidelines vary and may not always follow the visual guide presented here. Screened blocks should not be completed for this type of case.

BECAUSE THIS FORM IS USED BY VARIOUS GOVERNMENT AND PRIVATE HEALTH PROGRAMS, SEE SEPARATE INSTRUCTIONS ISSUED BY APPLICABLE PROGRAMS.

NOTICE: Any person who knowingly files a statement of claim containing any misrepresentation or any false, incomplete or misleading information may be guilty of a criminal act punishable under law and may be subject to civil penalties.

REFERS TO GOVERNMENT PROGRAMS ONLY

MEDICARE AND TRICARE PAYMENT: A patient's signature requests that payment be made and authorizes release of any information necessary to process the claim and certifies that the information provided in Blocks 1 through 12 is true, accurate and complete. In the case of a Medicare claim, the patient's signature authorizes any entity to release to Medicare medical and nonmedical information, including employment status, and whether the person has employer group health insurance, liability, no-fault, worker's compensation or other insurance which is responsible to pay for the services for which the Medicare claim is made. See 42 CFR 411.24(a). If item 9 is completed, the patient's signature authorizes release of the information to the health plan or agency shown. In Medicare assigned or TRICARE participation cases, the physician agrees to accept the charge determination of the Medicare carrier or TRICARE fiscal intermediary as the full charge determination of the Medicare carrier or TRICARE fiscal intermediary if this is less than the charge submitted. TRICARE is not a health insurance program but makes payment for health benefits provided through certain affiliations with the Uniformed Services. Information on the patient's sponsor should be provided in those items captioned in "Insured", i.e., items 1a, 4, 6, 7, 9, and 11.

BLACK LUNG AND FECA CLAIMS

The provider agrees to accept the amount paid by the Government as payment in full. See Black Lung and FECA instructions regarding required procedure and diagnosis coding systems.

SIGNATURE OF PHYSICIAN OR SUPPLIER (MEDICARE, TRICARE, FECA AND BLACK LUNG)

I certify that the services shown on this form were medically indicated and necessary for the health of the patient and were personally furnished by me or were furnished incident to my professional service by my employee under my immediate supervision, except as otherwise expressly permitted by Medicare or TRICARE regulations.

For services to be considered as "incident" to a physician's professional service, 1) they must be rendered under the physician's immediate personal supervision by his/her employee, 2) they must be an integral, although incidental part of a covered physician's service, 3) they must be of kinds commonly furnished in physician's offices, and 4) the services of nonphysicians must be included on the physician's bills.

For TRICARE claims, I further certify that I (or any employee) who rendered services am not an active duty member of the Uniformed Services or a civilian employee of the United States Government or a contract employee of the United States Government, either civilian or military (refer to 5 USC 5536). For Black-Lung claims, I further certify that the services performed were for a Black Lung-related disorder.

No Part B Medicare benefits may be paid unless this form is received as required by existing law and regulations (42 CFR 424.32).

NOTICE: Any one who misrepresents or falsifies essential information to receive payment from Federal funds requested by this form may upon conviction be subject to fine and imprisonment under applicable Federal laws.

NOTICE TO PATIENT ABOUT THE COLLECTION AND USE OF MEDICARE, TRICARE, FECA, AND BLACK LUNG INFORMATION
(PRIVACY ACT STATEMENT)

We are authorized by CMS, TRICARE and OWCP to ask you for information needed in the administration of the Medicare, TRICARE, FECA, and Black Lung programs. Authority to collect information is in section 205(a), 1862, 1872 and 1874 of the Social Security Act as amended, 42 CFR411.24(a) and 424.5(a) (6), and 44 USC 3101; CFR 101 et seq and 10 USC 1079 and 1086; 5 USC 8101 et seq; and 30 USC 901 et seq; 38 USC 613; E.O. 9397.

The information we obtain to complete claims under these programs is used to identify you and to determine your eligibility. It is also used to decide if the services and supplies you received are covered by these programs and to insure that proper payment is made.

The information may also be given to other providers of services, carriers, intermediaries, medical review boards, health plans, and other organizations or Federal agencies, for the effective administration of Federal provisions that require other third parties payers to pay primary to Federal program, and as otherwise necessary to administer these programs. For example, it may be necessary to disclose information about the benefits you have used to a hospital or doctor. Additional disclosures are made through routine uses for information contained in systems of records.

FOR MEDICARE CLAIMS: See the notice modifying system No. 09-70-0501, titled 'Carrier Medicare Claims Record,' published in the Federal Register, Vol. 55 No. 177, page 37549, Wed., Sept. 12, 1990, or as updated and republished.

FOR OWCP CLAIMS: Department of Labor, Privacy Act of 1974, "Republication of Notice of Systems of Records," Federal Register, Vol. 55 No. 40, Wed., Feb. 28, 1990, See ESA-5, ESA-6, ESA-12, ESA-13, ESA-30, or as updated and republished.

FOR TRICARE CLAIMS: PRINCIPLE PURPOSE(S): To evaluate eligibility for medical care provided by civilian sources and to issue payment upon establishment of eligibility and determination that the services/supplies received are authorized by law.

ROUTINE USE(S): Information from claims and related documents may be given to the Dept. of Veterans Affairs, the Dept. of Health and Human Services and/or the Dept. of Transportation consistent with their statutory administrative responsibilities under TRICARE/CHAMPVA; to the Dept. of Justice for representation of the Secretary of Defense in civil actions; to the Internal Revenue Service, private collection agencies, and consumer reporting agencies in connection with recoupment claims; and to Congressional Offices in response to inquiries made at the request of the person to whom a record pertains. Appropriate disclosures may be made to other federal, state, local, foreign government agencies, private business entities, and individual providers of care, on matters relating to entitlement, claims adjudication, fraud, program abuse, utilization review, quality assurance, peer review, program integrity, third-party liability, coordination of benefits, and civil and criminal litigation related to the operation of TRICARE.

DISCLOSURES: Voluntary; however, failure to provide information will result in delay in payment or may result in denial of claim. With the one exception discussed below, there are no penalties under these programs for refusing to supply information. However, failure to furnish information regarding the medical services rendered or the amount charged would prevent payment of claims under these programs. Failure to furnish any other information, such as name or claim number, would delay payment of the claim. Failure to provide medical information under FECA could be deemed an obstruction.

It is mandatory that you tell us if you know that another party is responsible for paying for your treatment. Section 1128B of the Social Security Act and 31 USC 3801-3812 provide penalties for withholding this information.

You should be aware that P.L. 100-503, the "Computer Matching and Privacy Protection Act of 1988," permits the government to verify information by way of computer matches.

MEDICAID PAYMENTS (PROVIDER CERTIFICATION)

I hereby agree to keep such records as are necessary to disclose fully the extent of services provided to individuals under the State's Title XIX plan and to furnish information regarding any payments claimed for providing such services as the State Agency or Dept. of Health and Humans Services may request.

I further agree to accept, as payment in full, the amount paid by the Medicaid program for those claims submitted for payment under that program, with the exception of authorized deductible, coinsurance, co-payment or similar cost-sharing charge.

SIGNATURE OF PHYSICIAN (OR SUPPLIER): I certify that the services listed above were medically indicated and necessary to the health of this patient and were personally furnished by me or my employee under my personal direction.

NOTICE: This is to certify that the foregoing information is true, accurate and complete. I understand that payment and satisfaction of this claim will be from Federal and State funds, and that any false claims, statements, or documents, or concealment of a material fact, may be prosecuted under applicable Federal or State laws.

Public reporting burden for this collection of information is estimated to average 15 minutes per response, including time for reviewing instructions, searching existing date sources, gathering and maintaining data needed, and completing and reviewing the collection of information. Send comments regarding this burden estimate or any other aspect of this collection of information, including suggestions for reducing the burden, to CMS, Office of Financial Management, P.O. Box 26684, Baltimore, MD 21207; and to the Office of Management and Budget, Paperwork Reduction Project (OMB-0938-0008), Washington, D.C. 20503.

Figure 6–7. Back side of the CMS-1500 Health Insurance Claim Form approved by the American Medical Association's Council on Medical Service.

MEDICAID
No secondary coverage

MEDICAID FISCAL INTERMEDIARY NAME
MAILING ADDRESS
CITY STATE ZIP CODE

1. MEDICARE	MEDICAID	CHAMPUS	CHAMPVA	GROUP HEALTH PLAN	FECA BLK LUNG	OTHER	1a. INSURED'S I.D. NUMBER	(FOR PROGRAM IN ITEM 1)
☐ (Medicare #)	☒ (Medicaid #)	☐ (Sponsor's SSN)	☐ (VA File #)	☐ (SSN or ID)	☐ (SSN)	☐ (ID)	276835090	

2. PATIENT'S NAME (Last Name, First Name, Middle Initial)	3. PATIENT'S BIRTH DATE	SEX	4. INSURED'S NAME (Last Name, First Name, Middle Initial)
ABRAMSON ADAM	02 12 1995	M ☒ F ☐	

5. PATIENT'S ADDRESS (No., Street)	6. PATIENT RELATIONSHIP TO INSURED	7. INSURED'S ADDRESS (No., Street)
760 FINCH STREET	Self ☐ Spouse ☐ Child ☐ Other ☐	

CITY	STATE	8. PATIENT STATUS	CITY	STATE
WOODLAND HILLS	XY	Single ☐ Married ☐ Other ☐		

ZIP CODE	TELEPHONE (include Area Code)		ZIP CODE	TELEPHONE (include Area Code)
12345	(555) 482 6789	Employed ☐ Full-Time Student ☐ Part-Time Student ☐		( )

9. OTHER INSURED'S NAME (Last Name, First Name, Middle Initial)	10. IS PATIENT'S CONDITION RELATED TO:	11. INSURED'S POLICY GROUP OR FECA NUMBER

a. OTHER INSURED'S POLICY OR GROUP NUMBER	a. EMPLOYMENT? (CURRENT OR PREVIOUS) ☐ YES ☒ NO	a. INSURED'S DATE OF BIRTH MM DD YY SEX M ☐ F ☐

b. OTHER INSURED'S DATE OF BIRTH MM DD YYYY M ☐ SEX F ☐	b. AUTO ACCIDENT? PLACE (State) ☐ YES ☒ NO	b. EMPLOYER'S NAME OR SCHOOL NAME

c. EMPLOYER'S NAME OR SCHOOL NAME	c. OTHER ACCIDENT? ☒ YES ☐ NO	c. INSURANCE PLAN NAME OR PROGRAM NAME

d. INSURANCE PLAN NAME OR PROGRAM NAME	10d. RESERVED FOR LOCAL USE	d. IS THERE ANOTHER HEALTH BENEFIT PLAN? ☐ YES ☐ NO *If yes*, return to and complete item 9 a-d.

READ BACK OF FORM BEFORE COMPLETING AND SIGNING THIS FORM.

12. PATIENT'S OR AUTHORIZED PERSON'S SIGNATURE I authorize the release of any medical or other information necessary to process this claim. I also request payment of government benefits either to myself or to the party who accepts assignment below.

SIGNED _____ DATE _____

13. INSURED'S OR AUTHORIZED PERSON'S SIGNATURE I authorize payment of medical benefits to the undersigned physician or supplier for services described below.

SIGNED _____

14. DATE OF CURRENT: ◄ ILLNESS (First symptom) OR INJURY (Accident) OR PREGNANCY (LMP) MM DD YYYY	15. IF PATIENT HAS HAD SAME OR SIMILAR ILLNESS GIVE FIRST DATE MM DD YYYY	16. DATES PATIENT UNABLE TO WORK IN CURRENT OCCUPATION FROM MM DD YYYY TO MM DD YYYY

17. NAME OF REFERRING PHYSICIAN OR OTHER SOURCE	17a. I.D. NUMBER OF REFERRING PHYSICIAN	18. HOSPITALIZATION DATES RELATED TO CURRENT SERVICES FROM MM DD YYYY TO MM DD YYYY

19. RESERVED FOR LOCAL USE	20. OUTSIDE LAB? ☐ YES ☒ NO $ CHARGES

21. DIAGNOSIS OR NATURE OF ILLNESS OR INJURY (RELATE ITEMS 1,2,3 OR 4 TO ITEM 24E BY LINE)

1. 931   3. _____
2. _____ 4. _____

22. MEDICAID RESUBMISSION CODE _____ ORIGINAL REF. NO. _____

23. PRIOR AUTHORIZATION NUMBER

24. A. DATE(S) OF SERVICE From MM DD YYYY To MM DD YYYY	B. Place of Service	C. Type of Service	D. PROCEDURES, SERVICES, OR SUPPLIES (Explain Unusual Circumstances) CPT/HCPCS MODIFIER	E. DIAGNOSIS CODE	F. $ CHARGES	G. DAYS OR UNITS	H. EPSDT Family Plan	I. EMG	J. COB	K. RESERVED FOR LOCAL USE
071420XX	23	1	99282	1	37 02	1		X		
071420XX	23	2	69200	1	49 93	1		X		

25. FEDERAL TAX I.D. NUMBER SSN EIN	26. PATIENT'S ACCOUNT NO.	27. ACCEPT ASSIGNMENT? (For govt. claims, see back)	28. TOTAL CHARGE	29. AMOUNT PAID	30. BALANCE DUE
71 32061XX ☒	030	☒ YES ☐ NO	$ 86 95	$	$ 86 95

31. SIGNATURE OF PHYSICIAN OR SUPPLIER INCLUDING DEGREES OR CREDENTIALS (I certify that the statements on the reverse apply to this bill and are made a part thereof.)	32. NAME AND ADDRESS OF FACILITY WHERE SERVICES WERE RENDERED (if other than home or office)	33. PHYSICIAN'S, SUPPLIER'S BILLING NAME, ADDRESS, ZIP CODE AND PHONE #
PEDRO ATRICS MD 071420XX SIGNED *Pedro Atrics MD* DATE	COLLEGE HOSPITAL 4500 BROAD AVENUE WOODLAND HILLS XY 12345 0001 HSC 43700F	COLLEGE CLINIC 4567 BROAD AVENUE WOODLAND HILLS XY 12345 0001 555 486 9002 PIN# GRP# HSC12345F

reference initials

Figure 6–8. A Medicaid case with no secondary coverage emphasizing basic elements and screened blocks that do not require completion.

MEDICARE
NO SECONDARY COVERAGE

MEDICARE FISCAL INTERMEDIARY NAME
MAILING ADDRESS
CITY STATE ZIP CODE

1. MEDICARE MEDICAID CHAMPUS CHAMPVA GROUP FECA OTHER	1a. INSURED'S I.D. NUMBER (FOR PROGRAM IN ITEM 1)
[X] (Medicare #) [ ] (Medicaid #) [ ] (Sponsor's SSN) [ ] (VA File #) [ ] HEALTH PLAN (SSN or ID) [ ] BLK LUNG (SSN) [ ] (ID)	123 XX 6789A

2. PATIENT'S NAME (Last Name, First Name, Middle Initial)	3. PATIENT'S BIRTH DATE MM DD YYYY SEX	4. INSURED'S NAME (Last Name, First Name, Middle Initial)
HUTCH BILL	05 07 1910 M[X] F[ ]	

5. PATIENT'S ADDRESS (No., Street)	6. PATIENT RELATIONSHIP TO INSURED	7. INSURED'S ADDRESS (No., Street)
8888 MAIN STREET	Self [ ] Spouse [ ] Child [ ] Other [ ]	
CITY STATE WOODLAND HILLS XY	8. PATIENT STATUS Single [X] Married [ ] Other [ ]	CITY STATE
ZIP CODE TELEPHONE (include Area Code) 12345 (555) 732 1544	Employed [ ] Full-Time Student [ ] Part-Time Student [ ]	ZIP CODE TELEPHONE (include Area Code) ( )

9. OTHER INSURED'S NAME (Last Name, First Name, Middle Initial)	10. IS PATIENT'S CONDITION RELATED TO:	11. INSURED'S POLICY GROUP OR FECA NUMBER NONE
a. OTHER INSURED'S POLICY OR GROUP NUMBER	a. EMPLOYMENT? (CURRENT OR PREVIOUS) [ ] YES [X] NO	a. INSURED'S DATE OF BIRTH MM DD YY SEX M [ ] F [ ]
b. OTHER INSURED'S DATE OF BIRTH MM DD YYYY SEX M [ ] F [ ]	b. AUTO ACCIDENT? PLACE (State) [ ] YES [X] NO	b. EMPLOYER'S NAME OR SCHOOL NAME
c. EMPLOYER'S NAME OR SCHOOL NAME	c. OTHER ACCIDENT? [ ] YES [X] NO	c. INSURANCE PLAN NAME OR PROGRAM NAME
d. INSURANCE PLAN NAME OR PROGRAM NAME	10d. RESERVED FOR LOCAL USE	d. IS THERE ANOTHER HEALTH BENEFIT PLAN? [ ] YES [ ] NO *If yes,* return to and complete item 9 a-d.

READ BACK OF FORM BEFORE COMPLETING AND SIGNING THIS FORM.

12. PATIENT'S OR AUTHORIZED PERSON'S SIGNATURE I authorize the release of any medical or other information necessary to process this claim. I also request payment of government benefits either to myself or to the party who accepts assignment below. SIGNED SOF DATE	13. INSURED'S OR AUTHORIZED PERSON'S SIGNATURE I authorize payment of medical benefits to the undersigned physician or supplier for services described below. SIGNED

14. DATE OF CURRENT: MM DD YYYY ◄ ILLNESS (First symptom) OR INJURY (Accident) OR PREGNANCY (LMP)	15. IF PATIENT HAS HAD SAME OR SIMILAR ILLNESS GIVE FIRST DATE MM DD YYYY	16. DATES PATIENT UNABLE TO WORK IN CURRENT OCCUPATION FROM MM DD YYYY TO MM DD YYYY
17. NAME OF REFERRING PHYSICIAN OR OTHER SOURCE GERALD PRACTON MD	17a. I.D. NUMBER OF REFERRING PHYSICIAN 46278897XX	18. HOSPITALIZATION DATES RELATED TO CURRENT SERVICES FROM MM DD YYYY TO MM DD YYYY
19. RESERVED FOR LOCAL USE		20. OUTSIDE LAB? $ CHARGES [ ] YES [X] NO
21. DIAGNOSIS OR NATURE OF ILLNESS OR INJURY (RELATE ITEMS 1,2,3 OR 4 TO ITEM 24E BY LINE) 1. 487 0 3. 2. 4.		22. MEDICAID RESUBMISSION CODE ORIGINAL REF. NO. 23. PRIOR AUTHORIZATION NUMBER

24. A DATE(S) OF SERVICE From To MM DD YYYY MM DD YYYY	B Place of Service	C Type of Service	D PROCEDURES, SERVICES, OR SUPPLIES (Explain Unusual Circumstances) CPT/HCPCS MODIFIER	E DIAGNOSIS CODE	F $ CHARGES	G DAYS OR UNITS	H EPSDT Family Plan	I EMG	J COB	K RESERVED FOR LOCAL USE
031 020 XX	11		99205	1	132 28	1			64	211067XX

25. FEDERAL TAX I.D. NUMBER SSN EIN 75 67321XX [ ] [X]	26. PATIENT'S ACCOUNT NO. 040	27. ACCEPT ASSIGNMENT? (For govt. claims, see back) [X] YES [ ] NO	28. TOTAL CHARGE $ 132 28	29. AMOUNT PAID $	30. BALANCE DUE $
31. SIGNATURE OF PHYSICIAN OR SUPPLIER INCLUDING DEGREES OR CREDENTIALS (I certify that the statements on the reverse apply to this bill and are made a part thereof.) BRADY COCCIDIOIDES 031020XX SIGNED *Brady Coccidioides MD* DATE	32. NAME AND ADDRESS OF FACILITY WHERE SERVICES WERE RENDERED (if other than home or office) SAME		33. PHYSICIAN'S, SUPPLIER'S BILLING NAME, ADDRESS, ZIP CODE AND PHONE # COLLEGE CLINIC 4567 BROAD AVENUE WOODLAND HILLS XY 12345 0001 555 486 9002 PIN# GRP# 3664021CC		

reference initials

Figure 6–9. Example of a completed CMS-1500 Health Insurance Claim Form for a basic Medicare case with no other insurance coverage. The physician has accepted assignment. Screened blocks should not be completed for a Medicare case with no other insurance.

MEDICARE/MEDICAID
(primary) (secondary)
Crossover claim

MEDICARE FISCAL INTERMEDIARY NAME
MAILING ADDRESS
CITY STATE ZIP CODE

1.	MEDICARE	MEDICAID	CHAMPUS	CHAMPVA	GROUP HEALTH PLAN	FECA BLK LUNG	OTHER	1a. INSURED'S I.D. NUMBER	(FOR PROGRAM IN ITEM 1)
	[X] (Medicare #)	[X] (Medicaid #)	☐ (Sponsor's SSN)	☐ (VA File #)	☐ (SSN or ID)	☐ (SSN)	☐ (ID)	660 XX 2715A	

2. PATIENT'S NAME (Last Name, First Name, Middle Initial)
JOHNSON KATHRYN

3. PATIENT'S BIRTH DATE
MM 09 DD 07 YYYY 1937   SEX M ☐ F [X]

4. INSURED'S NAME (Last Name, First Name, Middle Initial)

5. PATIENT'S ADDRESS (No., Street)
218 VEGA DRIVE

6. PATIENT RELATIONSHIP TO INSURED
Self ☐ Spouse ☐ Child ☐ Other ☐

7. INSURED'S ADDRESS (No., Street)

CITY
WOODLAND HILLS   STATE XY

8. PATIENT STATUS
Single ☐ Married [X] Other ☐

CITY   STATE

ZIP CODE
12345

TELEPHONE (include Area Code)
(555) 482 9112

Employed ☐ Full-Time Student ☐ Part-Time Student ☐

ZIP CODE   TELEPHONE (include Area Code) (   )

9. OTHER INSURED'S NAME (Last Name, First Name, Middle Initial)

10. IS PATIENT'S CONDITION RELATED TO:

11. INSURED'S POLICY GROUP OR FECA NUMBER
NONE

a. OTHER INSURED'S POLICY OR GROUP NUMBER

a. EMPLOYMENT? (CURRENT OR PREVIOUS)
☐ YES [X] NO

a. INSURED'S DATE OF BIRTH
MM DD YY   SEX M ☐ F ☐

b. OTHER INSURED'S DATE OF BIRTH
MM DD YYYY   M ☐ SEX F ☐

b. AUTO ACCIDENT?   PLACE (State)
☐ YES [X] NO

b. EMPLOYER'S NAME OR SCHOOL NAME

c. EMPLOYER'S NAME OR SCHOOL NAME

c. OTHER ACCIDENT?
☐ YES [X] NO

c. INSURANCE PLAN NAME OR PROGRAM NAME

d. INSURANCE PLAN NAME OR PROGRAM NAME

10d. RESERVED FOR LOCAL USE
MCD016745289

d. IS THERE ANOTHER HEALTH BENEFIT PLAN?
☐ YES ☐ NO *If yes,* return to and complete item 9 a-d.

READ BACK OF FORM BEFORE COMPLETING AND SIGNING THIS FORM.
12. PATIENT'S OR AUTHORIZED PERSON'S SIGNATURE I authorize the release of any medical or other information necessary to process this claim. I also request payment of government benefits either to myself or to the party who accepts assignment below.

SIGNED *Kathryn Johnson*   DATE *10/1/XX*

13. INSURED'S OR AUTHORIZED PERSON'S SIGNATURE I authorize payment of medical benefits to the undersigned physician or supplier for services described below.

SIGNED

14. DATE OF CURRENT: ILLNESS (First symptom) OR INJURY (Accident) OR PREGNANCY (LMP)
MM DD YYYY

15. IF PATIENT HAS HAD SAME OR SIMILAR ILLNESS GIVE FIRST DATE MM DD YYYY

16. DATES PATIENT UNABLE TO WORK IN CURRENT OCCUPATION
FROM MM DD YYYY   TO MM DD YYYY

17. NAME OF REFERRING PHYSICIAN OR OTHER SOURCE
BRADY COCCIDIOIDES MD

17a. I.D. NUMBER OF REFERRING PHYSICIAN
64211067XX

18. HOSPITALIZATION DATES RELATED TO CURRENT SERVICES
FROM MM DD YYYY   TO MM DD YYYY

19. RESERVED FOR LOCAL USE

20. OUTSIDE LAB? $ CHARGES
☐ YES [X] NO

21. DIAGNOSIS OR NATURE OF ILLNESS OR INJURY (RELATE ITEMS 1,2,3 OR 4 TO ITEM 24E BY LINE)
1. 172 7   3.
2.   4.

22. MEDICAID RESUBMISSION CODE   ORIGINAL REF. NO.

23. PRIOR AUTHORIZATION NUMBER
7680560012

24. A. DATE(S) OF SERVICE From MM DD YYYY To MM DD YYYY	B. Place of Service	C. Type of Service	D. PROCEDURES, SERVICES, OR SUPPLIES (Explain Unusual Circumstances) CPT/HCPCS | MODIFIER	E. DIAGNOSIS CODE	F. $ CHARGES	G. DAYS OR UNITS	H. EPSDT Family Plan	I. EMG	J. COB	K. RESERVED FOR LOCAL USE
100120XX	24		11600	1	195 06	1			50	307117XX

25. FEDERAL TAX I.D. NUMBER   SSN EIN
74 60789XX   ☐ [X]

26. PATIENT'S ACCOUNT NO.
050

27. ACCEPT ASSIGNMENT? (For govt. claims, see back)
[X] YES ☐ NO

28. TOTAL CHARGE
$ 195 06

29. AMOUNT PAID
$

30. BALANCE DUE
$

31. SIGNATURE OF PHYSICIAN OR SUPPLIER INCLUDING DEGREES OR CREDENTIALS (I certify that the statements on the reverse apply to this bill and are made a part thereof.)
COSMO GRAFF MD   100320XX
SIGNED *Cosmo Graff, MD* DATE

32. NAME AND ADDRESS OF FACILITY WHERE SERVICES WERE RENDERED (if other than home or office)
WOODLAND HILLS AMBULATORY CENTER
1229 CENTER STREET
WOODLAND HILLS XY 12345 0001
95 0513700

33. PHYSICIAN'S, SUPPLIER'S BILLING NAME, ADDRESS, ZIP CODE AND PHONE #
COLLEGE CLINIC
4567 BROAD AVENUE
WOODLAND HILLS XY 12345 0001
555 486 9002
PIN#   GRP# 3664021CC

reference initials

Figure 6–10. Example of a Medicare/Medicaid crossover claim. The CMS-1500 claim form is sent to Medicare (primary) payer) and then processed automatically by Medicaid (secondary payer). Screened blocks should not be completed for this type of case.

MEDICARE/MEDIGAP
(primary) (secondary)
Crossover claim

MEDICARE FISCAL INTERMEDIARY NAME
MAILING ADDRESS
CITY STATE ZIP CODE

1. MEDICARE ☒ (Medicare #)	MEDICAID ☐ (Medicaid #)	CHAMPUS ☐ (Sponsor's SSN)	CHAMPVA ☐ (VA File #)	GROUP HEALTH PLAN ☒ (SSN or ID)	FECA BLK LUNG ☐ (SSN)	OTHER ☐ (ID)	1a. INSURED'S I.D. NUMBER (FOR PROGRAM IN ITEM 1) 419 XX 7272A

2. PATIENT'S NAME (Last Name, First Name, Middle Initial)
BARNES AGUSTA E

3. PATIENT'S BIRTH DATE MM 08 DD 29 YYYY 1917 SEX M ☒ F ☐

4. INSURED'S NAME (Last Name, First Name, Middle Initial)

5. PATIENT'S ADDRESS (No., Street)
356 ENCINA AVENUE

6. PATIENT RELATIONSHIP TO INSURED
Self ☐ Spouse ☐ Child ☐ Other ☐

7. INSURED'S ADDRESS (No., Street)

CITY WOODLAND HILLS   STATE XY

8. PATIENT STATUS
Single ☒ Married ☐ Other ☐
Employed ☐ Full-Time Student ☐ Part-Time Student ☐

CITY   STATE

ZIP CODE 12345 0000   TELEPHONE (include Area Code) (555) 467 2646

ZIP CODE   TELEPHONE (Include Area Code) ( )

9. OTHER INSURED'S NAME (Last Name, First Name, Middle Initial)
SAME

10. IS PATIENT'S CONDITION RELATED TO:

11. INSURED'S POLICY GROUP OR FECA NUMBER
NONE

a. OTHER INSURED'S POLICY OR GROUP NUMBER
MEDIGAP 419167272

a. EMPLOYMENT? (CURRENT OR PREVIOUS)
YES ☐ NO ☒

a. INSURED'S DATE OF BIRTH MM DD YY   M ☐ SEX F ☐

b. OTHER INSURED'S DATE OF BIRTH MM DD YYYY   M ☐ SEX F ☐

b. AUTO ACCIDENT?   PLACE (State)
YES ☐ NO ☒

b. EMPLOYER'S NAME OR SCHOOL NAME

c. EMPLOYER'S NAME OR SCHOOL NAME

c. OTHER ACCIDENT?
YES ☐ NO ☒

c. INSURANCE PLAN NAME OR PROGRAM NAME

d. INSURANCE PLAN NAME OR PROGRAM NAME
CALFCA002

10d. RESERVED FOR LOCAL USE

d. IS THERE ANOTHER HEALTH BENEFIT PLAN?
YES ☐ NO ☐ *If yes,* return to and complete item 9 a-d.

READ BACK OF FORM BEFORE COMPLETING AND SIGNING THIS FORM.

12. PATIENT'S OR AUTHORIZED PERSON'S SIGNATURE I authorize the release of any medical or other information necessary to process this claim. I also request payment of government benefits either to myself or to the party who accepts assignment below.
SIGNED *Agusta E. Barnes*   DATE *11/21/XX*

13. INSURED'S OR AUTHORIZED PERSON'S SIGNATURE I authorize payment of medical benefits to the undersigned physician or supplier for services described below.
SIGNED *Agusta E. Barnes*

14. DATE OF CURRENT: MM DD YYYY ILLNESS (First symptom) OR INJURY (Accident) OR PREGNANCY (LMP)

15. IF PATIENT HAS HAD SAME OR SIMILAR ILLNESS GIVE FIRST DATE MM DD YYYY

16. DATES PATIENT UNABLE TO WORK IN CURRENT OCCUPATION
FROM MM DD YYYY TO MM DD YYYY

17. NAME OF REFERRING PHYSICIAN OR OTHER SOURCE
GASTON INPUT MD

17a. I.D. NUMBER OF REFERRING PHYSICIAN
32783127XX

18. HOSPITALIZATION DATES RELATED TO CURRENT SERVICES
FROM MM DD YYYY TO MM DD YYYY

19. RESERVED FOR LOCAL USE

20. OUTSIDE LAB? YES ☐ NO ☒ $ CHARGES

21. DIAGNOSIS OR NATURE OF ILLNESS OR INJURY (RELATE ITEMS 1,2,3 OR 4 TO ITEM 24E BY LINE)
1. 78659
2.
3.
4.

22. MEDICAID RESUBMISSION CODE   ORIGINAL REF. NO.

23. PRIOR AUTHORIZATION NUMBER

24. A DATE(S) OF SERVICE From MM DD YYYY — To MM DD YYYY	B Place of Service	C Type of Service	D PROCEDURES, SERVICES, OR SUPPLIES (Explain Unusual Circumstances) CPT/HCPCS MODIFIER	E DIAGNOSIS CODE	F $ CHARGES	G DAYS OR UNITS	H EPSDT Family Plan	I EMG	J COB	K RESERVED FOR LOCAL USE
112120XX	11		93350	1	183	31	1		67	805027XX
112120XX	11		93017	1	68	90	1		67	805027XX

25. FEDERAL TAX I.D. NUMBER 70 64217XX SSN ☐ EIN ☒

26. PATIENT'S ACCOUNT NO. 060

27. ACCEPT ASSIGNMENT? (For govt. claims, see back) YES ☒ NO ☐

28. TOTAL CHARGE $ 252 21

29. AMOUNT PAID $

30. BALANCE DUE $

31. SIGNATURE OF PHYSICIAN OR SUPPLIER INCLUDING DEGREES OR CREDENTIALS (I certify that the statements on the reverse apply to this bill and are made a part thereof.)
PERRY CARDI MD
SIGNED *Perry Cardi, MD* DATE 112220XX

32. NAME AND ADDRESS OF FACILITY WHERE SERVICES WERE RENDERED (if other than home or office)
SAME

33. PHYSICIAN'S, SUPPLIER'S BILLING NAME, ADDRESS, ZIP CODE AND PHONE #
COLLEGE CLINIC
4567 BROAD AVENUE
WOODLAND HILLS XY 12345 0001
555 486 9002
PIN#   GRP# 3664021CC

reference initials

Figure 6–11. Example of a completed CMS-1500 Health Insurance Claim Form for a Medicare (primary) and Medigap (secondary) crossover claim. Shaded blocks should not be completed for this type of case.

OTHER INSURANCE/MEDICARE-MSP
(primary)   (secondary)

OTHER INSURANCE COMPANY NAME
MAILING ADDRESS
CITY STATE ZIP CODE

1. MEDICARE	MEDICAID	CHAMPUS	CHAMPVA	GROUP HEALTH PLAN	FECA BLK LUNG	OTHER	1a. INSURED'S I.D. NUMBER	(FOR PROGRAM IN ITEM 1)
[X] (Medicare #)	☐ (Medicaid #)	☐ (Sponsor's SSN)	☐ (VA File #)	[X] (SSN or ID)	☐ (SSN)	☐ (ID)	609 XX 5523A	

2. PATIENT'S NAME (Last Name, First Name, Middle Initial)
BLAIR GWENDOLYN

3. PATIENT'S BIRTH DATE MM 09 DD 01 YYYY 1931 SEX M☐ F[X]

4. INSURED'S NAME (Last Name, First Name, Middle Initial)
BLAIR GWENDOLYN

5. PATIENT'S ADDRESS (No., Street)
416 RICHMOND STREET

6. PATIENT RELATIONSHIP TO INSURED
Self [X] Spouse ☐ Child ☐ Other ☐

7. INSURED'S ADDRESS (No., Street)
SAME

CITY WOODLAND HILLS STATE XY

8. PATIENT STATUS
Single ☐ Married [X] Other ☐
Employed [X] Full-Time Student ☐ Part-Time Student ☐

CITY   STATE

ZIP CODE 12345 0000   TELEPHONE (include Area Code) (555) 459 1519

ZIP CODE   TELEPHONE (include Area Code) ( )

9. OTHER INSURED'S NAME (Last Name, First Name, Middle Initial)

10. IS PATIENT'S CONDITION RELATED TO:

11. INSURED'S POLICY GROUP OR FECA NUMBER
7845931Q

a. OTHER INSURED'S POLICY OR GROUP NUMBER

a. EMPLOYMENT? (CURRENT OR PREVIOUS)
☐ YES [X] NO

a. INSURED'S DATE OF BIRTH MM DD YY SEX M☐ F☐

b. OTHER INSURED'S DATE OF BIRTH MM DD YYYY SEX M☐ F☐

b. AUTO ACCIDENT? PLACE (State)
☐ YES [X] NO

b. EMPLOYER'S NAME OR SCHOOL NAME
CITY LIBRARY

c. EMPLOYER'S NAME OR SCHOOL NAME

c. OTHER ACCIDENT?
☐ YES [X] NO

c. INSURANCE PLAN NAME OR PROGRAM NAME
ABC INSURANCE COMPANY

d. INSURANCE PLAN NAME OR PROGRAM NAME

10d. RESERVED FOR LOCAL USE

d. IS THERE ANOTHER HEALTH BENEFIT PLAN?
☐ YES ☐ NO *If yes,* return to and complete item 9 a-d.

READ BACK OF FORM BEFORE COMPLETING AND SIGNING THIS FORM.
12. PATIENT'S OR AUTHORIZED PERSON'S SIGNATURE I authorize the release of any medical or other information necessary to process this claim. I also request payment of government benefits either to myself or to the party who accepts assignment below.

SIGNED SOF   DATE

13. INSURED'S OR AUTHORIZED PERSON'S SIGNATURE I authorize payment of medical benefits to the undersigned physician or supplier for services described below.

SIGNED SOF

14. DATE OF CURRENT: MM DD YYYY ◄ ILLNESS (First symptom) OR INJURY (Accident) OR PREGNANCY (LMP)

15. IF PATIENT HAS HAD SAME OR SIMILAR ILLNESS GIVE FIRST DATE MM DD YYYY

16. DATES PATIENT UNABLE TO WORK IN CURRENT OCCUPATION FROM MM DD YYYY TO MM DD YYYY

17. NAME OF REFERRING PHYSICIAN OR OTHER SOURCE
GERALD PRACTON MD

17a. I.D. NUMBER OF REFERRING PHYSICIAN
46278897XX

18. HOSPITALIZATION DATES RELATED TO CURRENT SERVICES FROM MM DD YYYY TO MM DD YYYY

19. RESERVED FOR LOCAL USE

20. OUTSIDE LAB? $ CHARGES
☐ YES [X] NO

21. DIAGNOSIS OR NATURE OF ILLNESS OR INJURY (RELATE ITEMS 1,2,3 OR 4 TO ITEM 24E BY LINE)
1. 110 1
2.
3.
4.

22. MEDICAID RESUBMISSION CODE ORIGINAL REF. NO.

23. PRIOR AUTHORIZATION NUMBER

24. A DATE(S) OF SERVICE From MM DD YYYY To MM DD YYYY	B Place of Service	C Type of Service	D PROCEDURES, SERVICES, OR SUPPLIES (Explain Unusual Circumstances) CPT/HCPCS	MODIFIER	E DIAGNOSIS CODE	F $ CHARGES	G DAYS OR UNITS	H EPSDT Family Plan	I EMG	J COB	K RESERVED FOR LOCAL USE
031520XX	11		99243	25	1	103 51	1			54	022287XX
031520XX	11		11750		1	193 45	1			54	022287XX

25. FEDERAL TAX I.D. NUMBER SSN ☐ EIN [X]
62 74109XX

26. PATIENT'S ACCOUNT NO.
070

27. ACCEPT ASSIGNMENT? (For govt. claims, see back)
[X] YES ☐ NO

28. TOTAL CHARGE
$ 296 96

29. AMOUNT PAID
$ 100 00

30. BALANCE DUE
$

31. SIGNATURE OF PHYSICIAN OR SUPPLIER INCLUDING DEGREES OR CREDENTIALS (I certify that the statements on the reverse apply to this bill and are made a part thereof.)
NICK PEDRO DPM   031620XX
SIGNED *Nick Pedro, DPM* DATE

32. NAME AND ADDRESS OF FACILITY WHERE SERVICES WERE RENDERED (if other than home or office)
SAME

33. PHYSICIAN'S, SUPPLIER'S BILLING NAME, ADDRESS, ZIP CODE AND PHONE #
COLLEGE CLINIC
4567 BROAD AVENUE
WOODLAND HILLS XY 12345 0001
555 486 9002
PIN#   GRP# 3664021CC

reference initials

Figure 6–12. Template for a case in which another insurance company is the primary payer and Medicare is the secondary payer (MSP).

TRICARE
No secondary coverage

TRICARE FISCAL INTERMEDIARY
MAILING ADDRESS
CITY STATE ZIP CODE

1. MEDICARE MEDICAID CHAMPUS CHAMPVA GROUP HEALTH PLAN FECA BLK LUNG OTHER		1a. INSURED'S I.D. NUMBER (FOR PROGRAM IN ITEM 1)

1. MEDICARE (Medicare #) □   MEDICAID (Medicaid #) □   CHAMPUS (Sponsor's SSN) [X]   CHAMPVA (VA File #) □   GROUP HEALTH PLAN (SSN or ID) □   FECA BLK LUNG (SSN) □   OTHER (ID) □

1a. INSURED'S I.D. NUMBER (FOR PROGRAM IN ITEM 1): 581147211

2. PATIENT'S NAME (Last Name, First Name, Middle Initial): SMITH SUSAN J

3. PATIENT'S BIRTH DATE: MM 03 DD 16 YYYY 1976   SEX M □ F [X]

4. INSURED'S NAME (Last Name, First Name, Middle Initial): SMITH WILLIAM D

5. PATIENT'S ADDRESS (No., Street): 420 MAPLE STREET

6. PATIENT RELATIONSHIP TO INSURED: Self □ Spouse [X] Child □ Other □

7. INSURED'S ADDRESS (No., Street): SAME

CITY: WOODLAND HILLS   STATE: XY

8. PATIENT STATUS: Single □ Married [X] Other □

CITY: STATE:

ZIP CODE: 12345 0000   TELEPHONE (include Area Code): (555) 789 9898

Employed □ Full-Time Student □ Part-Time Student □

ZIP CODE: TELEPHONE (include Area Code): ( )

9. OTHER INSURED'S NAME (Last Name, First Name, Middle Initial):

10. IS PATIENT'S CONDITION RELATED TO:

11. INSURED'S POLICY GROUP OR FECA NUMBER

a. OTHER INSURED'S POLICY OR GROUP NUMBER

a. EMPLOYMENT? (CURRENT OR PREVIOUS): YES □ NO [X]

a. INSURED'S DATE OF BIRTH: MM 06 DD 12 YY 1974   SEX M [X] F □

b. OTHER INSURED'S DATE OF BIRTH: MM DD YYYY   M □ SEX F □

b. AUTO ACCIDENT? YES □ NO [X]   PLACE (State)

b. EMPLOYER'S NAME OR SCHOOL NAME: USN

c. EMPLOYER'S NAME OR SCHOOL NAME

c. OTHER ACCIDENT? YES □ NO [X]

c. INSURANCE PLAN NAME OR PROGRAM NAME: TRICARE/CHAMPUS

d. INSURANCE PLAN NAME OR PROGRAM NAME

10d. RESERVED FOR LOCAL USE

d. IS THERE ANOTHER HEALTH BENEFIT PLAN? YES □ NO [X]   If yes, return to and complete item 9 a-d.

READ BACK OF FORM BEFORE COMPLETING AND SIGNING THIS FORM.
12. PATIENT'S OR AUTHORIZED PERSON'S SIGNATURE I authorize the release of any medical or other information necessary to process this claim. I also request payment of government benefits either to myself or to the party who accepts assignment below.

SIGNED SOF   DATE

13. INSURED'S OR AUTHORIZED PERSON'S SIGNATURE I authorize payment of medical benefits to the undersigned physician or supplier for services described below.

SIGNED

14. DATE OF CURRENT: MM 10 DD 28 YYYY 20XX   ILLNESS (First symptom) OR INJURY (Accident) OR PREGNANCY (LMP)

15. IF PATIENT HAS HAD SAME OR SIMILAR ILLNESS GIVE FIRST DATE MM DD YYYY

16. DATES PATIENT UNABLE TO WORK IN CURRENT OCCUPATION: FROM MM 07 DD 21 YYYY 20XX TO MM 09 DD 17 YYYY 20XX

17. NAME OF REFERRING PHYSICIAN OR OTHER SOURCE: ADAM LANGERHANS MD

17a. I.D. NUMBER OF REFERRING PHYSICIAN: G05783X

18. HOSPITALIZATION DATES RELATED TO CURRENT SERVICES: FROM MM 08 DD 06 YYYY 20XX TO MM 08 DD 08 YYYY 20XX

19. RESERVED FOR LOCAL USE

20. OUTSIDE LAB? YES □ NO [X] $ CHARGES

21. DIAGNOSIS OR NATURE OF ILLNESS OR INJURY (RELATE ITEMS 1,2,3 OR 4 TO ITEM 24E BY LINE)
1. 650   3.
2.   4.

22. MEDICAID RESUBMISSION CODE   ORIGINAL REF. NO.

23. PRIOR AUTHORIZATION NUMBER

24. A. DATE(S) OF SERVICE From MM DD YYYY — To MM DD YYYY	B. Place of Service	C. Type of Service	D. PROCEDURES, SERVICES, OR SUPPLIES (Explain Unusual Circumstances) CPT/HCPCS | MODIFIER	E. DIAGNOSIS CODE	F. $ CHARGES	G. DAYS OR UNITS	H. EPSDT Family Plan	I. EMG	J. COB	K. RESERVED FOR LOCAL USE
080620XX	21	1	59400	1	1864 30	1				A01817X

25. FEDERAL TAX I.D. NUMBER: 72 57130XX   SSN □ EIN [X]

26. PATIENT'S ACCOUNT NO.: 080

27. ACCEPT ASSIGNMENT? (For govt. claims, see back) YES [X] NO □

28. TOTAL CHARGE: $ 1864 30

29. AMOUNT PAID: $

30. BALANCE DUE: $ 1864 30

31. SIGNATURE OF PHYSICIAN OR SUPPLIER INCLUDING DEGREES OR CREDENTIALS (I certify that the statements on the reverse apply to this bill and are made a part thereof.)
BERTHA CAESAR MD
SIGNED Bertha Caesar, MD   DATE 081020XX

32. NAME AND ADDRESS OF FACILITY WHERE SERVICES WERE RENDERED (if other than home or office)
COLLEGE HOSPITAL
4500 BROAD AVENUE
WOODLAND HILLS XY 12345 0001
95 0731067

33. PHYSICIAN'S, SUPPLIER'S BILLING NAME, ADDRESS, ZIP CODE AND PHONE #
COLLEGE CLINIC
4567 BROAD AVENUE
WOODLAND HILLS XY 12345 0001
555 486 9002
PIN# 7257130XX   GRP#

reference initials

Figure 6–13. Example of a completed CMS-1500 claim form, used when billing for professional services rendered in a TRICARE Standard case. Screened blocks should not be completed for this type of case.

CHAMPVA
No secondary coverage

CHAMPVA INSURANCE COMPANY NAME
MAILING ADDRESS
CITY STATE ZIP CODE

1. MEDICARE	MEDICAID	CHAMPUS	CHAMPVA	GROUP HEALTH PLAN	FECA BLK LUNG	OTHER	1a. INSURED'S I.D. NUMBER	(FOR PROGRAM IN ITEM 1)
☐ (Medicare #)	☐ (Medicaid #)	☐ (Sponsor's SSN)	☒ (VA File #)	☐ (SSN or ID)	☐ (SSN)	☐ (ID)	560 XX 4444	

2. PATIENT'S NAME (Last Name, First Name, Middle Initial)	3. PATIENT'S BIRTH DATE	SEX	4. INSURED'S NAME (Last Name, First Name, Middle Initial)
DEXTER BRUCE R	MM 03 DD 13 YYYY 1934	M ☒ F ☐	DEXTER BRUCE R

5. PATIENT'S ADDRESS (No., Street)	6. PATIENT RELATIONSHIP TO INSURED	7. INSURED'S ADDRESS (No., Street)
226 IRWIN ROAD	Self ☒ Spouse ☐ Child ☐ Other ☐	SAME

CITY	STATE	8. PATIENT STATUS	CITY	STATE
WOODLAND HILLS	XY	Single ☒ Married ☐ Other ☐		

ZIP CODE	TELEPHONE (include Area Code)		ZIP CODE	TELEPHONE (include Area Code)
12345 0000	(555) 497 1338	Employed ☐ Full-Time Student ☐ Part-Time Student ☐		( )

9. OTHER INSURED'S NAME (Last Name, First Name, Middle Initial)	10. IS PATIENT'S CONDITION RELATED TO:	11. INSURED'S POLICY GROUP OR FECA NUMBER
		023

a. OTHER INSURED'S POLICY OR GROUP NUMBER	a. EMPLOYMENT? (CURRENT OR PREVIOUS)	a. INSURED'S DATE OF BIRTH	SEX
	☒ YES ☐ NO	MM DD YY	M ☐ F ☐

b. OTHER INSURED'S DATE OF BIRTH	SEX	b. AUTO ACCIDENT?	PLACE (State)	b. EMPLOYER'S NAME OR SCHOOL NAME
MM DD YYYY	M ☐ F ☐	☐ YES ☒ NO		USAF

c. EMPLOYER'S NAME OR SCHOOL NAME	c. OTHER ACCIDENT?	c. INSURANCE PLAN NAME OR PROGRAM NAME
	☐ YES ☒ NO	

d. INSURANCE PLAN NAME OR PROGRAM NAME	10d. RESERVED FOR LOCAL USE	d. IS THERE ANOTHER HEALTH BENEFIT PLAN?
		☐ YES ☒ NO If yes, return to and complete item 9 a-d.

READ BACK OF FORM BEFORE COMPLETING AND SIGNING THIS FORM.
12. PATIENT'S OR AUTHORIZED PERSON'S SIGNATURE I authorize the release of any medical or other information necessary to process this claim. I also request payment of government benefits either to myself or to the party who accepts assignment below.

SIGNED SOF   DATE

13. INSURED'S OR AUTHORIZED PERSON'S SIGNATURE I authorize payment of medical benefits to the undersigned physician or supplier for services described below.

SIGNED

14. DATE OF CURRENT: ILLNESS (First symptom) OR INJURY (Accident) OR PREGNANCY (LMP)	15. IF PATIENT HAS HAD SAME OR SIMILAR ILLNESS GIVE FIRST DATE	16. DATES PATIENT UNABLE TO WORK IN CURRENT OCCUPATION
MM DD YYYY	MM DD YYYY	FROM MM DD YYYY TO MM DD YYYY

17. NAME OF REFERRING PHYSICIAN OR OTHER SOURCE	17a. I.D. NUMBER OF REFERRING PHYSICIAN	18. HOSPITALIZATION DATES RELATED TO CURRENT SERVICES
GERALD PRACTON MD	C01402X	FROM MM 07 DD 29 YYYY 20XX TO MM 07 DD 31 YYYY 20XX

19. RESERVED FOR LOCAL USE	20. OUTSIDE LAB?	$ CHARGES
	☐ YES ☒ NO	

21. DIAGNOSIS OR NATURE OF ILLNESS OR INJURY (RELATE ITEMS 1,2,3 OR 4 TO ITEM 24E BY LINE)	22. MEDICAID RESUBMISSION
1. 600 0 3.	CODE ORIGINAL REF. NO.
2. 4.	23. PRIOR AUTHORIZATION NUMBER

24. A. DATE(S) OF SERVICE		B. Place of Service	C. Type of Service	D. PROCEDURES, SERVICES, OR SUPPLIES (Explain Unusual Circumstances) CPT/HCPCS MODIFIER	E. DIAGNOSIS CODE	F. $ CHARGES		G. DAYS OR UNITS	H. EPSDT Family Plan	I. EMG	J. COB	K. RESERVED FOR LOCAL USE
From MM DD YYYY	To MM DD YYYY											
072920XX		21	2	52601	1	1193	53	1				C06430X

25. FEDERAL TAX I.D. NUMBER	SSN EIN	26. PATIENT'S ACCOUNT NO.	27. ACCEPT ASSIGNMENT? (For govt. claims, see back)	28. TOTAL CHARGE	29. AMOUNT PAID	30. BALANCE DUE
77 86531XX	☐ ☒	090	☒ YES ☐ NO	$ 1193 53	$	$ 1193 53

31. SIGNATURE OF PHYSICIAN OR SUPPLIER INCLUDING DEGREES OR CREDENTIALS (I certify that the statements on the reverse apply to this bill and are made a part thereof.)	32. NAME AND ADDRESS OF FACILITY WHERE SERVICES WERE RENDERED (if other than home or office)	33. PHYSICIAN'S, SUPPLIER'S BILLING NAME, ADDRESS, ZIP CODE AND PHONE #
GENE ULIBARRI MD 073020XX	COLLEGE HOSPITAL 4500 BROAD AVENUE WOODLAND HILLS XY 12345 0001 95 0731067	COLLEGE CLINIC 4567 BROAD AVENUE WOODLAND HILLS XY 12345 0001 555 486 9002
SIGNED Gene Ulibarri DATE		PIN# 7786531XX GRP#

reference initials

Figure 6-14. An example of a completed CMS-1500 Health Insurance Claim Form for a CHAMPVA case with no secondary coverage. Screened blocks should not be completed for this type of case.

WORKERS' COMPENSATION

WORKERS' COMPENSATION INSURANCE COMPANY NAME
MAILING ADDRESS
CITY STATE ZIP CODE

1. MEDICARE MEDICAID CHAMPUS CHAMPVA GROUP HEALTH PLAN FECA BLK LUNG OTHER	1a. INSURED'S I.D. NUMBER (FOR PROGRAM IN ITEM 1)
☐ (Medicare #) ☐ (Medicaid #) ☐ (Sponsor's SSN) ☐ (VA File #) ☐ (SSN or ID) ☐ (SSN) ☒ (ID)	667289

2. PATIENT'S NAME (Last Name, First Name, Middle Initial)	3. PATIENT'S BIRTH DATE MM DD YYYY SEX	4. INSURED'S NAME (Last Name, First Name, Middle Initial)
BARTON PETER A	11 14 1976 M ☒ F ☐	D F CONSTRUCTION

5. PATIENT'S ADDRESS (No., Street)	6. PATIENT RELATIONSHIP TO INSURED	7. INSURED'S ADDRESS (No., Street)
14890 DAISY AVENUE	Self ☐ Spouse ☐ Child ☐ Other ☒	1212 HARDROCK PLACE

CITY	STATE	8. PATIENT STATUS	CITY	STATE
WOODLAND HILLS	XY	Single ☐ Married ☐ Other ☐	WOODLAND HILLS	XY

ZIP CODE	TELEPHONE (include Area Code)		ZIP CODE	TELEPHONE (include Area Code)
12345 0000	(555) 427 7698	Employed ☒ Full-Time Student ☐ Part-Time Student ☐	12345 0000	(555) 427 8200

9. OTHER INSURED'S NAME (Last Name, First Name, Middle Initial)	10. IS PATIENT'S CONDITION RELATED TO:	11. INSURED'S POLICY GROUP OR FECA NUMBER
a. OTHER INSURED'S POLICY OR GROUP NUMBER	a. EMPLOYMENT? (CURRENT OR PREVIOUS) ☒ YES ☐ NO	a. INSURED'S DATE OF BIRTH MM DD YY SEX M ☐ F ☐
b. OTHER INSURED'S DATE OF BIRTH MM DD YYYY SEX M ☐ F ☐	b. AUTO ACCIDENT? ☐ YES ☒ NO PLACE (State)	b. EMPLOYER'S NAME OR SCHOOL NAME
c. EMPLOYER'S NAME OR SCHOOL NAME	c. OTHER ACCIDENT? ☐ YES ☒ NO	c. INSURANCE PLAN NAME OR PROGRAM NAME
d. INSURANCE PLAN NAME OR PROGRAM NAME	10d. RESERVED FOR LOCAL USE	d. IS THERE ANOTHER HEALTH BENEFIT PLAN? ☐ YES ☐ NO *If yes,* return to and complete item 9 a-d.

READ BACK OF FORM BEFORE COMPLETING AND SIGNING THIS FORM.

12. PATIENT'S OR AUTHORIZED PERSON'S SIGNATURE I authorize the release of any medical or other information necessary to process this claim. I also request payment of government benefits either to myself or to the party who accepts assignment below.

SIGNED _____ DATE _____

13. INSURED'S OR AUTHORIZED PERSON'S SIGNATURE I authorize payment of medical benefits to the undersigned physician or supplier for services described below.

SIGNED _____

14. DATE OF CURRENT: MM DD YYYY ◄ ILLNESS (First symptom) OR INJURY (Accident) OR PREGNANCY (LMP)	15. IF PATIENT HAS HAD SAME OR SIMILAR ILLNESS GIVE FIRST DATE MM DD YYYY	16. DATES PATIENT UNABLE TO WORK IN CURRENT OCCUPATION
01 04 20XX		FROM 01 04 20XX TO 03 27 20XX

17. NAME OF REFERRING PHYSICIAN OR OTHER SOURCE	17a. I.D. NUMBER OF REFERRING PHYSICIAN	18. HOSPITALIZATION DATES RELATED TO CURRENT SERVICES MM DD YYYY
		FROM TO

19. RESERVED FOR LOCAL USE		20. OUTSIDE LAB? ☐ YES ☐ NO $ CHARGES

21. DIAGNOSIS OR NATURE OF ILLNESS OR INJURY (RELATE ITEMS 1,2,3 OR 4 TO ITEM 24E BY LINE)	22. MEDICAID RESUBMISSION CODE ORIGINAL REF. NO.
1. 71831 3.	
2. 4.	23. PRIOR AUTHORIZATION NUMBER

24. A. DATE(S) OF SERVICE From MM DD YYYY To MM DD YYYY	B. Place of Service	C. Type of Service	D. PROCEDURES, SERVICES, OR SUPPLIES (Explain Unusual Circumstances) CPT/HCPCS MODIFIER	E. DIAGNOSIS CODE	F. $ CHARGES	G. DAYS OR UNITS	H. EPSDT Family Plan	I. EMG	J. COB	K. RESERVED FOR LOCAL USE
022720XX	11	1	29055	1	150 51	1				

25. FEDERAL TAX I.D. NUMBER SSN EIN	26. PATIENT'S ACCOUNT NO.	27. ACCEPT ASSIGNMENT? (For govt. claims, see back)	28. TOTAL CHARGE	29. AMOUNT PAID	30. BALANCE DUE
74 65412XX ☒	100	☐ YES ☐ NO	$ 150 51	$	$ 150 51

31. SIGNATURE OF PHYSICIAN OR SUPPLIER INCLUDING DEGREES OR CREDENTIALS (I certify that the statements on the reverse apply to this bill and are made a part thereof.)	32. NAME AND ADDRESS OF FACILITY WHERE SERVICES WERE RENDERED (if other than home or office)	33. PHYSICIAN'S, SUPPLIER'S BILLING NAME, ADDRESS, ZIP CODE AND PHONE #
RAYMOND SKELTON MD 022820XX SIGNED *Raymond Skelton, M.D.*	SAME	COLLEGE CLINIC 4567 BROAD AVENUE WOODLAND HILLS XY 12345 0001 555 486 9002 PIN# GRP# 3664021CC

reference initials

Figure 6–15. An example of a completed CMS-1500 Health Insurance Claim Form for a workers' compensation case. Screened blocks should not be completed for this type of case.

Electronic
Data Interchange (EDI)

7

- List prevention measures to retain computer confidentiality.
- Describe what is necessary when adopting a computer system.
- Explain the difference between carrier-direct and clearinghouse electronically transmitted claims.
- State the job duties of an electronic claims professional.
- Describe the use of patient encounter forms, crib sheets, and scannable encounter forms in electronic claim submission.
- Indicate some computer transmission problems.
- Name some types of interactive computer transactions.

OBJECTIVES*

After reading this chapter you should be able to:

- Specify differences between manual and electronic claim submission.
- Identify components of a computer system.
- Define computer terminology and interpret abbreviations.
- Explain how to manage and store computer data.

KEY TERMS

audit trail

back up

batch

bit

bug

byte

carrier-direct system

central processing unit (CPU)

clearinghouse

debug

down time

electronic claims processor (ECP)

electronic claim submission (ECS)

electronic data interchange (EDI)

electronic mail (e-mail)

encryption

file

format

gigabyte

hard copy

hardware

input

interactive transaction

interface

Internet

keypad

kilobyte

local area network (LAN)

megabyte

memory

modem

mouse

multipurpose billing form

output

Continued.

---

*Performance objectives and exercises for hands-on practical experience for this chapter appear in the *Workbook*.

History of an Electronic Claim

In the 1960s and early 1970s large hospitals began submitting electronic claims for payment to insurance carriers. An *electronic claim* is one that is submitted by means of central direct wire, dial-in-telephone, or personal computer upload or download. The transmission of such claims became known as **electronic data interchange (EDI).** This is a process by which understandable data are sent back and forth via computer linkages between two or more entities that function alternatively as sender and receiver. Electronic transmissions are sent encrypted so that they cannot be easily read if they are intercepted by a wrong individual. **Encryption** is used to assign a code to represent data and is done for security purposes. In encrypted (encoded) versions, the data look like gibberish to unauthorized users and must be decoded to be used or read.

In the mid-1970s the Medicare program expanded, thereby increasing the number of covered individuals. To reduce the number of paper claims and administrative costs, the Centers for Medicaid and Medicare Services (CMS) began to emphasize **electronic claims submission (ECS).** This system of transmission was practical only for hospitals and large medical practices, because some carriers required 25 or more claims per batch. A **batch** is a group of claims for different patients sent at the same time from one facility.

In 1981 the National Electronic Information Corporation (NEIC) was formed by 11 major insurance companies. This provided a national network to receive process, edit, sort, and transmit electronic claims to insurers. The NEIC system allows the physician to use one version of software to communicate with different insurers. Claims can be submitted directly to NEIC for routing or through a network of independent software vendors, clearinghouses, and billing centers. A **clearinghouse,** also referred to as a third-party administrator (TPA), is an entity that receives transmission of claims, separates the claims by carrier, performs software edits on each claim to check for errors, and sends claims electronically to the correct insurance payer.

CMS has a Medicare Transaction System (MTS) that is for Part A (hospital services) and Part B (outpatient medical services) claims processing. This system replaces the numerous software processing programs formerly used by Medicare's claims contractors with a national electronic standard program. The system is used for nearly all Medicare transactions, including claims submission called electronic medical claims (EMC), payment, direct deposit, online eligibility verification, coordination of benefits, and claims status.

Advantages of Electronic Claim Submission

Currently almost all insurance companies participate in electronic claim submission. Claims sent electronically require no signing or stamping, no searching for an insurance carrier's address, no postage fees or trips to the post office, and no storing or filing of claim forms in a file cabinet. Also they leave an **audit trail,** a chronological record of submitted data that can be traced to the source to determine the place of origin. Generally cash flow is improved and less time is spent processing claims, thereby freeing staff for other duties. Information goes from one computer to another, which reduces overhead by decreasing labor costs and human error. Payment from electronically submitted claims is received in 2 weeks or less. In comparison, payment from claims completed manually and sent by mail is received in 4 to

6 weeks. A proof of receipt is generated at the carrier's end, thus eliminating the insurance carrier's excuse, "We never received the claim, please resubmit."

Another important advantage of ECS is the online error-edit process that may be incorporated into the software in the physician's office, clearinghouse, or insurance company. This allows the person processing the claim to know of an error immediately so a correction can be made. The insurance carrier writes a check, returns the claim for more information, or sets it aside for manual review. Information about problem claims can be telecommunicated immediately, allowing quicker submission of corrected data.

Disadvantages of Electronic Claim Submission

A disadvantage of sending claims electronically is that each insurance company has its own standards and each provider requires billing software with the capability of converting the claims data to what the carrier wants. In addition, some carriers require local codes. With thousands of insurance companies, this is very confusing to software programmers and providers. Large manuals are required to read each carrier's claims denial codes.

HIPAA Compliance Alert

Health Insurance Portability and Accountability Act and Electronic Claims

As part of the Balanced Budget Act of 1997, the Health Insurance Portability and Accountability Act (HIPAA) was created to establish new standards and guidelines for insurance claims, patient privacy, security, and more. The first standard established was with insurance claims. The purpose of this was to eventually eliminate the requirement to send claims by paper and establish one standard for claims submission, claims payment, benefit verification, and more. Code sets, such as the American Medical Association's Current Procedural Terminology (CPT) and the World Health Organization's *International Classification of Diseases, 9th Revision, Clinical Modification* (ICD-9-CM), Volume 2 were established as the only code sets for providers and carriers to use. Local codes were eliminated. Covered entities, such as hospitals, providers, and health plans, must become compliant with these new standards. The target date for everyone to become compliant with this law was extended to October 16, 2003. Medicare will not pay any paper claim received after October 16, 2003.

Many carriers, to become compliant with the electronic portion of HIPAA, began establishing Internet Web sites so that providers can check eligibility, submit claims, and check claims status.

Only covered entities are required to become compliant with the HIPAA laws. An independent medical biller or medical billing company is not a covered entity. It is known as a Business Associate because it performs a service for the covered entity. However a Business Associate does have some responsibility to ensure compliance with HIPAA. If it sends claims, then its or the clearinghouse's software must be HIPAA compliant with the new standards. A Business Associate Agreement must be in place with each provider and with anyone to whom they send Personal Health Information (PHI). If it is sending accounts to a collection agency, the provider should have a Business Associate Agreement with the collection agency, even though the billing service or clearinghouse is sending patient information. This is because the contract with the collection agency is between the provider and the collection agency.

The Privacy portion of HIPAA became effective on April 15, 2003. This gives patients access to their health information. Covered entities and their Business Associates must take extra precautions to safeguard a patient's personal health information considering that most or all of this information is contained on computer systems and is sent electronically. Business Associates must ensure that the PHI they are provided is protected from unauthorized disclosure. Receive assurances from those to whom PHI are sent that they too are safeguarding this information. Develop Compliance Plans and Policies and Procedures outlining the protection of this information and the steps taken in the event there is an unauthorized disclosure. To assist in this someone should be assigned the duties of Privacy Officer and Security Officer. Perform a GAP Analysis of the business to find areas that might cause problems. Examples of a GAP Analysis would be to observe how PHI is distributed within the company. Are documents showing PHI left on desktops for others to see or take? Check trash cans and dumpsters to see what is being thrown out. Listen to phone calls to determine if PHI is being discussed in an unofficial setting. Check facsimile machines to see if cover sheets are marked to let the recipient know they are receiving PHI. Look to see where facsimile and copy machines are located. Can nonemployees access this area? Are employees talking about cases at the break room or lunch table? If coders are coding from home, how are they protecting the PHI they are taking with them? Is this information safe from theft or

Figure 7–1. Illustration of the hardware components of a computer system. The system consists of input devices (keyboard, 7, and mouse, 6), a central processing device (inside the system unit, 1), output devices (monitor, 3, and printer, 9), auxiliary storage devices (disk drives 4, 5, and 8, also located within the system unit), and a transmission device or modem (inside the system unit, 2).

damage? Can their family members access this information or is it secured when not working? Are computer systems safe from outside hackers? Are login and logout procedures required when an employee is not working at his or her desk? What does the employee do with the PHI when not at his or her desk? One has an idea where he or she stands once a GAP Analysis is performed. All one may have to do next is train the staff on HIPAA, continue creating policies and procedures, and monitor day-to-day operations.

In February 2003 the rules for the Security aspect of HIPAA were published. Covered entities and their Business Associates have until February 2005 to become compliant with this portion of the law.

Computer Components

When working in a business whether at an in-home office or a facility, equipment may have mechanical or technical problems at times. Thus one must know the workings of the *computer* as well as some of the *peripheral* devices. A computer is a machine that uses electricity to maneuver information according to programmed instructions in a larger volume and at a lower cost, faster, and more efficiently than can be done by hand (Fig. 7–1). Peripherals are input, output, and storage units that are attached to the computer by cables, such as zip drives, speakers, printer, and modems. A **modem** is a device (internal or external peripheral) used to transmit electronic information over a dedicated telephone line. A modem accomplishes the task of transmitting an electronic claim to the insurance carrier.

Hardware

Hardware represents the physical components of a computer system (e.g., display screen, hard disk, keyboard, and mouse) (Fig. 7–2). First, data must be **input** using a keyboard, which resembles a typewriter keyboard, or a **keypad,** which is used for numeric computation. A **mouse,** *track ball,* or scanning device can also be used to input information. The computer has a television-like screen attached to it, called a **video display terminal (VDT),** which displays the output of data, or **soft copy.** It is also known as a monitor, cathode ray tube (CRT), or liquid crystal display (LCD). The computer is set up to **interface** with a computer **output** device, a printer, which produces **hard copy** of data in readable form. Printer output can be produced by dot matrix, laser-generated copy, or ink jet.

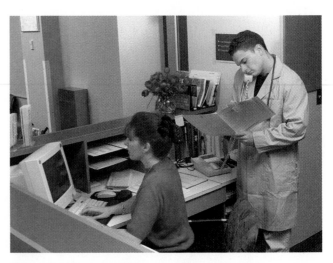

Figure 7–2. Insurance billing specialist's workstation.

Software

Software represents the **program** (computer instructions) necessary to make hardware perform a specific task. Although each insurer has different software, physicians typically select one that can interface with the insurance companies they deal with most. Software programs can be purchased or leased. Many types of software are used to perform medical insurance billing.

Memory

In addition to hardware and software a computer has a **central processing unit (CPU),** which acts as the brain of the computer system. It includes the computing capability and working memory. A computer contains two types of **memory: read-only memory (ROM)** and **random access memory (RAM).** Data stored in ROM can be read but not changed. ROM usually contains a permanent program. Whichever medical software program is used is stored in ROM. RAM allows data to be stored randomly and retrieved directly by specifying the address location. The data entered into the medical software are stored in RAM. If the computer is turned off and the data have not been saved, then the data are erased in RAM. Data always should be saved on the hard disk. They also can be saved on a magnetic storage device, such as a CD-ROM recordable disk, zip disk, or 3.5-inch disk (Fig. 7–3).

Computer storage capacity to save data in memory is measured in **bytes,** each of which consists of a group of eight **bits** (from "*bi*nary dig*its*"), the smallest unit of storage possible (Box 7–1). One byte of storage capacity holds one piece of information. Memory capacity is measured in kilobytes, megabytes, or gigabytes. One **kilobyte** stores 1024 bytes or characters, and one **megabyte** is equal to 1000 kilobytes. A **gigabyte** holds approximately 1 billion bytes or characters.

Networks

Local Area Network

Many business sites have more than one or two computer stations. A system setup, referred to as a **local area network (LAN),** is used to interlink multiple computers found, for example, in hospitals, clinics, and large medical practices. In a LAN setup computers that are contained within a room or building are connected by cables, allowing them to share files and devices such as printers.

Installing software on a LAN computer has different installation instructions then when installing software on a single computer terminal.

A

B

Figure 7–3. A, Components of a 3.5-inch disk. **B,** Components of a compact disk-read-only memory (CD-ROM) showing one of the concentric circles in which data are recorded.

In fact, many schools have the computers networked. Therefore this type of system setup may be encountered before actually beginning work as an insurance biller.

Wide Area Network

A *wide area network (WAN)* is a communications network that covers a wide geographic area. Examples of wide area networks are America Online, CompuServe, the worldwide airline reservation system, and in the medical field, MEDLINE and Physicians Online. MEDLINE was developed by the National Library of Medicine and is a database with access fees that provides 7 million references from approximately 4000 medical journals published worldwide.

BOX 7–1

Computer Storage Memory

Bit	0 and 1 (smallest storage unit)
Byte	8 bits
Kilobyte	1024 bytes
Megabyte	1000 kilobytes
Gigabyte	1000 megabytes or 1 billion bytes

The Internet and the World Wide Web

The **Internet** is a large interconnected message-forwarding system linking academic, commercial, government, and military computer networks all over the world. Applications available are **electronic mail (e-mail)**, online conversations (one-on-one or in chat rooms), information retrieval, and bulletin board systems (BBS) where messages may be posted via the World Wide Web facility on the Internet. Some insurers offer incentives to practitioners for using the Web to process medical claims, make referrals, and check claim status, patient eligibility, and deductibles. Incentives can consist of faster payment of claims, payment of claim transaction fees, and direct deposit of claim payments to the practice's bank account. A Uniform or Universal Resource Locator (URL) is the Web address or location of an organization, government or military network, commercial business, or academic or research site on the Internet (e.g., *http://www.ama-assn.org* [American Medical Association]).

Electronic Mail

E-mail is the transmitting, receiving, storing, and forwarding of text, voice messages, attachments, or images by computer from one person to another. Every computer user subscribing to an online service may establish an e-mail address (Example 7–1).

EXAMPLE 7–1

Electronic Mail (e-mail) Address

mason@aol.com means:

Mason	Individual user (Mason)
@	at
aol	site (America Online, an online service provider)
com	type of site (commercial business)

Because this is a more cost-effective and efficient method of sending a message to someone and obtaining a quicker response, one may be composing, forwarding, and responding by means of e-mail with staff in other locations, patients, and insurance billers (Fig. 7–4). One must set standards to follow when communicating via e-mail. The messages sent reflect one's professional image.

1. Identify the sender and the reason for the message.
2. Compose the message in a clear and concise manner using good grammar and proper spelling. Make sure it cannot be misconstrued.
3. Include a descriptive subject line. If a reply changes the topic, then change the subject line.
4. Do not put confidential information in an e-mail message (e.g., patient-identifiable information).
5. Encrypt (code) all files about patients and e-mail attachments and limit the size of attachments. Some users pay a per-minute connect time and download the attachment.
6. Recognize that all e-mail is discoverable in legal proceedings; therefore be careful with content and choice of words.
7. Do not use all capital letters for more than one word.
8. Insert a blank line between paragraphs.
9. Surround URLs (long Web addresses) with angle brackets [ ] to avoid problems occurring at the end of a line with the word wrap feature.
10. Do not use variable text styles (bold or italic) or text colors.
11. Quote sparingly when automatically quoting the original message in replies. Some programs allow the selection of text in the original message by pressing a keyboard shortcut, and only that text appears quoted in the reply. Insert quote marks to differentiate original and new text.
12. Avoid sending or forwarding junk messages (e.g., welcome messages, congratulation messages, jokes, and chain messages).
13. Avoid "emoticons," a short sequence of keyboard letters and symbols used to convey emotion, gestures, or expressions (e.g., :- for "smiley").
14. Do not respond immediately if someone's e-mail is angry or emotional. Put the message aside until the next day and then answer it diplomatically.
15. Do not write anything racially or sexually offensive.
16. Insert a short signature at the end of the message that includes name, affiliation, and e-mail or URL address.

Subj: **anesthesia modifiers**
Date: Thursday, August 17, 2000
To: apcmonitor@shore.net

Question: Is conscious sedation considered anesthesia in relationship to modifier -73 and -74? A speaker at a recent conference said "yes" but another said it had not yet been clarified by CMS. Our fiscal intermediary manual has an example that said modifier -52 would be used in conjunction with a colonoscopy with conscious sedation. What is correct?
brownm@aol.com

Figure 7–4. Electronic mail message to *The APCs Weekly Monitor* asking a question about use of modifiers.

Web Search Engine

One also may access the Internet and use a Web browser (search engine) to go to a specific address to obtain current legal and regulatory information from insurance programs and federal agencies, which may involve downloading data or attachments from the Web. Some Web sites to contact for current information about insurance regulations and code updates for insurance billing are given at the end of the chapter.

HIPAA Compliance Alert

Computer Confidentiality

Confidentiality Statement

The majority of information in patients' medical records and physicians' financial records is considered confidential and sensitive. Employees who have access to such computer data should have integrity and be well chosen because they have a high degree of responsibility and accountability. It is wise to have those handling sensitive computer documents sign an annual confidentiality statement, as recommended by the Alliance of Claims Assistance Professionals (Fig. 7–5). In this way the statement can be updated when an individual's responsibilities increase or decrease. The statement should contain the following:

◗ Written or oral disclosure of information pertaining to patients is prohibited.
◗ Disclosure of information without consent of the patient results in serious penalty (e.g., immediate dismissal).

An additional example of an employee confidentiality agreement that may be used by an employer when hiring an insurance biller is shown in Chapter 1, Figure 1–6.

YOUR COMPANY NAME
ADDRESS
PHONE/FAX

CONFIDENTIALITY STATEMENT

I, _____ , understand and acknowledge that as a
 (Type in individual's name)
principle/employee of _____(company name)_____ my position
as ___(job title)___ requires that I access and use computer equipment and
software applications owned or leased by___(company name)___ .
I understand that my position as a principle/employee of this company obligates me to abide by
the purchase, lease or rental agreements applicable to this equipment and software.

I understand and acknowledge that my position may require that I handle information regarding
the physicians and medical suppliers who are clients of___(company name)___ .
I understand and acknowledge that such client information, including financial data, fees,
corporate structure, etc., is privileged and confidential and that I am not at liberty to divulge or
discuss such information with unauthorized individuals within this company or to anyone outside
this company.

I understand and acknowledge that my duties may require me to access and/or process specific
patient data for individuals under the care of___(company name)___ client
physicians and/or medical suppliers. I understand and acknowledge that all patient's data is
protected under federal privacy legislation and that discussion or release of this information in any
form without the patient's express permission is prohibited by federal law and subject to
prosecution and civil monetary penalties for any violation.

I further understand that violations of this confidentiality agreement will result in termination of
employment with___(company name)___ .

My signature below is to verify my understanding and acceptance of the above data
confidentiality requirements and to signify my explicit agreement to abide by these requirements.

_____   _____ Date
  Signature

_____   _____
  Type Name   Title

Figure 7–5. Sample of confidentiality statement for an employee using computer equipment and software. (National Association of Claims Assistance Professionals, Inc., Downers Grove, IL.)

Prevention Measures

Employees can take a number of preventive measures to maintain computer security. Follow these guidelines:

1. Obtain a software program that stores files in coded form.
2. Never leave disks or tapes unguarded on desks or anywhere else in sight.
3. Use a privacy filter over the computer monitor so data may be read only when one is directly in front of the computer.
4. Log off the computer terminal before leaving a work station, especially if working in a LAN environment, which is used in most hospitals, clinics, or large offices.
5. Check and double-check the credentials of any consultant hired.
6. Read the manuals for the equipment, especially the sections entitled "Security Controls," and follow all directions.
7. Store confidential data on diskettes or zip disks rather than only to the computer's hard drive. Diskettes should be stored in a locked, secure location, preferably one that is fireproof and away from magnetic fields.
8. Make sure the computer system has a firewall installed and proper antivirus software. This can keep amateurs, but not professional hackers, from accessing an electronic system. Hackers can access digital copiers, laser printers, fax machines, and other electronic equipment that have internal memories. Some offices transmit and receive data during low-cost, low-volume hours. This means the modem is left on.
9. Develop passwords for each individual user and access codes to protect the data. A **password** is a combination of letters, numbers, or symbols that each individual is assigned to access the system. Passwords should be changed at regular intervals and never written down. A good password is composed of more than five characters and is case sensitive. *Case sensitive* means that the password must be entered exactly as stored using upper or lower case characters. Delete obsolete passwords from the system. Change any passwords known by an employee who is fired or resigns. Individuals with their own passwords allow the employer to distinguish work done by each employee. If errors or problems occur, focus may then be directed toward correcting the individual user who can learn from the mistakes.
10. Send only an account number (not the patient's name) when e-mailing a colleague with specific questions (e.g., about coding).

Records Management

Data Storage

A paperless office requires an organized and efficient system for keeping **files** that have been saved to the hard drive against accidental destruction. Keep financial records on disks or tapes and store them in an area that does not have temperature extremes or magnetic fields.

When data is keyboarded, it is wise to **back up** (save data) frequently. Automated back up is possible, and the computer regularly initiates the process. Most financial software programs display a screen prompt instructing the operator to back up before quitting the program. If there is no automated back up, remember to always back up files at the end of the day or several times a week so information is not lost during a power outage (e.g., surge, spike, blackout, brownout, and lightning), computer breakdown, or head crash. *Head crash* occurs when the read-write head on a disk drive strikes the surface of the disk, causing damage at the point of impact.

About once a week a verification process should be done that compares the original records with the copies. This can take 20% to 30% longer than ordinary back up, but if a comparison is not made there is no way to ensure that the data have been backed up. Store back-up copies away from the office in case of fire, flood, or theft.

Maintain a notebook (log) of the documents on disks or tapes with an index located at the front of the book. The log enables one to keep track of files and should list when the files were backed up last so they can be located quickly. Be sure another employee knows where this notebook is kept and is familiar with how to track down files through this system. Note the code for accessing these documents and date revisions when updating old documents. Do NOT put anything related to personal health information in this log, for example: 31403.DOC, Mrs. Private Patient Positive HIV Report.

Electronic Power Protection

Plug equipment into power surge suppressors or better yet, one with an uninterruptible power supply (UPS) to prevent computer and data file damage. In addition, the entire office should be protected by a surge suppressor installed near the electric circuit breaker panel. This device is called an all-office or whole-office surge suppressor.

Selection of an Office Computer System

A medical practice wishing to use an in-office computer or an individual wishing to set up his or her own business should consider the following:

1. What is the cost of the basic equipment and will it be purchased or leased?
2. What accessories will be necessary and what are their costs?
3. How much space will be necessary for the equipment and accessories for the office or home office business?
4. What type of electrical installation should be done to handle electronic transmission of data?
5. Should a computer fax or modem be obtained or should there be a separate fax line installed?
6. How much electrical energy will be used and how much additional cost will be necessary?
7. If the computer is on a time-sharing system with other users, how much will the telephone line cost when communicating online or directly to the computer?
8. What are the hardware maintenance costs and who will do the repair work?
9. What initial software will be necessary and will it be compatible with the operating system?
10. What is the estimated cost of software upgrades and will upgrades require an expanded operating system?
11. What are the software maintenance costs and who will provide technical support?
12. Should a document scanner be obtained?
13. What forms will be used as output from the computer? Also consider their size, design, acquisition, storage, waste, and cost.
14. What other supplies will be necessary and what will their costs be?
15. How many on the staff will operate the computer? Will recruitment be necessary? Who will train employees? How much training time is necessary?
16. Will there be financing when the equipment is purchased and, if so, what type?
17. Will there be insurance and a warranty on the system?
18. How much will the consulting costs be?
19. What is the backup support and response time when there is a system crash (software or hardware)? Who will respond to software problems and who will respond to hardware problems?
20. How much time will it take to convert the current accounting system to the computerized system, and who will be doing the conversion?

Computer Claims Systems

For a better understanding of how insurance claims are transmitted, know the two types of systems and how they work (e.g., carrier-direct and clearinghouse).

Carrier-Direct

Fiscal agents for Medicaid, Medicare, TRICARE, and many private insurance carriers use the **carrier-direct system.** With this system the medical practice must have its own computer and software or the physician must lease a terminal from the carrier to key-in claim data directly. The data are then transmitted via modem over a dedicated telephone line.

Clearinghouse

If the physician's system cannot be linked with the insurance carrier or the insurers do not accept claims directly from the physician's office, then the physician may use a *clearinghouse*, which forwards a batch of claims to the insurers. The insurance carrier may stipulate that the claims be sent on diskette or tape to a clearinghouse, which reformats the claims, performs an edit check, transmits them to the carrier, and charges the physician a fee.

As mentioned in earlier chapters the medical practice submits either paper claims (typed or computer generated) or electronic claims when using this system. Claims are submitted every day or once a week, dictated by need or volume.

Some clearinghouses have additional services, such as manually processing claims to carriers that are not online. This means that the physician's office can send all claims electronically to the clearinghouse rather than processing half of them electronically and printing and mailing the rest. Sufficient volume must exist with a particular insurer to make using a clearinghouse cost-effective. Clearinghouses may charge a flat fee per claim or charge a percentage of the claim's dollar volume. Some clearinghouses advance a certain amount determined by the contract before the carrier has paid the claims and then keep whatever it recovers. Figure 7–6 is a flow sheet illustrating electronic claim submission.

Electronic Claims Processor

An individual who converts insurance claims to standardized electronic format and transmits electronic claims data is known as an **electronic claims processor (ECP).** This individual can work in a physician's office, clinic setting, or billing center, or be self-employed. A knowledgeable and efficient ECP can expedite payment to the physician and reduce the number of rejected claims. One of the duties of an ECP is to perform a front-end edit (online error checking) to correct any errors before the claim is transmitted to the insurance carrier. A good software program can edit claims and indicate areas where data are missing.

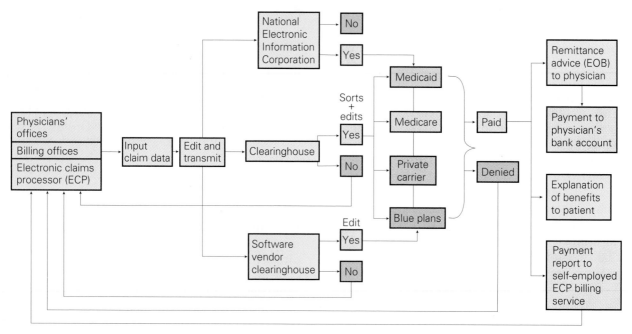

Figure 7–6. Flow sheet of electronic transmission systems showing path for claim payment via the National Electronic Information Corporation (NEIC), clearinghouse, and independent software vendor. Also indicates when payment is made to physician and depicts locations where claims may not pass an edit or are denied.

An important responsibility of an ECP is to make sure the software is always up-to-date. Diagnostic and procedural codes should be updated annually in the software as well as on the encounter form. This ensures that claims are always correctly submitted. Failure to do this can result in claims that are refused, denied, or downcoded.

The Alliance of Claims Assistance Professionals (ACAP) offers an examination to those eligible and interested in being certified as an ECP. Those who pass receive the title certified electronic claims professional (CECP). Information about certification is given in Chapter 17.

Electronic Data Interchange

A physician who plans to begin electronic billing must contact all major insurers and the fiscal intermediaries for each government or state program for a list of vendors approved to handle ECS. Each carrier has special electronic billing requirements and knows which systems can meet their criteria and are compatible in format. The field data requested are almost identical to that necessary on the CMS-1500 claim form. It is also important to request information from insurance carriers about how to submit an electronic bill for patients who have secondary coverage. Some carriers, such as Medicare fiscal intermediaries, may provide the software and training to encourage electronic submission.

Carrier Agreements

It is necessary to have a signed agreement with each carrier with whom the physician wishes to submit electronic claims. Look over the agreement carefully to make sure it will be accepted for ECS.

Signature Requirements

Physician

The physician's signature on the agreement is a substitute for his or her signature on the claim form.

Patient

For assigning benefits and release of medical information, each patient's signature must be obtained either once a month, once a year, or on a one-time basis, depending on the circumstance of each case, because there are no signatures on electronic claims (Fig. 7–7). An authorization and assignment release may be designed specifically for the purpose of obtaining signatures for transmitting electronic claims. The CMS-1500 Health Insurance Claim form also may be used for this purpose, and the patient should sign in Block 12 or 13. Some software programs ask a question whether the patient's signature is on file and require a "yes" or "no" answer. Other software systems do not have this requirement so it depends on how the software is set up.

PATIENT'S MEDICARE ELECTRONIC SIGNATURE MONTHLY AUTHORIZATION FORM

I authorize any holder of medical or other information about me to release to the Social Security Administration and Center for Medicare and Medicaid Services or its intermediaries or carriers any information needed for this or a related Medicare claim. I permit a copy of this authorization to be used in place of the original, and request payment of medical insurance benefits either to myself or to the party who accepts assignment.

_____   _____
Signature of Patient   Date

A

PATIENT'S MEDICARE ELECTRONIC SIGNATURE ONE-TIME AUTHORIZATION FORM

I request that payment of authorized Medicare benefits be made either to me or on my behalf to _____ for services furnished me by that physician or supplier. I permit a copy of this authorization to be used in place of the original and authorize any holder of medical information about me to release to the Center for Medicare and Medicaid Services or its agents any information needed to determine these benefits or the benefits payable for related services.

_____   _____
Signature of Patient   Date

B

Figure 7–7. Examples of patients' Medicare electronic signature authorization forms. **A,** Monthly form. **B,** One-time form.

Signatures must be maintained on file in the physician's record for 72 months (6 years) after the month in which the claim was submitted. Some Medicare fiscal intermediaries require annual renewal of signatures, so check with the local carrier.

Multipurpose Billing Forms

As mentioned in Chapter 2 a **multipurpose billing form** (also known as charge slip, communicator, encounter form, fee ticket, patient service slip, routing form, super bill, or transaction slip) is a form used to record information about the service rendered to a patient. It is personalized and custom-printed to the specialty of the physician. These forms may be printed by the computer and customized with specific patient information, thus saving outside printing expenses and time filling in patient data.

Crib Sheet Encounter Form

In 1992 when the CPT Evaluation and Management procedure codes were introduced, another routing slip method was designed by physicians. An abbreviated style is used, and the form is known as a crib sheet or charge slip. A *crib sheet* is a summary form listing key components of the Evaluation and Management (E/M) codes (Fig. 7–8). It aids the physician in determining the correct level of E/M service, ensures each component is addressed in the physician's dictation, and expedites data entry of professional services. The physician circles the codes, and the insurance billing specialist takes that information and enters it into the computer system. Because crib sheets are abbreviated and not in detail, they, along with other types of billing forms, cannot be used in place of documentation in the patient record and may not withstand an external audit.

Scannable Encounter Form

Some encounter forms are designed so that they may be scanned to input charges and diagnoses into the patient's computerized account (Fig. 7–9). Time is saved and fewer errors occur because no keystrokes are involved.

Keying Insurance Data for Claim Transmission

Manual claim completion is accomplished by obtaining patient and insurance data, looking up a diagnosis and procedure in an index, referring to medical and financial records, and following block-by-block guidelines for the CMS-1500 insurance claim form. Much of this source information is found on an encounter form that is used to post charges and payments.

When one is operating computer software, the encounter form also may be used to obtain information. A screen **prompt** (question) appears on the monitor, and the data are keyed in reply to the prompt. Reusable data are entered initially in a file and identified by a number. Each treating physician, referring physician, patient, and insurance carrier has a computer code number assigned; for example, Dr. Jones might be keyed in as 010; a patient, Jane Doe, might be input as an account number; and the ABC Insurance Company might be 003. This information is stored in the database and is the same as that necessary for completing a claim manually. It is automatically retrieved by the system when a computer code number is keyed in and used to generate a computerized claim or electronic claim. Because there are computer code numbers and prompts for each item, there is less chance for error or omitting mandatory information. The program checks to see that data are complete and in proper **format.**

Some entries are made using a *macro.* This technique involves a series of menu selections, keystrokes, or commands that have been recorded into memory and assigned a name or key combination. When the macro name is keyed in, the steps or

CHARGE SLIP

MC2 NAME: DATE:

CODE	HIST	EXAM	DEC	CODE	HIST	EXAM	DEC
99201	* NEW PAT. OFF.			99261	+ F.UP CONSULT — INPATIENT		
99202	* EPF	EPF	SF	99262	+ EPF	EPF	MC
99203	* D	D	LC	99263	+ D	D	HC
99204	* C	C	MC	99281	* EMERG.DEP.		
99205	* C	C	HC	99282	* EPF	EPF	LC
99211	+ EST.PAT.OFF.			99283	* EPF	EPF	L-MC
99212	+ PF	PF	SF	99284	* D	D	MC
99213	+ EPF	EPF	LC	99285	* C	C	HC
99214	+ D	D	MC	99291	CRITIC.CARE 1st Hr.		
99215	+ C	C	HC	99292	ADDIT. 30 MIN		
99221	* INIT.HOSP.VIS — NEW or ESTAB.			99301	* NURSING FACIL.		
99222	* C	C	MC	99302	* D	C	M-HC
99223	* C	C	HC	99303	* C	C	M-HC
99231	+ SUBSQ.HOSPIT.			99311	+ SNF SUBSEQ.		
99232	+ EPF	EPF	LC	99312	+ EPF	EPF	MC
99233	+ D	D	HC	99313	+ D	D	M-HC
99238	HOSPIT.DISCH.			99341	* HOME SERVICES — NEW PAT.		
99241	* CONSULT.OFF.			99342	* PF	PF	SF-LC
99242	* EPF	EPF	SF	99343	* EPF	EPF	MC
99243	* D	D	LC	99351	+ ESTAB.PATIENT		
99244	* C	C	MC	99352	+ EPF	EPF	MC
99245	*C	C	HC	99353	+ D	D	HC
99251	* INIT.CONSULT. — INPATIENT			DIAGNOSIS:		CPT CODES:	
99252	* EPF	EPF	SF				
99253	* D	D	LC				
99254	* C	C	MC				
99255	* C	C	HC				

KEY: PF: Probl.Foc. EPF: Expand.Probl.Foc D: Detail. C: Comprehens.
LC: Low Complex. MC: Moder.Complex. HC: High Complex.

Requirem.: *: 3 Key Components req. + : 2 out of 3 Key Compon. req.

Figure 7–8. Example of a crib sheet. This system of abbreviations has cut in half the time the physician spends in choosing the correct Evaluation and Management Current Procedural Terminology codes according to the three key components: history, physical examination, and medical decision making. The format shown here can be adapted to any specialty. (From Helmut O. Haar, MD, Ventura, CA.)

characters in the macro are executed from beginning to end, saving time and key strokes.

Some general guidelines for keying in data and billing electronic claims follow:

▶ Do not use special characters (dashes, spaces, or commas).

▶ Use the patient account numbers to differentiate between patients with similar names.

▶ Use correct numeric locations of service code, valid CPT, or Healthcare Common Procedure Coding System (HCPCS) procedure codes.

▶ Do not bill codes using modifiers -21 or -22 electronically unless the carrier receives documents (called attachments) to justify more payment.

▶ Print out an insurance billing worksheet or perform a front-end edit (online error checking) to look for and correct all errors before the claim is transmitted to the insurance carrier.

▶ Request electronic-error reports from the insurance carrier to make corrections to the system.

▶ Obtain and cross-check the electronic status report against all claims transmitted.

▶ After input is complete the information is stored in memory and a claim may be transmitted individually or in batches. Batched claims can be divided according to insurance type or date(s) of service and are ideally sent during low-volume times.

Electronically Completing the Claim

Coding Requirements

When one is electronically transmitting insurance claims, the following may be required:

1. ICD-9-CM diagnostic codes
2. CPT codes with modifiers

CFR

PAT 4140.0

( ) 985-6575 01/22/1936 F63
PRI: (Y) BLUE SHIELD ENVOY
201-XX-9969
SEC:

DOCTOR:	**2 FRANK CHI, M.D.**
ROOM:	
APPTLOC:	
APPTCD:	
REASON:	OX, F/U visit
LAST DX:	000.0 No diagnosis applicable
SSN/STA:	201-XX-9969, 1 Active
OVERLAY:	1 INTERNAL MEDICINE

APPT DATE:	**05/27/XX**
APPT TIME:	2:30 PM
APPT LEN:	10 min.
DEPT/LOC:	0, n/a
DSET/PRT:	1, 12
ACCT BAL:	75.00
PAT DUE:	0.00
VOUCHER:	7887

NEW PT OFFICE VISITS
①②③④Ⓟ/Ⓛ 99203 NP LEVEL THREE
①②③④Ⓟ/Ⓛ 99204 NP LEVEL FOUR
①②③④Ⓟ/Ⓛ 99205 NP LEVEL FIVE
EST PT OFFICE VISIT
①②③④Ⓟ/Ⓛ 99211 EST PT LEVEL ONE
①②③④Ⓟ/Ⓛ 99212 EST PT LEVEL TWO
①②③④Ⓟ/Ⓛ 99213 EST PT LEVEL THREE
①②③④Ⓟ/Ⓛ 99214 EST PT LEVEL FOUR
①②③④Ⓟ/Ⓛ 99215 EST PT LEVEL FIVE
①②③④Ⓟ/Ⓛ 00003 GLOBAL VISIT

OTHER PROCEDURES
①②③④Ⓟ/Ⓛ 99000 COLL & PREP/PAP TEST
①②③④Ⓟ/Ⓛ 93000 EKG WITH INTERPRETATION
①②③④Ⓟ/Ⓛ 82270 HEMOCCULT
①②③④Ⓟ/Ⓛ 81000 URINALYSIS

INJECTIONS
①②③④Ⓟ/Ⓛ ~FLU, FLU INJ/ADMIN/MCR
①②③④Ⓟ/Ⓛ ~9065 FLU INJ/NON MCR
①②③④Ⓟ/Ⓛ ~PNEU PNEUMO/ADMIN/MCR
①②③④Ⓟ/Ⓛ ~9073 PNEUMO INJ NON MCR

UNLISTED PROCEDURES

STOP FOR VERIFICATION
BREASTS
①②③④Ⓟ/Ⓛ 610.2 FIBROADENOSIS, BREAST
①②③④Ⓟ/Ⓛ 611.72 LUMP OR MASS IN BREAST

CARDIOVASCULAR
①②③④Ⓟ/Ⓛ 441.4 ABDOM AORTIC ANEURYSM
①②③④Ⓟ/Ⓛ 411.1 ANGINA
①②③④Ⓟ/Ⓛ 424.1 AORTIC VALVE DISORDER
①②③④Ⓟ/Ⓛ 427.31 ATRIAL FIBRILLATION
①②③④Ⓟ/Ⓛ 427.32 ATRIAL FLUTTER
①②③④Ⓟ/Ⓛ 427.61 ATRIAL PREMATURE BEATS
①②③④Ⓟ/Ⓛ 426.11 ATRIOVENT BLOCK-1ST DE
①②③④Ⓟ/Ⓛ 785.2 CARDIAC MURMURS NEC
①②③④Ⓟ/Ⓛ 429.3 CARDIOMEGALY
①②③④Ⓟ/Ⓛ 428.0 CONGESTIVE HEART FAILU
①②③④Ⓟ/Ⓛ 425.1 HYPERTR OBSTR CARDIOMY
①②③④Ⓟ/Ⓛ 414.01 ISCHEMIC CHR HEART DIS
①②③④Ⓟ/Ⓛ 426.2 LEFT BB HEMIBLOCK
①②③④Ⓟ/Ⓛ 424.0 MITRAL VALVE DISORDER
①②③④Ⓟ/Ⓛ 785.1 PALPITATIONS
①②③④Ⓟ/Ⓛ 427.0 PAROX ATRIAL TACHYCARD
①②③④Ⓟ/Ⓛ 427.1 PAROX VENTRIC TACHYCAR

CHEST
①②③④Ⓟ/Ⓛ 466.0 BRONCHITIS, ACUTE
①②③④Ⓟ/Ⓛ 491.0 BRONCHITIS, CHRONIC
①②③④Ⓟ/Ⓛ 493.20 CH OB ASTH W/O STAT AS
①②③④Ⓟ/Ⓛ 493.00 EXT ASTHMA W/O STAT AS

①②③④Ⓟ/Ⓛ 491.21 OBS CHR BRNC W ACT EXA
①②③④Ⓟ/Ⓛ 491.20 OBS CHR BRNC W/O ACT E

ENDOCRINE
①②③④Ⓟ/Ⓛ 250.61 DMI NEURO CMP CONTROLL
①②③④Ⓟ/Ⓛ 250.01 DMI WO CMP CONTROLLED
①②③④Ⓟ/Ⓛ 250.03 DMI UNCONTROLLED
①②③④Ⓟ/Ⓛ 250.60 DMII NEURO CMP CONTROL
①②③④Ⓟ/Ⓛ 250.00 DMII WO CMP CONTROLLED
①②③④Ⓟ/Ⓛ 250.02 DMII UNCONTROLLED
①②③④Ⓟ/Ⓛ 272.0 HYPERCHOLESTEROLEMIA
①②③④Ⓟ/Ⓛ 272.1 HYPERGLYCERIDEMIA
①②③④Ⓟ/Ⓛ 245.2 HYPOTHYROIDISM
①②③④Ⓟ/Ⓛ 278.01 MORBID OBESITY
①②③④Ⓟ/Ⓛ 241.0 THYROID NODULE

EXTREMITIES
①②③④Ⓟ/Ⓛ 782.3 EDEMA
①②③④Ⓟ/Ⓛ 440.22 LOWER EXT EMBOLISM
①②③④Ⓟ/Ⓛ 451.0 PHLEBITIS-LEG
①②③④Ⓟ/Ⓛ 440.21 PVD W/CLAUDICATION
①②③④Ⓟ/Ⓛ 454.9 VARICOSE VEIN OF LEG

GI
①②③④Ⓟ/Ⓛ 789.06 ABDMNAL PAIN EPIGASTRI
①②③④Ⓟ/Ⓛ 789.02 ABDMNAL PAIN LFT UP QU
①②③④Ⓟ/Ⓛ 789.04 ABDMNAL PAIN LT LWR QU
①②③④Ⓟ/Ⓛ 789.05 ABDMNAL PAIN PERIUMBIL
①②③④Ⓟ/Ⓛ 789.03 ABDMNAL PAIN RT LWR QU
①②③④Ⓟ/Ⓛ 789.01 ABDMNAL PAIN RT UPR QU
①②③④Ⓟ/Ⓛ 578.1 BLOOD IN STOOL
①②③④Ⓟ/Ⓛ 575.12 CHOLECYSTITIS, ACUTE
①②③④Ⓟ/Ⓛ 564.0 CONSTIPATION
①②③④Ⓟ/Ⓛ 787.91 DIARRHEA
①②③④Ⓟ/Ⓛ 562.11 DIVERTICULITIS
①②③④Ⓟ/Ⓛ 562.10 DIVERTICULOSIS
①②③④Ⓟ/Ⓛ 574.20 GALLSTONE(S), CHRONIC
①②③④Ⓟ/Ⓛ 535.00 GASTRITIS
①②③④Ⓟ/Ⓛ 530.81 GERD
①②③④Ⓟ/Ⓛ 455.3 HEMORRHOID, EXT W/O COM
①②③④Ⓟ/Ⓛ 455.0 HEMORRHOID, INT W/O COM
①②③④Ⓟ/Ⓛ 564.1 IRRITABLE COLON
①②③④Ⓟ/Ⓛ 787.01 NAUSEA WITH VOMITING
①②③④Ⓟ/Ⓛ 569.3 RECTAL & ANAL HEMORRHA
①②③④Ⓟ/Ⓛ 530.11 REFLUX ESOPHAGITIS
①②③④Ⓟ/Ⓛ V76.41 SCREEN COLORECTAL

GU
①②③④Ⓟ/Ⓛ 601.0 ACUTE PROSTATITIS
①②③④Ⓟ/Ⓛ 600 BPH
①②③④Ⓟ/Ⓛ 592.0 CALCULUS OF KIDNEY
①②③④Ⓟ/Ⓛ 592.1 CALCULUS OF URETER
①②③④Ⓟ/Ⓛ 595.0 CYSTITIS, ACUTE
①②③④Ⓟ/Ⓛ 595.1 CYSTITIS, CHRONIC
①②③④Ⓟ/Ⓛ 599.7 HEMATURIA
①②③④Ⓟ/Ⓛ 607.84 IMPOTENCE, ORGANIC ORI
①②③④Ⓟ/Ⓛ 791.0 PROTEINURIA

HEENT
①②③④Ⓟ/Ⓛ 380.4 CERUMEN, IMPACTED
①②③④Ⓟ/Ⓛ 372.02 CONJUNCTIVITIS
①②③④Ⓟ/Ⓛ 784.7 EPISTAXIS
①②③④Ⓟ/Ⓛ 784.0 HEADACHE
①②③④Ⓟ/Ⓛ 464.0 LARYNGITIS/TRACHEITI
①②③④Ⓟ/Ⓛ 465.0 LARYNGOPHARYNGITIS, A
①②③④Ⓟ/Ⓛ 780.4 LIGHT-HEADEDNESS
①②③④Ⓟ/Ⓛ 346.00 MIGRAINE
①②③④Ⓟ/Ⓛ 460 NASOPHARYNGITIS, ACUT
①②③④Ⓟ/Ⓛ 381.01 OTITIS MEDIA
①②③④Ⓟ/Ⓛ 462 PHARYNGITIS, ACUTE
①②③④Ⓟ/Ⓛ 477.0 RHINITIS ALLERGIC
①②③④Ⓟ/Ⓛ 461.0 SINUSITIS, ACUTE
①②③④Ⓟ/Ⓛ 780.2 SYNCOPE/VERTIGO

HEMATOLOGIC
①②③④Ⓟ/Ⓛ 280.0 CHR BLOOD LOSS ANEMI
①②③④Ⓟ/Ⓛ 280.1 IRON DEF ANEMIA DIET
①②③④Ⓟ/Ⓛ 281.0 PERNICIOUS ANEMIA

HYPERTENSION
①②③④Ⓟ/Ⓛ 404.12 BEN HY HT/REN/CHF
①②③④Ⓟ/Ⓛ 403.10 BEN HTN REN W/O REN
①②③④Ⓟ/Ⓛ 403.11 BEN HYP WITH REN FAI
①②③④Ⓟ/Ⓛ 401.1 BENIGN HYPERTENSION
①②③④Ⓟ/Ⓛ 401.0 MALIGNANT HYPERTENSI
①②③④Ⓟ/Ⓛ 458.0 ORTHOSTATIC HYPOTENS

NEURO
①②③④Ⓟ/Ⓛ 345.10 GEN CNV EPIL W/O INT
①②③④Ⓟ/Ⓛ 435.3 TIA
①②③④Ⓟ/Ⓛ 433.10 CAROTID STENOSIS
①②③④Ⓟ/Ⓛ 437.0 CEREBRAL ATHEREOSCLER

OB GYN
①②③④Ⓟ/Ⓛ 112.1 CANDIDAL VULVOVAGINI
①②③④Ⓟ/Ⓛ 627.2 MENOPAUSAL SYMPTOMS
①②③④Ⓟ/Ⓛ V76.2 SCREEN MAL NEOP-CERV

RHEUMATOLOGIC
①②③④Ⓟ/Ⓛ 723.1 CERVICAL PAIN
①②③④Ⓟ/Ⓛ 274.0 GOUT
①②③④Ⓟ/Ⓛ 724.2 LUMBAGO/BACK PAIN
①②③④Ⓟ/Ⓛ 729.5 PAIN IN LIMB
①②③④Ⓟ/Ⓛ 724.1 PAIN IN THORACIC SPI
①②③④Ⓟ/Ⓛ 714.0 RHEUMATOID ARTHRITIS
①②③④Ⓟ/Ⓛ 724.3 SCIATICA
①②③④Ⓟ/Ⓛ 710.0 SYST LUPUS ERYTHEMAT

MISC
①②③④Ⓟ/Ⓛ 780.6 FEVER UNKN ORGIN
①②③④Ⓟ/Ⓛ 054.9 HERPES SIMPLEX NOS
①②③④Ⓟ/Ⓛ 786.05 SHORTNESS OF BREATH

UNLISTED DIAGNOSIS
①②③④Ⓟ/Ⓛ STOP FOR VERIFICATION

---

①②③④Ⓟ/Ⓛ **REFERRALS** ①②③④Ⓟ/Ⓛ **LOCATIONS** ①②③④Ⓟ/Ⓛ **DOCTORS** ①②③④Ⓟ/Ⓛ **NEXT VISIT**
①②③④Ⓟ/Ⓛ ①②③④Ⓟ/Ⓛ ①②③④Ⓟ/Ⓛ ①②③④Ⓟ/Ⓛ _____ DAYS
①②③④Ⓟ/Ⓛ ①②③④Ⓟ/Ⓛ ①②③④Ⓟ/Ⓛ F. CHI, MD ①②③④Ⓟ/Ⓛ _1_ WEEKS
①②③④Ⓟ/Ⓛ ①②③④Ⓟ/Ⓛ ①②③④Ⓟ/Ⓛ A. SWERD, MD ①②③④Ⓟ/Ⓛ _____ MONTHS
①②③④Ⓟ/Ⓛ ①②③④Ⓟ/Ⓛ ①②③④Ⓟ/Ⓛ J. STEVEN, MD ①②③④Ⓟ/Ⓛ

Figure 7–9. Scannable encounter form. Primary service or procedure is marked (with a #2 pencil) in the #1 location and linked to the primary diagnosis, which also is marked in the #1 location. The secondary procedures are marked in the #2 location as is the secondary diagnosis. The primary linkage for all services and procedures is connected to the physician performing the service and the location in which it took place. (Form template from Pearson NCS, Inc., Bloomington, MN. Form data are fictitious and not a part of the template.)

3. Medicare HCPCS national and regional procedural codes for services, supplies, and procedures

Most insurers require the physician to be responsible for assigning diagnostic and procedural codes. Refer to Appendix B for the names and addresses of publishers of the code books.

Because the insurance billing specialist inputs the codes, claims examiners should not recode. This eliminates transposition of numbers or missing or added digits on transmitted claims. During the edit and error process, software code editors identify invalid codes, age conflicts, gender conflicts, procedural and diagnostic code conflicts, and other data before issuing payment. If certain information is submitted incorrectly (e.g., patient's name or insurance identification number is incorrect, a diagnosis code is missing a fifth digit, or a provider's identification number is omitted), the claim is rejected and must be resubmitted with correct data. Incorrect coding may be keying errors, or it may be a deliberate attempt to obtain fraudulent payment. The edit check allows immediate feedback about the status of an electronically transmitted claim.

Medicare requires certain information when submitting paper and electronic claims for some blocks of the CMS-1500 claim form. Carriers may return claims if this information is omitted. A list of mandatory information and conditional requirements is shown in Table 7–1.

The physician or the medical insurance billing specialist may revise coding on the medical record and on the claim to reflect the services more accurately up until the time at which the claim is transmitted for payment.

Encoder and Grouper

Encoders and groupers may be used when hospitals or large medical practices or clinics transmit an electronic claim. A computer-assisted *encoder* (computer software program that assigns a code to represent data) helps users assign the most accurate code by prompting them with a series of questions or choices leading to a specific code assignment or by affecting code assignment by displaying code-specific edits. However, there are cases in which an encoder would not accurately assign codes; therefore one must never be completely dependent on code-assist software. For example, if a patient has three thorns incised and extracted (removed), the CPT code 10120 *incision and removal of foreign body, subcutaneous tissue;* simple (integumentary system) might be generated by the encoder. But if internally audited, the case may warrant CPT code 27372 *removal of foreign body, deep, thigh region in knee* area (musculoskeletal system). Thus one learns that not all procedures involving the skin are found in the integumentary system and, if deeper skin layers are affected, a code may be found in another system. A *grouper* is software designed for use in a network that serves a group of users working on a related project that allows access to the same data.

Automated Coding

Still in its infancy but being developed is *automated coding.* This system does not make the coder go through questions or steps to assign a code. Instead, the system pulls data (diagnoses, procedures, and patient care information) that is linked to a code, and the code is assigned automatically. Thus complete and accurate documentation of clinical information must be input into the patient's medical record to ensure that an accurate code is generated.

Electronic Processing Problems

Some problems can occur in electronic claims submission. Usually a status report of claims is received electronically from the insurance company; it consists of an acknowledgment report and indicates assigned and not assigned claims, crossed over and not crossed over claims, claims accepted with errors, and rejected claims (Fig. 7–10). Data transmission problems arise periodically because of hardware or software problems.

Bug

An error in a program is called a **bug;** to remove the error is to **debug.** A static telephone line can impair transmission of claims, delaying transmission and resulting in rejected claims. Sometimes the computer malfunctions, resulting in a period known as **down time.** Peak load problems may occur, delaying access to the insurance carrier's computer. Claims should be submitted early in the morning or after hours to avoid "traffic jams" (logjams).

Virus

A **virus** is a destructive program that copies itself and attaches to other programs in the computer system. Some viruses destroy programs and data after a precise lapse of time. To help prevent a virus from infecting the computer, software designed to display a warning message when an infected disk has been found should be installed. Antiviral utility software programs must be updated frequently. The virus scan software should not be bypassed when booting up the computer. As an additional prevention measure, public domain software files should never be downloaded from electronic bulletin boards or other communication systems. E-mail from unfamiliar sources

| TABLE 7–1 | **Medicare Requirements When Submitting Paper and Electronic Claims** |

Mandatory Information

Block No.	Paper Claims	Electronic Claims
1A.	Insured ID number	Insured ID number
2.	Patient name	Patient last and first names
11.	Insured policy group number	Group number/Source of payment
13.	Patient signature source	Patient signature source/Release of information indicator
24a.	Dates of service	Service from/through dates
24b.	Place of service	Place of service
24d.	Procedures, services, and so on	HCPCS procedure code
24f.	$ charges	Line charges
24g.	Days or units of service	Units of service
31.	Provider signature indicator	Provider signature indicator
33.	Provider's billing name and address	Provider last and first names
		Payer organization, name
		Provider Medicare number (batch level)
		Provider's pay-to address 1
		Provider's pay-to city
		Provider's pay-to state
		Provider's pay-to ZIP code
		Provider's pay-to telephone number

Conditional Requirements

Block No.	Paper Claims	Electronic Claims
4.	Insured name	Insured last and first names
6.	Patient relationship to insured	Patient relationship to insured
7.	Insured address	Insured address-line 1 Insured city, state, ZIP code, and telephone number
9c.	Employer or school name	Insured employer name
9d.	Insurance plan or program name	Group name
14.	Date of current illness, and so on	Accident/symptom date
17.	Name or refer/ordering	Refer/ordering provider last name
17a.	ID no. of refer/ordering	Refer/ordering provider NPI, referring provider NPI
19.	Reserved for local use	Date last seen, supervising provider NPI, date of last x-ray
20.	Outside lab	Laboratory indicator, lab charges, purchased service indicator, purchased service charge
21.	Diagnosis	Diagnosis 1, 2, 3, 4
24d.		HCPCS modifier 1, 2, 3, 4
24k.	Reserved for local use	Rendering provider NPI
32.	Facility name and address	Facility/laboratory name and/or facility/laboratory NPI number, mammography certification no.

or questionable files from the Internet should never be downloaded. Bringing in a disk from outside the office (or classroom) should be avoided because the disk may be infected by a virus. A networked computer station can infect all of the other networked stations if it becomes infected with a virus.

Facsimile Communication Transmission

Insurance claims, as well as supporting documentation on a claim, may be sent to the carrier via a fax machine if the carrier's guidelines allow this. Even clearer transmission is accomplished if the office

computer has fax capabilities. The process is simple, fast, and accurate.

Digital fax claims are not considered as electronic claims. *Digital fax* is a claim that arrives at the insurance carrier via fax but is never printed on paper. The fax is encoded by optical character recognition (OCR) and transmitted into the claims processing system, bypassing manual data entry.

Some carriers require the medical office to complete a short test phase; claims may be faxed and processed after approval. A cover sheet may or may not be necessary; some carriers allow multipage claims or claims with attachments.

College Clinic
Practon, Gerald MD
4567 Broad Avenue
Woodland Hills, XY 12345-0001   12345-0000

                                                 XYZ INSURANCE COMPANY
|ι|ιιιιι||ιι||ι|ιιιι|ι||ιιιιιι||ιι||ι|ι|ιι|ιιι| MEDICARE ADMINISTRATION

ELECTRONIC CLAIMS ACKNOWLEDGMENT REPORT

DATE: 02-28-20XX

SUBMITTER CODE: 000002469

RECEIPT DATE: 02-28-20XX

THERE WERE NO EDIT ERRORS DETECTED AND THE CLAIMS WERE PASSED TO OUR
CLAIMS PROCESSING SYSTEM.

YOU SHOULD BE INFORMED OF THE STATUS OF ALL CLAIMS ON THE NEXT OUTPUT
REPORT YOU RECEIVE FROM US.

FOLLOWING ARE STATISTICS RELATED TO THE PROCESSING OF YOUR BATCH:

TOTAL CLAIMS SUBMITTED	50
TOTAL CLAIMS ACCEPTED	50
TOTAL CLAIMS REJECTED	0
TOTAL CLAIMS ACCEPTED WITH ERRORS	0
% OF ERRORS TO CLAIMS EDITED	0%
TOTAL CHARGES ACCEPTED:	$15,267.00
TOTAL ASSIGNED CHARGES:	$4,289.00
TOTAL NON ASSIGNED CHARGES:	$0.00
TOTAL CROSSOVER CHARGES:	$10,978.00
TOTAL CHARGES REJECTED:	$0.00
TOTAL BATCHES TRANSMITTED	1
TOTAL DETAIL LINES SUBMITTED	146

A

Figure 7–10. A, Electronic Claims Acknowledgment Report indicating status of all claims transmitted electronically to XYZ Insurance Company on February 28, 20XX.

Although most procedure codes no longer require reports, a few codes still need them. If the claim is transmitted electronically, "Report Sent" or "Report Faxed" should be indicated in the "Comments" field of the EMC claim format. The documentation then should be immediately mailed or faxed to the insurance carrier. Some insurance carriers set up a fax line specifically for electronic billers and may require that an agreement form be completed and signed (Fig. 7–11).

After receiving the claims, some carriers send a faxback report verifying acceptance of the submitted claims (Fig. 7–12). However the fax machine should be left on to ensure receiving the report.

Payments are received more quickly after claims have been faxed than after paper claims are sent via mail.

See Chapters 1 and 3 for legal information regarding faxing documents and confidentiality issues.

Some general fax guidelines for insurance claims follow:

▶ Purchase light blue-green or white unlined—NOT red—versions of the CMS-1500 claim form and NOT photocopies containing claim form lines.
▶ Use dark, distinct print.
▶ Select a fixed pitch font, such as sans serif, with a font size of 10 to 14 points.

XYZ INSURANCE COMPANY
MEDICARE ADMINISTRATION

ELECTRONIC CLAIMS BILLER OUTPUT REPORT ** DUE TO SYSTEM CHANGES THIS REPORT SHOWS ONLY ASSIGNED CLAIMS THIS WEEK **

CURRENT DATE: 03/04/20XX

SUBMITTER CODE: 000002469 MAIL

TAPE VOL. SER. NO.:

	ASSIGNED (NOT CROSSOVER)	ASSIGNED CROSSOVER	NOT ASSIGNED	TOTAL
CLAIMS:	105	114	0	219
TOTAL CHARGES	$47,647.00	$14,551.00	$0.00	$62,198.00
COMPLETED CLAIMS:	93	106	0	199
CLAIMS SETTLED BUT NOT PAID	0	0	0	0
CLAIMS PAID	88	51	0	139
CLAIMS APPLIED TO DEDUCTIBLE	5	2	0	7
CLAIMS DENIED	0	0	0	0
CLAIMS TRANSFERRED	0	0	0	0
CLAIMS SENT TO MEDICAID	0	53	0	53
TOTAL AMOUNT PAID	$15,493.57	$5,817.48	$0.00	$21,311.05
PENDING CLAIMS:	12	8	0	20
CLAIMS PENDING MANUAL REVIEW	9	4	0	13
CLAIMS PENDING CWF RESPONSE	0	4	0	4
CLAIMS PENDING DEVELOPMENT	3	0	0	3
TOTAL AMOUNT PENDING	$6,005.00	$1,500.00	$0.00	$7,505.00

INSURANCE BILLING COMPANY
230 MAIN STREET, SUITE J
WOODLAND HILLS XY 12345-0000

B

Figure 7–10, cont'd. B, Weekly report (Electronic Claims Biller Output Report) of assigned claims.
Continued.

▶ Properly align and center claim data.
▶ Do not use stamps or stickers or hand write information on the claim.
▶ Do not submit claims on continuous-feed paper unless the pages are separated.

Electronic Inquiry or Claims Status Review

Eligibility Verification

Smart Card

Cards similar to plastic credit cards are beginning to make their way into the insurance scene. A *smart card* is a wallet-sized, machine-readable card containing computer chips that allows the card to store a variety of information, such as payer information, coverage limits, eligibility status, and precertification requirements. As an extra service some hospitals supply cards containing the patient's medical record and history. This service is especially helpful for patients who have complex health histories, such as heart conditions, or for patients with serious allergies and those requiring special medication. These cards can function like self-contained minicomputers. Refer to Chapter 9 for information on how smart cards are used as credit and debit cards.

Swipe Card

A *swipe card* is a plastic machine-readable wallet-sized card with a magnetic strip containing small memory capacity. This card is used to hold small amounts of information, such as patient's eligibility and coverage.

Smart cards and swipe cards allow information to be transferred electronically and may be used for eligibility verification.

Computer Verification

Some insurance carriers can be accessed directly by computer and can give information electronically about patient eligibility. All that is necessary is to type demographic and insurance information about a patient into the computer and push a button. The information received on the computer screen is the

XYZ INSURANCE COMPANY
MEDICARE ADMINISTRATION

CLAIMS ACCEPTED WITH ERRORS
(PLEASE CORRECT FOR FUTURE TRANSMISSIONS)

REPORT DATE:	02-28-20XX
SUBMITTER CODE:	000005905
SUBMITTER NAME:	COLLEGE CLINIC
RECEIPT DATE:	02-28-20XX
PROVIDER CODE:	3664021CC
PROVIDER NAME:	COLLEGE CLINIC
PROVIDER ADDR:	4567 BROAD AVENUE
	WOODLAND HILLS XY 12345-0001

BENE'S NAME HIC NUMBER	DATE OF SVC	SUBMITTER FIELD DATA	LINE NO.	ERROR MESSAGE
KIRKORIAN C	02/19/20XX	KIRKOR0001	04	MODIFIER IS MISSING OR INVALID FOR DIAGNOSTIC TEST BILLED BY A PHYSICIAN
FOLEY D	02/27/20XX	FOLEY00001	01	SERVICE FROM DATE IS INVALID (093099)
			01	PLACE OF SERVICE IS INVALID (31)
				SUM OF THE DETAIL LINE CHARGES DOES NOT EQUAL TOTAL CHARGES FIELD (90.00)

C

Figure 7–10, cont'd. **C,** Weekly report showing claims accepted with errors to be corrected before retransmission.

same as the information that the insurance company's employee uses to verify and determine the patient's eligibility, insurance coverage, and benefits.

Interactive Transaction

Interactive transaction is back-and-forth communication between two computer systems. One requests information and the other provides information during what is referred to as online real time. It can involve eligibility verification, deductible status, claim inquiries, status of claims, and other insurance claim data. The patient's deductible status can be tracked from all providers the patient has seen during the year.

Other information also may be accessed, such as limiting charges, fee schedules, allowables, procedure codes, and postoperative days for specific procedures. Many insurance companies, such as Medicare fiscal intermediaries, provide access to information on assigned pending and paid claims. Additional information that may be determined includes whether the individual has other coverage and which insurance carrier should be billed as

primary. In addition, some insurance carriers deposit payments into the physician's bank account automatically via electronic funds transfer (EFT).

Remittance Advice Statements

An online transaction about the status of a claim is called an *electronic remittance notice*. This gives information on charges paid or denied and automatically posts the information to patients' accounts without data entry if the software has this feature. The computer tests the claims computer data against various guidelines or parameters known as *screens*. If the services billed on the claim exceed the screens, the claim is denied, returned to the physician for more information, or sent for review. If a claim is denied or rejected, the ECP receives a printout stating the reason. The missing, miscoded, or incomplete information should be added or corrected and the claim resubmitted; this process is more efficient than remaining on a telephone on hold or resubmitting a claim via mail.

The Medicare electronic remittance advice (RA), formerly known as Explanation of Medicare Benefits

```
                          XYZ INSURANCE COMPANY
                          MEDICARE ADMINISTRATION

                          REJECTED ELECTRONIC CLAIMS
                       (PLEASE CORRECT FOR FUTURE TRANSMISSIONS)


REPORT DATE:                            02-28-20XX
SUBMITTER CODE:                         000005905
SUBMITTER NAME:                         COLLEGE CLINIC
RECEIPT DATE:                           02-28-20XX


PROVIDER CODE:                          3664021CC
PROVIDER NAME:                          COLLEGE CLINIC
PROVIDER ADDR:                          4567 BROAD AVENUE
                                        WOODLAND HILLS XY 12345-0001
```

BENE'S NAME HIC NUMBER	DATE OF SVC	SUBMITTER FIELD DATA	LINE NO.	ERROR MESSAGE
LOREN B 278-26-6487-A	02/02/20XX	LOREN0000	2	DATE SUBMITTED IN THE FIELD BELOW WAS NOT IN EIGHT DIGIT FORMAT. FROM DATE OF SERVICE (9990420)
MARTINEZ A 550-10-0414-A	02/19/20XX	MARTINEZ	2	MEDICARE IS NOT IDENTIFIED AS A PAYOR ON THIS CLAIM
MOSS E 248-06-9870-A	02/22/20XX	MOSS0000	2	MEDICARE IS NOT IDENTIFIED AS A PAYOR ON THIS CLAIM

D

Figure 7–10, cont'd. D, Weekly report showing rejected electronic claims to be corrected and resubmitted.

(EOMB) is based on the American National Standards Institute (ANSI) Accredited Standards Committee X12 (ASC X12) Health Care Claim Payment/Advise (837), or "ANSI 837." A subcommittee, X12N, has developed standards for a variety of electronic transactions between third-party payers and health care providers.

The use of ANSI 837 Version 4010 generates an electronic Medicare remittance advice instead of the paper RA. To improve cash flow, ANSI 837 also allows EFT of Medicare payments to the physician's bank account, which is called *direct deposit.*

RESOURCES ON THE INTERNET

American Association of Professional Coders
www.aapcnatl.org
American Health Information Management Association's Clinical Coding Forum
www.ahima.org

Medical Association of Billers Coding and Billing Forum
www.e-medbill.com
American Medical Association
www.ama-assn.org
Blue Cross Blue Shield Association
www.bluecares.com
CHAMPVA
www.va.gov/hac/champva/champva.html
Federal Register
www.access.gpo.gov/su_docs/aces140.html
Health and Human Services Office of Inspector General
www.oig.hhs.gov/
Centers for Medicaid and Medicare Services
www.cms.gov
Medicaid
www.chcs.org/resource/state.html
Medicare
www.medicare.gov
Listing of all 50 State Insurance Commissioners
www.naic.org/1regulator/usamap.htm
TRICARE
www.mytricare.com

Figure 7–11. Example of a fax agreement between a physician and an insurance carrier.

PROVIDER AGREEMENT

This Agreement is made by and between Blue Shield of California, herein called "Carrier" and_____, herein called "Provider."
                                   (Provider Name/Provider Number)

It is understood that this Agreement is subject to modification, revision, or termination due to changes in the prime contract between the Carrier and the Center for Medicare and Medicaid Services or changes in federal laws or regulations pertaining to Medicare. This Agreement will be deemed modified, revised, or terminated, to comply with any change in the federal law or regulations or change in the aforesaid prime contract on the effective date of such change.

In consideration of the Carrier agreeing to permit Provider to Fax claims in lieu of written requests for payment, Provider agrees:

(1)   That claims will be submitted to the Carrier in the specific format required by the Carrier, as is described in the Blue Shield of California instructions to billers as they may be amended from time to time.

(2)   That the Secretary of the Center for Medicare and Medicaid Services, his or her designee(s) or agent(s), or the Carrier has the right to audit and confirm for any purposes any information submitted by the Provider and shall be permitted access to claim documentation records and original source documentation, including patient signatures, medical and financial records in the office of the Provider or any other place for that purpose. Any and all incorrect payments discovered, as a result of such audit, will be adjusted according to the applicable provisions of Title XVIII of the Social Security Act, as amended, Federal Regulations, or Supplementary Medical Insurance (Medicare Part B) Guidelines.

(3)   That the Provider accepts responsibility for any and all Medicare claims submitted to the Carrier to research and correct any and all billing or claim discrepancies submitted under this agreement and that the Carrier will be held harmless for any claims, costs, or damages incurred as a result of such discrepancies.

(4)   That all original source documents and source records (e.g., medical/financial records and/or billing statements) will be maintained in such a way that all faxed claims can be readily associated and identified by source documents, including patient's signatures or signatures on behalf of patient. All original source documents will be retained for a period of seventy-two months following the date of submission to the Carrier. Medical records shall be retained pursuant to applicable state law.

(5)   That all claims represent services or supplies actually furnished by the Provider identified on the faxed claims; that all claims have corresponding original source documents as referenced in this Agreement; and that no claims will be submitted to the Carrier which the Provider knows or has reason to know conflict with the Social Security Act, as amended, Federal Regulations, or Medicare guidelines.

(6)   That the submission of a faxed claim to the Carrier is a claim for Medicare payment, and that anyone who misrepresents or falsifies any record or other information essential to that claim or that is required pursuant to this Agreement may, upon conviction, be subject to fine and imprisonment under Federal law. That the required patient signatures or appropriate signatures on behalf of patients are on file in accordance with prescribed procedures. If assignment is accepted, the Provider agrees to accept the reasonable charge, as determined by the Carrier, as the full charge for services on the claim and to bill the patient for deductible, co-insurance, and noncovered services.

_____   _____
PROVIDER NAME   PROVIDER NUMBER

_____   _____
PROVIDER ADDRESS   TELEPHONE NUMBER

_____   _____
                                         PROVIDER FAX NUMBER

BY _____

DATE _____

CONTROL NUM	PATIENT NAME	HIC NUMBER	DATES OF SVC	TOTAL AMOUNT	PHYSICIAN
1094003000000	Herman, Louise	123456789A	1201XX123120	161.10	xxAxxxxxx
1094003000010	Hope, Hortense	951847623B	1201XX121720	91.29	xxAxxxxxx
1094003000020	Kamb, Charles	753869421C1	1229XX122920	128.88	xxAxxxxxx

BLUE SHIELD OF CALIFORNIA FAX SUBMISSION
450 W EAST AVE, CHICO, CA 95926
916-896-7195

DATE: 01/19/20XX

PROVIDER RID (FAX) NUMBER: XXX-XXXX

Figure 7–12. Example of a faxback report verifying receipt of three transmitted insurance claims.

TRICARE Support Office
www.tso.osd.mil
Workers' Compensation related links
www.comp.state.nc.us/ncic/all50.htm

STUDENT ASSIGNMENT LIST

✔ Study Chapter 7.
✔ Answer the review questions in the *Workbook* to reinforce the theory learned in this chapter and to help prepare for a future test.

✔ Complete the assignments in the *Workbook* to edit and correct insurance claims that have been transmitted and rejected with errors.
✔ Turn to the Glossary at the end of this textbook for a further understanding of the Key Terms used in this chapter.

Receiving Payments and Insurance Problem Solving

CHAPTER OUTLINE

- Explain reasons for claim inquiries.
- Define terminology pertinent to problem claims.
- State solutions for problem claims.
- Identify reasons for rebilling a claim.
- List four objectives of state insurance commissioners.
- Mention seven problems to submit to insurance commissioners.
- Describe situations for filing appeals.
- Name three levels of review under the TRICARE appeal process.
- State six levels of review and appeal in the Medicare program.
- Determine which forms to use for the Medicare review and appeal process.

OBJECTIVES*

After reading this chapter you should be able to:

- Identify three health insurance payment policy provisions.
- Name three claim management techniques.
- Identify purposes of an insurance company history reference file.
- Indicate time limits for receiving payment for manually versus electronically submitted claims.

---

*Performance objectives and exercises for hands-on practical experience for this chapter appear in the *Workbook*.

Follow-Up After Claim Submission

For an overall picture of where and when insurance claim problems occur after submission, all aspects of the insurance picture must be studied from beginning to end. This chapter begins with the provisions for payment in the insurance contract and explains how this affects the timeliness for payment. Then the text demonstrates how to interpret the document that accompanies the payment and learn how to manage and organize financial records. To improve cash flow, numerous problems that can occur are presented and some solutions are offered. Finally, the review and appeal processes are discussed for various programs.

With the development of proficient skills and experience in following up on claims, one can become a valuable asset to his or her employer and bring in revenue that might otherwise be lost to the business.

Claim Policy Provisions

Insured

Each health insurance policy has provisions relating to insurance claims. There is a provision that the claimant has an obligation to notify the insurance company of a loss within a certain period of time or the insurer has the right to deny benefits for the loss.

If the insured is in disagreement with the insurer for settlement of a claim, a suit must begin within 3 years after the claim was submitted. Another provision states that an insured person cannot bring legal action against an insurance company until 60 days after a claim is submitted.

Payment Time Limits

The health insurance policy also has a provision about the insurance company's obligation to pay benefits promptly when a claim is submitted. However, time limits vary in this provision from one insurance carrier or program to another. Specific time limits mentioned in insurance contracts should be read and noted. It is reasonable to expect payment as shown in Table 8–1. If a payment problem

develops and the insurance company is slow or ignores, denies, or exceeds time limits to pay a claim, then it is prudent to contact the insurance company. In the letter the contracted time limit should be stated, the reason the claim has not been paid should be asked, and a copy should be retained for the physician's files. If the problem persists and there is no favorable response, the state insurance commissioner should be contacted to see whether he or she can take action to improve the situation; a copy of the correspondence should also be mailed. Many state insurance commissioners have broad powers to regulate the insurance companies within their state; others have no powers at all. If the carrier is a self-insured plan, a Medicaid or Medicare HMO, or an ERISA–based plan, the insurance commissioner will not be able to assist with carrier issues. Claims may be submitted to the insurance company repeatedly with none of them ever being recorded. The one claim that will make it to the insurance company is the one that arrives after the self-determined timely filing deadline. If the provider has no contract with the carrier, the provider is not obligated to the carrier's deadline. Their denial should be appealed and payment demanded.

Managed care plans usually process claims on a daily basis, but some plans release payments quarterly. There are plans that withhold a percentage that is reserved in a pool and distributed at the end of the fiscal year. In some states, managed care plans do not come under the jurisdiction of the state insurance commissioner but of another agency. The state medical society should be contacted to find out who is the responsible entity. Because managed care plans vary considerably in payment policies and administrative procedures, Chapter 10 details follow up on procedures and problem-solving techniques.

Explanation of Benefits

An **explanation of benefits (EOB)/remittance advice (RA)** is a document issued stating the status of the claim; whether it is paid, suspended (pending), rejected, or denied. A **suspended claim** is one that is processed by the insurance carrier but is held in an indeterminate (pending) state about payment either

TABLE 8–1	Time Limit for Receiving Insurance Reimbursement	
Program	**From Date Claim Was Manually Submitted (by mail)**	**From Date Claim Was Electronically Submitted**
Private insurance companies	4–6 weeks	2 weeks or less
TRICARE standard	8–12 weeks	2 weeks or less
Medicare	4–6 weeks	2 weeks for participating physicians
		3 weeks for nonparticipating physicians
Workers' compensation	4–8 weeks	2 weeks or less

because of an error or the need for additional information. The EOB also states the allowed and disallowed amounts by the insurance carrier. The allowed amount is the maximum dollar value the insurance company assigns to each procedure and service on which payment is based. Typically a percent (e.g., 80%) of the allowed amount is paid by the insurance carrier. If benefits have been assigned, the physician receives a copy of the EOB/RA along with a payment check, also called a voucher. If benefits have not been assigned, payment goes to the patient and the physician may have a difficult time obtaining this payment and EOB.

Components of an EOB

At first glance, the form may seem difficult to understand. Unfortunately, there is no standard format for EOBs from one carrier to the next, but information contained in each one usually is the same. If one line at a time is read, the description and calculations for each patient may be understood easily. The EOB breaks down how payment was determined and contains the following information in categories or columns:

1. Insurance company's name and address
2. Provider of services
3. Dates of services
4. Service or procedure code numbers
5. Amounts billed by the providers
6. Reduction or denial codes. Comment codes (reason, remarks, or notes) indicating reasons payments were denied, asking for more information to determine coverage and benefits, or stating amounts of adjustment because of payments by other insurance companies (coordination of benefits)
7. Claim control number
8. Subscriber's and patient's name and policy numbers
9. Analysis of patient's total payment responsibility (amount not covered, copayment amount, deductible, coinsurance, other insurance payment, and patient's total responsibility)
10. Copayment amount(s) due from the patient
11. Deductible amounts subtracted from billed amounts
12. Total amount paid by the insurance carrier

Refer to Figure 8–1, which illustrates an EOB for a private insurance carrier, and identify each component mentioned in the preceding list.

Interpretation of an EOB

Reading and interpreting an EOB has become a complicated procedure for a number of reasons. If several patients' claims are submitted to an insurance carrier, the EOB may reflect the status of all of those claims and one check may be issued. If the physician has signed a contract agreeing to discount fees with a number of insurance carriers and managed care plans, payment amounts may vary along with the percentage of the fee that is adjusted off of the account. In addition, if more than one physician is in the medical practice and the practice is submitting claims using one group tax identification number, more than one physician's patients' claims may appear on a single EOB. The explanation of benefits shown in Figure 8–1 should be read line by line to interpret the meanings under each category or column, and the numbered explanations should be referred to when necessary.

Posting an EOB

When an EOB is received in the physician's office, the claim(s) should be pulled or the patient's computerized account should be referred to, and every payment against the applicable insurance contract should be checked to find out whether the amount paid is correct. Refer to the step-by-step directions for posting to a patient's financial accounting record in Chapter 2 and see Figure 2–17.

If services are reimbursed and are not clearly described on an EOB, ask the patient to send a copy of the EOB he or she received from the carrier. The patient's copy often differs from the physician's copy and may have a better explanation of what was or was not paid.

Claims paid with no errors are put into a file designated for closed claims. An EOB for a single payment may be stapled to the claim form and then filed with the closed claims according to the date the payment was posted. EOBs that have many patients' payments listed may be filed in an EOB file. Some offices prefer to make copies of each multiple EOB, highlight the appropriate patient account, and attach the copy to the individual claim or file it in each patient's financial record.

Additional information and examples of documents may be found in the following chapters: Chapter 10 explains a Statement of Remittance for managed care systems, Chapters 7 and 11 explain both a Medicare electronic RA and a hard copy RA, and Chapter 13 shows a Summary Payment Voucher for the TRICARE program.

State Insurance Commissioner

Commission Objectives

The insurance industry is protected by a special exemption from the Federal Trade Commission (FTC) under the McCarran Act (named for the late

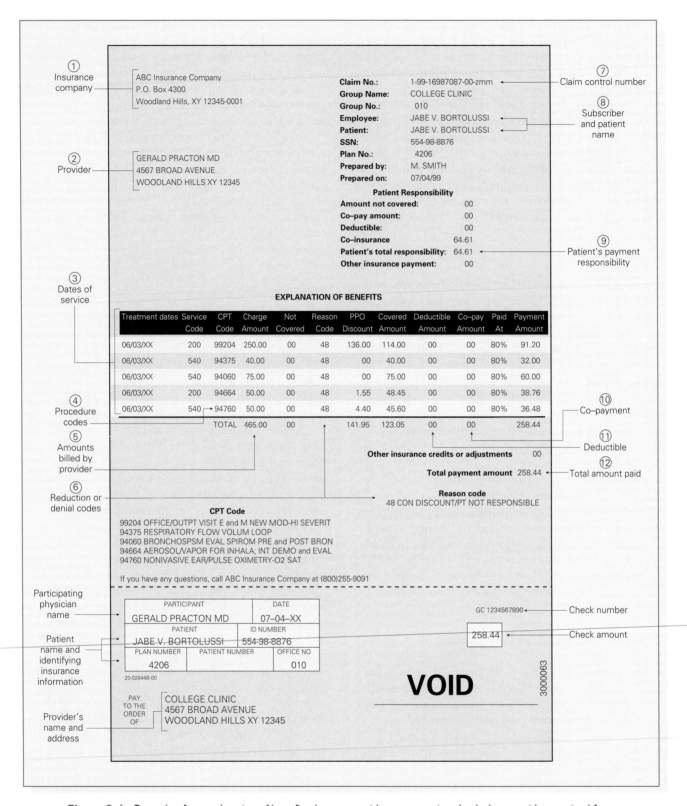

Figure 8–1. Example of an explanation of benefits document with accompanying check that provider received from a private insurance company.

Senator Pat McCarran of Nevada). Under the exemption the FTC cannot attack unfair or deceptive practices if there is any state law about such practices. The regulations vary widely from state to state, and by no means are all 50 states equally strict. If a complaint arises about an insurance policy, medical claim, or insurance agent or broker, the insurance department of the state of residence or the state where the insurance company's corporate office is headquartered should be contacted. Sometimes this department is referred to as the insurance commission of the state. State insurance departments usually have various objectives, including the following:

▶ To make certain that the financial strength of insurance companies is not unduly diminished

▶ To monitor the activities of insurance companies to make sure the interests of the policyholders are protected

▶ To verify that all contracts are carried out in good faith

▶ To make sure that all organizations authorized to transact insurance, including agents and brokers, are in compliance with the insurance laws of that state

▶ To release information on how many complaints have been filed against a specific insurance company in a year

▶ To help explain correspondence related to insurance company bankruptcies and other financial difficulties

▶ To assist if a company funds its own insurance plan

▶ To help to resolve insurance conflicts

The insurance commissioner can hold a hearing to determine whether licensed insurers, agents, or brokers are in compliance with the insurance laws of the state, but the commissioner does not have the authority vested in a court of law to order an insurance company to make payment on a specific claim.

The insurance commissioner reviews the policy to see whether the denial of a claim by the insurance company was based on legal provisions of the insurance contract and advises the patient if there is an infraction of the law. If there is an infraction the patient should consult an attorney to determine whether the claim should be submitted to a court of law.

Types of Problems

The types of problems that should be submitted to the insurance commissioner are as follows:

1. Improper denial of a claim or settlement for an amount less than that indicated by the policy, after proper appeal has been made
2. Delay in settlement of a claim, after proper appeal has been made
3. Illegal cancellation or termination of an insurance policy
4. Misrepresentation by an insurance agent or broker
5. Misappropriation of premiums paid to an insurance agent or broker
6. Problems about insurance premium rates

7. Two companies that cannot determine who is primary

Commission Inquiries

Requests to the insurance commissioner must be submitted in writing. An example of an insurance complaint form showing pertinent necessary information when making a request for assistance from the state insurance commissioner is shown in Figure 8-2. In some states the insurance commissioner requires that the complaint come from the patient even if an assignment of benefits form has been signed. In such a case a letter or form should be prepared for the patient to sign and then submitted. Depending on the situation of the case, one may wish to send copies to the state medical association or an attorney. Mail may be sent certified, return receipt requested. The request should contain the following information:

1. The inquiring person's (patient) or policyholder's name, because the commissioner's responsibility is to the patient (the consumer), not the physician
2. The policyholder's address
3. The policyholder's telephone number
4. The insured's name
5. Name, address, and title of the insurance agent or official of the insurance company
6. A statement of the complaint including, if possible, a copy of the policy, medical bills, unpaid medical insurance claim, canceled checks, and any correspondence from the company pertaining to the claim
7. The patient's signature
8. The name and address of the insurance company, agent, or broker, or name and address of the finance company if the premium was financed
9. The policy or claim number
10. The date of loss
11. The date the patient signed the complaint form

If an insurance company is continually a slow payer, a method to speed up payments is to include a note to the carrier that reads, "Unless this claim is paid or denied within 30 days, a formal written complaint will be filed with the state insurance commissioner."

Another method is to send a letter to the insurance commissioner with a copy notation inserted at the end to the insurance company. It might read, "The attached claim has been submitted to the XYZ Insurance Company. It has not been paid or denied. Please accept this letter as a formal written complaint against the XYZ Insurance Company."

INSURANCE COMPLAINT FORM

To: State Insurance Commissioner
Address
City, State, ZIP code

1. ──→ Your Name ___Grace T. O'Neal___

2. ──→ Address ___4572 Southport St.___

___Woodland Hills, XY 12345___

3. ──→ Day Telephone No. ___555-421-0733___

4. ──→ Insured: ___Grace T. O'Neal___

___XYZ Insurance Company___ ←── 8.
(Agent or Company Complaint Against)

Policy No. ___531 OK 492___ ←── 9.

Date of Loss: ___10-11-20XX___ ←── 10.

Claim or File No. _____

Is this the only complaint you have filed with the insurance commissioner concerning this matter?
Yes ___X___ No _____

5. ──→ Have you taken up this problem with an official of the company, agent, or broker: If yes, give name, address, and title. Yes ___X___ No _____

___John Knave, Insurance Agent___
_____

The following is a brief statement of what the agent or company has done, or failed to do:

6. ──→ Insurance payment has been denied by insurance company as a noncovered service, but policy covers professional procedure performed.

7. ──→ _Grace T. O'Neal_ ___12-15-20XX___ ←── 11.
Signature of Patient   Date

Attach a copy of the insurance policy, related documents, correspondence, etc.

Figure 8–2. Insurance complaint form, showing pertinent necessary information when stating a complaint and making a request for assistance from the state insurance commissioner.

Insurance companies are rated according to the number of complaints received about them, so they do not want the insurance commissioner to be alerted to any problems. Some states have information available to the public on how many claims have been submitted against a company if this information is needed. Refer to Appendix A to contact the state insurance commissioner for assistance or information about state laws.

Claim Management Techniques

Insurance Claims Register

Chapter 2 contained follow-up procedures for insurance claims by logging the completed claims onto an insurance claims register (see Fig. 2–23). A log like this also could be developed and updated with little effort using a spreadsheet software program, which would allow statistical data to be retrieved quickly and easily. Most medical software programs offer practice management reports that can

be used to track insurance payments. Regardless of the method used, ease of tracking quickly and accurately should be the goal in setting up a system.

After logging into a register, place a copy of all insurance claims in a pending file labeled for each month of service so that the unpaid claims can be retrieved for easy follow-up. Or place a copy of the insurance claim in an alphabetical file by insurance company name. This method permits an inquiry on multiple outstanding claims in one letter to the insurance carrier each month rather than many letters covering individual claims. Place the insurance claims register in a loose-leaf notebook indexed according to the various insurance companies. When referring to a claims register, delinquent claims can be quickly located by simply looking through the book under the Date Claim Paid column. If that column is blank, check the Date Claim Submitted column and follow up as needed.

When referring to a report generated by a medical software program, claims are aged according to date submitted, allowing easy reference for timely follow up. Send a claim tracer when no payment has been received from the insurance company.

When a payment is received, pull all copies of claims that correspond with the payments and attach the EOB/RA. Post payment received and the contracted adjustment to the patient's financial accounting record and to the day sheet or the computerized financial record. File the EOB/RA and deposit the payment check in the physician's bank account. Draw a line through the pertinent information in the claim register, but do not obscure data. When all claims on the page have been paid, draw a diagonal line across the page. Pages may be retained for future reference.

Tickler File

An alternate method used to track pending or resubmitted insurance claims is a *tickler file*. This file is also called a *suspense* or *follow-up file*. A type of tickler file is also used to remind patients of upcoming or missed appointments (see Chapter 2, Fig. 2–21). Tickler files also can be set up in computer systems that prompt the insurance billing specialist to telephone or send inquiries about unpaid insurance claims.

To set up this reminder system, divide active claims by month and file them in chronological order by date of service. Subdivisions also can be made by patient name or in numerical order by account number. Maintain the active file (unpaid claims) for the calendar year and put inactive resolved claims (older than 1 year) in storage that is accessible.

To incorporate this system into the billing process, start by printing two completed CMS-1500 claim forms or copy completed claim forms. Send the original to the payer and file the copy in the tickler file by date of service. After receiving the payment check and EOB/RA, pull all claims noted on the EOB/RA from the tickler file. Post the payment to the patient's account (financial accounting record) and day sheet or financial record in the computer system. Compare the charges made on each claim to the payments listed on the EOB/RA. Refer to the insurance contract, if necessary. If a patient has received many services and the claim was submitted on several forms, determine whether services on all forms were processed for payment. After performing this reconciliation process, attach a copy of the EOB/RA to the claim and put it in a paid file. Each claim should be referenced with the date of payment posted to the patient's account.

Delinquent claims remaining in the tickler file and exceeding the contract time limits should be traced. Complete the insurance claim tracer form shown in Figure 8–3. If a claim has been denied, send a letter to the appeals division of the insurance company as shown in Figure 8–4. Attach a copy of the tracer or letter to the claim and refile it in the tickler file. It is recommended to send a copy of correspondence marked "For your information," to the patient. Follow-up procedures for claim inquiries are discussed next in detail.

Insurance Company Payment History

Medical practices that employ computer software to handle the financial end of the business refer to monthly computerized reports used to track the payment history of insurance companies. This is an easy method to discover which companies pay slowly or pay less on certain services, and provides excellent reports for tax purposes.

To manually obtain this information, make a file of 3 × 5-inch index cards or 8 × 11-inch three-hole punched sheets in a loose-leaf binder listing the insurance companies or managed care plans that send claim payments directly to the physician. Every time a payment is received, pull out the card or the loose-leaf sheet for that company and update the information. The following information is necessary for tracking:

▶ Insurance company name and regional office addresses
▶ Claims filing procedures
▶ Payment policies (provisions) for each plan
▶ Time limits to submit claims
▶ Time limit for receiving payments
▶ Dollar amount for each procedural code number
▶ Names of patients covered and their policy and group numbers

If the patients' names and group policy numbers are listed, this file is helpful when discussing with the patient what the insurance company may be expected to pay for certain services. Remember that group numbers may change annually as benefits increase or decrease, so be sure to keep the policy numbers current.

An insurance company payment history system can help avoid potential problems and pinpoint requirements that must be met to help secure additional payment on a reduced or denied claim.

Claim Inquiries

An **inquiry,** sometimes called a **tracer** or follow up, is made to an insurance company to locate the status of an insurance claim or inquire about payment determination shown on the EOB/RA. As mentioned, claim status can be accessed easily by means of computer or teledigital response systems, thus speeding up inquiry time. It also may be accessed with a telephone call or by mail. Here are some reasons for making inquiries.

COLLEGE CLINIC
4567 Broad Avenue
Woodland Hills, XY 12345-0001
Telephone (555) 486-9002
Fax (555) 487-8976

INSURANCE CLAIM TRACER

INSURANCE COMPANY NAME American Insurance   DATE: 09/14/XX   .

ADDRESS   P.O. Box 5300, New York, New York 12000   .

Patient name: Marcella Austin

Date of birth: May 25, 1970

Employer: TC Corporation

Insured: Marcella Austin

Policy/certificate No.   9635 402-A

Group name/No.   B0105

Date of initial claim submission: 08/02/XX

Date(s) of service: 07/02/XX to 07/10/XX

Total charges submitted: $536.24

An inordinate amount of time has passed since submission of our original claim. We have not received a request for additional information and still await payment of this assigned claim. Please review the attached duplicate and process for payment within 7 days.

DETAILS OF INQUIRY

Please check the claim status and return this letter to our office. Thank you.

- ☐   No record of claim.
- ☐   Claim received and payment is in process.
- ☐   Claim is in suspense (comment please).
- ☐   Claim is in review (comment please).
- ☐   Additional information needed (comment please)
- ☐   Applied to deductible. Amount: $ _____
- ☐   Patient not eligible for benefits.
- ☐   Determination issued to beneficiary.
- ☐   Claim paid. Date: _____   Amount: $ _____   To whom: _____
- ☐   Claim denied (comment please).

Comments: _____

_____

Thank you for your assistance in this important matter. Please contact the insurance specialist named below if you have any questions regarding this claim.

Insurance Specialist: Katelyn Chang   (555) 486-9002 Ext. 236   .

Treating Physician: Gene Ulibarri, MD   State license number C1480XX   .

Provider Number: 256788831XX   Provider's IRS number 77-86531XX .

Figure 8–3. Insurance claim tracer showing how a form may be set up to follow up on a delinquent claim.

- ▸ There was no response to a submitted claim.
- ▸ Payment was not received within the time limit for the plan or program.
- ▸ Payment is received but the amount is incorrect.
- ▸ Payment is received but the amount allowed and the patient's responsibility are not defined.
- ▸ Payment received was for a patient not seen by the physician. It is possible to receive a payment check made out to a payee's name that is different from

ABC MEDICAL GROUP, INC.

123 Main Street
Woodland Hills, XY 12345-0239
Tel. 555/487-4900
Fax. No. 555/486-4834

September 12, 20XX

Ms. Jane Hatfield
Appeals Division
XYZ Managed Care Plan
100 South H Street
Anytown, XY 12345-0001

Dear Ms. Hatfield:

Re: Claim number: A0958
       Patient: Carolyn B. Little
       Dates of service: August 2–10, 20XX

Recently I received a denied claim from your office (see enclosure). A
review of the contract I have with your managed care plan shows that these
services should have been approved and paid according to your fee
schedule.

Enclosed is a photocopy of my chart notes for the professional services
rendered to the patient on these dates. I have seen Ms. Little five times in
the last nine days and each service was medically necessary by the specific
complaints expressed by the patient.

On examination, I found the complaints by the patient were valid.

If after review of this claim you still feel reimbursement is not
appropriate, please forward this request to the Peer Review Committee for
a final determination.

If you need additional information, please telephone, fax, or write my
office.

Sincerely,

John Doe, MD

mtf
Enclosures

Figure 8–4. A letter asking for a review about a claim submitted and denied by a managed care plan.

the patient's name. Making a call may quickly clarify for whom the payment is being made.

In addition to nonpayment or reduced payment, there are other reasons for inquiries to an insurance company, including:

▶ EOB/RA shows that a professional or diagnostic code was changed from what was submitted.
▶ EOB/RA shows that the service was disallowed. The claim should be revised and resubmitted. Check to see whether the procedure codes were correct and that the services listed were described fully enough to justify the maximum, allowable benefits.
▶ There is an error on the EOB/RA.
▶ The check received was made out to the wrong physician.

Inquire about the claim if any of these situations occurs. If the inquiry is submitted in writing, some

programs require special forms completed with a copy of the claim attached. Figure 8–4 is an example of a letter used when asking for a review about a denied claim that was submitted to a managed care plan. If a claim must be reviewed after payment has been rendered, send in the letter as shown in Figure 8–5. When calling, document the name of the person spoken to, date and time of call, department or extension of the person, and an outline of the conversation.

Problem Claims

Types of Problems

There are many types of problem claims (e.g., delinquent, in suspense [pending], lost, rejected, denied, downcoding, partial payment, payment lost

COLLEGE CLINIC
4567 Broad Avenue
Woodland Hills, XY
12345-0001
Telephone 555/486-9002
Fax (555) 487-8976

Committee on Physician's Services

Re: Underpayment
Identification No.: _____ M18876782
Patient: Peaches Melba
Type of Service: Plastic & Reconstructive Surgery
Date of Service: 1 - 3 - XX
Amount Paid: $ 75.00
My Fees: $ 180.00

Dear Sirs:

Herewith a request for a committee review of the above-named case, since I consider the allowance paid very low having in mind the location, the extent, the type, and the necessary surgical procedure performed: The skin graft, one inch in diameter, included the lateral third of eyebrow and was full thickness to preserve hair follicles.

Operative report for the surgery has been sent to you with the claim.

Considering these points I hope that you will authorize additional payment in order to bring the total fee to within reasonable and customary charges.

Sincerely,

Cosmo Graff, M.D.

Cosmo Graff, M.D.

mf
enclosure

Figure 8–5. A letter appealing a fee reduction. This letter lists important data and is sent to the insurance carrier after payment has been received that the physician believes should be increased.

in the mail, payment paid to patient, and overpayment). These problems require some type of follow-up action. The claim status may be indicated on an EOB; however sometimes a claim is submitted and no status is reported. As mentioned, sending a claim inquiry form (tracer) is often the quickest way of determining the status of a claim (Fig. 8–3).

To prevent repeated claims errors, the office manager should identify the source of the errors within the medical office. Often a claim may be denied because of an error that occurred when collecting registration information at the front desk or when posting charges to the account. Other errors occur because of wrong procedure or diagnostic codes, incorrect provider numbers, and a variety of situations mentioned in prior chapters. A large number of claims are denied for wrong gender and wrong year of birth. The more unusual or foreign-sounding a name is, the more denials occur based on gender.

The individual handling the front desk must collect insurance information accurately and update this information routinely (e.g., insurance

identification number and address). The person posting to accounts must be certain to post to the correct account and see that supplemental insurers are billed after the primary insurance carrier has paid. Identified errors should be brought to the attention of the individual(s) responsible to improve accuracy of outgoing claims and avoid future problems.

Delinquent, Pending, or Suspense

The following are specific claim problems and possible solutions.

Problem: The term **delinquent claim** means payment is overdue from a nonpayer. The nonpayer can be an insurance company, managed care plan, or intermediary for the Medicaid, Medicare, or TRI-CARE programs. Sometimes nonpayment is caused by a claim in review or in **suspense** because of an error or the need for additional information. The carrier may be investigating a claim because of preexisting conditions or possibly because the patient may have a work-related injury.

Solution: Use claim management techniques (e.g., insurance claims register, tickler file, insurance company payment history) to keep on top of delinquent claims, so that follow up can be accomplished in a timely manner. If the office handles a large volume of claims, divide the unpaid claims into four groups, one for each of the three largest insurers and the fourth for all others. Work on one group each week so the work is spread out over the 4 weeks in the month. Write a follow-up letter to the insurance company asking for payment and enclose a copy of the original claim form or complete and send in the insurance claim tracer shown in Figure 8–3.

Lost Claims

Problem: When an insurance claim is received by the insurance company, the claim is date stamped usually within 24 hours, assigned a claim number, and logged into the payer system. However if there is a backlog of claims it may take 7 to 15 days or longer to be logged into the system. If one calls to find out the status of the claim during that time, one may be told it has not been received or it may be considered a **lost claim.**

Solution: Ask if there is a backlog of claims to resolve the situation. This indicates that the claim probably has not been logged into the system. Always verify that the patient is insured by the insurance carrier and is covered for the basic benefits claimed. If it is determined to be lost, then submit a copy of the original claim referencing it "copy of the original claim submitted on *(date)*." Before sending it verify the correct mailing address (e.g., post office box number, ZIP code). There are several ways to track the claim if there have been various problems with the same insurance company. Send it by certified mail with return receipt or fax the claim and ask for a confirmation. Another method available to show proof that a special communication was sent by a deadline is to obtain and complete a Certificate of Mailing form from the post office. The form is initialed and postmarked at the post office and returned to the insurance biller for office file records. Because the post office does not keep a record of the mailing, this certificate costs less than certified mail. If there is verifiable information of a lost claim, call or write to the provider relations department or member services and explain the problem. Possibly check the time limit in the contract with the payer in question. Some contracts have a clause that specifies any claims not paid within a certain number of days (e.g., 30 days) after receipt will be paid at an increased rate or in full. If there may be mishandling of claims, gather documentation and send a letter to the state insurance commission with a letter to the insurance carrier about the action taken.

Rejected Claims

Chapter 6 expressed some common reasons why claims are rejected or delayed. A **rejected claim** is one submitted that does not follow specific insurance carrier instructions or contains a technical error (Fig. 8–6). Such claims may be disproved or discarded by the system and returned to the biller. Technical errors consist of missing or incorrect information and are found through computer edits, screening processes for benefit provisions, and proofreading. Medicare-mandated prepayment screens are discussed in Chapter 11.

Problem: Claim rejections occur because of the following:

- Transposed numbers
- Missing, invalid, or incorrect procedure codes and modifiers
- Missing or invalid place of service
- Mismatch of place of service to type of service
- Missing referring physician when billing tests
- Missing or invalid provider number when the patient was referred
- Incorrect, invalid, nonspecific, or missing diagnostic code numbers
- Incorrect dates of service
- Incorrect year of service
- Incorrect number of days in the month (e.g., February)
- Code description does not match services rendered
- Duplicate dates of service
- Duplicate charges

Solution: If a claim is rejected and returned, add the missing or incomplete information and resubmit a corrected claim for regular claims processing. Do not send a corrected claim for review or appeal.

Figure 8–6. Insurance billing specialist troubleshooting a rejected claim.

Problem: Claim submitted for several services and one service is rejected for incomplete information and other services are paid.

Solution: Complete a new CMS-1500 claim form including all information and resubmit for the rejected services only. Note in Block 19 that it is a resubmission.

Problem: Insurance carrier requests further information or information about another carrier.

Solution: Verify primary and secondary insurance information with the patient and call or mail the information to the insurance company. Identify the subscriber, subscriber number, and date of service on all correspondence.

Problem: Resubmitted claim is returned a second time.

Solution: Review the EOB/RA statement to see if there is a denial code or narrative explanation. Examine the claim for missing, incomplete, or incorrect information and, if found, correct it. Evaluate the claim to determine if it is a candidate for the appeal process. Determine if a specific appeal form must be submitted. Submit chart notes, a detailed summary, or a copy of the operative or pathology report, as applicable, to clearly identify the procedure or service. Enclose a cover letter with the resubmitted data.

Denied Claims

A **denied claim** is one that may be denied because of medical coverage policy issues or program issues. Insurance companies save money when a claim is denied, and only a small percentage of individuals pursue appeals. State laws require insurance companies to notify the insured of a denial and state why the claim was denied. It is possible that payment can be received even after a claim has been denied in whole or in part.

When a claim is denied and the patient has not been contacted by the insurance company, notify the patient by telephone or mail as soon as possible to keep him or her informed. Always retain the correspondence from the insurance company so it can be quickly retrieved in the event a patient inquires and has additional questions. The recourse to a denied claim is to appeal and request a review in writing. The appeals process varies between insurance carriers. A Medicare claim may be appealed by requesting a review in writing, and federal laws require that an explanation be given for each denied service. In Medicare Part B hearing cases, carriers have been instructed to pay an appealed claim if the cost of the

hearing process is more than the amount of the claim.

Some reasons why claims are not paid because of denial include the following:
- Payable only for selected diagnoses
- Frequency limitations or restrictions per benefit period
- Procedure performed by ineligible specialty provider (e.g., podiatrist would not be paid for neurosurgery)
- Bundled with other services
- Payable only in certain locations (e.g., outpatient only)
- Prior approval needed and not obtained
- Diagnosis did not justify the service or procedure rendered

One cannot simply change the information and resubmit to resolve the problem. Some additional examples with suggested solutions are as follows:

Problem: Service was not a policy or program benefit (e.g., routine physical examination, routine tests, routine foot care, routine dental care, cosmetic surgery, custodial care, eye or hearing examinations for glasses or hearing aids, and some immunizations). Plastic surgery is considered a general exclusion in many insurance policies.

Solution: Send the patient a statement with a notation of the response from the insurance company. Better yet, always verify coverage for routine physical examinations or tests and services that are in question as to whether they will be paid by the insurance policy.

Problem: Treatment given for a preexisting condition. (Currently some policies do not include this exclusion.)

Solution: When a patient is referred, ask the referring physician to forward information on all preexisting conditions that may be relevant to the surgery or procedure to be performed. Request verification of insurance coverage from the insurer for the surgery or procedure with regard to preexisting conditions. Request authorization for the surgical procedure or diagnostic tests. If authorization is denied, have the physician discuss other treatment or payment options with the patient (e.g., rendering minimum level of interim care until the preexistence period, usually 6 months, has expired). If the physician believes that the patient's condition is not preexisting, send an appeal to the insurance company. Otherwise bill the patient, noting the insurance company's response on the statement.

Problem: Insurance coverage canceled before service.

Solution: Send the patient a statement with notation of the insurance determination on the bill.

Problem: Insurance coverage lapsed beyond renewal date for service rendered.

Solution: Send the patient a statement with notation of the response from the insurance company on the bill.

Problem: Service provided before coverage was in effect.

Solution: Send the patient a statement with notation of the response from the insurance company on the bill.

Problem: Service provided when the patient was no longer a member of the insurance plan.

Solution: Send the patient a statement with notation of the response from the insurance company on the bill.

Problem: Insurance company indicates provided service was not medically necessary.

Solution: Determine under what circumstances the insurance carrier considers the service medically necessary. The problem may be that the diagnostic code does not properly support the procedural codes being reported. It is vital that the physician's documentation be specific enough to support the necessity of the services provided. If the physician believes the patient's condition supported the medical necessity for the service, send an appeal for review to the insurance company, explaining in detail the reasons why. Or have the insurance physician write to the patient and advise what might have been a better course of treatment. Keep a list of codes that have been denied for medical necessity and what further determinations were made in the insurance company payment history. Check the insurance contract to determine if the patient may be billed. Consider asking patients to sign a Waiver of Liability form before treatment. Bill the patient if payment may be denied.

Problem: Service was for an injury that is considered as compensable under workers' compensation.

Solution: Locate the carrier for the industrial injury, request permission to treat, and send the carrier a report of the case with a bill. Notify the patient's health insurance carrier monthly about the status of the case.

Problem: Service was not precertified for a surgery, hospitalization, or diagnostic procedure.

Solution: Ask the patient to bring in his or her insurance policy for review to determine whether precertification was necessary for the service or whether any sanctions are imposed. If there were problems or difficulties about the case leading to the reason precertification was not obtained, write a letter of appeal noting the history.

Problem: Patient did not pay premium.

Solution: Verify insurance coverage before treatment begins, especially for procedures and surgery. Change patient's account to "cash" if insurance is not in force.

Problem: Service or procedure is experimental.

Solution: Verify if procedure is approved by the insurance company before procedure is done.

Problem: Deductible was not met.

Solution: Ask patient when he or she arrives at the office about status of deductible. Collect from patient if deductible has not been met. Consider holding the claim if several services are performed during the same time period and the patient paid the deductible at another office but it has not been recorded by the insurance company.

Problem: Services are considered cosmetic.

Solution: Appeal claim if the problem was treated because of a medical condition, not for cosmetic reasons.

Denied Claims Summary

Remember, prevention measures to avoid denied claims are as follows:

1. Include progress notes and orders for tests for extended hospital services.
2. Submit a letter from the prescribing physician documenting necessity when ambulance transportation is used.
3. Clarify the type of service (e.g., primary surgical services versus assist-at-surgery services).
4. Use modifiers to further describe and identify the exact service rendered.
5. Keep abreast of the latest policies for the Medicare, Medicaid, and TRICARE programs by reading local newsletters.
6. Obtain current provider manuals for Medicaid, Medicare, and TRICARE so these are available for

quick reference. When bulletins or pages are received from these programs during the year, keep the manuals up-to-date by inserting the current material.

Downcoding

Lowered reimbursement is the result of downcoding. As mentioned in Chapter 5, downcoding occurs for the following reasons:

Problem: Coding system used on a claim does not match the coding system used by the insurance carrier receiving the claim. Computer software is designed to convert the code submitted to the nearest code in use. However, payment may be less.

Solution: Monitor reimbursements and monitor downcodes to discover which codes are affected. Then telephone the insurance carrier and ask which code system is in use, obtain the proper book, and use the appropriate system.

Problem: Insufficient diagnostic information on a claim.

Solution: Be sure each procedure listed on the claim form is linked to an appropriate diagnosis. Refer to the medical record if necessary.

Problem: Unspecified diagnoses are listed on the claim form. Routine use of too many nonspecific diagnostic codes (ICD-9-CM codes that have number "9" as the fourth or fifth digit) result in denials or downcoding, especially if extensive or specific surgery is involved.

Solution: Make sure the physician dictates specific diagnoses and does not circle nonspecific diagnoses on an encounter form. Always code to the highest level of specificity. Refer to the patient's medical record when necessary.

Payment Paid to Patient

Problem: Sometimes an insurance payment may be sent in error to the patient after an assignment of benefits has been signed and sent in with the insurance claim. In some cases a clause may be in the insurance policy that payment may be made only to the insured.

Solution: Call the insurance company to verify whether the payment was made and to whom. If the account is substantially overdue, ask for a copy of the endorsed check or EOB/RA statement that indicates where payment was sent. If the carrier refuses, ask for help from the supervisor of the provider or customer relations department. There are two different courses of action to take after this has been verified.

1. Call the patient explaining that the insurance company sent payment to him or her in error and ask when full payment can be expected. Document the commitment in the patient's financial record. If not able to reach the patient by telephone, send a letter by certified mail to the patient. If the patient still refuses to pay, inform the patient that the provider is forced to write off the debt, that the money is considered taxable income to the patient, and the undeclared income the patient received will be reported to the Internal Revenue Service on the 1099 form. This may assist in getting the debt paid. If not discuss with the physician whether he or she wishes to discharge the patient from the practice. It is also advisable to send the information to the credit bureau.

2. Send a letter to the insurance company including a copy of the claim with EOB/RA indicating payment was made to the patient and a copy of the assignment of benefits. Demand payment from the insurance company, stating the need to honor the assignment. The insurance company must recover the payment from the patient. If a dead end is reached after pursuing reimbursement from the insurance company, then file a complaint with the state insurance commissioner. After receiving the physician's complaint, the commissioner will write to the insurance company and request a review of the claim. If the insurance company admits that there is an assignment of benefits and that it inadvertently paid the patient, the insurance company must pay the physician within 2 to 3 weeks and honor the assignment even before it recovers its money from the patient. The insurance company will then file for payment from the patient.

Two-Party Check

Problem: Patient cashes a two-party check. A **two-party check** is a check that is made out to the physician and the patient. Although not legal, the patient may be successful in cashing it without the endorsement of the physician.

Solution: Do not allow time to pass. Immediately advise the insurance company of the fraud so it may recover the money from the person who accepted the check without proper endorsement.

Problem: A check is received made out to both the physician and the hospital and only part of the sum is the physician's payment.

Solution: Call the insurance company and ask how much should be retained by the physician. Ask whose tax identification number will be used on the 1099 form for reporting income to the Internal Revenue Service. The hospital's income should not be reflected on the physician's 1099 form. To avoid another problem like this, inquire why the insurance company paid in this manner. Sometimes a participating agreement may exist that the physician did not know about.

Overpayment

An **overpayment** is a sum of money paid by the insurance carrier or patient to the provider of service that is more than the bill or more than the allowed amount. Overpayments may be discovered immediately, called to one's attention by the patient or insurance carrier, or not discovered for several months or years. First determine if an overpayment exists by reviewing the available financial documents on the case in question. Then decide how to handle the overpayment.

It is wise to develop an overpayment policy and procedure for each type of insurer, program, or managed care plan and for every type of overpayment situation that may occur.

Problem: Overpayment. Scenarios that may occur are as follows:

▶ Receiving more than one's fee from an insurance carrier
▶ Receiving more than the contract rate from a managed care plan
▶ Receiving payments that should have been paid to the patient
▶ Receiving duplicate payments from two or more insurance carriers or from the patient and one or more third-party payers
▶ Receiving payment made for someone who is not the provider's patient

Solution: In any type of overpayment situation, always cash the third-party payer's check and make out a provider's refund check. In case of an audit this establishes documentation showing the problem has been resolved.

Refund checks usually are written once a month by the bookkeeper. Make sure this office policy is clearly stated and adhered to in all cases. If the patient pays and a third party pays and the overpayment must be refunded to the patient, always write a check—never refund in cash. If the patient pays by credit card, wait until the charges have cleared to draft a check.

If the patient cannot be located to return the money, send a check by registered mail to the patient's last known address. When it comes back marked "undeliverable," retain the document as legal proof that an honest effort was made to return the overpayment. The money should be listed as taxable income and put in the bank.

Commercial Carriers

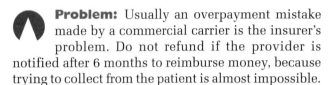 **Problem:** Usually an overpayment mistake made by a commercial carrier is the insurer's problem. Do not refund if the provider is notified after 6 months to reimburse money, because trying to collect from the patient is almost impossible.

Solution: First call and notify the patient; then proceed cautiously before refunding money. If two or more insurance carriers send duplicate payments, write a letter to each explaining the situation and let them straighten it out. Then send a refund to the correct insurance carrier after receiving a letter explaining to whom the money should be sent.

Managed Care Plan

 Problem: Discovering an overpayment from a managed care plan.

Solution: Develop a policy about overpayments and have it documented in the provider's contract. Allow the plan 60 days to audit its payments.

Medicare

 Problem: If an overpayment has been made from Medicare, refund the money immediately. If it is not paid back, future claims may be held up and past claims may be reviewed.

Solution: Check the billing and medical records to see whether the provider made any mistakes. If an error has been made by the insurance carrier, send a letter with documentation to appeal and prove the provider's case.

Rebilling

If a claim has not been paid, *do not* **rebill (resubmit)** the insurance carrier by sending in a monthly claim. Such claims are considered duplicate claims, and the insurance company may audit the physician's practice for trying to collect duplicate payment. Instead, follow up on the claim as indicated in the previous section. If it is discovered that an error has been made in billing a case, then send in a *corrected* claim.

Generally if a bill has not been paid, the physician rebills the patient every 30 days. Bill patients on a monthly basis, even when insurance payment is expected. Clearly identify on the statement that the insurance biller has submitted an insurance claim as well as what action is expected from the patient. If collection becomes a problem, action can be referenced to the date of service if the patient has been billed consistently. See Chapter 9 for the wording of notations on statements and in the collection process.

Review and Appeal Process

An **appeal** is a request for payment by asking for a review of an insurance claim that has been inadequately or incorrectly paid or denied by an insurance company. Usually there is a time limit for appealing a claim. Always check every private insurance carrier, Medicare, TRICARE, and workers' compensation payment against the appropriate fee schedule or customary profile to determine whether the benefits were allowed correctly. To find out this information, read the EOB/RA document or refer to provider manuals for the various programs.

An appeal on a claim should be based not only on billing guidelines but also on state and federal insurance laws and regulations. A bimonthly newsletter that links to regulatory information online is available at *www.integsoft.com/appeals/tal.* A software program designed to help providers generate effective insurance appeal letters is available from Appeal Solutions. To locate this company, see Appendix B, Collections.

There may be a discrepancy in the way the physician or physician's staff and insurance company interpret a coding guideline. The decision to appeal a claim should be based on several factors. The provider should determine that there is sufficient information to back up his or her claim, and the amount of money in question should be sufficient in the physician's opinion. Ultimately the decision to appeal often rests in the physician's hands, not the insurance billing specialist. It takes a team effort to appeal a claim successfully. To proceed, make a telephone call to the insurance company. It may save time and money and an expert who is able to solve the problem may be reached. The following are some basic guidelines:

▶ Assemble all documents needed (e.g., patient's medical record, copy of the insurance claim form, and EOB/RA).
▶ Remain courteous at all times.
▶ Obtain the name and extension number of the insurance claims representative or adjuster and keep this with the telephone records. After developing rapport, one may wish to call on him or her in the future for help. Ask for any toll-free numbers that the company may have, and keep these for future reference.

▶ Listen carefully. Jot down the date and take notes of how to solve the problem. This may be of help if another problem of the same type occurs.

An appeal is filed in the following circumstances:

▶ Payment is denied and the reason for denial is not known.
▶ Payment is received but the amount is incorrect. Perhaps there was an excessive reduction in the allowed payment.
▶ The physician disagrees with the decision by the insurance carrier about a preexisting condition.
▶ Unusual circumstances warranted medical treatments that are not reflected in payment.
▶ Precertification was not obtained within contract provisions because of extenuating circumstances, and the claim was denied.
▶ Inadequate payment was received for a complicated procedure.
▶ "Not medically necessary" is stated as the reason for denial and the physician disagrees.

PROCEDURE: Filing an Official Appeal

The following are basic steps to file an official appeal:

1. Send a letter explaining the reason why the provider does not agree with the claim denial listed on the EOB/RA.
2. Abstract excerpts from the coding resource book and attach a photocopy of the article or pertinent information showing the name of the article, coding resource, and date of publication.
3. Send copies of similar cases with increased reimbursement from the same insurance company, if available from the insurance company payment history file.
4. Call the insurance company and speak to the individual responsible for appeals, explaining what the resubmission is trying to accomplish. Direct the correspondence to this person.
5. Retain copies of all data sent for the physician's files.

If the appeal is won but copies of the same documents must be submitted each time this issue arises, ask the insurance carrier how future claims with the same issue may be handled.

Appeals must be in writing, but some programs require completion of special forms. Always send a copy of the original claim, EOB/RA, and any other documents to justify the appeal.

Remember that it is always important to keep track of the status after inquiry or appeal until payment for the case is resolved. Use the insurance claims register shown in Chapter 2 or a separate active file labeled "Appeals Pending."

If an appeal is not successful, the physician may want to proceed to the next step, which is a peer review. A **peer review** is an evaluation done by a group of unbiased practicing physicians to judge the effectiveness and efficiency of professional care rendered. This group determines the medical necessity and subsequent payment for the case in question. Some insurance companies send a claim for peer review routinely for certain procedures that have been done for particular diagnoses.

Additional information on tracing delinquent claims, appealing or reviewing a claim, or submitting a claim for a deceased patient can be found in the chapters on Medicaid, Medicare, TRICARE, and workers' compensation.

Medicare Review and Appeal Process

A physician or beneficiary has the right to appeal a claim after payment or denial. The Medicare program has six levels of appeal and special guidelines to follow. The steps (levels) follow:

1. Inquiry
2. Review
3. Fair hearing
4. Administrative law judge (ALJ) hearing
5. Appeals council review
6. Federal district court hearing

Table 8–2 illustrates the Medicare Part B appeals process.

Inquiry (Level 1)

If the claim was denied because of a simple error made by the insurance biller, such as omission of the National Provider Identifier (NPI) of the referring physician or failure to code a diagnosis, then resubmit a corrected claim. Include only the denied services and indicate in Block 19 "resubmission, corrected claim." In the event the insurance carrier made an error—for example, a procedure code was different from what was submitted or the date of service was entered incorrectly from the paper claim into the carrier's computer—then resubmit the claim with an attachment explaining the error. If response to the resubmission indicates that the claim has been "processed" previously, then go to the next appeal level.

Review (Level 2)

The physician may ask for a **review** when a claim is assigned. The request must be within 6 months from the date of the original determination shown on the RA. Figure 8–7 shows Form CMS-1964, which may be used in requesting a review of Medicare Part B claims. However, some carriers have developed their own request forms. Contact the carrier to find out the necessary form. Review the RA for the denial code or narrative stating why the claim has been denied. Check the claim for accuracy of diagnostic, procedural, or HCPCS codes or missing modifiers, as well as any other item that might be incorrect or missing.

A form on the physician's letterhead must include the following information:

1. Current date
2. Medicare provider number

TABLE 8–2	Medicare Part B Appeals Process			
Step (Level)	Time Limit for Request	Amount in Controversy	Jurisdiction	Form
1. Inquiry		None	Carrier	CMS 1500 (possible attachment)
2. Review	6 months from date of initial determination	None	Carrier	CMS 1964
3. Fair Hearing	6 months from date of review determination	$100	Fair Hearing Officer, Medicare Fiscal Agent	CMS 1965
4. Administrative Law Judge Hearing	60 days from receipt or review decision	>$500	Carrier Social Security Bureau of Hearings and Appeals	CMS 1965
5. Appeals Council Review	60 days from receipt of hearing decision or dismissal	$500	Bureau of Hearings and Appeals	HA 520
6. Federal District Court Review	60 days from receipt of Appeals Council decision	$1000	US District Attorney Court	

DEPARTMENT OF HEALTH AND HUMAN SERVICES
HEALTH CARE FINANCING ADMINISTRATION

FORM APPROVED
OMB No. 0938-0033

REQUEST FOR REVIEW OF PART B MEDICARE CLAIM
Medical Insurance Benefits – Social Security Act

NOTICE—Anyone who misrepresents or falsifies essential information requested by this form may upon conviction be subject to fine and imprisonment under Federal Law.

1 Carrier's Name and Address

Medicare Blue Cross and
Blue Shield of Texas, Inc.
P.O. Box 660031
Dallas, TX 75266-0031

2 Name of Patient

Jose F. Perez

3 Health Insurance Claim Number

032-XX-6619

4 I do not agree with the determination you made on my claim as described on my Explanation of Medicare Benefits dated:
3-2-20XX

5 MY REASONS ARE: (Attach a copy of the Explanation of Medicare Benefits, or describe the service, date of service, and physician's name—NOTE.—If the date on the Notice of Benefits mentioned in item 3 is more than six months ago, include your reason for not making this request earlier.)

01-21-20XX Electrocardiographic monitoring; 24 hours (93224)

Physician: Gerald Practon, MD

6 Describe Illness or Injury: Heart palpitations, tachycardia, & light headedness (near syncopal episode). Although patient

had a previous Holter monitor within the 6 mo time limitation, it did not provide any clinical evidence of disease.

Patient underwent recent monitoring after experiencing additional symptoms that were more severe than the initial

symptoms.

7
[X] I have additional evidence to submit. (Attach such evidence to this form.)

[ ] I do not have additional evidence.

COMPLETE ALL OF THE INFORMATION REQUESTED. SIGN AND RETURN THE FIRST COPY AND ANY ATTACHMENTS TO THE CARRIER NAMED ABOVE. IF YOU NEED HELP, TAKE THIS AND YOUR NOTICE FROM THE CARRIER TO A SOCIAL SECURITY OFFICE, OR TO THE CARRIER. KEEP THE DUPLICATE COPY OF THIS FORM FOR YOUR RECORDS.

8 SIGNATURE OF **EITHER** THE CLAIMENT **OR** HIS REPRESENTATIVE

Claimant	Representative *Gerald Practon, MD*
Address	Address 4567 Broad Avenue
City, State, and ZIP Code	City, State, and ZIP Code Woodland Hills, XY 12345
Telephone Number	Date	Telephone Number 555-486-9002	Date 6-5-20XX

FORM CMS-1964 (9/91)

CARRIER'S COPY

Figure 8–7. Request for Review of Part B Medicare Claim Form CMS-1964. This form can be used by the Medicare beneficiary or physician when requesting a review of a submitted claim.

3. RA number or claim number
4. Date of RA
5. Patient's name
6. Patient's health insurance claim number (HICN)
7. Date of service

8. Place of service
9. Procedure code(s)
10. Amount billed
11. Amount approved
12. Amount paid

13. Denial reason (action code description from the RA)
14. Brief statement of why service should be reviewed

Attach the following with the review request:

15. Copy of the original insurance claim
16. Copy of the RA showing the denial
17. Photocopy of other documents such as operative or pathology report or detailed summary about the procedure with appropriate words highlighted to help the reviewer
18. Cover letter explaining the procedure indicating justification for the services and the reason the provider should receive more reimbursement. Include the physician's NPI in the letter (Fig. 8–8).

Mail the documents by certified mail with return receipt requested and retain copies of all documents sent to the carrier in the provider's pending file.

If a claim is unassigned the beneficiary (patient) can pursue the review or appoint the physician as an authorized representative. The patient completes forms CMS-1964 and SSA-1696 (Figs. 8–7 and 8–9) and obtains the physician's acceptance signature. Decisions on unassigned claims are sent to the patient.

Send all requests to the review department. Most insurance carriers have an address or post office box for review requests that is different from initial claim submissions, so be sure to send it to a correct current address. A review usually is completed by the insurance carrier within 30 to 45 days. Make a follow-up inquiry if no response is received in that time frame.

If certain procedures are consistently denied, ask the carrier what information is necessary to process the claim. If the provider is not satisfied with the results of the review, move to the next level and request a fair hearing.

Figure 8–8. A cover letter for a Medicare review request to be sent with photocopies of documents pertinent to a claim.

PHYSICIAN'S LETTERHEAD

January 2, 20XX

Committee on Physician's Services
Medicare
Street address of fiscal intermediary
City, State, ZIP Code

Dear Madam or Sir:

Re: Underpayment

Identification No.:	1910-2192283-101
Patient:	Mrs. Sarah C. Nile
Type of Service:	Exploratory laparotomy
Date of Service:	December 1, 20XX
Amount Paid:	$000.00
My Fees:	$0000.00

Herewith a request for a committee review of the above-named case, since I consider the allowance paid very low having in mind the patient's condition prior to surgery, the location, the extent, the type, and the necessary surgical procedure performed.

Enclosed are photocopies of the history and physical showing the grave status of the patient prior to surgery, operative report, pathology report, and discharge summary. The Medicare Remittance Advice and the Medicare CMS-1500 claim originally submitted are also enclosed.

Considering these points, I hope that you will authorize additional payment in order to bring the total fee to a more reasonable amount.

Sincerely,

Hugh R. Aged, MD
NPI# 73542109XX

mf

Enclosures (6)

DEPARTMENT OF
HEALTH AND HUMAN SERVICES
CENTERS FOR MEDICARE & MEDICAID SERVICES

NAME (Print of Type)	H.I. CLAIM NUMBER
Carol T. Usner	432-XX-9821
WAGE EARNER (if different)	SOCIAL SECURITY NUMBER

Section I   **APPOINTMENT OF REPRESENTATIVE**

I appoint this individual <u>Gene Ulibarri, MD 4567 Broad Ave., Woodland Hills, XY 12345</u>
(Print or type name and address of individual you want to represent you)

to act as my representative in connection with my claim or asserted right under Titles XI, or XVIII of the Social Security Act. I authorize this individual to make or give any request or notice; to present or to elicit evidence; to obtain information; and to receive any notice in connection with my claim wholly in my stead.

SIGNATURE (Beneficiary)	ADDRESS
Carol T. Usner	530 Hutch Street, Woodland Hills, XY 12345
TELEPHONE NUMBER (555) 386-0122 (Area Code)	DATE August 3, 20XX

Section II   **ACCEPTANCE OF APPOINTMENT**

I, <u>Gene Ulibarri, MD</u> , hereby accept the above appointment. I certify that I have not been suspended or prohibited from practice before the Social Security Administration; that I am not, as a current or former officer or employee of the United States, disqualified from acting as the claimant's representative; and that I will not charge or receive any fee for the representation unless it has been authorized in accordance with the laws and regulations referred to on the reverse side hereof. In the event that I decide not to charge or collect a fee for the repesentation, I will notify the Social Security Administration. (Completion of Section III satisfies this requirement.)

I am a/an <u>medical doctor</u>
(Attorney, union representative, relative, law student, etc.)

SIGNATURE (Representative)	ADDRESS 4567 Broad Ave., Woodland Hills, XY 12345
TELEPHONE NUMBER (555)-486-9002 (Area code)	DATE August 3, 20XX

Section III (Optional)   **WAIVER OF FEE OR DIRECT PAYMENT**
(Note to Representative: You may use this portion of the form to waive a fee or to waive direct payment of the fee from withheld past-due benefits.)

I waive my right to charge and collect a fee for representing _____
_____ before the Social Security Administraion or the Centers for Medicare & Medicaid Services.

SIGNATURE	DATE

(See important information on reverse)
Form SSA-1696-U4 (3-88)

Figure 8–9. Form SSA-1696-U4 completed by a Medicare patient appointing the physician as his or her authorized representative.

Fair Hearing (Level 3)

If the physician feels the review is unfair and wishes to request a hearing, obtain and complete the CMS-1965 form Request for Hearing Part B Medicare Claim (Fig. 8–10) from either the Medicare carrier or local Social Security Administration office. Two conditions must be met to proceed to this level:

1. A fair hearing must be requested within 6 months from the date of the Medicare review determination letter.

HOW TO COMPLETE THIS FORM

Print or type your full name and your Social Security Number.

Section I—APPOINTMENT OF REPRESENTATIVE

You may appoint as your representative an attorney or any other qualified individual. You may appoint more than one person, but see "The Fee You Owe The Representative(s)." You may NOT appoint as your representative an organization, the law firm, a group, etc. For example, if you go to a law firm or legal aid group for help with your claim, you may appoint any attorney or other qualified individual from that firm or group, but NOT the firm or group itself.

Check the block(s) for the program in which you have a claim. Title II, check if your claim concerns disability or retirement benefits, etc. Title XVI, check if the claim concerns Supplemental Security Income (SSI) payments. Title IV FMSHS (Federal Mine Safety and Health Act), check if the claim is for black lung benefits. Title XVIII, check only in connection with a proceeding before the Social Security Administration involving entitlement to medicare coverage or enrollment in the supplementary medical insurance plan (SMIP). More than one block may be checked.

Section II—ACCEPTANCE OF APPOINTMENT

The individual whom you appoint in Section I above completes this part. Completion of this section is desirable in all cases, but it is mandatory only if the appointed individual is not an attorney.

Section III—WAIVER OF FEE

This section may be completed by your representative if he/she will not charge any fee for services performed in this claim. If you had appointed a co-counsel (second representative) in Section I and he/she will also not charge you a fee, then the co-counsel should also sign this section or give a separate waiver statement.

GENERAL INFORMATION

1. When you have representative:

   We will deal directly with your representative on all matters that affect your claim. Occasionally, with the permission of your representative, we may deal directly with you on the specific issues. We will rely on your representative to keep you informed on the status of your claim, but you may contact us directly for any information about your claim.

2. The authority of your representative:

   Your representative has the authority to act totally on your behalf. This means he/she can (1) obtain information about your claim the same as you; (2) submit evidence; (3) make statements about facts and provisions of the law; and (4) make any request (including a fee request). It is important, therefore, that you are represented by a qualified individual.

3. When will the representative stop:

   We will stop recognizing or dealing with your representative when (1) you tell us that he/she is no longer your representative; (2) your representative does any one of the following; (a) submits a fee petition, or (b) tells us that he/she is withdrawing from the claim, or (c) he/she violates any of our rules and regulations, and a hearing is held before an administrative law judge (designated as hearing officer) who orders your representative disqualified or suspended as representative of any Social Security claimant.

4. The fee you owe the representative(s):

   Every representative you appoint has a right to petition for a fee. To charge you a fee, a representative must first file a fee petition with us. Irrespective of your fee agreement, you never owe more than the fee we have authorized in a written notice to you and representative(s). (Out-of-pocket expenses are not included). If your claim went to court, you may owe an additional fee for your representative's service before the court.

5. How we determine the fee:

   We use the criteria on the back of the fee petition (Form SSA 1560-U4), a copy of which your representative must send you.

6. Review of the fee authorization:

   If you or your representative disagrees with the fee authorization, either of you may request a review. Instructions for filing this review are on the fee authorization notice.

7. Payment of fees:

   If past-due benefits are payable in your claim, we generally withhold 25 percent of the past-due benefits toward possible attorney fees. If no past-due benefits are payable or this is an SSI claim, then payment of the fee we have authorized is your responsibility.

8. Penalty for charging an unauthorized fee:

   If your representative wants to charge and collect from you a fee that is greater than what we had authorized, then he/she is in violation of the law and regulations. Promptly report this to your nearest Social Security office.

Form SSA-1696-U4 (3-88)

Figure 8–9, cont'd.

2. The amount in controversy (AIC) must be at least $100. This amount may represent a single claim or a combination of several smaller claims involving common billing issues.

The request for an appeal must include the patient's name, Medicare health insurance card number, all carrier control numbers involved, date of review determination, NPI, reason for requesting the hearing, and type of hearing (in-person, by telephone, or on-the-record). Address the request to the fair hearing officer in care of the Medicare fiscal agent. The mailing address of the hearing usually is different from the review request address. The provider may request that a physician of his or

DEPARTMENT OF HEALTH AND HUMAN SERVICES CENTERS FOR MEDICAIRE & MEDICAID SERVICES		Form Approved OMB No. 0938-0034

REQUEST FOR HEARING
PART B MEDICARE CLAIM
Medical Insurance Benefits–Social Security Act

NOTICE—Anyone who misrepresents or falsifies essential information requested by this form may upon conviction be subject to fine and imprisonment under Federal Law.

CARRIER'S NAME AND ADDRESS	**1** NAME OF PATIENT
Medicare Blue Cross Blue Shield of North Dakota 4510 13th Avenue, S.W. Fargo, ND 58121-0001	Deborah P. Sawyer **2** HEALTH INSURANCE CLAIM NUMBER 481-XX-6491

3 I disagree with the review determination on my claim and request a hearing before a hearing officer of the insurance carrier named above.

MY REASONS ARE: *(Attach a copy of the Review Notice. NOTE.—If the review decision was made more than 6 months ago include your reason for not making this request earlier.)*

Complications arose during the surgical procedure requiring additional procedures performed. See attached chart notes and medical reports.

4 CHECK ONE OF THE FOLLOWING:

[X] I have additional evidence to submit. (Attach such evidence to this form or forward it to the carrier within 10 days.)

[ ] I do not have additional evidence.

CHECK ONLY ONE OF THE STATEMENTS BELOW

[ ] I wish to appear in person before the Hearing Officer.

[X] I do not wish to appear and hereby request a decision on the evidence before the Hearing Officer.

5   **EITHER THE CLAIMANT OR REPRESENTATIVE SHOULD SIGN IN THE APPROPRIATE SPACE BELOW**

SIGNATURE OR NAME OF CLAIMANT'S REPRESENTATIVE	CLAIMANT'S SIGNATURE
Gaston Input, MD	*Deborah P. Sawyer*
ADDRESS 4567 Broad Avenue	ADDRESS 1065 Evans Road
CITY, STATE, AND ZIP CODE Woodland Hills, XY 12345	CITY, STATE, AND ZIP CODE Woodland Hills, XY 12345
Telephone Number 555-486-9002 / Date 10-11-20XX	TELEPHONE NUMBER 555-742-1821 / DATE 10-11-20XX

(Claimant should not write below this line)

ACKNOWLEDGEMENT OF REQUEST FOR HEARING

Your request for a hearing was received on _____. You will be notified of the time and place of the hearing at least 10 days before the date of the hearing.

SIGNED   DATE

FORM CMS-1965 (8-79)

Figure 8–10. Request for Hearing: Part B Medicare Claim Form CMS-1965.

her specialty review the case to offer advice or opinion to the fair hearing officer.

An acknowledgment should be received within 10 days, and the provider may either attend the hearing or waive the right to appear. When choosing the latter, inform the fair hearing officer in writing and enclose any additional documents that should be considered at the hearing. The fair hearing officer will send a written decision based on Medicare regulations, which may be full reversal of the initial claim ruling; adjustment of the review level decision giving more reimbursement; or complete denial. If not satisfied, proceed to the next level.

Administrative Law Judge Hearing (Level 4)

A request for a hearing before an administrative law judge (ALJ) may be made if the amount still in question is $500 or more (usually in combined claims). The request must be made within 60 days of receiving the fair hearing officer's decision. It may take 18 months to receive an ALJ assignment. Proof of the claim represents an unusual case and warrants special consideration, which may lead to a successful conclusion. However, the decision might be reversed, allow partial adjustment of the carrier's payment, or deny payment. If the final judgment is not satisfactory, then proceed to the next level.

Appeals Council Review (Level 5)

The Appeals Council is part of the Office of Hearings and Appeals of the Social Security Administration. A request must be made within 60 days of the ALJ decision; if there is a question that the final judgment was not made in accordance with the law, the council by its own election may review the ALJ decision. If the council denies a review, the provider may file a civil action for a federal district court hearing.

Federal District Court Hearing (Level 6)

At this highest level, the amount in controversy must be $1000 or more, and an attorney must be hired to represent the provider and manage the case. The case may be filed where the physician's business is located. Contact the local medical society for suggestions of names of attorneys experienced at this level of the appeals process.

CMS Regional Offices

One final suggestion (and this can be done with steps for a hearing or a review) is to write or telephone the medical director at one of the CMS regional offices. Sometimes a regional officer intercedes or takes steps to correct problems or inequities. CMS regional offices may be located by accessing the Medicare Web site; see Resources on the Internet at the end of this chapter.

Medigap

Insurance companies that sell Medigap policies must be certified before being allowed to sell in each state. The certification can be lifted from any insurer that does not honor its contract agreements. Only the state insurance commissioner can exert pressure on Medigap insurance companies. If payment is slow in coming or is not received from a Medigap insurer, tell the insurer, "If I do not receive payment, I will have no alternative but to contact the state insurance commissioner."

Document complete follow-up information on each Medigap insurer (firm name, address, telephone number, and policy numbers) of every patient seen.

TRICARE Review and Appeal Process

 Before appealing a TRICARE claim, an inquiry should be sent to verify claim status and attempt to resolve the problem. Figure 8–11 shows an example of a form that may be used for inquiring about a TRICARE Standard claim. TRICARE appeals procedures applicable to the routine processing of TRICARE Standard claims are described here. However, TRICARE managed care contracts have been adopted throughout the United States and the appeals procedures that TRICARE contractors use in these areas may vary. For information on how to file reviews and appeals for those contracts, ask the contracting insurance carrier for instructions and forms.

Three levels for review under TRICARE Standard appeal procedures exist:

1. *Reconsideration* (conducted by the claims processor or other TRICARE contractor responsible for the decision in a particular case)
2. *Formal review* (conducted by TRICARE headquarters)
3. *Hearing* administered by TRICARE headquarters but conducted by an independent hearing officer

Reconsideration

Participating providers may appeal certain decisions made by TRICARE, requesting reconsideration. Providers who do not participate may not appeal, but TRICARE Standard patients and parents or guardians of patients younger than 18 years of age who seek care from nonparticipating providers may file appeals. Providers who do not participate may not receive any information about a particular claim without the signed authorization of the patient or the patient's parent or guardian.

Matters that can be appealed include the following:

1. Medical necessity disagreements (inappropriate care, level of care, investigational procedures)
2. Factual determinations (hospice care, foreign claims, provider sanction cases)
   a. Denials or partial denials of requests for preauthorization for certain services or supplies
   b. Coverage issues—notification that TRICARE will not pay for services before or after a certain date

TRICARE CLAIM INQUIRY

Date: _____

TO: TRICARE
Address of fiscal intermediary
City, State, Zip Code

FROM: Provider's name   Telephone number
Address   Fax number
City, State, Zip Code

RE: Sponsor's Social Security Number _____

Sponsor's Name _____

Patient's Name _____

Patient's Mailing Address:

_____

Street   City   State   Zip Code

Dates of service claim: _____

Total charges billed on claim: _____

Claim number that appears on TRICARE Explanation of Benefits
(leave blank if the claim has not been paid and information is not available)

_____

A. _____   I have submitted a claim, but have not received any payment
or other notification from you.

B. _____   I have received notification or payment concerning the claim,
but feel it may have been processed incorrectly.

C. _____   Deductible Status. Please confirm that individual and family
deductibles have been applied correctly.

D. _____   Coverage for this patient is under

                     _____ **TRICARE**   _____ **CHAMPVA**

E. _____   Additional information or explanation that will assist
reviewing or processing the claim is attached to this letter or
written in this area.

Figure 8–11. A TRICARE Standard claim inquiry form that may be completed to obtain a quick reply. Mail to the TRICARE fiscal intermediary for your region.

Matters that cannot be appealed include the following:

1. Denial of services received from a provider not authorized to provide care under TRICARE
2. A specific exclusion of law or regulation
3. Allowable charges for particular services
4. Issues relating to the establishment and application of diagnosis-related groups
5. Decisions by the claims processor to ask for additional information on a particular case
6. A determination of a person's eligibility as a TRICARE beneficiary

The TRICARE department handling appeals collects and organizes all information necessary to review the case effectively. Usually a determination decision is made within 60 days from receipt of the appeal. Disagreements about the amount allowed for a particular claim may be reviewed by the claims processor to determine whether it was calculated correctly. However, an individual cannot appeal the amount that the TRICARE contractor determines to be the allowable charge for a certain medical service.

Requests must be sent to the claims processor of the state in which services were provided and must be postmarked within 90 days of the date the provider receives the Summary Payment Voucher (formerly referred to as an EOB). Include photocopies of the claim, Summary Payment Voucher, and other supporting documents with the request form or letter. The claim identification number assigned by the claims processor should be included in any inquiry concerning payment of the claim. If TRICARE denies the initial request, then the other two levels of review, formal review and hearing, may be pursued.

Formal Review

A formal review must be done within 60 days from the date on the reconsideration decision notice. Include photocopies of the notice as well as any other information or documents to support why there is a disagreement in the TRICARE decision. The case is reviewed again and a formal review decision is issued. The formal review decision is final if the amount in dispute is less than $300.

Hearing

An independent hearing may be pursued if the amount in dispute is $300 or more. The request must be postmarked or received within 60 days from the date of the formal review decision. A hearing is conducted by an independent hearing officer at a location convenient to both the requesting party and the government.

VIDEO RESOURCE

MEDICAL ASSISTANT VIDEO SERIES, TAPE 6: "The CMS Files: A Case for Medical Billing Accuracy."
This video is an interesting and entertaining presentation about what happens to rejected claim forms. It gives reasons why claims are denied and ways to avoid such problems. It gives excellent reinforcement of material learned in this chapter, especially when viewed after the chapter has been read. An assignment is presented in the *Workbook* for completion after viewing this video.

RESOURCES ON THE INTERNET

Medicare forms may be downloaded and printed and regional offices may be located at:
www.medicare.gov
A bimonthly newsletter that links to regulatory information online is located at:
www.integsoft.com/appeals/tal

STUDENT ASSIGNMENT LIST

✔ Study Chapter 8.
✔ Answer the review questions in the *Workbook* to reinforce the theory learned in this chapter and to help prepare you for a future test.
✔ Complete the assignments in the *Workbook* to fill in a form for tracing a delinquent claim, locate errors on a returned claim, and complete a form to appeal a Medicare case.
✔ Turn to the Glossary at the end of this textbook for a further understanding of the Key Terms used in this chapter.

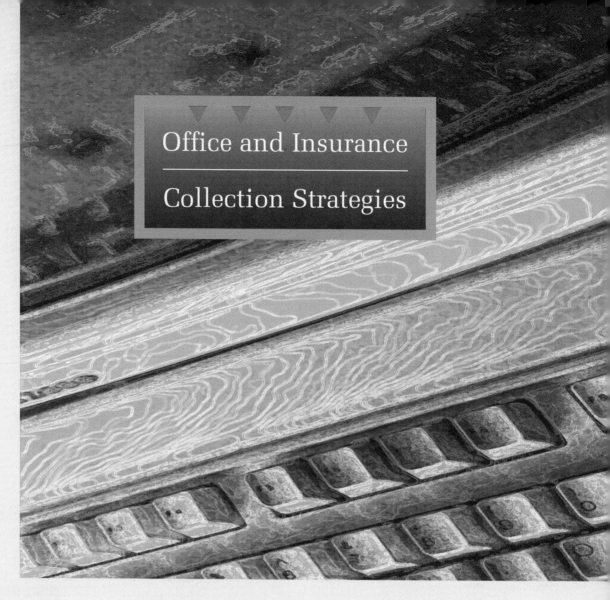

Office and Insurance
Collection Strategies

9

CHAPTER OUTLINE

- Define accounts receivable and explain how it is handled.
- Recite types of fee adjustments available to patients.
- Enumerate credit options available to patients.
- Perform oral and written communication collection techniques.
- State the role of a billing service, collection agency, and credit bureau in the collection process.
- List possible solutions to collection problems.
- Explain the purpose of small claims court in the collection process.
- Name basic actions in tracing a debtor who has moved and left no forwarding address.

OBJECTIVES*

After reading this chapter you should be able to:

- Define credit and collection terminology.
- Translate collection abbreviations.
- Describe office billing procedures.
- Define aging analysis.
- Discuss ways to determine fees and describe an office's fee policies.
- Summarize credit laws applicable to a physician office setting.

KEY TERMS

accounts receivable

age analysis

automatic stay

balance

bankruptcy

cash flow

collateral

collection ratio

computer billing

credit

credit card

creditor

cycle billing

debit card

debt

debtor

discount

dun message

estate administrator

estate executor

fee schedule

financial accounting record

garnishment

insurance balance billing

itemized statement

lien

manual billing

netback

no charge (NC)

nonexempt assets

professional courtesy

reimbursement

secured debt

Continued.

---

*Performance objectives and exercises for hands-on practical experience for this chapter appear in the *Workbook*.

Cash Flow Cycle

The practice of medicine is both a profession and a business. Although the physician decides what type of medicine he or she will practice, it is often the multiskilled health practitioner (MSHP) who is responsible for the business portion of the practice. It is extremely important for the physician and insurance specialist to work together to provide all patients the best possible medical care and ensure that the physician is paid fairly for services rendered.

Today this process has become increasingly difficult. Physician office and billing practices have evolved from the barter system of days past; and since the Great Depression, the availability of credit and credit cards have become a common feature of the financial marketplace. The word **credit** comes from the Latin **credere,** which means "to believe" or "to trust." This trust is in an individual's business integrity and his or her financial ability to meet obligations when they become due. For many, the idea of credit has changed and may simply mean to put off paying today what one can pay tomorrow.

A large percentage of **reimbursement** to physicians' offices is generated from third-party payers (private insurance, government plans, managed care contracts, and workers' compensation). The physician, the MSHP responsible for financial affairs, and the patient must understand these insurance contracts, which list reimbursement provisions, medical services not covered, the portion of the bill the patient is responsible for, and the process for reimbursing the office.

Accounts Receivable

Accounts receivable (A/R) include the unpaid balances due from patients for services that have been rendered. Each medical practice has a policy about handling A/R. The effectiveness of this policy and its enforcement are reflected in the practice's **cash flow.** The cash flow is the ongoing availability of cash in the medical practice. When charges are collected at the time of service, the A/R is zero. In an ideal situation all outstanding balances are paid within 60 days; however, this is not possible for the following reasons:

1. Health care expenses have increased and exceed the expenses the patient pays for everyday living.
2. The public feels it is a right, rather than a privilege, to receive the best possible health care. Therefore care of the indigent becomes an unreimbursable expense in the medical office.
3. Legal proceedings often delay the payment of medical expenses.
4. Insurance carriers do not pay claims in a timely manner, resulting in further delays in the collection of patient copayments.

By monitoring the A/R, the insurance billing specialist is able to evaluate the effectiveness of the collection process. The formula for finding out the A/R ratio is to divide the month-end A/R balance by the monthly average charges for the prior 12-month period. An average total A/R (all monies not collected at the time of service) should be one and one-half to two times the charges for 1 month of services (Example 9–1).

EXAMPLE 9–1

Formula

Physician's Charges Monthly Total	$50,000 × 1.5 = $75,000 or	Total Outstanding Accounts Receivable
	$50,000 × 2.0 = $100,000	

Total outstanding A/R should range from $75,000 to $100,000.

Accounts that are 90 days or older should not exceed 15% to 18% of the total A/R. To calculate this figure divide the total amount of A/R by the amount of accounts that are 90 days old and older (Example 9–2).

EXAMPLE 9–2		
Formula for Determining Percentage of Accounts over 90 Days		
Amount of A/R over 90 days	A/R Total	Percentage of A/R over 90 days
$12,000	× $75,000	= 16%

The best way to keep the A/R down is to verify insurance benefits before sending claims, collect copays and deductibles at the time of service, obtain authorizations for noncontracted HMO patients, and monitor the A/R on a weekly basis. Electronic claims that have not been paid within 30 days and paper claims unpaid within 45 days of submission have problems that can range from the carrier asking for additional information from the patient to the patient not being one of the carrier's insured.

The **collection ratio** is the relationship of the amount of money owed to a physician and the amount of money collected on the physician's A/R. A collection rate of 90% to 95% should be a goal for the MSHP managing collections in the physician's office. To calculate the collection rate for a 1-month period, divide the amount of monies collected during the current month by the total amount of the A/R.

Patient Education

Information should be provided about office fees and payment policies during the initial contact with the patient. This decreases the number of billing statements sent and increases collections. Never allow a patient to believe that he or she is not responsible for the bill. Discuss copayment requirements (see Chapter 2) with patients who are enrolled in managed care plans, and convey the office policy of collecting this amount when registering the patient for the office visit. A new patient information pamphlet or brochure and confirmation letter (Fig. 9–1) may be sent to welcome the new patient to the practice. This letter informs the patient about the practice, clearly outlines payment expectations, provides collection policies and procedures in printed form, establishes a contact person, invites questions, and confirms all specific details discussed.

Patient Registration Form

There is no substitution for good information-gathering techniques at the time of initial patient registration. Always obtain complete and accurate information from the patient on the first visit. Chapter 2 describes what data should be obtained from the patient; Figure 2–7 is an example of a patient registration information form, also called a patient information sheet. Have the guarantor agree in writing to pay for all medical treatment. By obtaining the guarantor's signature, he or she is then bound by contract to pay the bill.

Learn as much as possible about the patient before any services are provided. This is when the patient is likely to be the most cooperative. Information provided on the patient information sheet will prove critical to any billing and collection efforts. The patient should be instructed to answer all questions and indicate any spaces on the form that do not apply by marking "N/A" (not applicable). Review of the completed patient information sheet ensures that all blanks have been addressed and accurate information has been collected. It also alerts office staff of an account that may be a future problem. Items often overlooked are the street address, when a post office box is given; an apartment or mobile home number; and a business telephone number with department and extension. These help to trace a patient who has moved. If a patient refuses to divulge any information, invoking the privacy laws, it should be policy to require payment for services at the time care is rendered. A potential nonpaying patient may be recognized at this time. Some indications to look for follow:

▶ Incomplete information on the registration form
▶ Multiple changes of residence
▶ Questionable employment record
▶ No business or home telephone
▶ Post office box listed with no street address
▶ Motel address
▶ Incomplete insurance information
▶ No referral information or authorization from a primary care physician for patients enrolled in a managed care plan

Employers are changing health plans with increasing frequency and patients are more transient than ever, so update this form whenever the patient is seen or every 6 months. This can be done by printing out a data sheet or having the patient review a copy of his or her registration form and inserting changes or corrections with a red pen. New information also can be obtained using an updated or abbreviated form (see Chapter 2, Fig. 2–9).

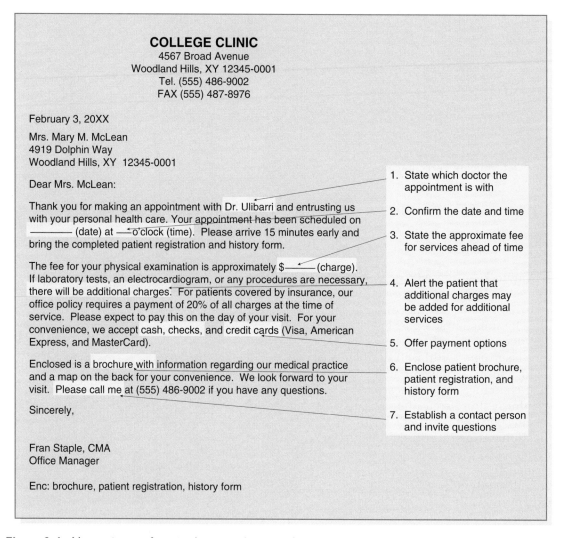

COLLEGE CLINIC
4567 Broad Avenue
Woodland Hills, XY 12345-0001
Tel. (555) 486-9002
FAX (555) 487-8976

February 3, 20XX

Mrs. Mary M. McLean
4919 Dolphin Way
Woodland Hills, XY 12345-0001

Dear Mrs. McLean:

Thank you for making an appointment with Dr. Ulibarri and entrusting us with your personal health care. Your appointment has been scheduled on ————— (date) at —‡o'clock (time). Please arrive 15 minutes early and bring the completed patient registration and history form.

The fee for your physical examination is approximately $—‡—(charge). If laboratory tests, an electrocardiogram, or any procedures are necessary, there will be additional charges‡ For patients covered by insurance, our office policy requires a payment of 20% of all charges at the time of service. Please expect to pay this on the day of your visit. For your convenience, we accept cash, checks, and credit cards (Visa, American Express, and MasterCard).

Enclosed is a brochure with information regarding our medical practice and a map on the back for your convenience. We look forward to your visit. Please call me at (555) 486-9002 if you have any questions.

Sincerely,

Fran Staple, CMA
Office Manager

Enc: brochure, patient registration, history form

1. State which doctor the appointment is with

2. Confirm the date and time

3. State the approximate fee for services ahead of time

4. Alert the patient that additional charges may be added for additional services

5. Offer payment options

6. Enclose patient brochure, patient registration, and history form

7. Establish a contact person and invite questions

Figure 9–1. New patient confirmation letter emphasizing information to incorporate when writing to a new patient.

Fees

Fee Schedule

Most medical practices operate with more than one fee schedule. As discussed in Chapter 5, a **fee schedule** is a listing of accepted charges or established allowances for specific medical procedures. Determine which fee schedule applies to a patient before quoting fees and stating policies about the collection of fees. Under federal regulations, a list of the most common services the physician offers, including procedure code numbers, with a description of each service and its price, must be available to all patients, and a sign must be posted in the office advising patients of this.

Occasionally, a physician assigns a fee for a service that is not on the fee schedule, such as an uncanceled appointment (referred to as a "no show"), completion of an insurance form, a long-distance telephone consultation, a narrative medical report for an insurance company, or interest assessed on a delinquent account. It is advisable to inform patients before billing for any such services to preserve the patient–physician relationship.

If the fee schedule is increased at a later date, a notice should be placed in the reception room and communicated to patients via their monthly billing statements.

Fee Adjustments

Discounted Fees

A physician may choose to discount his or her fees for various reasons, but it is ill-advised. A **discount** is a reduction of the normal fee based on a specific amount of money or a percentage of the charge. When a physician offers a discount, it must apply to the total bill, not just the portion that is paid by the patient (copayment or coinsurance amount). By following this rule, the physician is giving a discount to the patient and the insurance company but the same discount must be given to each member of the insurance plan. This practice could reduce the physician's profile with the insurance company and trigger a reduction in the physician's allowable reimbursement schedule; therefore the physician should consider the outcome of discounting fees. All discounts must be noted on the patient's **financial accounting record**/ledger card (Fig. 9–2), and any financial reasons or special circumstances should be documented in the patient's medical record. This ensures complete record keeping and safeguards any questions that may be brought up during a financial audit.

Cash Discounts

Cash discounts may be offered (5% to 20%) to patients who pay the entire fee, in cash, at the time of service. If a cash discount system is offered, this policy should be posted in the office and every active patient sent notification. Research your state laws because some states do not allow cash discounts.

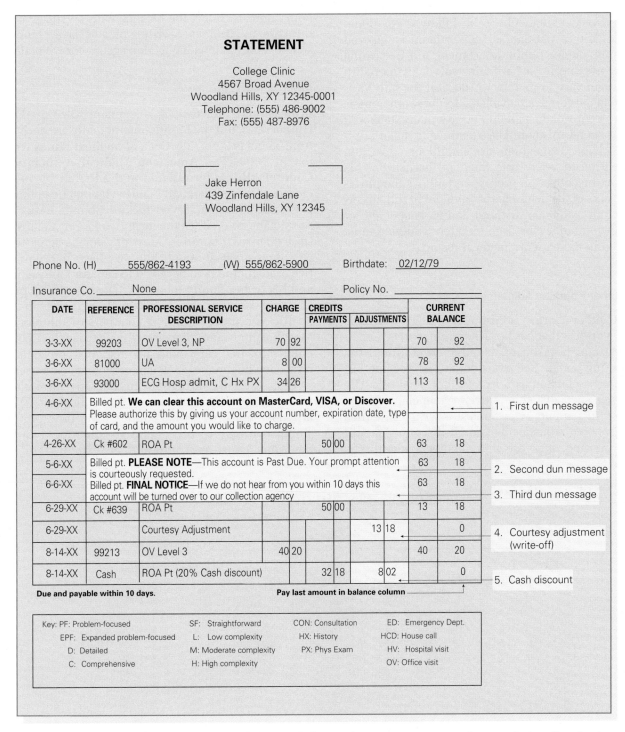

Figure 9–2. Financial accounting record (ledger card) showing dun messages, courtesy adjustment (write-off), and cash discount.

Financial Hardship

Financial hardship cases are the most difficult for the physician to determine. The insurance billing specialist should never assume anything about a patient's financial status, nor judge a patient's ability to pay by his or her appearance. The Department of Health and Human Services has published a 1999 guideline on poverty income (Fig. 9–3), which is used to determine eligibility for uncompensated services under the Hill-Burton program, the Community Services Block Grant program, and the Head Start program. Physicians may choose to follow these guidelines to direct patients to government-sponsored programs, obtain public assistance, and determine who is eligible for a hardship waiver. A hardship waiver can vary from 25% to 100% of the bill. Various financial forms are available to obtain this information; a copy of the patient's wage and tax statement (W2) or tax return should be examined to make a reliable decision. The patient also should sign a written explanation to verify true financial hardship. This helps in the collection process and allows the physician to accept the insurance as payment in full, in certain circumstances, without being suspected of insurance fraud. The reason for a fee reduction must be noted in the patient's medical record.

Write-off or Courtesy Adjustment

A write-off or courtesy adjustment (preferred term) is an asset or debt that has been determined to be uncollectable and is taken off (subtracted/credited) the accounting books. It is considered lost income but may not be claimed as a loss for tax purposes. The insurance specialist should obtain financial information on all patients who request a write-off. Office policies about adjustments and all discounts should be in writing, and all staff members should be

informed. The physician must approve the portion of the charge to be credited to the financial record before the debt is forgiven. There are three circumstances when a write-off can be performed. The first is as stated in the preceding, when the patient has proved a financial hardship. The second is when it will cost more to bill the balance than what is owed. For example, the balance may be $1.05. It will cost the practice more to collect this than what it is worth. This type of write-off is known as a small balance write-off. The last situation is when the provider has made a good faith effort to collect the balance with no success. In this case, the balance is written off and the account is sent to a professional collection agency for collection.

Professional Courtesy

Professional courtesy is a concept attributed to Hippocrates, but the foundations actually are derived from Thomas Percival's **Code of Medical Ethics** written in 1803. The **American Medical Association Code of Ethics,** formulated and adopted in 1847, closely mirrored Percival's code. The practice of professional courtesy served to build bonds between physicians and reduce the incentive for physicians to treat their own families. Most physicians agree that one of the greatest honors and privileges in the practice of medicine is to be asked to care for a physician and his or her family members. The practice of professional courtesy often was extended to others in the health care profession and members of the clergy. Most hospitals and many surgeons have given up the practice of free care today because most physicians now have insurance coverage for medical expenses.

Professional courtesy means making no charge to anyone, patient or insurance, for medical care. The law does not provide exceptions that allow professional courtesy to physicians in situations where the same courtesy could not be extended to all

2002 GUIDELINES ON POVERTY INCOME

Size of family unit	48 contiguous states and D.C.	Alaska	Hawaii
1	$ 8,860	$11,080	$10,200
2	$11,940	$14,930	$13,740
3	$15,020	$18,780	$17,280
4	$18,100	$22,630	$20,820
5	$21,180	$26,480	$24,360
6	$24,260	$30,330	$27,900
7	$27,340	$34,180	$31,440
8	$30,025	$38,030	$34,980
For each additional person add:	$ 3,080	$ 3,850	$ 3,540

Figure 9–3. Department of Health and Human Services 2002 guidelines on poverty income; published in the *Federal Register.*

patients. Physicians must examine their policies on professional courtesy to ensure that they do not violate the contractual terms in private or managed care insurance policies or Medicare/Medicaid laws and regulations. If the treating physician does not bill the physician-patient for services rendered, the third-party payer is relieved of its contractual obligation. If the treating physician waives the deductible and copayment, the physician may be accused of not treating others with the same insurance coverage in an equal manner. Although there may be some situations in which it is defensible to not charge for services to health care professionals, the physician should ensure that this professional courtesy is not linked to patients who have been referred to the practice. There are laws that prohibit any inducement or kickbacks from physicians (or others) that could influence the decision of a physician (or other) to refer patients or that may affect a patient's decision to seek care.

Copayment Waiver

Waiving copayments is another way physicians have reduced the cost of medical care for patients in the past. In doing so the physician accepts the insurance payment only. In most situations both private insurers and the federal government ban waiving the copayment; therefore it is not recommended. Waiving copayments could violate the contract between the patient and insurance company. Some insurance companies look at this as a means of recouping its losses by undergoing litigation against the provider or demanding the return of all payments made to the provider.

No Charge

No charge (NC) means waiving the entire fee for professional care. This is permitted as long as it is not part of a fraudulent scheme and is offered to all patients. All "NC" visits must be fully documented in the clinical portion of the patient's medical record and the financial record. A physician or insurance specialist cannot assess a fee for services for which the insurance company does not approve as a way of trying to satisfy a patient's deductible.

Another instance when "no charge" occurs on a patient's account is when follow-up visits are posted after a patient undergoes surgery considered under a surgical package or Medicare global fee structure. When posting such charges in a computer system, CPT procedure code 99024 (postoperative follow-up visit included in global fee) may be used.

Reduced Fee

Precautions should be taken before reducing the fee of a patient who dies. The doctor's sympathy in this case could be misinterpreted and result in a malpractice suit. A fee reduction should never be based on a poor result in the treatment of a patient.

If a patient is disputing a fee and the physician agrees to settle for a reduced fee, the agreement should be in writing with a definite time limit for payment and the words "without prejudice" inserted. By doing this the physician protects the right to collect the original sum if the patient fails to pay the reduced fee. The physician and patient should sign the agreement and each should receive a copy.

Communicating Fees

People have a difficult time asking each other for money and talking about financial obligations. Financial arrangements should be discussed up front and in great detail before any services are provided (Fig. 9–4). Many medical practices create their own collection problems by not being clear about how and when they expect to be paid. If patients are not told that payment is due at the time of service, most assume they can pay at a later time. Following are some guidelines to help communicate effectively about money:

1. Be courteous at all times but express a firm, businesslike approach that will not offend the patient.
2. Never badger or intimidate a patient into paying; merely state the payment policy and educate the patient.
3. Inform the patient of the fee and any deductible and balance due in a clear manner.
4. Verify the patient's copayment listed on his or her insurance card and collect this amount before the patient's office visit.
5. Make it easier for the patient to pay rather than leave without making payment.
6. Do not give the patient an option by asking if he or she would like to pay now or have a bill sent.

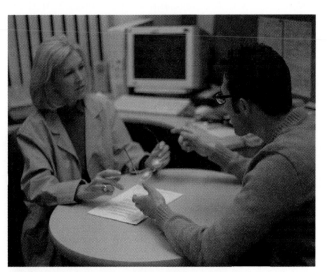

Figure 9–4. Insurance billing specialist discussing fees with the patient.

7. Motivate the patient to pay by appealing to his or her honesty, integrity, and pride.

The following are examples of communicating in a positive manner and letting the patient know exactly what is expected:

▶ "The office visit is $62, Mrs. Smith. Would you like to pay by cash, check, or credit card?"

▶ "Your copayment is $10, Mr. Jones. I will collect it before your office visit."

▶ "Your insurance policy shows a $100 deductible that is your responsibility and currently has not been met, Miss Rodriguez. You must pay the full fee today, which is $75."

▶ "Mrs. Merryweather, I must collect $4.77 today for your vitamin B$_{12}$ injection. The injection is not covered by your insurance policy."

▶ "We look forward to seeing you on Tuesday, March 3, at 10 AM., Mr. Gillespie. The consultation fee will be approximately $150 and payment is expected at the time of service. We accept cash, check, or credit cards for your convenience."

Collecting Fees

Payment at the Time of Service

Do not miss the opportunity to ask for payment at the time of service. Collect all fixed copayments before the patient is seen to alleviate billing for small amounts. Patients do not make health care bills a priority, so the importance of collecting outstanding bills, coinsurance amounts, and money from cash-paying patients up front should be communicated to office staff. One-on-one communication is the best way to motivate a **debtor.** Each patient's account **balance** (amount due) should be reviewed before his or her appointment. If the appointment schedule is on a computer system, print the account balance by each patient's name. If an appointment book is used, make a copy of the page showing the day's schedule. Write overdue balances by the patient's name after obtaining overdue amounts from each patient's financial accounting record card. This information also should be recorded on the transaction slip for that day's visit and may be "flagged" when the transaction slips are printed or written. Treat this information confidentially and keep it out of view of other patients. When a patient arrives whose name is "flagged," alert the Patient Accounts Manager.

To do effective preappointment collection counseling, the patient should be led to a quiet area away from the general activity of the office. Sit down with the patient and discuss the situation. Use an understanding attitude and helpful nature while verbalizing phrases such as "I understand" and "I can help." Ask direct questions to learn exactly what problems the patient is facing. Answers to questions such as, "When do you expect your next paycheck?" and,

"How much are you able to pay today?" help determine the strategy. The goal should be to try and collect the full amount. If that is not possible, try to collect a portion of the balance. Get a promise to pay for the remaining balance by a specific date. If the patient is unable to comply, set up a payment plan. The chances of reaching a mutually satisfactory resolution are greatly improved when the two parties are face to face.

A personal interview is better than a telephone interview because a financial agreement can be signed when the debtor is present (Fig. 9–5), resulting in a better follow-up response. Let the patient know that the practice is willing to help and that the debtor should inform the insurance specialist if he or she runs into further problems making the payment. This personal contact helps if a renegotiation of the agreement is needed. A medical practice cannot refuse to let an established patient see the doctor because of a **debt,** but the office staff has every right to ask for payment while the patient is in the office (Fig. 9–6). Some practices are placing automated teller machines (ATMs) in their waiting rooms. ATMs are almost everywhere today and they help generate a small income for having the ATMs in place. Putting an ATM machine in the waiting room gives the reluctant patient a means of obtaining funds to pay the medical bill while in the office. If the patient gives every excuse to keep from paying then and there, the patient will never pay the bill.

Encounter Forms

Multipurpose billing forms (see Chapter 2) are known by many names, including encounter form. They are helpful when collecting fees at the time of service. Encounter forms can be given to patients to bill their insurance companies, used to inform patients of current charges and outstanding balances, and used as receipts for payment (Fig. 9–7).

Patient Excuses

Nonpayers show a tendency to dismiss financial arrangements with curt remarks. Look directly at the patient, confidently expecting payment. Demonstrate to the patient the right to request payment. Be ready if excuses are offered. Table 9–1 shows examples of patients' excuses and possible responses.

When a patient chatters nervously, it may be a way of setting up reasons to rationalize not paying. Do not let this be distracting. Pause after asking for payment and do not say another word until the patient responds. Many people feel uncomfortable with silence, but pauses may work to advantage and help complete a transaction. The cash flow and collection ratio are increased by taking this approach, while decreasing billing chores and collection costs. The quick identification of nonpayers may be obtained and the person responsible for collections notified.

FINANCIAL AGREEMENT

Left margin notes:

1. Total amount of the debt; wording "cash price" must be used according to Regulation Z
2. Amount of down payment
3. Finance charge; must be in capital letters and stand out
4. Interest rate expressed as an annual percentage; must be in capital letters and stand out
5. Amount of each payment
6. Date each payment is due
7. Date final payment is due; itemized payment record allows tracking of payments and balance owed
8. Signature of patient and physician with copies retained by both; narrative must be included

For professional SERVICES rendered or to be rendered to:

Patient __Keenan Kellog__ Daytime phone __555-486-0132__

Parent if patient is a minor _____

1. Cash price for services... $ 5000.-
2. Cash down payment.. $ 300.-
3. Charges covered by insurance service plan................. $ 4000.-
4. Unpaid balance of cash price................................. $ 700.-
5. Amount financed (the amount of credit provided to you)... $ 700.-
6. **FINANCE CHARGE** (the dollar amount the credit will cost you)........ $ -0-
7. **ANNUAL PERCENTAGE RATE** (the cost of credit as a yearly rate)..... $ 0%
8. Total of payments (5 + 6 above – the amount you will have paid when you have made all scheduled payments)................. $ 700.-
9. Total sales price (1 + 6 above – sum of cash price, financing charge and any other amounts financed by the creditor, not part of the finance charge)................. $ 5000.-

You have the right at anytime to pay the unpaid balance due under this agreement without penalty. You have the right at this time to receive an itemization of the amount financed.

[X] I want an itemization   [ ] I do not want an itemization

Total of payments (#8 above) is payable to Dr. __Astro Parkinson__ in __7__ monthly installments of $__100.__ each and __-0-__ installments of $__-0-__ each. The first installment being payable on __Feb. 15__ 20 __XX__ and subsequent installments on the same day of each consecutive month until paid in full.

NOTICE TO PATIENT

Do not sign this agreement if it contains any blank spaces. You are entitled to an exact copy of any agreement you sign. You have the right at any time to pay the unpaid balance due under this agreement.

The patient (parent or guardian) agrees to be and is fully responsible for total payment of services performed in this office including any amounts not covered by any health insurance or prepayment program the responsible party may have. See your contract documents for any additional information about nonpayment, default, any required prepayment in full before the scheduled date and prepayment refunds and penalties.

Signature of patient or one parent if patient is a minor:

X ____ *Keenan Kellog* ____

Doctor's Signature ____ *Astro Parkinson, MD* ____

SCHEDULE OF PAYMENT

No.	Date due	Amount of installment	Date paid (Ck #)	Date paid	Amount paid	Balance owed
		Total amount				700 –
D.P			Ck #			
1	2/15	100 –	572	2/10	100 –	600 –
2	3/15	100 –	598	3/13	100 –	500 –
3	4/15	100 –				
4	5/15	100 –				
5	6/15	100 –				
6	7/15	100 –				
7	8/15	100 –				
8						
9						
10						
11						
12						
13						
14						
15						
16						
17						
18						
19						
20						
21						
22						
23						

Figure 9–5. Financial Agreement Form (#1826) used for financial payment plans. By completing this form the physician provides full disclosure of all information required by the Truth in Lending Act, Regulation Z. (From SYCOM, A Division of New England Business Service, Inc., Groton, MA.)

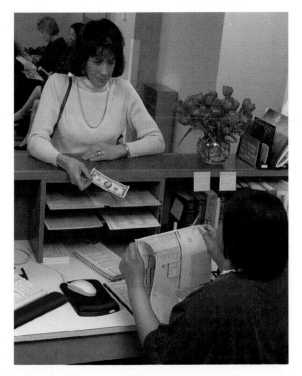

Figure 9–6. Receptionist collecting copayment from the patient.

Payment by Check

Check Verification

Check verification requires the insurance specialist to become familiar with the appearance of a good check. A personal check is the most common method of payment in most medical offices, but it is not a personal guarantee of payment. A driver's license and one other form of identification always should be required. Check these against existing records. Call the bank to verify all out-of-state and suspicious checks. A verification service, which is a private company with resources to quickly identify patient information over the telephone, or a check authorization system, may be worthy of consideration for clinics and larger group practices.

Check Forgery

Forgery is false writing or alteration of a document to injure another person or with intent to deceive (e.g., signing another person's name on a check to obtain money or pay off a debt without permission). To guard against forgery, always check to be sure the

TAX ID #3664021CC
Medicaid #HSC12345F
Medicare DME #34007

COLLEGE CLINIC
4567 Broad Avenue
Woodland Hills, XY 12345-0001
Tel. (555) 486-9002
FAX (555) 487-8976

CO-PAY: ___$10.00___
CO. NAME: Quality Care
IPA: _____

1. Insurance identifying data

☐ PRIVATE　　☐ BLUE CROSS　　☐ MEDI-CAL　　☐ MEDICARE　　☒ HMO　　☐ PPO

ACCOUNT #	PATIENT'S LAST NAME	FIRST	INITIAL	TODAY'S DATE
3794	McDonald	Lydia	P.	5/6/ XX

ASSIGNMENT: I hereby assign payment directly to College Clinic of the surgical and/or medical benefits, if any, otherwise payable to me for his/her services as described below.
SIGNED (Patient, or Parent, if Minor) *Lydia McDonald*　　　　　DATE:5/6/ XX

2. Assignment of medical benefits

ICD-9	DESCRIPTION							
789.0	Abdominal pain	433.1 ✔	Coronary A. dis.	401.	Hypertension	353.2	Radiculopathy, cervical	
995.3	Allergic reaction	733.	Costochondritis	242.90	Hyperthyroidism	353.4	Lumbar	
290.10	Alzheimer's	430.	CVA	790.6	Hyperuricemia	592.0	Renal stone	
285.	Anemia	595.0	Cystitis	276.8	Hypokalemia	714.0	Rheumatoid arthritis	
413.9	Angina	311.	Depression	244.	Hypothyroid	724.3	Sciatica	
300.4	Anxiety reaction	692.	Dermatitis	244.	Hypothyroidism	461.	Sinusitis	
414.0	ASHD	250.0	Diabetes mell	564.1	Irritable bowel synd.	V45.0	Stat post pacemaker	
493. ✔	Asthma bronchial	562.11	Diverticulitis	386.	Labyrinthitis	780.2	Syncope	
491.2 ✔	Asth broncho-chr.	427.9	Ectopy or VPC's	724.5	Low back pain	727.	Tendonitis	
781.2	Ataxia	782.3	Edema	780.7	Malaise and fatigue	531.	Ulcer	
427.31	Atrial fib	610.1	Fibrocystic breast	424.0	Mitral valve prolapse	465.	URI	
586	Azotemia	535.	Gastritis	728.85	Muscle spasm	599.	Urin. tract inf.	
600	BPH	558.	Gastroenteritis	410.	Myocardial infar.	616.10	Vaginitis	
466.0	Bronchitis acute	274.	Gout	715.80	Osteoarthritis	079.	Viral syndrome	
490.	Bronchitis chr.	784.0	Headache	733.	Osteoporosis			
426.50	Bundle BR block	389.9	Hearing loss	382.	Otitis media			
786.50	Chest pain	578.1	Hematochezia	785.1	Palpitations			
428.0	CHF	599.7	Hematuria	462	Pharyngitis			
575.1	Cholecystitis	455.6	Hemorrhoids	486	Pneumonitis			
564.1	Colitis	553.3	Hernia hiatal	511.	Pleurisy			
416.	COPD	550.	Hernia inguinal	601.	Prostatitis			
		274.4	Hyperlipidemia	696.1	Psoriasis			

3. Additional diagnostic codes

4. Additional procedure codes

✔	DESCRIPTION	CPT-4/MD	FEE	✔	DESCRIPTION	CPT-4/MD	FEE	✔	DESCRIPTION	CPT-4/MD	FEE
	OFFICE VISIT–NEW PATIENT				OFFICE PROCEDURES				X-RAY		
	Intermediate	99203	60.00	✔	EKG 12 lead	93000	55.00		Chest	71020	55.00
	Extended	99204	95.00		2DM mode echo	99307	500.00				
✔	Compreh.	99205	195.		Doppler	93320	250.00				
	Consultation	99245	250.00		Color doppler	93325	200.00				
	OFFICE VISIT–ESTAB. PATIENT				Treadmill	93015	295.00				
	Intermediate	99213	55.00		Stress echo	93350-YB			IMMUNIZATIONS/INJECTIONS		
	Extended	99214	65.00		Oximetry w/Exercise	94761	75.00	✔	Flu	90724	20.00
	Compreh.	99215	195.00		Aspiration major jt.	20610	60.00		Pneumococcal	90732	20.00
					Intermediate jt.	20605	45.00		Injection	907	
	MISCELLANEOUS				Trigger point/ten. inj.	20550	45.00		LABORATORY: See attached requisition sheet		
					Sigmoidoscopy-flex.	45330	145.00		Collection and handling	36415	9.00
					Slow flow loop	94375	35.00		Urinalysis	81000	10.00
					Spirometry	94010	50.00				
					w/Bronchodilator	94060	65.00				
					Cerumen removal	69210	40.00				

RETURN APPOINTMENT INFORMATION
_____WEEKS ___3___MONTH(S)

SET UP FOLLOWING TESTS

DOCTOR'S SIGNATURE: *P Cardi MD*

PLEASE REMEMBER THAT PAYMENT IS YOUR OBLIGATION REGARDLESS OF INSURANCE OR OTHER THIRD PARTY INVOLVEMENT.

REC'D BY:
☐ BANK CARD
☑ CASH
☐ CHECK
_____

PREVIOUS BALANCE	-0-
TODAY'S FEE	270.00
AMOUNT REC'D/CO-PAY	10.00
BALANCE	260.00

5. Patient's previous balance

6. Total charges and payments received

Figure 9–7. Encounter form; diagnostic codes from *International Classification of Diseases, 9th revision, Clinical Modification* (ICD-9-CM), and procedural codes for professional services from *Current Procedural Terminology* (CPT). (From Bibbero Systems, Inc., Petaluma, CA.)

endorsement on the back of the check matches the name on the front. Be suspicious if the beneficiary or provider states that he or she did not receive the check but the insurance company shows it as being cashed, or if the payee of the check claims that the signature is not his or hers.

Payment Disputes

Problem checks appear in many forms. One is the check for partial payment when the debtor (the patient) writes "payment in full" on the check. If the **creditor** (the physician) cashes the check, it may be argued that the debt is paid in full. A legal theory

TABLE 9–1	**Responses to Patients Avoiding Payment Response**
Excuse	**Response**
"Just bill me"	"As we explained when we made your appointment, Mr. Barkley, our practice bills for charges more than $50. Amounts under $50 are to be paid at the time of the visit. That will be $25 for today's visit, please."
"I have insurance to cover this."	"We will be billing your insurance for you, Miss Butler, but your policy shows a deductible in the amount of $300 that still must be met. We must collect the full fee for today's visit, which is $150 to meet that deductible responsibility."
"I get paid on Friday; you know how it is."	"I understand. Why don't you write the check today and postdate it for Saturday. We will hold the check and deposit it on the next business day" (depending on office policy).
"If I pay for this I won't be able to pay for the prescription."	"Our payment policy is very much like the pharmacy; we expect payment at the time of service. Let me check and see if the doctor can dispense some medication samples to last until you can get your prescription filled."
"I don't have that much with me."	"How much can you pay, Mrs. Fish? I can accept $10 now and give you an envelope to send us the balance within the week, or I can put it on your credit card." (Get a commitment and write the balance due under the sealing flap of the envelope. Also write the date on a tickler calendar or the patient's financial accounting record while the patient is watching.)
"I'll take care of it."	"I know you will, Mr. Stone; I just need to know when that will be so I can document your intentions for our bookkeeper." (Get a commitment and write down the date on a tickler calendar or on the patient's financial accounting record card while in view of the patient. Hand him an envelope with the amount due written under the sealing flap.)
"I forgot my checkbook."	"We take Visa, MasterCard, and American Express, Mr. Storz." (If the patient still does not pay, provide him with a self-addressed envelope and write the patient's name, account number, date of service, amount due, and expected payment date under the sealing flap. Restate the expected payment date as you hand the patient the envelope. Note the date on a tickler calendar or on the patient's financial accounting record card while the patient is watching.)

called "accord and satisfaction" may apply to this situation if the debt is truly disputed by the debtor. If the check is retained (and cashed) by the physician, it can be considered "accord and satisfaction," and the physician cannot procure the balance from the patient. The operative words are "truly disputed." If there is a legitimate, genuine dispute over the amount of the bill, and an amount less than the full amount of the bill is accepted, the physician could be precluded from seeking the balance. However, acceptance of payment does not necessarily mean acceptance of the "paid in full" remark. A good safeguard is to read the state's accord and satisfaction laws; the Uniform Commercial Code, Articles 3, 4, and 9; and the Retail Installment Sales Act and Escheats Law. Even if a check marked "paid in full" is accidentally cashed, 90 days may be available to rectify the situation by returning the fund to the patient and informing him or her that the accord and satisfaction is not acceptable.

Unsigned Checks

Another problem is unsigned checks. First ask the patient to come to the office and sign the check or send a new one. If unable to reach the patient or if there is a transportation or time limitation problem, write the word "over" or "see reverse" on the signature line on the front of the check. On the back of the check, where the endorsement should appear, write "lack of signature guaranteed," the practice's name, and one's own name and title. This endorsement in effect is a guarantee that the practice will absorb the loss if the patient's bank or the patient does not honor the check.

Returned Checks

When the physician's office receives notice that a check was not honored, the reason should be stated on the back of the check. The most common reason is nonsufficient funds (NSF). Call the bank or patient to see if they suggest redepositing it. It may be an oversight or miscalculation by the patient. If it is not worth redepositing, or a second NSF notice is received, call the patient immediately. Be courteous but straight to the point. Check the state laws about NSF checks. There is a time limit for making the check good, and there are additional charges (up to 10% of the value of the check) that the patient must make to restore the check. If the patient does not respond, the matter may be turned over to the State Attorney or satisfaction may be obtained through small claims court. Send an NSF demand letter (Fig. 9–8) by certified mail with return receipt requested, and include the following:

1. Check date
2. Check number
3. Bank the check is drawn on
4. Name of person the check was payable to
5. Check amount

Figure 9–8. Demand letter for returned check. This letter serves as a formal notice to collect payment and notifies a patient of impending legal action.

COLLEGE CLINIC
4567 Broad Avenue
Woodland Hills, XY 12345-0001
Tel. (555) 486-9002
FAX (555) 487-8976

August 15, 20XX

Mrs. Maxine Holt
444 Labina Lane
Woodland Hills, XY 12345-0001

Dear Mrs. Holt:

The following check has been dishonored by the bank and returned without payment:

Date:	08/04/20XX
Check No.:	755
Amount:	$106.11
Payable to:	Perry Cardi, MD
Bank:	Woodland Hills National Bank
Reason:	Nonsufficient funds

This is a formal notice demanding payment in the amount of $106.11 within 15 days from today's date or your account will be considered for legal action.

Please make payment immediately by cash, cashier's check, or money order at the above address. Your immediate attention will be appreciated.

Sincerely,

Delores Yee, CMA-A

Patient Accounts Manager
for Perry Cardi, MD

---

6. Any allowable service charge
7. Total amount due
8. Number of days the check writer has to take action

Once a patient has been informed of the returned check, explain that the facility will no longer be able to accept checks as payment. Future payments should be in the form of cash, money order, or a cashier's check. If the patient wishes the check returned, be sure to photocopy it and keep it in the financial record because it serves as an acknowledgment of the debt. The bad check may be returned to the patient after it has been replaced with a valid payment. Place a notation on the patient's record to this effect.

Larger facilities may consider a check authorization system to guard against bad checks. With such a system the company supplies a terminal that gives an approval number for each check that is taken in and guarantees payment on the checks authorized. If no approval is given, another form of payment is necessary. The check guarantee service receives a percentage for the checks that they approve and collects all bad check charges from the patient. One way to help discourage bad checks is to charge a penalty for returned checks. This information should be included in the new patient brochures and posted in the office for all patients to view. Perhaps make reference to the particular section of the state Civil Code's provisions about checks for nonsufficient funds if it is desired to collect more than the face value of the check.

If notified that the checking account is closed, do not waste time trying to contact the patient. Send a demand letter immediately. In most states legal action can be taken if the patient does not respond in 30 days. Consider filing a claim in small claims court. Most states have written codes or statutes pertaining to bad checks. Often legislation allows the creditor to add punitive damages to the amount of the debt being collected, sometimes up to three times the amount of the check.

When a patient stops payment on a check, it is usually done to resolve a good faith dispute. In this case, the patient believes that he or she has legal entitlement to withhold payment. The physician may want to contact a lawyer to discuss his or her legal rights and responsibilities before sending a demand letter and trying to collect.

Itemized Statements

Every patient receives an **itemized statement** (Fig. 9–9) of his or her account showing the dates of service, a list of detailed charges, copayments and deductibles

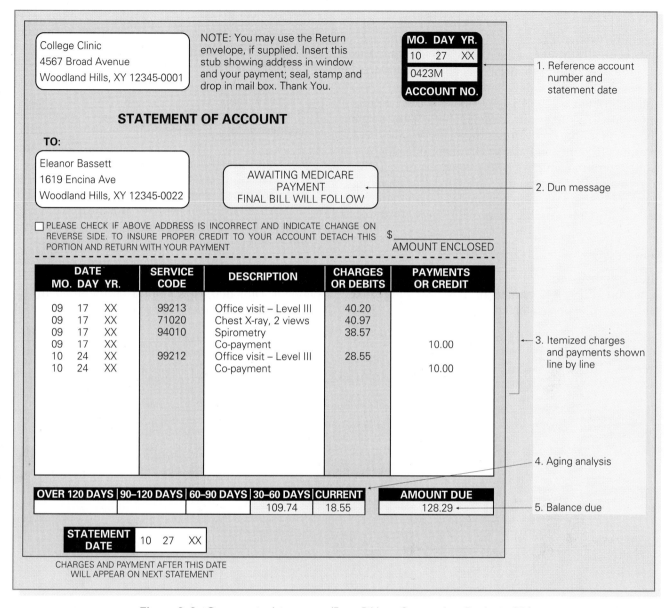

Figure 9–9. Computerized statement. (From Bibbero Systems, Inc., Petaluma, CA.)

paid, the date insurance claim was filed (if appropriate), applicable adjustments, and the account balance. These items also are listed on the patient's account or financial accounting record card (see Chapter 2, Fig. 2–17; and Fig. 9–2). Timeliness, accuracy, and consistency have a significant effect on the cash flow and collection process when sending itemized statements.

Professional bills are a reflection of the medical practice. The billing statement should be patient oriented and easy to read and understand. Avoid technical terms and abbreviations that might lead to misunderstandings and confusion. Enclose a return envelope. Addressed envelopes should contain the statement "Forwarding Service Requested" so the postal service can forward the mail and provide the physician's office with a notice of the patient's

new address. When this notice is received in the physician's office, it should be circulated to all necessary departments to record the new information.

Patients can be oriented to the billing process by having the insurance specialist generate a printed statement when they are ready to leave the office and explaining pertinent information, such as account number, dates of service, payments, procedures, interest fees, copayments, and deductibles. Patient information pamphlets about common health concerns such as blood pressure, cholesterol, or back pain can be sent along with the bill to convey a caring attitude.

The office is likely to experience an increase in telephone calls from inquiring patients when statements go out in the mail. One person or one department should handle all billing questions, ensuring a consistent response.

Age Analysis

Age analysis is a term used for the procedure of systematically arranging the A/R by age from the date of service. Accounts are usually aged in time periods of 30, 60, 90, and 120 days and older, as shown at the bottom of Figure 9–9. An aging analysis can be done automatically in a computer system. This helps collection follow up by providing easy recognition of overdue accounts and allows the insurance specialist to determine which accounts need action in addition to a regular statement. A decision tree showing time frames for sending statements and telephone calls is presented in this chapter in Figure 9–10.

Dun Messages

Dun messages are used on statements to promote payment (Figs. 9–2 and 9–9). The best and most effective collection statements include a handwritten note; however this is seldom possible. Dun messages also can be printed by the computer system or applied with brightly colored labels. Some examples of dun messages are:

- "If there is a problem with your account, please call me at (555) 486-0000—Marlayn."
- "This bill is now 30 days past due. Please remit payment."
- "This bill is now 60 days past due. Please send payment immediately."
- "Your account is 90 days past due. Please remit payment now to avoid collection action."
- "FINAL NOTICE: If we do not hear from you within 10 days, this account will be turned over to our collection agency."

Do not send intimidating, impatient, or threatening statements. These only serve to antagonize patients. Dun messages should be included in different languages and sent to patients who speak

COLLECTION DECISION TREE

Figure 9–10. Collection decision tree. This is a quick reference used to help determine when to send statements, make telephone calls, and send accounts to a collection agency.

English as a second language. Some examples follow:

▸ "No payment yet; your payment by return mail will be appreciated."
▸ "No hemos recibido pago. Agraciéramos remita por correo."
▸ "Payment needed now. No further credit will be extended."
▸ "Se requiere pago hoy. No se le estendera mas credito."

Manual Billing

Manual billing is usually done by photocopying the patient's financial accounting record and placing it in a window envelope. The financial accounting record becomes the statement and should be clear and readable with no crossouts or misspellings. Typewritten statements may be used by small offices and generally are typed on continuous form paper. The completed statements are separated, folded, and placed into billing envelopes.

A coding system with metal clip-on tabs or peel-off labels that are placed on the financial accounting record card can be used with a manual system. Each time the account is billed a different color tab or label is placed on the financial accounting record card, which shows at a glance how many times the account has been billed. It also provides aging of accounts, although if a report is desired it must be done manually in addition to this process.

Computer Billing

Computer billing is made possible by installing software that controls the A/R. All charges, payments, and adjustments are posted into the computer system by a medical assistant; these figures can be used to generate a hard copy, that is, statements and reports (Fig. 9–9). The computer program usually offers choices of billing types, including patient billing, **insurance balance billing,** discounted billing, and no bill. The insurance specialist can instruct the computer to print all bills of a specific type. The computer also can be instructed to print bills according to specific accounts, dates, and insurance types. Accounts are automatically aged, and standard messages can be printed on the statements for each of the aged dates (30, 60, 90, or 120 days). Some systems allow personalized messages to be inserted that override the standard messages.

Billing Services

Billing services are employed by many medical practices to reduce administrative paperwork by taking over the task of preparing and mailing patient statements. These services also may be employed to prepare and mail insurance claim forms or send them electronically. They may provide data entry of patients' demographic and billing information, charges, receipts, and adjustments; tracking of payments from patients and third-party payers; production of management reports, purging of inactive accounts, and collection of accounts.

Some advantages of billing services are advanced technology, professional and understandable bills, experts answering all billing-related telephone inquiries, and no downtime caused by vacations, or medical or personal leave. This service allows the medical office to have fewer disruptions and the freedom from worry about financial matters when trying to provide medical care.

Billing services are paid by a flat fee per account or a percentage of the collection. If a percentage is charged, the billing service is not paid until the account is collected; this provides an additional incentive to promote collection.

The physician's office sends billing and receipt information into the system daily. This may be done in writing or through a computer system. The billing service then prepares the bills, mails them, and may also receive payments. A periodic report is sent to the physician summarizing the transactions. This service also may be called a statement service, centralized billing, or outsourcing (when the owner of a medical practice transfers the ownership of a partial or full process [billing, transcription, coding] to a supplier). When choosing a billing service, make a list of important questions and visit the facility. Also visit a medical practice that has used the service for at least 3 years. The service's past performance is probably the best indicator of what can be expected in the future.

Billing Guidelines

Billing procedures are determined by the size of the practice, the number of accounts, and the number of staff members assigned to the collection process. Adopt a specific method of handling accounts and decide which billing routine best fits the practice. Check insurance and managed care contracts carefully to determine which circumstances allow for patients to be billed. Be sure to conform to federal guidelines if there is a need to bill managed care patients.

PROCEDURE: Seven-Step Billing and Collection Guidelines

1. Present the first statement at the time of service. This can be a formal statement or a multipurpose billing form.

2. Mail the second itemized statement within 30 days of treatment. The phrase "due and payable within 10 days" should be printed on each statement. Local paycheck issuing patterns should be considered before selecting a date statements are to be mailed. Choose which billing routine the office will use:

   a. Monthly Billing. Using the monthly billing system, all statements are mailed at the same time during the month. Choose a mail-out day at the beginning of the month so the patient will receive the bill near the 15th, or send statements near the end of the month, so the patient receives the bill on the 1st.

   b. Cycle Billing. **Cycle billing** is a system of billing accounts at spaced intervals during the month based on a breakdown of accounts by alphabet, account number, insurance type, or date of first service. This relieves the pressure of having to get all the statements out at one time and allows collection at a faster, more organized rate than accounts collected at random. It also allows continuous cash flow throughout the month and distributes the influx of incoming calls from patients about problem accounts. The number of cycles may be determined by how the collector wishes to divide the workload. Using two cycles per month, statements would be sent on the 25th to arrive by the 1st, and on the 10th to arrive by the 15th of the month. Using four cycles per month, statements should be sent every Tuesday or Wednesday to arrive at the end of the week. If a cycle that was established by the first date of service is used, and the patient was first seen on the 11th of the month, then every month on the 11th he or she should receive a bill.

3. Send the third statement 30 days after the second statement was sent. Indicate that the payment is past due.

4. Place the first telephone call to the patient. Ask if there is a problem. Ask for a payment commitment and set up a suspense file. Accounts are put in a suspense file for active follow up. Action must be taken within the time frame mentioned, after the patient has been so advised.

5. Check for payment as promised. Allow 1 day for mail delay. Place the second telephone call to the patient and ask for payment. Set up a new payment date. Allow 5 days.

6. Check for payment as promised. Send a 10-day notice advising the patient that unless payment is received in 10 days, the account will be turned over for legal action.

7. Check for payment. Promptly surrender the account for collection or legal action.

Figure 9–10 shows a collection decision tree to be used when determining when to send statements, 10-day notices, and accounts to a collection agency; and make telephone calls.

Credit Arrangements

Although payment at the time of service is ideal, many patients do not have funds available to pay at the time of the office visit. Alternative payment methods may be offered to help continuous cash flow and reduce collection costs.

Payment Options

Credit Card Billing

Credit card payment is an option that provides patients with an alternative to clear their account balances. Credit cards are issued by organizations that entitle the cardholder to credit at their establishments. This method of payment may be most useful as a down payment on uninsured or elective procedures. According to a survey by American Express, 33% of patients said they would use a credit card to pay for health care–related expenses if the option is given. Credit cards can help manage the A/R by improving cash flow, reducing billing costs, lowering overhead, and reducing the risk of bad debts. If a practice accepts credit cards, advise all patients in the following ways: display a credit card acceptance sign, include an insignia or message on the statement, include the credit card policy in the new patient brochure, and have staff members verbalize to patients that this option is available. Patients may prefer to clear a debt immediately and make monthly payments to the credit card company instead of owing money to their doctor.

Verifying Credit Cards

A one- or two-physician office may have a simple credit card imprinter in the office. The insurance specialist should check credit card warning bulletins to make sure that the card has not been canceled or stolen. Large practices may have an electronic credit card machine that allows the insurance specialist to swipe the card through the machine that is linked to the credit card company. Transactions then are approved, processed, and deposited into a bank account, usually in 2 working days. These machines may be rented or purchased.

Verifone terminals also are used for credit card authorization. They are small computers with built-in software and modems for communicating with other computers over telephone lines. They have a small alphanumeric keypad and a small display screen that can show a line or two of data. This device reads the information off the magnetic card as it is swiped through the machine, dials a telephone number, connects with another computer, verifies the patient's credit, and displays a message.

Verifying Credit Card Holders

Always verify the cardholder by asking for photo identification such as a driver's license. Examine the card carefully and observe the following guidelines:

▶ Accept a credit card only from the person whose name is on the card.

▶ Match the name on the card with the patient's other identification and make sure the expiration date has not passed.

▶ Look on the back of the card for the word "void." This is an alert that the card has been heated, which is a method used to forge a signature.

▶ Check the "hot list" for problem cards.

▶ Verify all charges regardless of the amount and get approval from the credit card company.

▶ Complete the credit card voucher (Fig. 9–11) before asking for a signature.

▶ Compare the signature on the credit card voucher against the signature on the card.

▶ Record the credit card number in the patient's financial file for future use if the patient's account has to be traced or transferred to a collection agency.

Credit Card Fees

Most banks directly deposit the credit card voucher and subtract the monthly fees from the practice's bank account. A statement from the bank indicates how much has been credited to the account. The fees can be negotiated based on volume, but usually range from 2% to 5%. Do not issue cash or check refunds for any payments made by credit card. Credit vouchers (Fig. 9–11) used for crediting a credit card account, are available at local banks. Patients who want to make payments may have their credit cards charged for each scheduled payment.

Credit Card Options

Other cards also are used for credit in a physician's office. ATM cards sometimes are accepted for medical care if the practice has a credit card scanner. Private-label cards are credit vehicles that can be used only to pay for health care. Some large practices offer their own private-label health cards. Smart cards also are used in some locations. They are small credit or debit cards that contain a computer chip that can store money in the form of electronic data. Special use smart cards for phone calls, gas stations, and fast food are now in use, as are common cards having multiple uses.

Visa offers a credit card service unique to the health care market. It has a Pre-Authorized Health Care Form that allows patients to authorize the

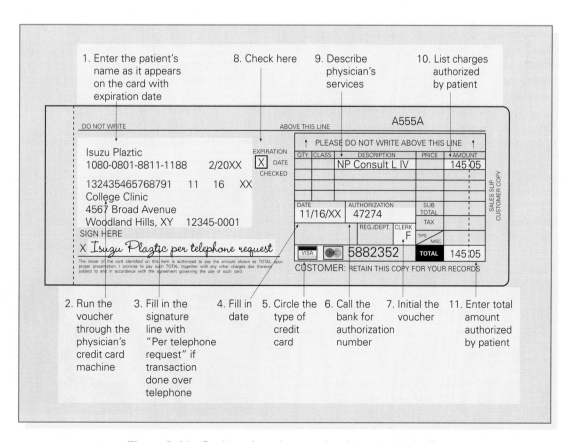

Figure 9–11. Credit card voucher completed in a physician's office.

medical office to bill their account directly for copayments and the balance not covered by insurance. Patients who need a series of treatments, such as allergy injections or chemotherapy, can fill out one form designating these services, which authorizes the staff to charge the patient's account directly.

A national medical card is now available for use by any professional or medical organization and enables the physician to offer a prearranged line of credit or an installment loan agreement by having the company take over the billing, accounting, and collecting for all patients who are approved for this service.

The convenience for patients and amount of reduced A/R should be weighed against the cost of setting up and operating this type of credit before making a decision about the use of credit cards in a medical practice.

Debit Cards

A **debit card** is a card permitting bank customers to withdraw cash at any hour from any affiliated ATM in the country. The holder also may make cashless purchases from funds on deposit without incurring revolving finance charges for credit. A small fee is charged to the customer's checking account when the card is used; however this fee is usually applied only once a month (if the debit card is used), regardless of how many times the card is used during the month. Medical practices offering credit card payment may use the same electronic credit card machine to swipe the debit card for verification and approval. Separate debit card machines are also available for businesses that do not accept credit cards. Debit cards take the place of check writing; however, once the debit card is approved for a certain amount, the bank that issued the debit card is responsible for paying the funds that were approved. There are no returned checks for non-sufficient funds with this method of payment.

E-Checks

Another payment option that is becoming popular is by e-check. With an e-check the patient gives his or her checking account information, such as account number, and bank routing number. No signature is necessary, and the check is deposited as though it were sent by the patient.

Payment Plans

Payment plans are another way of offering the patient a way of paying off an account by spreading out the amount due over a period of time. Caution should be taken when offering patients payment plans. The Truth in Lending Consumer Credit Cost Disclosure law (see Credit and Collection laws), also referred to as Regulation Z, requires full written disclosure about the finance charges for large payment plans involving

PAYMENT PLAN SCHEDULE

Balance due amount	Minimum monthly payment	Time frame for full payment
$0 – $200	$35	6 months
$201 – $500	$50	1 year
$500 – $1,000	$100	1 year
$1,001 – $3,000	$125	2 years
$3,001 – $5,000	$150	2 years
>$5,001*	$200	5 years

*Accounts over $5,000 must complete credit card application to certify minimum required payment and are subject to approval by office manager.

Figure 9–12. Payment plan schedule showing balance due amounts, minimum monthly payment, and payment time frames; used in the physician's office to negotiate monthly payments.

four or more installments, excluding a down payment. However, this regulation does not apply if the patient agrees to pay in one sum or in fewer than four payments and then decides independently to make drawn-out partial payments. Patients often think that if they make any amount of payment, the physician is required to accept that payment and not take any additional action. This is incorrect. The physician can take action, including sending the account to a collection agency. Have a written payment plan schedule when working with accounts in which payment plans may be offered. Figure 9–12 illustrates sample guidelines that may be used or revised according to individual practice and management policies (Fig. 9–13).

Credit and Collection Laws

The following laws are important because they provide the legal framework within which the insurance specialist must execute the physician's

Figure 9–13. Insurance billing specialist setting up a payment plan with a patient.

collection policy. In addition, each state may have specific collection laws that are necessary to research and obey.

Statute of Limitations

A formal regulation or law setting time limits on legal action is known as a **statute of limitations.** In regard to collections the statute of limitations is the maximum time during which a legal collection suit may be rendered against a debtor. However, for a lawsuit to be successful, a concerted effort should be made to collect on an account from the time services are rendered. The patient should receive regular statements indicating that if the insurer does not pay the patient will be held responsible.

Refer to Figure 9–14 to find out the statute of limitations for your state. Statutes vary according to

STATE OF LIMITATIONS		
State	**Open Accts.**	**Contracts Written/Oral**
Alabama	3	10
Alaska	6	6
Arizona	3	6/4
Arkansas	3	5/3
California	4	4/2
Colorado	6	6
Connecticut	6	6/3
Delaware	3	3
D.C.	3	3
Florida	4	5/4
Georgia	4	6/4
Hawaii	6	6
Idaho	4	5/4
Illinois	5	10/5
Indiana	6	10/6
Iowa	5	10/5
Kansas	3	5/3
Kentucky	5	15/5
Louisiana	3	10
Maine	6	20/6
Maryland	3	3
Massachusetts	6	20/6
Michigan	6	6
Minnesota	6	6
Mississippi	3	3/3
Missouri	5	10/5
Montana	5	8/5
Nebraska	4	5/4
Nevada	4	6/4
New Hampshire	6	3
New Jersey	6	6
New Mexico	4	6/4
New York	6	6
North Carolina	3	3
North Dakota	6	6
Ohio	6/15*	15/6
Oklahoma	3	5/3
Oregon	6	6
Pennsylvania	6	6/4
Rhode Island	10	10
South Carolina	3	3
South Dakota	6	6
Tennessee	6	6
Texas	4	4
Utah	4	6/4
Vermont	6	6
Virginia	3	5/3
Washington	3	6/3
West Virginia	5	10/5
Wisconsin	6	6
Wyoming	8	10/8

*6 oral/15 written

Figure 9–14. Individual state time limits (statute of limitations on civil actions) for collection of open accounts and oral or written contracts. (From Summary of Collection Laws, American Collectors Association, Inc., 2002.)

three kinds of accounts:

1. Open book accounts (also called open accounts): Accounts that are open to charges made from time to time. Payment is expected within a specific period but credit has been extended without a formal written contract. Physicians' patient accounts usually are open book accounts.
2. Written contract accounts: Accounts having a formal written agreement in which a patient signs to pay his or her bill in more than four installments (see Truth in Lending Act).
3. Single-entry accounts: Accounts having only one entry or charge; usually these are for a small amount.

Equal Credit Opportunity Act

The Equal Credit Opportunity Act (which is a federal law) prohibits discrimination in all areas of granting credit. If credit is offered, credit must be available fairly and impartially to all patients who request it. Obtaining detailed credit information before performing services will prevent accusations of credit discrimination. New patients can be informed that payment is due at the time of service, and they should arrive 20 minutes early to fill out a credit application if they would like to establish credit for possible future treatment. Check all information with a credit bureau that will verify data such as the patient's address, previous addresses, length of residence, employment history, and approximate wage. The report will also contain the patient's name changes, the patient's bill-paying history, and any history of bankruptcy. If the patient has a poor credit rating, credit may be denied and the patient then has 60 days to request the reason in writing. The law prohibits discrimination against any applicant for credit for the following reasons:

▶ Age, color, marital status, national origin, race, religion, or sex
▶ He or she has exercised rights under consumer credit laws
▶ An applicant is receiving income from any public assistance program

Fair Credit Reporting Act

Agencies who either issue or use reports on consumers (patients) in connection with the approval of credit are regulated by the Fair Credit Reporting Act. The act states that credit reporting agencies can only provide reports when:

▶ A court order is issued.
▶ The report is requested by the consumer (patient) or instructions are given by the patient to provide the report.
▶ There is a legitimate business need for the information.

If credit is refused, the physician must provide the patient with a reason credit was denied. Specific information about what the report contains is not necessary and should not be given. The provider also must give the name and address of the agency from which the report came. The patient must have an opportunity to correct any inaccuracies if they occur.

Fair Credit Billing Act

Per the Federal Trade Commission, the Fair Credit Billing Act (FCBA) applies to "open end" credit accounts, such as credit cards, and revolving charge accounts for department store accounts. It does not cover installment contracts such as loans or extensions of credit you repay on a fixed schedule. Consumers often buy cars, furniture, and major appliances on an installment basis, and repay personal loans in installments as well. The FCBA settlement procedures apply only to disputes about "billing errors," for example: unauthorized charges. Federal law limits your responsibility for unauthorized charges to $50; charges that list the wrong date or amount; charges for goods and services you did not accept or were not delivered as agreed; math errors; failure to post payments and other credits, such as returns; failure to send bills to the current address—provided the creditor receives the change of address, in writing, at least 20 days before the billing period ends; and charges for which an explanation or written proof of purchase along with a claimed error or request for clarification are requested.

To take advantage of the law's consumer protections, write to the creditor at the address given for "billing inquiries," not the address for sending payments, and include one's name, address, account number, and a description of the billing error. Send the letter so that it reaches the creditor within 60 days after the first bill was mailed that contained the error. Send the letter by certified mail, return receipt requested, for proof of what the creditor received. Include copies (not originals) of sales slips or other documents that support the position. Keep a copy of the dispute letter. The creditor must acknowledge the complaint in writing within 30 days after receiving it, unless the problem has been resolved. The creditor must resolve the dispute within two billing cycles (but not more than 90 days) after receiving the letter. Payment may be withheld on the disputed amount (and related charges) during the investigation. Any part of the bill not in question must be paid, including finance charges on the undisputed amount. The creditor may not take any legal or other action to collect the disputed amount and related charges (including finance charges) during the investigation. Although the account cannot be closed or restricted, the disputed amount may be applied against the credit limit. If the creditor's investigation determines the bill is correct, one must be told promptly and in writing how much is owed and why. Copies of relevant documents may be requested. At this point the disputed amount is owed plus any finance charges that accumulated while the amount was in dispute. The minimum amount that was missed because of the dispute may have to be paid. If the results of the investigation are disputed, the creditor may be written to within 10 days after receiving the explanation, and the disputed amount may be refused. At this point, the creditor may begin collection procedures. Any creditor who fails to follow the settlement procedure may not collect the amount in dispute, or any related finance charges, up to $50, even if the bill turns out to be correct. For example, if a creditor acknowledges the complaint in 45 days—15 days too late—or takes more than two billing cycles to resolve a dispute, the penalty applies. The penalty also applies if a creditor threatens to report, or improperly reports, one's failure to pay to anyone during the dispute period.

Truth in Lending Act

The federal Truth in Lending Act (TILA) of 1969 is a consumer protection act that applies to anyone who charges interest or agrees on payment of a bill in more than four installments, excluding a down payment. When a specific agreement is reached between patient and physician, Regulation Z of this act requires that a written disclosure of all pertinent information be made, regardless of the existence of a finance charge (Fig. 9–5). This full disclosure must be discussed at the time the agreement is first reached between patient and physician and credit is extended. It is essential to include the following items:

1. Total amount of the debt
2. Amount of down payment
3. Finance charge
4. Interest rate expressed as an annual percentage
5. Amount of each payment
6. Date each payment is due
7. Date final payment is due
8. Signature of patient and physician with copies retained by both

According to the Federal Trade Commission (FTC), the Truth in Lending provision is not applicable and no disclosures are necessary if a patient decides on his or her own to pay in installments or whenever convenient.

Late Payment Charges

Medical practices that implement late payment charges that meet the criteria defined in the TILA as a finance charge must comply with a host of requirements that revolve around proper disclosure to patients.

Charges must meet the following criteria to qualify as late payment charges:

1. The account balance must be paid in full at the time of initial billing.
2. The account is treated as delinquent when unpaid.
3. The charge is assessed to a patient's account only because of his or her failure to make timely payments.
4. Installments are limited to no more than three.
5. The creditor (physician or insurance specialist) makes a "commercially reasonable" effort to collect these accounts.

When a physician continues to treat a patient with an overdue account, the courts have viewed this as continuation of care and an extension of credit. Patients who fall into this delinquent status should be referred elsewhere. See Chapter 3 for instructions on sending a discharge letter. After the patient has paid the overdue amount, the patient can be taken back and treated on a cash-only basis.

Truth in Lending Consumer Credit Cost Disclosure

The Truth in Lending Consumer Credit Cost Disclosure is similar to the Federal Truth in Lending Act. It requires businesses to disclose all direct and indirect costs and conditions related to the granting of credit. All interest charges, late charges, collection fees, finance charges, and so forth must be explained up front, before the time of service. Include the following on all statements to charge interest and bill the patient monthly:

◗ Amount of each payment
◗ Due date
◗ Unpaid balance at the beginning of the billing period
◗ Finance charges
◗ Date balance is due

Fair Debt Collection Practices Act

The Fair Debt Collection Practices Act (FDCPA) was designed to address the collection practices of third-party debt collectors and attorneys who regularly collect debts for others. Although this act does not apply directly to physician practices collecting for themselves, a professional health care collector must avoid the actions that are prohibited for collection agencies. The main intent of the act is to protect consumers from unfair, harassing, or deceptive collection practices. Refer to the guidelines in Box 9-1, which are taken from the FDCPA to help avoid illegalities, enhance collections, and maintain positive patient relations. For more information

BOX 9–1

Fair Debt Collection Practices Act Guidelines

1. Contact debtors only once a day; in some states, repeated calls in 1 day or the same week could be considered harassment.
2. Place calls after 8 AM and before 9 PM.
3. Do not contact debtors on Sunday or any other day that the debtor recognizes as a Sabbath.
4. Identify yourself and the medical practice represented; do not mislead the patient.
5. Contact the debtor at work *only* if unable to contact the debtor elsewhere; no contact should be made if the employer or debtor disapproves.
6. Contact the attorney if an attorney represents the debtor; contact the debtor only if the attorney does not respond.
7. Do not threaten or use obscene language.
8. Do not send postcards for collection purposes; keep all correspondence strictly private.
9. Do not call collect or cause additional expense to the patient.
10. Do not leave a message on an answering machine indicating that you are calling about a bill.
11. Do not contact a third party more than once unless requested to do so by the party or the response was erroneous or incomplete.
12. Do not convey to a third party that the call is about a debt.
13. Do not contact the debtor when notified in writing that a debtor refuses to pay and would like contact to stop, except to notify the debtor that there will be no further contact or that there will be legal action.
14. Stick to the facts; do not use false statements.
15. Do not prepare a list of "bad debtors" or "credit risks" to share with other health care providers.
16. Take action immediately when stating that a certain action will be taken (e.g., filing a claim in small claims court or sending the patient to a collection agency).
17. Send the patient written verification of the name of the creditor and the amount of debt within 5 days of the initial contact.

about collection laws in your state, contact your state attorney general's office. The stricter law prevails if there is a conflict between state and federal laws.

The Collection Process

For collections to be handled effectively staff members should be trained in collection techniques. Most insurance specialists can be trained to be efficient collectors when given the correct tools. New collectors need time to gain confidence which is an important aspect of being a good collector.

Office Collection Techniques

Telephone Debt Collection

Telephone collections are made easier if the insurance billing specialist is convinced that he or she can collect before trying to convince the patient to pay. Two important factors to consider are the insurance specialist's ability to contact the patient and the patient's ability to pay the bill. Contact the patient in a timely manner at the first sign of payment delay. Prepare before making a telephone collection call by reviewing the account and noting anything unusual. Determine where the patient is employed (if unemployed). Decide what amount will be settled for if payment cannot be made in full. Make the first call count. Act in a calm, businesslike manner and combine empathy with diligence. Be positive and persuasive. Listen to what the patient has to say, even if he or she gets angry and raises his or her voice. Lower the volume of one's voice and respond in a composed manner. Try to pick up clues from what the patient is saying; he or she may be giving the real reason for nonpayment. Ask questions, show interest, and let the patient know that he or she is being listened to. Respond in a respectful manner and carefully word the reply; when patients are distressed they do not always make sense. The goal is to encourage the patient to pay, not agitate the patient. Use all resources and learn to negotiate.

Use an organized approach to determine which collection calls to make first. Print out the A/R by age and target the accounts that are in the 60- to 90-day category. The most effective results come from this group. If financial accounting record cards are used, pull all the cards with tabs or labels that indicate the patient has received two or three statements, depending on office protocol. Start with the largest amount owed and work the accounts in decreasing amounts owed. After this category has been completed, move on to the 90- to 120-day accounts. Finally, go after accounts that are more than 120 days old.

According to collection experts the best time to telephone is between 5:30 PM and 8:30 PM on Tuesdays and Thursdays and 9 AM to 1 PM on Saturdays. However, regardless of when the call is made, track the times when the most patients are contacted and adjust the calling schedule accordingly. Perhaps the physician's office hours should be increased to include one evening a week or Saturday mornings to make collection calls. Another option is the use of flex time in which the employee can choose his or her own working hours from within a broad range of hours approved by management. Use a private phone away from the busy operations of the office to eliminate interruptions. Patients may be embarrassed about not being able to pay their bills, and patient confidentiality must be maintained. Follow the rules stated in the Fair Debt Collection Practices Act.

Be alert for new ideas or approaches to collection by watching how banks and other retailers implement sophisticated collection skills. Decide if any of these could be used to the medical practice's advantage and present the techniques to the office manager. Keep abreast of improvements made to collection software that improve collection results and allow more collectors to work from their homes. Other advances (e.g., call block, which is an expanded telephone service) have made it more difficult to make collection calls. This service was originally intended to screen out unwanted telemarketing calls by intercepting blocked, unlisted, or unknown numbers. Standard numbers are usually allowed to go through. The key to averting a block is to make sure the number the call is being placed from is listed and within the patient's area. Telephone company's services vary, so research to discover all expanded services used in your area.

P R O C E D U R E : Telephone Collection Plan

Following are steps to assist in making the first collection call:

1. Set the mood of the call by the manner of speech and tone of voice. The first 30 seconds of the call set the scene for the relationship with the patient.
2. Identify the patient. Be certain the debtor is being spoken to before revealing the nature of the call.
3. Identify oneself and the facility.
4. Verify the debtor's address and any telephone numbers.
5. State the reason for the call.
6. Take control of the conversation and establish urgency by asking for full payment now; disclose the full amount owed.
7. Ask when payment will be made, how it will be made, and if it will be sent by mail or in person.
8. Pause for effect. This turns the conversation back to the patient to respond to the demand or explain why payment has not been made. Never assume that if a patient does not respond, it means no.
9. Find out if the patient needs clarification of the bill.
10. Inquire if the patient has a problem. Ask if the practice can be of assistance, especially when the patient is unable to give a reason for nonpayment.
11. If the patient is reluctant to agree to an amount, question him or her by asking one of the following: "How much are you willing to pay?" "Do you have a regular paycheck?" "Will payment be made through a checking account?"
12. Obtain a promise to pay with an agreeable amount and a due date; be clear how and when payment is expected, but give the patient a choice of action.
13. Ask for half of the amount if full payment is not possible.
14. Discuss a payment plan if the patient is not able to pay half of the balance owed. Be realistic and reasonable. It is self-defeating to set up payment arrangements the patient cannot afford. Advise the patient that the entire balance will become due and payable if the payment is even 1 day late. Ask the patient to please call before the due date with an explanation if any problems arise to prevent payment.
15. Restate the importance of the agreement.
16. Tell the patient to write down the amount and due date.
17. Document the agreement on the patient's financial accounting record, in the computer, or in a collection telephone log. Note the time the patient was spoken to.
18. Send confirmation of the agreement (Fig. 9–15).
19. Check the account the day after the payment was due; allow 1 day for mail delay. If the patient fails to make payment as promised, make another telephone call and ask the patient if there is still a problem. Get a new commitment to pay and confirm again. If the patient continues to avoid payment, advise the patient that the account will be turned over to a collection agency and follow through as stated.

Telephone "Don'ts"

The following is a list of **do nots** for telephone collections:

- Do not raise your voice and antagonize the patient.
- Do not accuse the patient of dishonesty or lying.
- Do not act like a "tough guy" or threaten a patient.
- Do not consent to partial payments until payment in full has been asked for and do not agree to a long string of small partial payments.
- Do not engage in a debate.
- Do not report a disputed account to a collection agency or bureau until the patient's dispute is disclosed as part of the record.

Telephone collection calls also are effective the day before patients are due for their appointments. State the date and time of the appointment and then remind the patient of the balance owed and ask if he or she would please bring payment to the appointment.

Figure 9–15. Telephone confirmation letter sent to remind patient of the payment terms agreed to in a telephone conversation.

COLLEGE CLINIC
4567 Broad Avenue
Woodland Hills, XY 12345-0001
Tel. (555) 486-9002
FAX (555) 487-8976

October 2, 20XX

Mr. Leonard Blabalot
981 McCort Circle
Woodland Hills, XY 12345-0001

Dear Mr. Blabalot:

I am glad we had an opportunity to discuss your outstanding balance with our practice during our phone conversation on October 1, 20XX. This will confirm and remind you that you agreed to pay $100 on your account on or before October 15, 20XX.

A return envelope is enclosed for your convenience.

Sincerely,

Charlotte Rose Routingham
Business Office

Enc. envelope

Telephone Collection Scenarios

The most difficult part of one-on-one collections is preparing for the many situations that may be encountered and the various responses the patient may make. Following are some statements patients make for not paying an account and examples of responses the insurance specialist can make:

Statement: "I can't pay anything now."
Response: "Are you employed? Are you receiving unemployment compensation, welfare, or Social Security benefits?"

You are determining the patient's ability to pay.

"Are you paying some of your bills?"

You are uncovering the fact that the patient is paying certain bills. You can then tell the patient that the bill must be taken care of, also, even if only a small amount at a time.

Statement: "I can't pay the whole bill now."
Response: "How long will it take you to pay this bill?"

Ask this instead of, "How much can you pay?"

Statement: "I can pay, but not until next month."
Response: "When do you get paid?"

Ask for payment the day after payday.
"Do you have a checking account?"

Ask for a postdated check.

Statement: "I have other bills."
Response: "This is also one of your bills that should be paid now. Let's talk about exactly how you plan payment."

Statement: "How about $10 a month (on a $350 bill)?"
Response: "I'd like to accept that, but our accountant does not allow us to stretch out payments beyond 90 days, which would be $105 a month."

This adheres to (Truth in Lending Law) regulations for collecting payment in installments without a written agreement. If the patient tries to cooperate, then compromise. If not, turn the account over to a collection agency.

Statement: "I sent in the payment."
Response: "When was the payment sent? To what address was it sent? Was it a check? On what bank was it drawn and for what amount? What is the canceled check number?"

Investigate to see if the check was posted to a wrong account. If not, call the patient back and ask if he or she would call his or her bank to see if it cleared; if it has not, the patient should stop payment. Ask the patient to call back and verify the status of the check. If the patient is lying, he or she will not follow through. Ask for a new check and tell the patient that a refund will be made if the other one shows up.

Statement: "I cannot make a payment this month."

Response: "The collection agency picks up all our delinquent accounts next Monday. I don't want to include yours, but I need a check today."

Statement: "The check's in the mail."

Response: "May I have the check number and date it was mailed?"

Call back in 3 days if not received.

Statement: "I'm not going to pay the bill because the doctor didn't spend any time with me."

Response: "May I confirm the doctor you saw, the date, and time? For what reason did you see the doctor? Do you still have the problem for which you saw the doctor?"

Get as much information as possible and research the office schedule the day the patient was seen. Let the doctor know about the patient's complaint and inquire how he or she would like to handle the complaint.

Statement: "I thought the insurance company was paying this."

Response: "Your insurance paid most of the bill; now the balance is your responsibility.

Please send your check before Friday to keep your account current."

Explain why (deductible, copayment benefit) the service is not covered under the insurance plan.

Collection Letters

Collection letters are another method of reaching patients and reminding them of their debt. Knowledge of the patient base and of individual patients may help determine the effectiveness of collection letters. Every facility is unique, and the number of accounts, the geographic spread of patients, the staff size, and the amount of time collectors have to spend on individual accounts helps determine which collection method best suits the practice.

Some positive aspects of collection letters are the following: They can reach a large number of patients rapidly and the cost is relatively low (especially if form letters are used; Fig. 9–16).

Collection letters have some negative aspects: Letters usually take 2 or 3 days to reach the patient and may lie unopened for a week or more; letters are one-way communication, thus lacking the ability to provide the reason for nonpayment; the response and recovery through letters are relatively poor; and manual preparation takes time (especially if a decision must be made before sending each letter).

Figure 9–16. Collection form letter sent to all patients who have not responded after two billing cycles.

COLLEGE CLINIC
4567 Broad Avenue
Woodland Hills, XY 12345-0001
Tel. (555) 486-9002
FAX (555) 487-8976

November 13, 20XX

Miss Melanie Markham
1001 Swallow Lane
Woodland Hills, XY 12345-0001

Dear Miss Markham:

It is the office policy of College Clinic to contact patients who have received two billing statements but have not responded. We realize this could be an oversight on your part, not a willful disregard of an assumed obligation. If you have a financial problem or a question about your account, please call me at (555) 486-9002 extension 443 or stop by our office.

We would like to thank you in advance for your cooperation in attending to this matter.

Sincerely,

Shirley Summer, CMA
Clarence Cutler, MD

The insurance specialist is often the one to compose collection letters and devise a plan for collection follow up. A series of collection letters may be written using varying degrees of forcefulness, starting with a gentle reminder. When a collection letter is written, use a friendly tone and ask why payment has not been made. Imply that the patient has good intentions to pay. This may be done by suggesting that the patient has overlooked a previous statement. Communicate the doctor's sincere interest in the patient. Always invite the patient to explain the reason for nonpayment in a letter, telephone call, or office visit. It should sound as though the patient is anxious to clear the debt.

When collection letters are sent toward the end of the year, include a statement letting the patient know that if the account is paid in full by the end of the year, the medical expense may be used as an income tax deduction. Another tactic is to send a notice advising the patient that he or she may skip December's payment because of increased expenses during the holidays. This tactic may be used as an opportunity to build patient relationships, but the collector must be firm and clear when offering such leeway. Collection letters sent after the first of the year can suggest that the patient clear the debt by using an income tax refund check.

Types of Collection Letters

There are several styles of collection letters. A form letter saves time and can go out automatically at specific times during the billing cycle (Fig. 9–16). Letters with checklists are a type of form letter (Fig. 9–17) that makes it easier for the patient to choose a payment option. Personally typed letters can be individualized to suit any situation. Collection letters should contain the following information:

▶ Full amount owed
▶ Services performed
▶ What action the patient should take
▶ Time frame in which the patient should respond
▶ How the patient should take care of the bill
▶ Why the patient should take care of the bill
▶ Address to which patients send payment
▶ Telephone number to contact the office
▶ Contact person's name
▶ Signature, which can be listed as "Financial Secretary," "Insurance Specialist," "Assistant to Doctor _____," or one's name and title with the physician's name below.

When pursuing collection, the insurance specialist should stay within the authorization of the physician. All letters should be noted on the back of the financial accounting record, in the collection log, or in the computer comment area. Abbreviations can be used to indicate which letter was sent (Table 9–2) along with the date the letter was mailed. Letters can be sent in brightly colored envelopes to attract attention.

The envelope should include "Address Service Requested" or "Forwarding Service Requested" on the outside to ensure the letter is forwarded if the patient has moved so that the office will be notified of the patient's new address. Always include a self-addressed stamped envelope.

Collection Abbreviations

Collection abbreviations can be used to save time and space while documenting efforts to collect and patients' responses. A few of the most common abbreviations are listed in Table 9–2. Always use standard abbreviations so anyone working on the account will know exactly what attempts have been made to collect and what action has been taken. Figure 9–18 illustrates some abbreviated collection entries, with interpretations, on the back of a financial accounting record.

Insurance Collection

Most patients carry some form of insurance; however, filing an insurance claim is only the first step in collecting fees owed. Good follow-up techniques (see Chapter 8) are necessary to ensure payment from the insurance carrier and copayment or coinsurance payment from the patient.

First, affirm that a clean insurance claim was sent with all necessary precertification, preauthorization, and documentation for services. Next, follow up in a timely manner with telephone calls and written tracers. Track all denials to learn what services are being denied and which insurance companies are denying payment. It is worth investing money and staff resources to identify the cause of claim denials. Send all high-dollar claims by certified mail to alleviate the problem of the insurance company saying that "it was never received." This saves time and is cost-effective.

History of Accounts

If the insurance company seems to be ignoring all efforts to trace the claim, an exact history of the account may be the best weapon with which to proceed. A history of the account is a chronological record of all events that have occurred. Keep all communications received from the insurance company, note all telephone calls, and keep copies of all documents sent. Send a copy of the history of the account directly to the insurance company and demand a reply. This may also be done in the case of an insurance company dispute or a refusal to pay.

Coinsurance Payments

Use a letter or statement to collect from patients who have insurance coverage. Clearly indicate to the patient that the insurance biller has submitted

---

COLLEGE CLINIC
4567 Broad Avenue
Woodland Hills, XY 12345-0001
Tel. (555) 486-9002
FAX (555) 487-8976

March 16, 20XX

Mr. Frank Lincoln
3397 Westminster Avenue
Woodland Hills, XY 12345-0001

Account No.   593287
Amount Due: $ _____

Dear Mr. Lincoln:

The care of our patients is more important than writing letters about overdue accounts. Yet, as you must realize, the expense of furnishing care can only be met by payments from appreciative patients.

Your account is seriously past due and has been removed from our current files because of its delinquent status. Our office policy indicates that your account should be placed with a collection agency. However, we would prefer to hear from you regarding your preference in this matter.

Enclosed is a current statement of your account. Please indicate your payment choice.

☐   I would prefer to settle this account immediately. Please find payment in full enclosed.

☐   I would prefer to make monthly payments (up to six months). To exercise this option
    please call and make arrangements to come into our office to sign a financial agreement.

☐   Please charge the full amount to my credit card. (We accept American Express, MasterCard,
    and Visa). To exercise this option, please telephone our office or fill in the enclosed form
    and return it with the envelope provided.

_____
        Signature   Date

Please select one of the three options above, sign the form, and return this notice within 10 days from the date indicated in the letter. A postmarked return envelope is provided. Failure to respond will result in an automatic referral to our collection agency. Please do not hesitate to call if you have any questions regarding this matter.

Sincerely,

Gil Steinberg
Office Manager

Enc. Envelope, Credit Card Agreement Form

Figure 9–17. Multipurpose collection letter with checklist. This advises patient of a seriously past due account, offers the patient three payment options, and warns the patient that failure to respond will result in a referral to a collection agency.

an insurance claim and advise the patient what action is expected. The status of the insurance claim should be noted on all statements. Notify patients promptly when insurance payment has been received. Ask patients to get involved in the insurance process or to pay the bill within 10 days if a problem exists. Following are examples of notations on statements for patients with insurance coverage:

▶ "We have received payment from your insurance company. The balance of $_____ is now your responsibility."

▶ "Your insurance company has paid its share of your bill. This statement is for the amount payable directly by you."

▶ "Your insurance company has paid $_____ for the above services. The remaining portion of $_____ is now your responsibility."

▶ "The balance of this account is your share of the cost. Please remit today. For questions, call 486-9002."

▶ "Your insurance company has not responded. The account is due and payable. Please contact your insurance company about payment. Thank you for your assistance."

TABLE 9–2	**Collection Abbreviations**			
ATTY	Attorney		NSN	No such number
B	Bankrupt		OFC	Office
Bal	Balance		OOT	Out of town
Bk*	Bank		OOW	Out of work
BLG	Belligerent		PA	Payment arrangement
BTTR	Best time to reach		PH or PH'D	Phoned
CB	Call back		Ph/Dsc*	Phone disconnected
CLM	Claim		PIF	Payment in full
DA*	Directory assistance		PIM	Payment in mail
DFB	Demand for Balance		PMT	Payment
DNK	Did not know		POE	Place of employment
DSC	Disconnected		POLK†	Polk directory
EMP	Employment		POW	Payment on way
EOM	End of month		PP	Promise to pay or partial payment
EOW	End of Week		PT	Patient
FA	Further action		RCD	Received
FN	Final notice		R/D*	Reverse directory
H	He (or husband)		RE	About
HHCO	Have husband call office		RES	Residence
HSB	Husband		S	She (or wife)
HTO	He telephoned office		SEP	Separated
HU	Hung up		SK*	Skip or skipped
INS	Insurance		SOS	Same old story
LI, L2	Letter one, letter two (sent)		SP/DEL*	Special delivery
LB	Line busy		STO	She telephoned office
LD	Long distance		T	Telephoned
LM	Left message		TB	Telephoned business
LMCO	Left message, call office		TR	Telephoned residence
LMVM	Left message, voice mail		TT	Talked to
LTR	Letter		TTA	Turned to agency
MR	Mail return		UE	Unemployed
NI, N2	Note one, note two (sent)		U/Emp	Unemployed
NA	No answer		UTC	Unable to contact
N/B*	Nearby or neighbors (no phone listing)		VFD	Verified
NFA*	No forwarding address		Vfd/E	Verified employment
NHD*	Never heard of debtor		Vfd/I	Verified insurance
NI	Not in		W/	Will
NLE	No longer employed		WCO	Will call office
NPL	No phone listed		WCIO	Will come in office
NPN	Nonpublished number		W/I	Walk-in
NR	No record		WVO	Will visit office
NSF	Not sufficient funds		X	By

*Used in skip tracing.
†Directories used to locate patients by street address or telephone number.

Insurance Checks Sent to Patients

Send a letter immediately to notify patients who receive insurance checks (see Chapter 8). Advise such patients that they have received payment from their insurance company and that their account is due and payable within 10 days. Do not send continuous monthly bills; instead speed up the collection process. If the patient refuses to pay and the physician does not want the patient to return, send a 10-day notification advising the patient that the account will go to a collection agency; if no response, discharge the patient from the practice.

Managed Care Organizations

When a medical practice deals with several managed care organizations, trying to remember all the contract information can be confusing. A managed care desk reference (see Chapter 10)

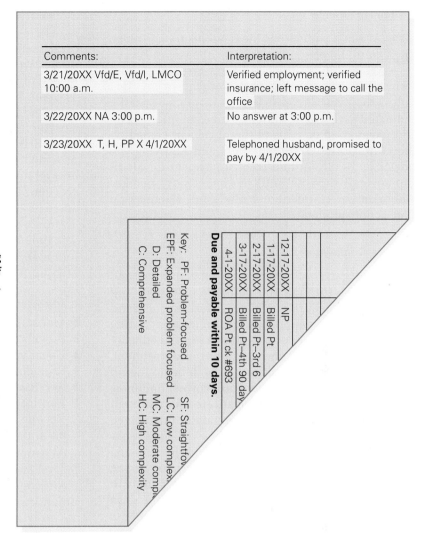

Figure 9–18. The back of a financial accounting record (ledger card) that shows examples of abbreviated collection entries with interpretation.

can help staff members find information quickly. "Promised payment date" along with all the other information on the desk reference grid or matrix can be easily referred to by the insurance specialist when trying to collect from managed care organizations.

Make sure all referral authorizations are in place before the patient is to be seen. If a patient shows up without a referral, offer to reschedule or inform the patient that the visit must be paid for in cash before leaving the office. If the patient has no money, a promissory note may be executed, but this action is not preferred and would be carried out as a last option.

When dealing with managed care contracts, do not sign any contract that holds a third party "harmless." The "hold harmless" clause is a way for one party to shift financial responsibilities to another party. Such "hold harmless" clauses often include phrases that state that the third party is "held harmless" to pay claims, liabilities, costs, expenses, judgments, or damages awarded by any court to all patients who bring any legal action against the medical practice. If the third party goes out of business or goes bankrupt before the contract is honored, the physician cannot collect

any money from the patient that the third party was to have paid. To avoid such possibilities, make sure payments from all managed care organizations are current.

Check to see that all third-party payers are insured by a federal agency. Such insurance would pay the physician in the event the managed care organization could not. We discuss more about managed care bankruptcy in Chapter 10.

Medicare

A provider must make genuine collection efforts to collect the unpaid deductible and coinsurance amounts from all Medicare patients. Reasonable efforts must include subsequent billings, telephone calls, and in-person collection efforts done in the same manner as with all patients. Accounts may not be written off until sequential statements (spaced 15 to 30 days apart) have been sent with an increasing intensity in the collection message. A telephone call should be placed to the debtor asking for payment, as well as requesting payment when the patient is seen in person.

Medigap Insurance

When a patient has Medigap insurance, make sure the patient's signature appears in Blocks 12 and 13 of the CMS-1500 insurance claim form. Do not routinely enter "signature on file" unless the insured has signed an insurance-specific statement authorizing release of medical information and payment of benefits to the physician named on the claim form. A signed statement allowing the physician to bill for and receive payment for Medigap-covered services until the beneficiary revokes authorization is preferred. A Medicare "signature on file" is not sufficient.

Workers' Compensation

Verify the validity of work-related injury and illness through the patient's employer and obtain accurate billing information. Send timely bills and reports using the correct coding system and fee schedule. Always keep the adjuster assigned to the case informed of ongoing treatment. The patient and employer should both be notified if a problem exists. Document all correspondence, including telephone authorizations for treatment and any tracing efforts. Any disputed or unresolved workers' compensation cases may be revised to self-pay, or be referred to a Financial Service Representative or the proper state-level authority. The physician may file for mediation on behalf of the patient if proper authorization was obtained and a claim form sent at the time of the patient's treatment. A claim also may be filed with the state labor board naming the patient's employer and workers' compensation carrier whenever there is difficulty getting full payment. The industrial board has the employer pressure the carrier to resolve the matter. If an insurance company has not paid or has sent a written notice of nonpayment, the provider may file a request for default judgment from the state authority. If the judgment is in the provider's favor, the payer is ordered to pay in full. See Chapter 14 for more information on delinquent workers' compensation claims.

Suing an Insurance Carrier

As stated under Statute of Limitations, there are time periods during which an insured person may sue the insurance company to collect the amount the claimant believes is owed. An insured person may not initiate a legal action against the insurer until 60 days after the initial claim has been submitted. A lawsuit against the insurer must be filed within 3 years of the date the initial claim was submitted for payment.

When the insurance company does not respond to reason or negotiation after the physician's office has tried to collect from an insurance plan, the only alternatives are surrender or litigation. A lawsuit may be worthwhile if a high-dollar claim is in question. Insurance carriers may be sued for payment under two circumstances: claim for plan benefits or breach of contract and claim for damages.

Claim for plan benefits is used when the claim is governed by the Employee Retirement Income Security Act (ERISA), a Federal Employee Health Benefit Act (FEHBA). ERISA governs health insurance that is provided as a benefit of employment. FEHBA governs all health insurance provided as a benefit to federal employees. An insured person is entitled to appeal a denied claim under these two federal laws. A timely request must be filed to sue for payment. The time limit for ERISA is within 60 days of denial; for FEHBA the time limit is within 6 months. Federal laws apply across the country and overrule all state laws. Suits based on claims for plan benefits may be made when denial is based on the following:

▶ Medical necessity
▶ Preexisting condition
▶ Usual and customary rate issues
▶ Providers or facilities that are not covered
▶ Services that fall within an exclusion to coverage
▶ Failure to offer Consolidated Omnibus Budget Reconciliation Act (COBRA) coverage by a plan administrator

When the claim falls outside of the scope of these federal laws, it is possible to sue if the conduct of the payer constitutes a violation of state laws relating to unfair insurance practices.

Suing on the basis of claim for damages falls entirely under state law. This is most likely to occur if the patient has no plan benefit but the patient or physician's office is led to believe so by the insurer or plan administrator. Examples may include the following:

▶ Insurer misquoting benefits during a verification of those benefits
▶ Denial of payment because of lack of medical necessity when preauthorization of treatment was obtained

Collection Agencies

Delinquent accounts should be turned over to a collection agency only after all reasonable attempts have been made to collect by the physician's office. Knowing when to turn accounts over helps determine the success of the collection agency. The longer the unpaid balance remains in the physician's office, the less chance the agency has to collect the account, so the determination that an account is uncollectable should be made quickly. Some guidelines follow:

▶ When a patient states that he or she will not pay or there is a denial of responsibility
▶ When a patient breaks a promise to pay

▶ When a patient makes partial payments and 60 days have lapsed without payment

▶ When a patient fails to respond to the physician's letters or telephone calls

▶ When payment terms fail for no valid reason

▶ When a check is returned by the bank because of insufficient funds and the patient does not make an effort to rectify the situation within 1 week of notification

▶ When delinquency coexists with marital problems, divorce proceedings, or child support agreements

▶ When a patient is paid by the insurance company and does not forward the payment to the physician (this constitutes fraud and may be pursued with legal action)

▶ When a patient gives false information

▶ When a patient moves and the office has used all resources to locate the patient

Not all accounts should go to a collection agency. Such accounts include those of personal friends, elderly widows or widowers living on pensions, and accounts with balances under $25. Many physicians prefer to adjust small bad debts off of the books rather than increase administrative costs. All disputed accounts should be reviewed and approved by the physician before they are sent to collection. There should be a systematized approach for turning accounts over to a collection agency that still allows room for an exception, should one occur.

Choosing an Agency

A collection agency should be chosen with great care because it is a reflection of the medical practice. Choose a reputable agency that is considerate and efficient with a high standard of ethics. The agency should specialize in physician accounts and have an attitude toward debtors with which the physician agrees. Find out how long the agency has been in business and request a list of at least 10 references and statistics on their collection effectiveness. The average collection rate varies greatly but falls between 20% and 60% on assigned accounts. Be sure the report rate includes all accounts more than 1 year old and does not exclude accounts with small balances.

An agency's performance can be evaluated by the amount collected, less the agency's fees, which is called the "**netback.**" For instance, if the collector recovered 25% of $5000 ($1250) and takes a 50% commission, the physician's netback is $625. If the collector recovered 25% of the $5000 ($1250) and charged a 30% commission, the netback is $375. Although the second agency collected less, its lower commission afforded the physician more money.

When choosing a collection agency, make sure: (1) to set up a separate PO Box or Lock Box for the collection project; (2) to set up a separate bank account for the collection project; (3) that the contract stipulates that all correspondence is sent to the PO Box. (no correspondence is to be sent to the collection agency's physical or payment address); (4) all e-checks and credit card receipts are deposited into the physician's bank account; and (5) under no circumstance is the collection agency to receive any payments. If money goes to the collection agency (whether insured, bonded, registered, or licensed) there is nothing to stop the collection agency from stealing the physician's money. The collection agency also could have a hidden lawsuit against them or an income tax lien, and the physician will lose all of his or her money if it is in the agency's bank account. *Do not* put "hold harmless" clauses in contracts. Hold the collection agency responsible for their actions. Many states do not regulate collection agencies. Many simply require the collection agency to be registered. In addition to checking references, check with the state's Department of Corporations to see whose name is on the collection agency's registration, if the tax identification number is correct and current, and if the address listed is different than the one the agency gave. Contact the circuit court and see if there are any lawsuits and judgments against the collection agency. Find out how many of their employees will be assigned to the account. Then monitor them once the contract is signed. They may have the best credentials and references and belong to all the correct organizations, but if they acquire an increasing number of accounts and the amount of recoupment remains constant each month or is less than the national average, they may be cherry picking the accounts. This is especially true when they are overanxious to receive a new file. If this happens, consider looking for another collection agency. Make sure an account can be recalled without a penalty. The patient may have coverage with a carrier already contracted with, so find out if the collection agency has the ability to resend a claim or if the billing company or office staff handle this. If so, does the contract have provisions for this, and does the collection agency receive recoupment for obtaining insurance information?

The biggest key to the agency's effectiveness is the doctor's own credit and collection policy. A comprehensive patient registration form, along with verifying employment, turning accounts over quickly when they qualify, and giving the agency all the available information, helps the agency pick up the paper trail and secure payment. A good collection agency has membership in a national collection society and the approval of the local medical society. Review the agency's financial statement and make sure the agency is licensed, bonded, and carries "hold harmless clause" insurance. If a patient should sue because of harassment, this insurance will protect the physician from being sued as well. The local bar association and state licensing bureaus can be contacted to see if any complaints have been lodged against the agency or law firm. Find out if the agency reports uncollectable debtors ("deadbeats") to a credit agency and investigate which one is used.

Types of Agencies

There are local, regional, and national agencies. National agencies and ones that use the Internet may have better results tracing skips (patients who owe balances on their accounts and move without leaving a forwarding address). Local agencies are more aware of the socioeconomic status of patients. Some agencies pay their staff commissions and bonuses for high productivity, and others are low-key and more customer-oriented. Find out the experience level of the staff and make sure the agency values the physician's business.

Another option is to use a collection service such as CollectNet. CollectNet gives small and mid-sized facilities with limited budgets the collection capabilities of large collection systems by connecting to databases. The medical practice is able to make calling lists, print collection letters, search for telephone numbers and addresses, access patient credit reports, write and format reports, monitor collection progress, and set automatic callback reminders. Optional features include BankruptcyNet, SkipNet, LetterNet, and BureauNet. Collection agencies use this service, but it is also available to large groups and clinics.

Agency Operating Techniques

Collection agencies must follow all the laws stated in the Fair Debt Collection Practices Act. They may not "harass" the debtor or make false threats and may not use letters that appear to be legal documents. A provision should be included for the agency to seek permission from the physician's office before suing a debtor in municipal court and charging a percent of the judgment. A progress report should be provided to the physician's office on a regular basis at least monthly. The agency also should return any uncollectable accounts to the physician's office within a reasonable time and not charge for these accounts. If a debtor moves, ask if the account is forwarded to another collection office. All procedures used to make collections should be shown to the physician's office, including collection letters and telephone script. The physician's office should be aware if the agency uses a personalized or standard approach. A personal visit to the premises of the collection agency can provide a first-hand view of its operating techniques.

Agency Charges

Agencies may be paid a flat rate on all accounts according to volume. Some agencies may leave the accounts in the control of the physician's office where the staff speaks with the patient and posts all delinquent incoming monies. Other agencies charge a commission based on a percentage of an account, and the physician's office refers all calls to the agency once the account is turned over to it. The fixed cost an agency pays to collect on an account is $3.96. A standard rate for most agencies to break even is one third of all monies collected, and an average rate charged is 50%. Make sure the commission is based on how much is collected on the overdue accounts and not the total amount of overdue accounts turned over to the agency.

Agency Assigned Accounts

Patients' accounts turned over to a collection agency should have a letter of withdrawal sent by certified mail (see Chapter 3, Fig. 3–24). Place a note on all financial accounting records indicating the date the account was assigned. Once an account has been given to a collection agency, it is illegal to send the patient a monthly statement. Financial management consultants usually recommend that the patient's balances be written off of the A/R at the time the account is assigned. A portion of the account balance can be written back on if and when the agency collects on the debt. Accounts also should be listed in a separate journal to help track the effectiveness of the agency. Allow enough columns to show the future date, amount, and percentage of an account collected by the agency, as well as the total account balance.

Flag or insert a full sheet of brightly colored paper in the patient's chart noting the date the account was assigned to collection. This will alert all medical staff of the situation if the patient calls on short notice or walks in to be seen. If the patient sends payment to the physician's office after the account has been turned over to an agency, notify the collection agency immediately. Any calls about accounts that have gone to collection should be referred to the agency.

Credit Bureaus

Collection agencies also can offer the services of a credit bureau. Credit bureaus gather credit information from many sources and make it available for a fee to members of a credit bureau service. Credit reports can be issued on new patients enabling the physician's office to verify credit. The information may consist of the patient's residence and moving habits (a measure of permanency), number of dependents, verification of employment and approximate salary, the patient's payment history on other merchant accounts, and any history of bankruptcy or use of an alias. This report can be obtained over the telephone or provided in written form.

The Fair Credit Reporting Act of 1971 allows a person to see and correct his or her credit report. The credit report can be checked for negative credit information, disputed information, mistakes, and out-of-date information. If credit is denied based in whole or in part on an adverse credit report, a letter should be sent advising the patient the name and address of the agency and stating that credit has been denied because credit requirements have not been met. The insurance specialist need not reveal data or specify the exact nature of the information obtained from the credit bureau but must name the bureau. A copy of the letter should be kept in the patient's file.

Credit Counseling

A consumer credit counseling service is a nonprofit agency that assists people in paying off their debts. The insurance specialist may have to refer patients for this service if continued medical care is being provided and the patient becomes overwhelmed by the cost. The patient may also contact his or her own bank or credit union, which may provide counseling at no charge. Care must be given with such referrals; use only legitimate agencies and warn patients that many private commercial debt consolidators may charge high fees. Dissatisfied patients may blame the physician or the insurance specialist if satisfactory financial arrangements are not made.

A patient seeking medical care who is unable to pay for services and is ineligible for state aid should be directed to the local hospital that services recipients under the Hill-Burton Act of 1946. These hospitals obtained federal construction grants to enlarge their facilities in exchange for their provision of health care for needy patients. The Department of Health and Human Services will furnish the names of local hospitals that participate in this service. Patients must complete financial applications to determine eligibility before care is rendered.

Small Claims Court

Small claims court is a part of our legal system that allows lay people to have access to a court system without the use of an attorney. Some advantages are a modest filing fee, minimal paperwork, exclusion of costly lawyers, and a short time frame from filing the action to trial date. Incorporated physicians usually must be represented by an attorney, and the agency must file in a municipal or justice court if an account has already been sent to a collection agency.

Most states have small claims courts (also called conciliation, common-pleas, general-sessions, justice courts, or people's court). Each state has monetary limits on the amount that can be handled in small claims court, and accounts should be reviewed for eligibility. The dollar amount varies from state to state and sometimes from one county to another. The average maximum amount generally ranges from $2000 to $3000; however a recent effort has been supported to raise the dollar limit for small claims courts to $20,000. There are several legislative bills being considered by U.S. Senate and House committees that address raising the dollar limit. Several states already have had such bills signed into law. The new limits in these states vary from $3,000 to $10,000. There also may be limits on the number of claims filed per year that are more than a specific dollar amount.

When filing a claim, the person filing the petition (the physician's office) is referred to as the plaintiff and the party being brought to suit (the patient) is called the defendant. It is generally recommended that the plaintiff send a written demand to the defendant before filing a lawsuit to give the defendant a last opportunity to resolve the claim.

PROCEDURE: Filing a Claim

1. Obtain a Claim of Plaintiff or Plaintiffs Original Petition form to notify the patient that action is being filed. This can be obtained from the clerk's office located at the municipal or justice court.
2. File the papers with the small claims court; make sure to have the patient's correct name and street address.
3. Pay the clerk the small filing fee.
4. Make arrangements to serve the defendant. The summons or citation can be served on the patient by a sheriff or court-appointed officer by paying a small fee plus mileage for the constable who serves it. The person serving the defendant must fill out a proof of service form.

A trial date will be set, and both plaintiff and defendant will be ordered to appear before the judge. Often a postcard is sent notifying the plaintiff when the defendant has been served. If the amount of delinquent debt is more than the monetary limit for the small claims court, consider "cutting the claim to fit" the limit. For example, if the amount of a debt is $2757 and the state limit is $2500, consider waiving (giving up) the $257 (difference) to bring the amount down to the limit. The claim cannot be divided into two different suits of $1378.50, and one cannot sue twice on the same claim.

Claim Resolutions

The plaintiff has four options after he or she is served:

1. Pay the claim. The court clerk will receive the money and forward it to the physician's office, but the filing fee or service charges will not be refunded.

2. Ignore the claim. The judge may ask the physician's representative to state the physician's side, but the physician will win by default and the judgment will be awarded in the physician's favor, usually including court costs.

3. Answer the petition. A contested court hearing will be held. The plaintiff (physician) has the burden of proving his or her claim to the court. A counterclaim may be filed by the patient at this time.

4. Demand a jury trial. The case will be taken out of small claims court and the physician will be notified by the county clerk to file a formal complaint in a higher court. An attorney must represent the physician if this occurs.

Trial Preparation

The plaintiff and defendant must both appear on the trial date or the claim will be dismissed and cannot be refiled. Instead of attending the trial in person, the doctor may send a representative, such as his or her assistant or bookkeeper. If the claim is settled before trial, a dismissal form should be dated, signed, and filed with the clerk.

Preparation for the trial is essential and can mean the difference between success and failure. Decide what the judge should hear to conclude in the physician's favor. Although one cannot be represented in court by a lawyer, a lawyer can be asked for advice before going to court. Following are recommendations to help prepare for trial:

1. Be on time; otherwise the court may give a judgment in the defendant's favor.

2. Be ready to submit the basic data required by the court: the physician's name, address, and telephone number; the patient's name and address; the delinquent amount being claimed; and a brief summary of the claim.

3. Show all dates of service and amounts owed, the date the physician's bill was due (if a series of treatments is involved), the date of the last visit, the date of the last payment (if any payment was made), and the amount still unpaid.

4. Include all attempts to collect the debt and organize all exhibits in chronological order. Include documentation such as copies of statements, letters, notes, receipts, contracts, dishonored checks, telephone calls, other discussions with the patient, and other evidence to present to the court. A timeline showing the sequence of events may be useful.

5. Speak slowly and clearly, present the case in a concise manner, and use a businesslike approach. Answer all questions accurately but briefly.

6. Present a witness if live testimony is relevant. A notarized statement from a witness is admissible but not as effective.

7. Try to anticipate the opposing party's evidence and arguments so a rebuttal may be prepared. Keep in mind that a third party will be making the decision.

The judge will question the physician or representative and the patient, review the evidence, and then make a ruling. Winning the case gives the physician the right to attach a debtor's bank assets, salary, car, personal assets, or real property. The small claims office can show the assistant how to execute a judgment. Judgments usually are effective for many years. There is a small charge if the physician decides to execute against the patient's assets, but the charge is recoverable from the defendant.

A losing defendant may appeal and request a new trial in superior court. The defendant may ask the judge to make small installment payments, but not all judges will order this alternative. If the defendant fails to pay, a writ of execution may be obtained from the clerk's office to enforce judgment. This writ of execution permits the marshal to obtain funds from a losing party's bank account or take items of the losing party's property to satisfy the judgment.

Federal Wage Garnishment Laws

Federal wage garnishment laws provide a limit on the amount of employee earnings withheld in a work week or pay period when a debtor's future wage is seized to pay off a debt. It also protects the employee from being dismissed if his or her pay is garnished for only one debt regardless of the number of levies that must be made to collect. This law is enforced by the compliance officers of the Wage and Hour Office of the U.S. Department of Labor. The law does not apply to federal government employees, court-ordered support of any person, court orders in personal bankruptcy cases, or state or federal tax levies. The patient's employer becomes involved as the "trustee" because the employer owes money to the debtor for wages earned.

Once a **garnishment** has been ordered by the court, an employer has to honor it by satisfying the terms of garnishment before wages can be paid to the debtor. Only a percentage of the wage (usually 25%) is garnished and paid to the creditor. This amount is determined from the employee's disposable earnings. Disposable earnings is the amount left after Social Security and federal, state, and local taxes are deducted. The statute resulting in the smaller garnishment applies when state garnishment laws conflict with federal laws. This method of collection should be considered a last resort for the medical office and used only with large bills.

Tracing a Skip

A patient who owes a balance on his or her account and moves but leaves no forwarding address is called a **skip.** In these cases an unopened envelope is returned to the office marked "Returned to Sender, Addressee Unknown." Instead, place the words "Forwarding Service Requested" below the doctor's return address on the envelope, and the post office will make a search and forward the mail to the new address. The physician's office will be informed of this new address for a nominal fee. Complete a Freedom of Information Act Form at the post office if the address is a rural delivery box number, and the United States Postal Service will provide the physical location of a person's residence. When patients send payments by mail, precautions must be taken to avoid discarding envelopes with a change of address. Always match the address on the envelope, along with the check, against the patient's account. One staff person should have the responsibility of updating all patients' addresses in all locations to prevent this problem.

Skip Tracing Techniques

Once it is determined that a patient is a skip, tracing should begin immediately. Office policies should be established stating how the skip should be traced, whether he or she is to be traced in the office, or at what point the account should be sent to a collection agency. Some offices choose to make only one attempt, whereas others prefer to do most of the detective work themselves. Box 9–2 lists techniques that can be used to initiate the search for the debtor.

Never state one's business with the patient when trying to make any of these contacts. Keep all information confidential. A good skip tracer must be patient and have the ability to pursue all necessary steps with tenacity and tact. A good imagination, a detective's instincts, and the ability to get along with people help in this tedious job.

Skip Tracing Services

There are several outside services from which to choose. Some agencies offer customized service with several levels of skip tracing available. Each level is more extensive and costly. The physician's office decides at which level it would like the search conducted. The first level usually involves verifying the patient's information and checking for typographical errors. The highest level uses every resource available to find the patient. The age of the account, the account balance, and the cost of the level of skip tracing service are all considerations when deciding which level to choose. A collection agency or credit bureau (as mentioned) also may offer the services of skip tracing.

Search via Computer

Another method of skip tracing is to use electronic databases or online services. "Information wholesalers" also exist that cater to bill collectors and

---

BOX 9–2

Search Techniques Used to Trace a Debtor

1. Cross-check the address on the returned envelope with the patient registration form and account to ensure it was mailed correctly.
2. Check the ZIP code directory to see if the ZIP code corresponds with the patient's street address or post office box.
3. File a request with the local post office to try to get a new or corrected address.
4. Look in the local telephone directory. Call people with names that are spelled the same. Check Information for a new or current listing.
5. Call the primary care physician for updated information when investigating for a physician specialist or any referring practice.
6. Determine if the patient has been seen at the hospital; if so, speak to someone in the accounts department.
7. Inquire at the patient's place of employment. If the patient is no longer employed, ask to speak to the personnel department in an effort to locate the patient. Do not divulge the reason for the call.
8. Contact persons listed on the patient registration form, including personal referrals.
9. Request information from the Department of Motor Vehicles if a driver's license number is available.
10. Obtain information from street directories, city directories, and cross-index directories (available at many public libraries) for a new address or the names and telephone numbers of neighbors, relatives, or landlords.
11. Telephone the local moving company or moving rental service and ask for the patient's new address.
12. Request information from utility companies.
13. Inquire at the patient's bank to see if he or she is still a customer.
14. Obtain the services of a local credit bureau to check reports and receive notification if the patient's Social Security number shows up under a different name or at a new address.
15. Contact the Board of Education when the patient has children or is a student, to find out the patient's school district and the school closest to his or her former residence. Request a forwarding address.
16. Call the police department if it is suspected that the patient may have a criminal record.
17. Check public records such as tax records, voter registration, court records, death and probate records, hunting and fishing licenses, and marriage licenses.

---

similar interested parties. Currently there are a number of bills pending in Congress aimed at restricting the flow of personal data in cyberspace. Perhaps in the future this information will not be so easy to obtain; however, conducting a successful electronic search is relatively easy at present. Following are several methods used to search electronic databases to locate a debtor's address and home telephone number.

- Surname scan. This can be done locally, regionally, or nationally based on data banks that have been compiled from public source documents.
- Address search. This provides property search and any change of address from all suppliers of data to the database, including the U.S. Postal Service. Names of other adults in the household also may be included who may have the debtor's telephone number listed under their name.
- Electronic directory. This allows access to the regional telephone operating company's screen of information.
- Credit holder search. This is used to establish occupation.
- Phone number search. This permits access to the names of other adults within the same household who have a telephone number.
- Neighbor search. This displays the names, addresses, and telephone numbers of the debtor's former neighbors.
- ZIP code search. This provides the names, addresses, and telephone numbers of everyone within that ZIP code who has the same last name as the debtor.
- City search. This locates everyone with the same last and first name within a given city, as well as all people who live in that city.
- State search. This finds all people with the same last name or same last and first name within the state and lists their addresses and telephone numbers.
- National search. This operates the same way as the state search. It is recommended for people with unusual last names.
- Business search. This lists all the names of the businesses in the neighborhood of the patient's last known residence. This search may help find where the patient has relocated or verify the patient's place of employment.

Refer to the end of the chapter for a listing of some of the larger directories used on the Internet and explore several directories to cross-check results because of frequent data change. Information is not secure when using the Internet. The patient's right to privacy must never be violated.

Special Collection Issues

Bankruptcy

Bankruptcy laws are federal laws applicable in all states that ensure equal distribution of the assets of an individual among the individual's creditors. There are two kinds of bankruptcy petitions: voluntary and involuntary. A voluntary petition is one filed by a person asking for relief under the Bankruptcy Reform Act (the Code). An involuntary petition is one filed against a person by his or her creditors requesting that a person obtain relief under the Code.

When a patient files for bankruptcy, he or she becomes a ward of the court and has its protection. The patient is granted an **automatic stay** against creditors, which means that the physician may contact patients only for the name, address, and telephone number of their attorney. The insurance specialist should no longer send statements, make telephone calls, or attempt to collect the account. A creditor can be fined for contempt of court if he or she continues to proceed against the debtor. If a collection agency has the account and has been notified of the bankruptcy, the situation is the same as if the physician has been notified. If the physician is notified first, the collection agency should be called and informed of the fact. Notification of bankruptcy does not have to be in writing; verbal communication is valid (e.g., if a patient telephones the doctor's office to inform him or her of the bankruptcy). Bankruptcy remains part of the debtor's permanent credit record for 10 years.

After a patient informs the physician's office of the bankruptcy, determine what type of bankruptcy the debtor has filed. Refer to Table 9–3 for a listing of the five types of bankruptcy cases.

Bankruptcy Rules

Under the bankruptcy rules an unsecured creditor must file proof of claim in Chapter 7 or Chapter 13 bankruptcies within 90 days after the first date set for the meeting of creditors. When filing a claim, the proper form may be obtained from a stationery store or by writing to the presiding judge of the bankruptcy court. If a creditor fails to file a claim, the creditor will lose his or her right to any proceeds from the bankruptcy. A plan for payment will be approved by the court. The trustee may be contacted from time to time to check the status of the claim and the payments that should be expected. Once a patient has filed for bankruptcy there must be a time lapse of 6 years before he or she can file again. The only exception to this is Chapter 13 bankruptcy.

Terminally Ill Patients

Although it may be difficult to collect from patients who are about to die, it is usually harder to collect from the estate after they are gone. When a patient is too sick or scared to communicate necessary information, speak to family members and stress to the need for help. Approximately 50% of the time terminally ill patients want to do the right thing. Call the patient before he or she comes in to receive service. Make sure the patient is aware of the existing balance and try to work with the patient to eliminate at least a portion of the balance before the next appointment. Estimate costs and prepare a plan that is agreeable to both the physician and the patient.

| TABLE 9–3 | **Types of Bankruptcy Cases** |

Chapter 7 Case	
This is sometimes called a *straight petition in bankruptcy* or *absolute bankruptcy*. In this case, all of the **nonexempt assets** of the bankrupt person are liquidated and are distributed according to the law to the creditors. Secured creditors are first in line for payment of all **secured debt.** Unsecured creditors are last. A person declares those to whom he or she owes money and is not required to make payment, thus eliminating all of the debtor's outstanding legal obligations for **unsecured debt.** Most medical bills are considered unsecured debt because they are not backed by any form of **collateral.** The only debt that is discharged in Chapter 7 bankruptcy is the debt that had been incurred up to the point of filing	for protection under Chapter 7. So, if a patient files before services are rendered, the bankruptcy laws do not apply for the treatment provided. A Chapter 7 bankruptcy does not necessarily result in the discharge of all debts. If the patient lies about his or her financial status, the debt may not be dischargeable. If the debt incurred was for a luxury service (e.g., facelift), immediately preceding the filing, it is possible that it may not be discharged. Consult the practice's attorney before adjusting the debt off the books in such a situation. All creditors are notified by the Administrator in Bankruptcy as to the proceedings and may choose either to attend the proceedings or make a claim against whatever assets remain.

Chapter 9 Case	**Chapter 12 Case**
This case is used for reorganization proceedings when a city or town is insolvent or unable to meet its debts. A plan is put into effect to adjust such debts.	This case is used for reorganization when a farmer is unable to meet his or her debts.

Chapter 11 Case	**Chapter 13 Case**
This case is used for reorganization of a business enterprise when the company is unable to meet its debts but would like to continue business and would be unable to do so if creditors took away its assets. A plan of arrangement is confirmed by the court, and each class of creditor must accept the plan or receive at least that which it would receive on liquidation of the company.	This is sometimes called a *wage earner's bankruptcy*. It is designed to protect the wage earner from creditors while allowing the wage earner to make arrangements to repay a portion of his or her bills (about 70%) over a 3- or 5-year period. The debtor pays a fixed amount agreed upon by the court to the trustee in bankruptcy. A claim needs to be filed as directed by the debtor's attorney.

Estate Claims

Great care and sensitivity should be taken when trying to collect on a deceased patient's account. The entire probate system was set up to help protect families from painful involvement in estate settlements. Do not offend the deceased's family by making contact during the time of bereavement. However, a claim should be filed after the first or second week so the physician's name can be added to the list of creditors.

PROCEDURE: Filing an Estate Claim

Following are steps to take when filing a claim on an estate.

1. Confirm the date and place of death with the hospital, nursing home, or funeral home.

2. Pursue payment from all third-party payers first.
3. Contact the Register of Wills' office in the county where the patient lived or the probate department of the superior court, County Recorder's Office. Request a Statement of Claim form or the county's proper document to formally register a claim against an estate.
4. File the claim according to the instructions received with the claim form. When probate is filed, a notification will be sent advising the court of probate, the attorney representing the estate, and the **estate executor** or **estate administrator.** Perhaps a small fee should be included for court costs.
5. Send an itemized statement by certified mail, return receipt, to the attorney and copies to the executor and the court. If the physician treated the deceased patient's last illness, that fact should be clearly indicated on the statement.
6. Allow the legal system to take its course. A call to the executor can be made periodically to check on the status of the estate.

The claim is then denied or accepted. If accepted, an acknowledgment of the debt is sent to the physician's office. Many delays arise because of the legal complications of settling an estate, but the debts are paid according to a priority system when the estate is settled. Usually funeral expenses are paid first; following in order are estate administration expenses, claims due for the deceased person's last illness, and taxes and other debts. Any amounts left are divided among family members. A lien or lawsuit may be filed against the estate in the rare case of a rejection of the claim.

Various state time limits and statutes govern the filing of a claim against an estate. Check with the county court in your state to obtain filing deadlines. Deadlines may range from 2 months to 3 years but must be adhered to for successful collection from an estate.

Litigation

A difficult question arises when the physician is advised that a patient is involved in a pending litigation related to the services provided to the patient. It may not be necessary to wait until the litigation is resolved to pursue payment. Assess whether the patient has the ability to pay before possibly receiving a settlement in a lawsuit. Before withholding collection activity, the medical practice should get a guarantee that the physician will be paid in full before the patient (debtor) receives money out of a settlement. The agreement must be guaranteed by the lawyer representing the patient. If the patient is working, regular payments should be required pending the settlement of the patient's litigation. It is always advisable to contact a malpractice attorney in such cases.

Liens

A **lien** is a claim on the property of another as security for a debt. This may include a claim on a future settlement of a lawsuit. The physician may be asked to accept a lien by a patient or the patient's attorney when the patient has been involved in an automobile accident and is awaiting a settlement (Fig. 9–19). In litigation cases, a lien is a legal promise to satisfy a debt owed by the patient to the physician out of any proceeds received on the case. See Chapter 14 for further details about industrial cases.

Patient Complaints

It is generally in the physician's best interest to resolve patient complaints and billing disputes quickly, accurately, and amicably. Always address collection complaints seriously. Listen to the patient with an open mind. Note specifically what the patient is saying and what the patient wants to do. Look beyond the complaint to determine what caused the problem. The source of the problem should be resolved, not just the result of the problem. A patient complaint form may be adapted to prompt staff to pay close attention to positive customer relations. This form may help screen poor collection techniques by staff members, pinpoint billing department problems, and identify policies and procedures that need improvement.

The patient may refuse to pay the physician if the patient's complaint is not addressed. Following are some guidelines to follow when a patient calls or writes a letter complaining about the physician or the medical practice:

1. Listen carefully (or read the letter carefully) and establish exactly what the patient complaint is and what the patient wants done about it.
2. Thank the person for calling (or writing); demonstrate appreciation of his or her input into the situation.
3. Apologize, regardless of whether the patient is right or wrong.
4. Answer the complaint. Explain what happened, if applicable, and state what is being done about it.
5. Use a professional and sincere approach. If the patient is wrong, state that the complaint is unjustified. Do not be sarcastic, condescending, or insulting.
6. Take all complaints seriously. Do not respond in a lighthearted manner or use humor; it will only serve to upset the patient.
7. Respond in letter form. Whether the complaint has been received by telephone or by letter, take the time to write to answer the complaint. This indicates that the matter is not being taken lightly.
8. Be cordial and sincere. Express to the patient the hope of continuing a friendly relationship, but that payment is needed. Treat the patient with respect, good will, and sincere appreciation. Often kindness can turn a negative into a positive. The complaint can be turned into a payment.
9. Follow up after the complaint has been resolved by looking at the root of the problem and taking the necessary time to communicate this to the office manager. This will allow for a plan of action that will help prevent the same type of problem from recurring.

Collection Controls

All collections should be carefully controlled to prevent lost checks and embezzlement. See Chapter 1 for a complete description of the different types of bonding insurance and precautions to take when processing monies and insurance claims in the physician's office.

REQUEST FOR ALLOWANCE OF LIEN
ASSIGNMENT AND AUTHORIZATION

WHEREAS, I have a right or cause of action out of personal injury, to wit:

I, _____hereby authorize_____ ,
       patient's name   physians name

to furnish upon request, to my attorney,_____ , any and all medical records, or reports of examination, diagnosis, treatment, or prognosis but not necessarily limited to those items as set forth herein, in addition to an itemized statement of accounts for services rendered therefore or in connection therewith, which my attorney may from time to time request in connection with the injuries described above and sustained by me on the_____day of_____, 20XX.

I hereby irrevocably authorize and direct my said attorney set forth herein to pay to _____all charges for attendance in court,
          patient's name
if required as an expert witness whether he testifies or not; reports or other data supplied by him; depositions given by said doctor; medical services rendered or durgs supplied; and any other responsible and customary charges incurred by my attorney as submitted by_____and in
                                    physicians name

connection with said injury. Said payment or payments are to be made from any money or monies received by my attorney whether by judgment, decree, or settlement of this case, prior to disbursement to me and payment of the amount as herein directed shall be the same as if paid by me. This authorization to pay the aforementioned doctor shall constitute and be deemed as assignment of so much of my recovery I receive. It is agreed that nothing herein relieves me of the primary responsibility and obligation of paying my doctor for services rendered, and I shall at all times remain personally liable for such indebtedness unless released by the aforementioned doctor or by payment disbursed by my attorney. I accept the above assignment:

Dated:_____ Patient:_____

As the attorney of record for the above-named, I hereby agree to observe the terms of this agreement, and to withhold from any award in this case such sums as are required for the adequate protection of Dr._____

Date:_____ Attorney:_____

Figure 9–19. A patient's authorization to release information to an attorney and grant lien to the physician against proceeds of settlement in connection with accident, industrial, or third-party litigation cases.

RESOURCES ON THE INTERNET

Web sites to help you search for a debtor
Anywho
     www.anywho.com
Bigfoot
www.bigfoot.com/
Database America
     www.databaseamerica.com
InfoSpace
     www.infospace.com
Info USA
     www.infousa.com
People Finder
     www.lookupusa.com/

Search-It-All
     www.searchitall.net/peoplefinder.asp
Switchboard
     www.switchboard.com
WhoWhere?
     www.whowhere.com/
Yahoo People Search
     www.yahoo.com/search/people/
411Locate
     www.411locate.com
Web site for small claims court
     www.halt.org

STUDENT ASSIGNMENT LIST

✔ Study Chapter 9.
✔ Answer the review questions in the *Workbook* to reinforce the theory learned in this chapter and to help prepare you for a future test.
✔ Complete the assignment in the *Workbook* to give you hands-on experience in selecting a dun message, posting a courtesy adjustment and insurance or patient payment, composing a collection letter, and completing a credit card voucher and a financial agreement.
✔ Turn to the Glossary at the end of this textbook for a further understanding of the Key Terms used in the chapter.

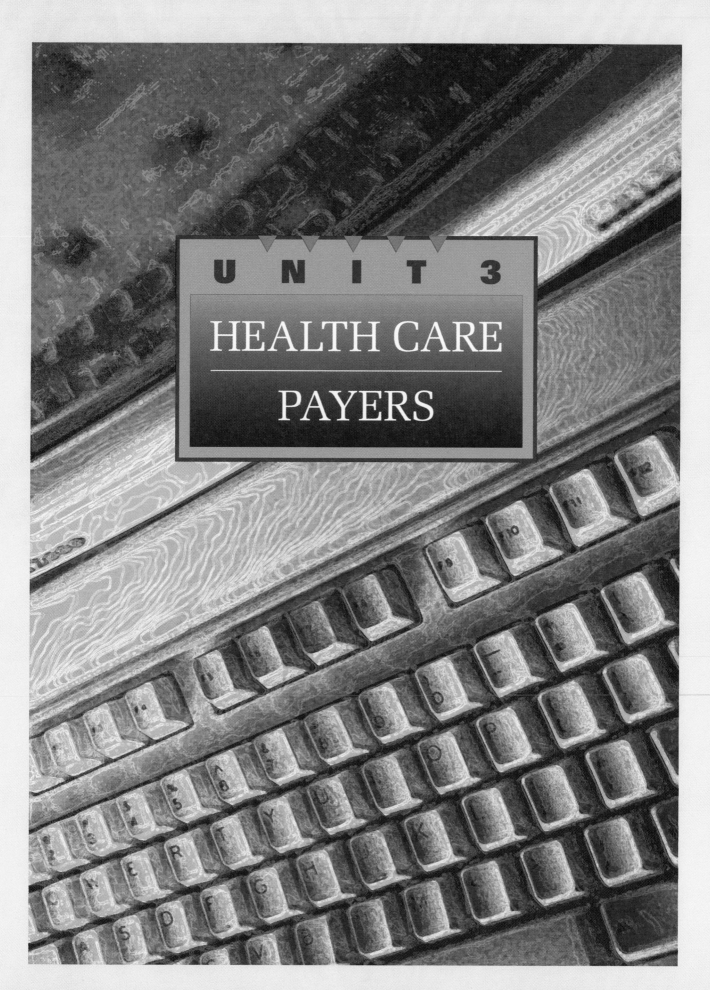

UNIT 3

HEALTH CARE
PAYERS

Private Insurance and Managed Care Systems

CHAPTER OUTLINE

■ Explain health
maintenance organization
benefits and eligibility
requirements.
■ State reasons for
professional review
organizations.
■ Define independent
practice associations.
■ Name the elements of
preferred provider
organizations.
■ Identify four types of
authorizations for medical
services, tests, and
procedures.

OBJECTIVES*

After reading this chapter, you
should be able to:

■ Define a prepaid health
plan (PHP).
■ Identify types of managed
care health plans.
■ List two types and two
different functions of
foundations.
■ State the provisions of the
Health Maintenance
Organization Act of 1973.

*Performance objectives and exercises for hands-on practical experience for this chapter
appear in the *Workbook*.

KEY TERMS—cont'd

service area

staff model

stop loss

tertiary care

turfing

utilization review (UR)

verbal referral

withhold

Private Insurance

Numerous private insurance companies across the United States offer health insurance to individuals and groups. Most offer a variety of managed care plans. This chapter describes the difference between private insurance and managed care. Fee-for-service reimbursement was discussed in previous chapters. This chapter explains managed care capitation as a form of reimbursement.

Blue Cross/Blue Shield (BCBS) plans are pioneers in private insurance and had a nonprofit status that made them unique among all private insurance carriers for many years. Blue Cross/Blue Shield is the largest insurance company in the United States. Carriers are independent owned and operated in each state but work together in a network similar to a spider Web. Originally Blue Cross plans were developed to cover hospital expenses and Blue Shield plans were primarily established to cover physician services. Today different plans have been developed that allow members to seek treatment from Blue Cross/Blue Shield providers anywhere in the United States. There are so many different plans that it is difficult for the medical biller to know which type the member is enrolled in. The patient may have a traditional plan or a managed care plan (e.g., preferred provider organization [PPO], point-of-service [POS plan], independent [or individual] practice association [IPA], health maintenance organization [HMO], or Medicare HMO). Plans are different and may have diverse names in each state. This chapter describes these managed care systems.

Nationally the Blue Cross/Blue Shield Association is a single corporation covering hospital expenses, outpatient care, other institutional services, home care, dental benefits, and vision care. Most of the affiliated organizations have converted to for-profit status and operate in much the same way as other private insurance carriers. In some areas they are separate organizations, and in some situations they may compete against each other. Now that they are similar to other private insurance companies, they do not have nationally recognized rules and regulations or standardized claim form guidelines. In addition, Blue Cross/Blue Shield may act as a Medicare fiscal intermediary in certain regions. An experienced medical biller should be aware of the many problems these circumstances cause. For example, the policy number may require the claim to be sent to the home plan, or the policy number may require the claim to be sent through the provider's state carrier. Blue Cross/Blue Shield realizes this is a problem, so the organization is developing a product called Blue Plan that incorporates all products. The intent is to help the patient avoid making payments.

There are other unique situations with Blue Cross/Blue Shield in regard to contracts. Blue Cross/Blue Shield would like to have contracts with both medical groups and the providers that work for the group. This poses unique problems when the group and provider are contracted, when the group is contracted and the provider is not, and when there is no contract with either the provider or group. Each situation has a different effect on claims processing and payment.

Because Blue Cross/Blue Shield contracts like other types of private and managed care plans, in this textbook the organization is not listed separately in the description of types of fee structures, network physicians, managed care plans, and guidelines for completing the CMS-1500 insurance claim form.

Managed Care

Until the early 1970s most health insurance was delivered through traditional fee-for-service plans. This scenario has changed from high-cost, old-fashioned indemnity plans to less-expensive managed health care plans, such as HMOs. In this chapter the health care reforms of the past and present are defined and explained. In addition to HMOs, other types of prepaid group practice models that use a managed care approach and are operated by **managed care organizations (MCOs)** are discussed.

In prepaid group plans, patients join the plan and pay monthly medical insurance premiums individually or through their employer. The physician renders service to the patient, and the patient usually pays a small copayment and occasionally a deductible as required by the plan. Providers that join the plan are paid using the capitation method. **Capitation** is a system of payment used by managed care plans in which physicians and hospitals are paid a fixed per capita amount for each patient enrolled over a stated period of time, regardless of the type and number of services provided.

Prepaid Group Practice Health Plans

The *Ross-Loos Medical Group* in Los Angeles was America's oldest privately owned prepaid medical group. It was founded in 1929 by Drs. Donald E. Ross and H. Clifford Loos and existed only in southern California, where it expanded to 17 medical group locations. In 1975 the Ross-Loos Medical Group formed a corporation and received a federal grant to develop a health care system under the federal Health Maintenance Organization Act of 1973. In 1980 INA Healthplan, Inc., of Philadelphia merged with Ross-Loos. Ross-Loos is now known as CIGNA *Healthplans of California.*

Most CIGNA patients are served under a prepayment group plan by which they pay a monthly premium and receive hospital, surgical, and professional benefits from a CIGNA staff physician or CIGNA Health Care Center. Several thousand other CIGNA patients are private and are treated on a fee-for-service basis. In the case of an emergency when the patient is outside the area of a CIGNA Health Care Center, he or she may seek professional or hospital care in other facilities, but CIGNA must be notified as soon as possible. A dental plan and Medicare supplemental plan also are available through CIGNA.

Another pioneer of the prepaid group practice concept is the *Kaiser Permanente Medical Care Program.* It began in 1933 when Dr. Sidney R. Garfield and a few physicians working for him gave combined industrial accident and personal medical care to approximately 5000 workers building a freshwater aqueduct across the California desert to Los Angeles. Dr. Garfield charged the insurance carriers $1.50 per man per month and the workers 5 cents a day. In return he provided comprehensive health care. Then in 1938 Henry J. Kaiser and his son Edgar started a joint venture to complete the Grand Coulee Dam in Washington and invited Dr. Garfield to form a medical group to furnish care to the workers for 7 cents a day prepaid by the employer. The group expanded to include the workers' wives and children.

Kaiser Permanente now has centers in 12 regions covering 16 states. Patients are served under a prepayment group plan and receive hospital, surgical, and professional benefits from physicians located at the Kaiser Permanente Medical Care Centers. In most regions the Kaiser Permanente Medical Plan is a **closed panel program** composed of multispecialty physicians, and the plan limits the patient's choice of personal physicians to those practicing in one of the 12 geographic regions.

In January 1994 Kaiser Permanente announced a venture with Pacific Mutual Life Insurance Company to give Kaiser's 4.6 million California patients a less cost-effective option of using physicians and medical facilities outside the vast Kaiser network. This was the first time that Kaiser allowed certain member groups of its two California health maintenance organizations to seek medical help from non–Kaiser physicians and is termed a POS option (see discussion later in this chapter). In this option Kaiser pays up to a specified amount and the patient pays the rest, depending on the contract. Kaiser does not provide care on a fee-for-service or cost reimbursement basis.

In emergency situations when patients cannot reach a Kaiser Center, they may seek the services of outside facilities or physicians. They are transferred to a Kaiser facility when their condition stabilizes.

Health Maintenance Organization Act of 1973

An HMO is a prepaid group practice that can be sponsored and operated by the government, medical schools, clinics, foundations, hospitals, employers, labor unions, community or consumer groups, insurance companies, hospital medical plans, or the Veterans Administration.

In 1973 Congress passed the Health Maintenance Organization Act of 1973 (Public Law 93-222), creating authority for the federal government to assist HMO development in a number of ways, including: (1) providing grants, loans, and loan guarantees to offset the initial operating deficits of new HMOs that meet federal standards (e.g., are federally qualified); and (2) requiring most employers to offer an HMO to their employees as an alternative to traditional health insurance.

Eligibility

Those who have voluntarily enrolled in an HMO plan from a specific geographic area (**in-area** or **service area**) or who are covered by an employer who has paid an established sum per person to be covered by the plan are eligible. The law states that an employer employing 25 or more persons may offer the services of an HMO as an alternative health treatment plan for employees. Medicare and Medicaid beneficiaries also may become members of managed care plans whether retired or employed. The federal government reimburses the HMOs on a **per capita** basis, depending on the size of the enrollment. This means that the HMO is paid a fixed per capita amount (also known as capitation) for each patient served without considering the actual number or nature of services provided to each person.

To qualify as an HMO an organization must present proof of its ability to provide comprehensive health care. To retain eligibility an HMO must render periodic performance reports to the offices of the Department of Health and Human Services. Thus accurate and complete medical records are imperative to the survival and cost control of an HMO.

Primary Care Physician

Most managed care plans use a **primary care physician (PCP)** as a gatekeeper. A **gatekeeper** is a physician who controls patient access to specialists and diagnostic testing services. PCPs usually are physicians who practice in the fields of internal medicine, family practice, general practice, or pediatrics. Although obstetrics/gynecology is considered specialty care, the obstetrician/gynecologist may be contracted as a PCP, and when not it is common for MCOs to allow self-referral by members to obstetricians/gynecologists for certain services (e.g., Pap smears).

Identification Card

Each enrollee of a managed care plan is given an identification card as shown in Chapter 2, Figure 2–10. The card usually lists the patient's name, member number, group number, and primary care physician's name. The name of the MCO and type of plan with the amount of copayment for various outpatient services (e.g., office visit, emergency department, urgent care center, and pharmacy) also are included.

Both sides of the patient's card should be photocopied because the insurance address, telephone numbers used for inquiries and authorizations or other important information may be listed on the front or back of the card.

Benefits

Benefits under the HMO Act fall under two categories: basic and supplemental health service, which are listed in Box 10–1.

Health Care Reform

Over the past 60 years leaders of the United States from Presidents Roosevelt to Clinton have announced reforms of the health care system. Medical practices have made transitions from rural to urban, generalist to specialist, solo to group practice, and fee-for-service to capitation, and have expanded to a number of health care delivery systems that try to manage the cost of health care. Before capitation, **fee-for-service** was the usual method of billing by physicians in private practice. A professional service was rendered by the physician to the patient, and the physician expected to receive a fee for the service provided.

A major restructuring of the United States health care system was needed during the 1990s for the following reasons:

▶ A growing percentage of Americans were not covered by private or government insurance.

BOX 10–1

Health Maintenance Organization Act Benefits of 1973

Basic Health Services

Alcohol, drug abuse, and addiction medical treatment
Dental services (preventive) for children younger than age 12 years
Diagnostic laboratory, x-ray, and therapeutic radiology services
Emergency health services in or out of the HMO service area
Family planning and infertility services
Health education and medical social services
Home health services
Hospital services (inpatient and outpatient)
Mental health services on an outpatient basis, short-term (not to exceed 20 visits) ambulatory, evaluative, and crisis intervention
Physicians' services and consultant or referral services without time or cost limits
Preventive health services (e.g., physical examinations for adults, vision and hearing tests for children through age 17 years, well-baby care, immunizations, and health education)

Supplemental Health Services

Dental care not included in basic benefits
Extended mental health services not included in basic benefits
Eye examinations for adults
Intermediate and long-term care (nursing facilities and nursing homes)
Prescription drugs
Rehabilitative services and long-term physical medicine (e.g., physical therapy)

▶ Employers had to pay escalating health care premiums and did not want to cut wages to cover these costs.

▶ Government needed to reduce the deficit by keeping down increases in the Medicare and Medicaid programs.

▶ Physicians and hospital costs soared with no end in sight because of inflation, high-tech equipment, expensive medications, and so on.

▶ Patients spent more and more money for less and less care and coped with a system riddled with inefficiency and fraud.

Integrated health care delivery systems have been formed in many states in the past decade to reduce costs. These have included MCOs, physician–hospital organizations, and group practices accepting a variety of MCOs and fee-for-service patients. These systems allow for better negotiations for contracts with large employers and managed care plans, as well as with medical and office suppliers for discounts. Each type of organization differs in ownership, purpose, governance, management, and type of services provided. Even before the government released its health care reform proposal, some states began establishing laws implementing managed care for the general populations, as well as for Medicaid patients and those injured on the job (workers' compensation cases). Hawaii has had a statewide universal health insurance plan since 1974. Many regions have large groups of Medicare-eligible people who have opted to belong to an HMO or other prepaid plans.

In 1994 California put together the first working alliance in the nation, followed by Florida's voluntary purchasing group, the Community Health Purchasing Alliances. In California the alliance is formally known as the Health Insurance Plan of California. This allows firms with 5 to 50 workers to offer their employees a wide choice of different insurance programs. All plans must offer the same benefits, but some physicians and hospitals are more desirable than others. The company must pay an amount equal to at least half of the cost of the lowest-priced plan; the worker pays the remainder.

In the future those on Medicaid, younger than age 65 years, and not receiving either Aid to Families with Dependent Children (AFDC) or Supplemental Security Income (SSI) may no longer be part of Medicaid. They might obtain their health benefits like everyone else. AFDC and SSI recipients would be covered under a Medicaid plan, but Medicaid would pay a capitated premium (payment per capita) to the alliance. The recipient would pick a low-cost plan from the state alliance. Some states have pilot projects in certain communities to determine whether this is feasible for the entire state.

Managed Care Systems

Health Maintenance Organizations

The oldest of all the prepaid health plans is the **HMO.** An HMO is a plan or program by which specified health services are rendered by participating physicians to an enrolled group of persons. Fixed periodic payments are made in advance to providers of services **(participating physicians)** by or on behalf of each person or family. If a health insurance carrier administers and manages the HMO, it contracts to pay in advance for the full range of health services to which the insured is entitled under the terms of the health insurance contract.

HMO Models

There are important differences in the structure of various HMOs that influence the way physicians practice and, perhaps, the quality of medical care delivered. Following are several types of HMO models.

Prepaid Group Practice Model

The **prepaid group practice model** delivers services at one or more locations through a group of physicians who contract with the HMO to provide care or through its own physicians who are employees of the HMO. For example, Kaiser Permanente is a prepaid group practice model where physicians form an independent group (Permanente) and contract with a health plan (Kaiser) to provide medical treatment to members enrolled by the plan. Although the physicians work for a salary, it is paid by their own independent group, not by the administrators of the health plan. This is designed to permit the physicians to concentrate on medicine.

Staff Model

The **staff model** is a type of HMO in which the health plan hires physicians directly and pays them a salary instead of contracting with a medical group.

Network HMO

A *network HMO* contracts with two or more group practices to provide health services.

Write to the Office of Health Maintenance Organizations for further information on HMOs.*

---

*Centers for Medicaid and Medicare Services, Room 4350, Cohen Building, 330 Independence Ave, SW, Washington, DC 20201.

Exclusive Provider Organizations

An **exclusive provider organization (EPO)** is a type of managed care plan that combines features of HMOs (e.g., enrolled population, limited provider panel, gatekeepers, utilization management, capitated provider reimbursement, authorization system) and PPOs (e.g., flexible benefit design, negotiated fees, and fee-for-service payments). It is referred to as exclusive because employers agree not to contract with any other plan. The member must choose medical care from network providers with certain exceptions for emergency or out-of-area services. If a patient decides to seek care outside the network, generally he or she is not reimbursed for the cost of the treatment. Technically many HMOs can be considered EPOs. However, EPOs are regulated under insurance statutes rather than federal and state HMO regulations.

Foundations for Medical Care

A **foundation for medical care (FMC)** is an organization of physicians sponsored by a state or local medical association concerned with the development and delivery of medical services and the cost of health care. The first Foundation for Medical Care was established in 1954 in Stockton, California. Foundations have sprung up across the United States, and some comprehensive foundations have assumed a portion of the underwriting risk for a defined population. Foundations deal primarily with various groups—employer groups, government groups, and county and city employees. Some plans are open to individual subscribers, but these instances usually represent a small percentage of the foundation activity.

There are basically two types of foundations for medical care operations and each functions differently: (1) a **comprehensive type of foundation,** which designs and sponsors prepaid health programs or sets minimum benefits of coverage; and (2) a **claims-review type of foundation,** which provides evaluation of the quality and efficiency of services by a panel of physicians to the numerous fiscal agents or carriers involved in its area, including the ones processing Medicare and Medicaid. Reviews are done for services or fees that exceed local community guidelines.

A key feature of the foundation is its dedication to an incentive reimbursement system. For a participating physician, income is received in direct proportion to the number of medical services delivered (e.g., fee-for-service) rather than payment through capitation. The FMC offers a managed care plan fee schedule to be used by member physicians. In some areas foundation physicians agree to accept the foundation allowance as payment in full for covered services. The patient is *not* billed for the balance. However, the patient is billed for nonbenefit items, a deductible, and coinsurance.

The patient may select any member or nonmember physician he or she wishes. Member physicians agree to bill the foundation directly, and a nonmember physician may wish to collect directly from the patient. Many foundations submit claims on the CMS-1500 form, and others transmit data electronically. The foundation movement has a national society, the American Managed Care and Review Association (AMCRA),* which can provide further information on AMCRA or foundations in an individual state.

Independent Practice Associations

Another type of MCO is the **IPA,** in which the physicians are not employees and are not paid salaries. Instead they are paid for their services on a capitation or fee-for-service basis out of a fund drawn from the premiums collected from the subscriber, union, or corporation by an organization that markets the health plan. A discount of up to 30% is withheld to cover costs of operating the IPA. IPA physicians make contractual arrangements to treat HMO members out of their own offices. A participating physician may also treat non–HMO patients.

Preferred Provider Organizations

A **PPO** is another type of managed care plan. A PPO contracts with a group of providers (designated as "preferred") to deliver care to members. PPO members have the freedom to choose any physician or hospital for services, but they receive a high level of benefits if the preferred providers are used. There are usually coinsurance requirements and deductibles, and claims have to be filed. Occasionally the PPOs pay 100% of the cost but most do not. As with major medical policies, coinsurance requires the patient to pay 20% to 25% of the allowed amount up to a certain point and then the PPO pays 100% of the balance. Predetermination of benefits may be required, as well as fee limits, quality control, and utilization review. Some hospital indemnity plans pay fixed fees for various services. The patient pays the difference if the charges are higher.

Physician Provider Groups

A **physician provider group (PPG)** is a physician-owned business entity that has the flexibility to deal with all forms of contract medicine and still offer its

---

*1227 25th St, NW, #610, Washington, DC 20037 (formerly known as the American Association of Foundations for Medical Care).

own packages to business groups, unions, and the general public. One division may function as an IPA under contract to an HMO. Another section may act as the broker or provider in a PPO that contracts with hospitals, as well as other physicians, to market services or medical supplies to employers and other third parties. Still another portion might participate in joint ventures with hospitals, freestanding imaging centers and laboratories, purchase of diagnostic equipment, retail medical equipment as a corporate subsidiary, and so on. The sideline businesses do not pay dividends but provide income to make future assessments to participating physicians unnecessary. The difference between an IPA and a PPG is that an IPA may not be owned by its member physicians, whereas a PPG is physician owned.

The ability of the PPGs to combine services (joint purchasing, marketing, billing, collections, attorneys, and accountant fees) is an advantage because it cuts down on the cost of running a business and allows each physician to retain his or her own practice in addition to these joint ventures. The physicians turn over a small percentage of their income to the PPG for expenses. Patients call one telephone number to make appointments, and the billing is done in one location.

Point-of-Service Plans

The typical **POS plan** combines elements of an HMO and a PPO while offering some unique features. It is basically an HMO consisting of a network of physicians and hospitals that provides an insurance company or an employer with discounts on its services. In a POS program members choose a primary care physician who manages specialty care and referrals. A POS plan allows the covered individual to choose service from a participating or nonparticipating provider, with different benefit levels. The POS program pays members a higher level of benefits when they use program (network) providers. The member may use providers outside the network, but higher deductibles and coinsurance percentages for out-of-network services give members incentives to stay within the network.

The POS plan may also provide nonparticipating benefits through a supplemental major medical policy. The key advantage of POS programs is the combination of HMO–style cost management and PPO–style freedom of choice.

Triple-Option Health Plan

This type of plan allows members to select from three choices: HMOs, PPOs, or indemnity insurance. Some of these plans allow the employee to change plans more often than traditional arrangements. They incorporate cost containment measures, such as precertification for hospital admission, hospital stays, and second surgical opinions.

Table 10–1 gives an overview or summary of five of the most common types of managed care plans.

Medical Review

Professional Review Organizations

A *professional review organization (PRO)* determines and assures the quality and operation of health care through a process called *peer review. Peer review* is an evaluation of the quality and efficiency of services rendered by a practicing physician or physicians within the specialty group. Practitioners in a managed care program may come under peer review by a

TABLE 10–1	**Managed Care Plans**				
Plan	**Network**		**Copay**	**Payment**	**Authorization**
	In	**Out**	**Deductible**	**Method**	**Required**
HMO	X		Fixed copay	Capitated Fee-for-service (carve outs)	X
PPO	75/25% 80/20% 90/10%	60/40% 70/30%	Fixed copay Deductible	Fee-for-service	X
IPA	Limit Large group		Fixed copay	Capitated Fee-for-service (carve outs)	X
EPO	X		Fixed copay	Fee-for-service Capitated	X
POS	X	X	Fixed copay Deductible	Fee-for-service Capitated	X

PRO. In this type of review one or more physician(s) working with the federal government under federal guidelines evaluate(s) another physician in regard to the quality and efficiency of professional care. The review may be used to examine evidence for admission and discharge of a hospital patient and to settle disputes on fees (see Chapter 8, Fig. 8–4). PROs are not restricted to MCO programs but also play a role in Medicare inpatient cases.

Utilization Review or Management

A management system called **utilization review (UR)** is necessary to control costs in a managed care setting. UR is a formal assessment of the cost and use of components of the health care system. The utilization review committee reviews individual cases to determine medical necessity for medical tests and procedures. It also watches over how providers use medical care resources. If medical care, tests, or procedures are denied, the patient must be informed of the need for the denied service and the risks of not having it. The written reasons for denial let the patient know his or her rights to receive the service and obligation to pay before obtaining such services.

Emphasis is placed on seeing a high volume of patients in a performance-based reimbursement system. **Churning** is when a physician sees a patient more than medically necessary and is done to increase revenue through an increased number of services. Churning may be seen in fee-for-service as well as some managed care environments. **Turfing** is to transfer the sickest, high-cost patients to other physicians so the provider appears to be a low utilizer. **Buffing** is to make this practice look justifiable to the plan. All of these situations may affect utilization review.

Management of Plans

Contracts

Obtain nationwide data from Medirisk, Inc.* to make a knowledgeable financial decision on how a managed care plan will impact an existing medical practice. Data supplied by this company can be used to evaluate existing fees, negotiate with managed care firms, and weigh practice expansions (e.g., add partners or a satellite office). A physician should have the contract reviewed by an attorney before signing a contract with a managed care plan. Additional information on managed care contracts is found in Chapter 10 under Management of Plans.

*5901 Peachtree Dunwoody Rd, NE, Suite 455, Building B, Atlanta, GA 30328.

Carve Outs

When an MCO contracts with a physician group, several important considerations are as follows:

1. How many patients will the MCO provide?
2. What is the per capita rate (capitation amount per patient)?
3. What services are included in the capitated amount?

Medical services not included in the contract benefits are called **carve outs** (not included within the capitation rate) and may be contracted for separately. For example, if an internist contracts with an MCO, all Evaluation and Management services, as well as ECGs, spirometries, hematocrits, fasting blood sugar tests, and urinalyses, might be included in the capitation amount that is received per person, per month, regardless of whether any of these services were rendered. However, sigmoidoscopies and hospital visits might be "carved out" of the contract and paid on a fee-for-service basis. Generally physicians prefer carve outs for expensive procedures when contracting with MCOs.

Preauthorization or Prior Approval

Some managed care plans require preauthorization for certain services or referral of a patient to see a specialist. The following are several types of referrals that a plan may use.

1. **Formal referral.** An authorization request is required by the MCO contract to determine medical necessity. This may be obtained via telephone or a completed authorization form mailed or transmitted via fax (Fig. 10–1).
2. **Direct referral.** An authorization request form is completed and signed by the physician and handed to the patient. Certain services may not require completion of a form and may be directly referred (e.g., obstetrical care, dermatology).
3. **Verbal referral.** Primary care physician informs the patient and telephones the referring physician that the patient is being referred for an appointment.
4. **Self-referral.** The patient refers himself or herself to a specialist. The patient may be required to inform the primary care physician.

Patients may be unaware of preapproval requirements. A good precaution is to ask the patient about insurance coverage at the time the appointment is made. If the patient is a member of a managed care plan, carefully review the patient's preauthorization requirements. If approval is necessary for certain situations, inform the patient of this before he or she sees the physician. If a patient has obtained the

Mary Jo Smith
College Clinic
4567 Broad Avenue, WH
Telephone No.: (555) 486-9002
Fax No.:(555) 487-8976

MANAGED CARE PLAN AUTHORIZATION REQUEST

☐ Health Net   ☐ Met Life
☐ Pacificare   ☐ Travelers
☐ Secure Horizons ☐ Pru Care
☐ Other

Member/Group No.: _54098XX_

**TO BE COMPLETED BY PRIMARY CARE PHYSICIAN
OR OUTSIDE PROVIDER**

Patient Name: ____Louann Campbell____ Date: _7-14-20XX_

☐ Male   ☐ Female   Birthdate: ___4-7-1952___ Home Telephone Number: __(555) 450-1666__

Address: _____2516 Encina Avenue, Woodland Hills, XY 12345-0439_____

Primary Care Physician:____Gerald Practon, MD____ Provider ID #:____TC 14021____

Referring Physician: ____Gerald Practon, MD____ Provider ID #:____TC 14021____

Referred to: ____Raymond Skeleton, MD____ Office Telephone number: __(555) 486-9002__

Address: __4567 Broad Avenue, Woodland Hills, XY 12345__

Diagnosis Code: _724.2_ Diagnosis __Low back pain__

Diagnosis Code: _722.10_ Diagnosis __Sciatica__

Treatment Plan: _____Orthopedic consultation and evaluation of lumbar spine; R/O herniated disc L4-5_____

Authorization requested for: ☐ Consult only   ☐ Treatment only   ☐ Consult/Treatment

☐ Consult/Procedure/Surgery   ☐ Diagnostic Tests

Procedure Code: _99244_ Description: __New patient consultation__

Procedure Code:_____ Description:_____

Place of service: ☒ Office ☐ Outpatient ☐ Inpatient ☐ Other   Number of Visits: _1_

Facility: _____ Length of Stay:_____

List of potential future consultants (i.e., anesthetists, surgical assistants or medical/surgical):

Physician's Signature: _____Gerald Practon, MD_____

TO BE COMPLETED BY PRIMARY CARE PHYSICIAN

PCP Recommendations: _See above_ PCP Initials: _GP_

Date eligibility checked: _7-14-20XX_ Effective Date: __1-15-20XX__

TO BE COMPLETED BY UTILIZATION MANAGEMENT

Authorized:_____ Auth. No._____ Not Authorized_____

Deferred: _____ Modified:_____

Comments:_____

Figure 10–1. A managed care plan treatment authorization request form completed by a primary care physician for preauthorization of a professional service.

written authorization approval, remind him or her to bring the form at the time of the scheduled visit. Even if preapproved *the treatment must be medically necessary* or payment may be denied after submission of a claim. If an authorization is delayed and the patient comes in for the appointment, the plan provided should be called to obtain a verbal authorization. The date, time, and name of the authorizing person should be documented; otherwise the patient's appointment may have to be rescheduled. A referral recommendation must be documented in the patient's record and, if applicable, sent to the referring physician.

A tracking system such as a referral tracking log should be in place for pending referrals so care may be rendered in a timely manner and patients do not

AUTHORIZATION REQUEST LOG								
Date requested	Patient name	Procedure/ consult	Insurance plan	1st F/U	2nd F/U	3rd F/U	Approved	Scheduled date
2/8/XX	Juan Percy	Bone scan- full body	Health Net	2/20			J. Smith	2/23/XX
2/8/XX	Nathan Takai	MRI-L-knee	Pru-Care	2/20	3/3			
2/9/XX	Lori Smythe	Consult Neuro G. Frankel MD	FHP	2/22			T. Hope	2/26/XX
2/10/XX	Bob Mason	Cervical collar	Secure Horizons	2/22	3/5	3/19		

Figure 10–2. An authorization request log to be used as a system for tracing referral of patients for diagnostic testing, procedures, and consultations.

get lost in the system (Fig. 10–2). This log should include the date the authorization is requested, patient's name, procedure or consultant requested, insurance plan, dates of follow-up, name of person who approved or denied the request, and appointment date for consult or procedure. Sometimes authorization approvals are sent to the primary care physician and not to the referring or ordering physician. In these cases, follow-up must be made with the primary care physician. A maximum 2-week turnaround time should be allowed and all authorization requests tracked.

If a managed care plan refuses to authorize payment for a recommended treatment, tests, or procedures, have the primary care physician send a letter to the plan that is worded similarly to that shown in Figure 10–3. Then send a letter such as that shown in Figure 10–4 to the patient informing him or her of this fact and asking the patient to appeal the denial of benefits.

In some managed care plans, when a primary care physician sends a patient to a specialist for consultation who is *not* in the managed care plan, the specialist bills the primary care physician. This is done because the primary care physician receives a monthly capitation check from the plan and any care for the patient must come from the capitation pool. This type of plan encourages primary care physicians not to refer patients so he or she can retain profits.

If a specialist recommends referral to another specialist **(tertiary care)**, be sure the recommendation is in writing. Call the specialist at a later date to see whether the recommendation was acted on. If the patient refuses to be referred, be sure this is documented. If a referral form is necessary, *do not* telephone or write a letter. The managed care plan may refuse payment if the proper form is not completed.

When a referral authorization form is received, make a copy of the form for each approved office visit, laboratory test, or series of treatments. Then use

the form as a reference to bill for the service. All copies being used indicates that all the services that the patient's plan has approved are completed. Ask the primary care physician or the managed care plan for a new authorization to continue treatment on the patient. The request should be generated in a timely manner so that treatment is not delayed.

Diagnostic Tests

Many managed care plans require that patients have laboratory and radiology tests performed at plan-specified facilities. These are referred to as *network facilities*. Obtain the necessary authorizations for such services and allow sufficient time to receive the test or x-ray results before the patient's return appointment.

Inform the patient ahead of time when there is doubt about coverage for a test or the managed care plan indicates a test is not covered. Disclose the cost and have the patient sign a waiver agreement to pay for the service, thus enabling the billing of the patient for the service. If an authorization is denied because a test is deemed "medically unnecessary" and the physician wishes to appeal, the physician can present clinical reasons to the MCO's medical director to receive approval and bring attention to possible expansion of benefits for future patients.

Managed Care Guide

To help you keep up with the growth of local managed care plans and remember which physician belongs to which plan in the practice, create a grid or matrix of all MCOs that the practice has contracts with. Use a sheet of paper and list each plan with billing address vertically in a column to the left; then list significant data horizontally across the top. Suggested titles for column categories are: eligibility telephone numbers, copayment amounts,

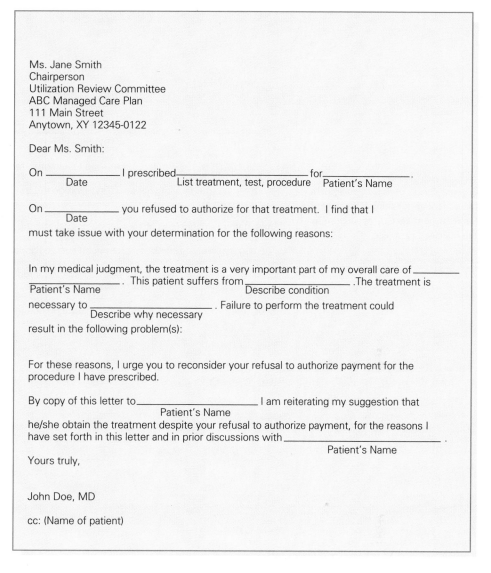

Figure 10–3. A letter to a managed care plan when there is a refusal to authorize payment for a recommended treatment, test, or procedure.

Ms. Jane Smith
Chairperson
Utilization Review Committee
ABC Managed Care Plan
111 Main Street
Anytown, XY 12345-0122

Dear Ms. Smith:

On _____ I prescribed_____ for_____ .
　　　Date　　　　　　　　　　List treatment, test, procedure　Patient's Name

On _____ you refused to authorize for that treatment. I find that I
　　　Date
must take issue with your determination for the following reasons:

In my medical judgment, the treatment is a very important part of my overall care of_____
_____ . This patient suffers from _____ .The treatment is
Patient's Name　　　　　　　　　　　　　　　Describe condition
necessary to _____ . Failure to perform the treatment could
　　　　　　　Describe why necessary
result in the following problem(s):

For these reasons, I urge you to reconsider your refusal to authorize payment for the
procedure I have prescribed.

By copy of this letter to_____ I am reiterating my suggestion that
　　　　　　　　　　Patient's Name
he/she obtain the treatment despite your refusal to authorize payment, for the reasons I
have set forth in this letter and in prior discussions with _____ .
　　　　　　　　　　　　　　　　　　　　　　　　　　Patient's Name
Yours truly,

John Doe, MD

cc: (Name of patient)

preauthorization requirements, restrictions on tests frequently ordered, participating laboratories, participating hospitals, and the contract's time limit for promised payment. Referring to this grid will provide specifics at a glance about each plan's coverage and copayment amounts (Fig. 10–5).

Plan Administration

Patient Information Letter

Inform managed care subscribers in writing what is expected from them and what they can expect in turn. The patient information letter should outline possible restrictions, noncovered items, expectations for copayment, and names of the managed care plans in which the physician is presently participating. Note if the patient neglects to notify the office of any change about eligibility status in the plan, such as **disenrollment;** the patient is then held personally responsible for the bill. Also mention that the managed care patient must inform the office if

hospitalization, surgery, or referral to a specialist is necessary. State that because of restrictions, failure to do so will make the patient liable for denied services. Post a sign in the waiting room advising managed care patients to check with the receptionist about participating plans.

Figure 10–6 is a sample letter of appropriate wording and content. File a copy of the letter given to the patient in the patient's medical record. Document in the medical record if the patient refuses to agree with managed care policy. Reimbursement may depend on the documentation.

Medical Records

Medical record management may differ when handling multiple managed care contracts. Place colored adhesive dots on patient file folder labels or color code managed care files by using a different colored chart for each EPO, HMO, IPA, and PPO patient. This decreases confusion and saves time

Mr. Avery Johnson
130 Sylvia Street
Anytown, XY 12345-0022

Dear Mr. Johnson:

On _____ I prescribed _____ for you. On _____ ,
      Date   Treatment, test, procedure   Date

_____ refused to authorize for same. On that basis,
   Name of Managed Care Plan

you have informed me of your decision to forego the treatment I have prescribed. I
expressed my concerns regarding your decision during our discussion on _____ about
                                                                 Date

the potential ramifications of your refusal to undergo the treatment.

The purpose of this letter is to recommend that you appeal _____
                                                Name of Managed Care Plan's

denial of benefits and reconsider your decision to forego the treatment in light of the
potential consequences of your refusal.

Should you wish to discuss this further, please do not hesitate to contact me.

Sincerely yours,

John Doe, MD

Figure 10–4. A letter to inform the patient about refusal of payment for treatment, test, or procedure by the managed care plan.

MANAGED CARE PLAN REFERENCE GUIDE

Plan name/address	Telephone eligibility	Copay	Preauthorization requirements	Test restrictions	Contracted lab(s) radiology	Contracted hospital(s)	Promised payment
Aetna PPO POB 43 WH XY 12345	555-239-0067	$5	hosp/surg/all dx tests	PE 1/yr	ABC Labs	College Hosp	30 days
Blue PPO POB 24335 WH XY 12345	555-245-0899	$8	referral specialist	PE 1/yr	Main St. Lab	St. John MC	30 days
Health Net POB 54000 WH XY 12345	555-408-5466	$5	hosp/surg see check list referrals	Mammo-gram 1/yr	Valley Lab	St. Joseph MC	45 days
Travelers MCO POB 1200 WH XY 12345	555-435-9877	$10	surg/hosp admit referrals	Pap >50 q3yr <50 q1yr	College Hosp. Metro Lab	College Hosp	30 days

Figure 10–5. Managed care plan quick reference guide to help keep track of specifics for each managed care plan in which the physician participates.

XYZ MEDICAL GROUP, INC.
1400 Avon Road, Suite 200
Woodland Hills, XY 12345

January 1, 20XX

TO: OUR PATIENTS

RE: PREFERRED PROVIDER ORGANIZATIONS

The following is a list of the PPOs and health insurance plans that we are members of and, therefore, will bill for you:

1. Georgia County Foundation
2. VIP Health Plan
3. Blue Cross Prudent Buyer Plan
4. Georgia County PPO
5. Northwest PPO
6. Blue Shield PPO

We are participating providers in several different PPOs. In order that we may maintain proper records for referrals and/or hospitalization, we request that each patient who is enrolled in a specific PPO keep our office currently informed regarding his or her eligibility status in that plan. Each time you are in the office for a visit, please verify with the receptionist that we have the correct coverage information.

If you have not informed us of changes in the status of your eligibility within the plan, you will be held responsible for any outstanding balance on your account due to that change.

Additionally, when your physician feels it is necessary to either hospitalize you or refer you to another physician outside this group, it is your responsibility to inform your physician that you belong to a specific PPO, as there may be restrictions imposed by that PPO regarding admission and referrals. If you fail to inform your physician at the time of referral or admission, our group may not be held responsible for noncoverage charges due to these restrictions.

If you have any questions regarding the above, please ask to speak to our insurance specialist.

I have read and understand the above text.

Signed: _____ Date: _____
               Patient (subscriber)

Figure 10–6. Letter to preferred provider organization subscribers outlining restrictions and noncovered services.

in identifying individual plans so that coverage, copayment, billing, and authorization requirements are met.

Scheduling Appointments

Screen patients when they call for appointments to determine whether they belong to the same prepaid health plan as the physician. Ask the patient to read from the insurance card to determine whether the physician's name is listed as the patient's primary care physician. Keep on hand an alphabetical list and profile of all plans with which the practice has a signed contract. It might also be useful to have a list of plans to which the practice does not belong. If the patient is not in a participating plan and still wishes to schedule a visit, inform him or her that payment at the time of the appointment is necessary and the amount is determined by the private fee schedule. This is an excellent idea if the patient is not a member of an HMO. In some states, Florida for example, an HMO patient cannot be billed for services that are covered. The provider must obtain authorization to treat the patient if the person is an HMO patient and the provider is not a participating provider because collecting from the HMO patient could backfire on the provider. The patient will pay for the visit, then send a copy of the receipt to his or her HMO. The HMO could file a complaint with the appropriate HMO regulatory agency because the provider treated their client without authorization and billed their client for the balance. The HMO could request a claim form from the provider and the provider would enter his or her private fee, which is more than the provider billed the HMO for another patient. This would open the door to possible fraud and abuse charges. The HMO could contact the patient, stating it should not have had to pay for the visit because the patient was in an HMO. Finally, the patient could demand a refund, and the provider would have no choice but to refund the money because the patient could turn the provider over to the HMO regulatory agency.

Encounter Form

Many managed care plans use an internal document on which the services rendered to the patient are checked off (charge ticket, encounter form, routing slip). It also may be used as a billing statement. The original is forwarded to the health plan's administrative office, and a copy is retained in the physician's files. Some plans require such documentation on a CMS-1500 Health Insurance Claim form. Examples of encounter forms are shown in Chapters 2, 7, and 9, Figures 2–14, 7–9, and 9–7.

Financial Management

Payment

Deductibles

Usually there is no **deductible** for a managed care plan. However, if there is one, be sure to ask patients if they have met their deductibles and collect them in the early months of the year (January through April).

Copayments

In a managed care plan a **copayment** is a predetermined fee paid by the patient to the provider at the time service is rendered. It is commonly referred to as a *copay* and is a form of cost sharing because the managed care plan or insurance company pays the remaining cost. Always collect the copay when the patient arrives for his or her appointment. Billing for small amounts is not cost-effective, and it is easy to forget to ask for payment when the patient is leaving the office. Copays are commonly made for office visits, prescription drugs, inpatient mental health services, urgent care visits, and emergency department visits. However, the amount may vary according to the type of service.

Payment Mechanisms

Payment mechanisms in managed care plans vary and can range from fee for service and capitation to salaried physicians. Following are some details about other payment mechanisms.

Contact Capitation

Contact capitation is based on the concept of paying physicians for actual patient visits or "contacts." A scenario under this payment method is when a patient is referred to a specialist for care. A "contact" occurs when the patient visits the specialist for treatment. The patient is assigned to the specialist for a defined period of time called the contact period. The length of the contact period is set in advance for each type of specialty by the participating specialty physician panel and MCO and may be tailored to the demographic and practice needs of the group. Each new patient visit during a contact period initiates a "contact point." Contact points determine how much to pay each physician. The average contact point value is determined by dividing the net specialty capitation pool or total amount of money set aside to be used for a particular specialty by the number of contacts in a certain time period. The average contact value is used to determine the amount paid to each specialist during each month in the contact period.

Case Rate Pricing

For specialists another payment method is *case rate pricing*. This means the specialist contracts with the managed care plan for an entire episode of care. This may be done for certain high-volume, expensive surgical procedures (e.g., knee surgery, cataracts, and bypass surgery).

Stop-Loss Limit

Some contracts have a "**stop-loss**" section, which means that if the patient's services are more than a certain amount, the physician can begin asking the patient to pay (fee for service). Monitor each patient's financial accounting record in those instances.

Contract Payment Time Limits

Usually state laws dictate the time limit within which a managed care plan must pay. The contract may or may not state the terms of payment, time limits, and late payment penalties, all of which can vary from one plan to another. Prompt payment laws require payment within 30, 45, 55, or 60 days. To diminish late payment of claims, a contract can specify that late claims accrue interest (e.g., 5% interest for claims paid after the payment time limit has elapsed). Some states have enacted laws enforcing interest penalties for late payment for either or both private payers as well as managed care plans. Therefore know the laws for the pertinent state. A time limit payment provision is an important factor to consider when reviewing a contract before a medical practice participates.

Monitoring Payment

Monitor payments made from all managed care plans and note whether the payment received is less than the agreed amount as stated in the contract. If payment has been reduced, send a letter to the plan citing, "As per contract see page about the fee for the consultation."

Sometimes a procedure (e.g., angioplasty with an assistant) may be done and the plan will not pay for an assistant, stating that it is not usual practice. However, perhaps the standard practice in a specific region is to always use an assistant for an angioplasty. When this is emphasized, the plan may remit additional payment.

Some states may have screening fees for emergency services and may or may not require prior approval for such services as defined by the Consolidated Omnibus Budget Reconciliation Act of 1985 (COBRA). There are also states that have adjudication laws with penalties if the managed care plan does not pay promptly. Take the following steps if claims are not paid in a timely manner (30 days):

1. Write to the plan representative and list the unpaid claims, claims paid after the payment time limit, and claims paid in error.

2. Send a statement to the director of the managed care plan notifying him or her that if the bill is not paid, the employer's benefits manager or patient will be contacted and alerted to outstanding, slow-paying accounts. Say that this will prevent the physician from renewing the plan's contract, and ask the recipient to contact the plan's representative. The consumer has a choice of managed care plans; if the present plan does not fulfill his or her intent to pay, the managed care plan loses members because of dissatisfaction.

3. Take examples and statistics to the next renegotiating session when the physician's contract is expiring.

Chapters 8 and 9 present information on how to handle slow or delinquent managed care plan payers.

Statement of Remittance

Managed care plans pay by either a capitation system (monthly check for the number of patients in the plan) or based on the services given to the patient (monthly check with a statement of remittance or explanation of benefits [EOB]).

In the capitation system a monthly check arrives written out for the total amount of monthly capitation. The accompanying paperwork lists all eligible patients being paid for on a per capita basis divided into two groups, commercial and senior. Patients categorized as commercial are usually younger than age 65 and are paid at a lesser rate because their risk

is lower (e.g., they do not need to see the doctor frequently). The senior patient category includes those older than age 65; these are paid at a higher rate because of the increased risk. Always verify the individual capitated amounts listed by each name on the accompanying paperwork against the monthly eligibility list to balance the amount of the check. Contact the MCO if an error appears. If a specialist is capitated, there may be thousands of patients on the capitation plan and a list of patients will not be provided. The capitation amount for a specialist may be only a few cents per month calculated according to the risk of the patient needing specialty services.

In the system when payment is based on services rendered and an EOB is generated, such statements itemize services that have been rendered to patients and usually indicate the amount billed, amount allowed, amount paid, and any copayment to be made by the patient (Fig. 10–7). Generally patients under managed care plans do not receive an EOB. Payments are checked against the managed care contract for verification and then posted to the patients' accounts. An error should be brought to the attention of the plan's administrator and, depending on the circumstances, appealed.

Accounting

Managed care plans vary in their financial reimbursement structure, and careful accounting procedures are required. Accounting can become a confusing issue because of mixture of private and managed care patients with copayment requirements, coinsurance amounts, deductibles, and withholds.

Fee-for-Service

Some medical practices handle managed care patient accounts the same as fee-for-service patient accounts. If coinsurance payment is necessary at the time of service, post first the charge and then the coinsurance prepayment, calculated on the percentage of the charge the plan allows. Finally, post an adjustment entry of the disallowed amount, which is calculated on a percentage of the MCO's allowable charge to balance the account (Fig. 10–8). An overpayment should be shown as a refund or credit to the account.

Year-End Evaluation

Withhold

Depending on the contract, a managed care plan may retain a percentage of the monthly capitation payment or a percentage of the allowable charges to physicians until the end of the year to cover operating expenses. This is known as **withhold.** A Statement of Remittance from the MCO shows the

STATEMENT OF REMITTANCE

PATIENT NAME (ID NUMBER)	SERVICE DATE MO. DAY YR	P O S	NO SVC	PROCEDURE NUMBER AND DESCRIPTION	AMOUNT BILLED	AMOUNT ALLOWED	RISK WITHHELD	CO PAY	AMOUNT PAID	ADJ. CODE
380224171-01 ALAN E.				CLAIM NO. 62730406 ACCOUNT NO.						
	092620XX	03	1	81000 URINALYSIS-ROUTINE	1000	1000	100	0	900	
	092620XX	03	1	82270 OCCULT BLOOD ANY S	1200	1200	120	0	1080	
	092620XX	03	1	99243 COMPRE RE-EXAM OR	6500	6500	650	0	5850	
	092620XX	03	1	36415 VENIPUNCTURE W/CEN	1700	1700	170	0	1530	
				CLAIM TOTALS =	10400	10400	1040	0	9360	
558700321-01 RONALD B.				CLAIM NO. 62730407 ACCOUNT NO.						
	092520XX	03	1	90050 LIM EXAM EVAL A/O	3000	3000	300	300	2400	
				CLAIM TOTALS =	3000	3000	300	300	2400	
473760096-01 DORMA L.				CLAIM NO. 62730408 ACCOUNT NO.						
	092520XX	03	1	90050 LIM EXAM EVAL A/O	3000	3000	300	300	2400	
				CLAIM TOTALS =	3800	3000	300	380	3120	

VENDOR SUMMARY: TOTAL AMOUNT PAID $1,638.96   TOTAL WITHHELD $194.39

AMOUNT PAID YEAR-TO-DATE: $42,411.95   AMOUNT WITHHELD YEAR-TO-DATE $5,109.94

Adjustment Code Legend
A = Adjusted: Billed amount exceeds VIP allowed.
O = Claim for service denied. Charges for this service included in other benefit payment. No patient liability.

Figure 10–7. Statement of remittance or explanation of benefits for noncapitated patients or contracted fee for service indicating the amount billed, amount allowed, amount paid, and any copayment that is to be made by the patient.

risk amounts withheld for each patient's visit in Column 8 of Figure 10–7. The withhold plus interest is returned to the physician at the end of the plan year if the budgeted services for the plan are not overused. However, the withhold or a portion of it is retained by the plan if services are overutilized. Thus the physicians share in any surplus or pay part of any deficit at year's end. This risk sharing creates an incentive for limiting care by the gatekeeper and limiting referrals to specialists, thereby keeping medical costs down. The withhold can cover all services or be specific to hospital care, **ancillary services** (laboratory/x-ray usages), or specialty referrals.

A managed care plan that withholds a percentage of the allowable charge must be tracked in the physician's accounts receivable so it is not prematurely written off as a bad debt. To do this, develop a capitation accounting worksheet listing the dates of service, patients' names, CPT code for the service rendered, fee-for-service charges, withheld amounts, and disallowed amounts (Fig. 10–9). Then total all columns. The total of the withheld column is a debit entry that indicates what the managed care plan owes to the medical practice pending its year-end reconciliation. If and when the withheld amount arrives, the accounting worksheet can be compared with the amount withheld during the year. The amount of withholds that are not returned to the physician is adjusted once withholds are settled.

The total of the column for disallowed amounts shows the amount written off by the medical practice. Combine the withheld returned amount with the managed care payment for the year to determine whether it is worthwhile for the practice to participate in the plan. Some practices can use the information to renegotiate increased fees when the managed care contract is to be renewed.

Capitation versus Fee-for-Service

Financial management reports are generated via computer and are the responsibility of the manager or accountant in most medical practices. However, it can be an asset for an insurance biller to have some knowledge of the content of these reports. Most medical practices monitor plan payments for profit or loss by comparing actual income from managed care patients with what would have been received from fee-for-service plans. To do this one designs a capitation accounting sheet for each capitated plan. This sheet shows a listing of dates of service and professional service descriptions (procedures, injections, and laboratory work), as well as charges and payments (Fig. 10–10). As managed care plan patients receive services, actual service fees are posted in a charge column from the office fee schedule as if the patient were a private payer. In a payment column, office visit, copayments, and the monthly capitation payment are posted. Then all columns are

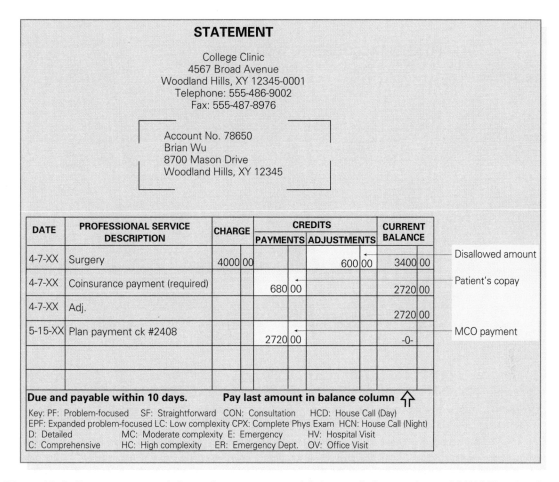

STATEMENT

College Clinic
4567 Broad Avenue
Woodland Hills, XY 12345-0001
Telephone: 555-486-9002
Fax: 555-487-8976

Account No. 78650
Brian Wu
8700 Mason Drive
Woodland Hills, XY 12345

DATE	PROFESSIONAL SERVICE DESCRIPTION	CHARGE	CREDITS		CURRENT BALANCE	
			PAYMENTS	ADJUSTMENTS		
4-7-XX	Surgery	4000 00		600 00	3400 00	← Disallowed amount
4-7-XX	Coinsurance payment (required)		680 00		2720 00	← Patient's copay
4-7-XX	Adj.				2720 00	
5-15-XX	Plan payment ck #2408		2720 00		-0-	← MCO payment

Due and payable within 10 days.   Pay last amount in balance column ⇧

Key: PF: Problem-focused   SF: Straightforward   CON: Consultation   HCD: House Call (Day)
EPF: Expanded problem-focused LC: Low complexity CPX: Complete Phys Exam HCN: House Call (Night)
D: Detailed   MC: Moderate complexity E: Emergency   HV: Hospital Visit
C: Comprehensive   HC: High complexity   ER: Emergency Dept.   OV: Office Visit

Figure 10–8. Posting to a patient's financial accounting record (ledger card) showing charge of $4000. The plan allows $3400; therefore the patient's prepaid coinsurance amount is $680 (20% of $3400). The managed care plan sent a check for $2720 (80% of $3400) and the disallowed amount ($600) is adjusted off of the account, which brings the account balance to zero.

totaled. It is necessary to apply a discount to the total charged amount for a realistic comparison because the physician usually is paid on an allowed amount rather than an actual charge. Calculate the difference between the actual charge and the average allowed amount to do this.

Compare the capitated payment amounts plus copayment amounts to the total discounted charges at the end of the year. This gives an accurate idea of whether the capitated payment received is adequate for the services the physician performed. Compiling monthly records and

DEBIT

Date	Patient	Service	Charge	Withhold	Disallow	
5/15/20XX	Mason	99204	106.11	5.94	21.22	Disallowed
5/15/20XX	Mason	93000	34.26	1.92	3.43	amounts
5/15/20XX	Mason	81000	8.00	.38	2.40	
5/15/20XX	Self	93501	1500.00	240.00	300.00	
Total			1648.38	248.24	327.05	Total withheld amount owed by MCO

Figure 10–9. A managed care plan when payment is on a fee-for-service basis. Note the disallowed portion of the charge, which is based on the plan's allowable charge. A portion of the allowable charge is withheld.

CAPITATION ACCOUNTING WORKSHEET

NAME OF PLAN ABC Managed Care Plan

DATE OF SERVICE	PROFESSIONAL SERVICE DESCRIPTION	CHARGES	PAYMENTS		
		Services Fees	Capitation	Copay	
20XX 1/15	Capitation (105 members) @ $8 ea		840.00 ←		Capitation payment
2/15	Capitation (115 members)		920.00		
2/20	Sanchez OV/Copay	35.00		5.00 ←	Copayment amount
2/22	Jones OV/Copay	35.00		5.00	
2/23	Davis OV/Copay	35.00 ←		5.00	Actual fee-for-service charge
3/6	Evans OV/Copay	35.00		5.00	
3/15	Capitation (130 members)		1040.00		
4/10	Wu OV/Copay	35.00		5.00	
4/15	Capitation (135 members)		1080.00		
	May through December are not shown				
END OF YEAR TOTALS		3500.00	6880.00	500.00	

Figure 10–10. An accounting sheet for a capitation plan from January through April showing dates of service, professional service descriptions, members' charges, and capitation payments and copayments received by the medical practice. Charges and payments columns may be totaled at the end of the year to compare capitation with fee-for-service earnings.

reviewing them at the end of the year helps a medical practice assess the gain or loss of each capitation plan.

Bankruptcy

If an MCO declares bankruptcy, such as a Chapter 11 filing, it is obligated to pay for all bills incurred after the filing. If the patient had treatment before the filing, a delay in getting reimbursed may occur because the MCO cannot repay debts incurred before its filing until it has worked out a reorganization plan. Physicians under contract with the MCO are obligated to honor their contractural commitments. If their contracts expire or if they have escape clauses, they may be required to continue accepting patients depending on the contract provisions.

Some clauses allow a physician to withdraw from seeing managed care patients or leave if the MCO is in bankruptcy proceedings for more than 4 months. However, bankruptcy courts have broad powers to prevent physicians from leaving MCOs in bankruptcy proceedings if the court deems such actions to be detrimental to the rehabilitation of the debtor.

In some states, laws such as California's Knox-Keene Health Care Service Plan Act of 1975 prohibit hospitals and physicians under contract to an MCO from billing patients. Other states do not have such protection but may have emergency insurance funds to limit the financial liability of enrollees in bankrupct MCOs. If the insurance commissioner is written to, he or she will refer the letter to the MCO. However, letters make insurance commissioners aware of problems that have developed.

Chapter 9 contains information on the topic of bankruptcy.

Conclusion

In summary, the medical biller should be aware that no matter what the type of plan, it is either purchased by an individual or paid by an employer. This is extremely important to know because if the plan is paid by the employer it is regulated by the Employee Retirement Income Security Act, also known as ERISA. This law regulates all managed care insurance paid by the employer or supplemented by the employee for the employee's spouse or children, which today is about 85% of the claims that are non–Medicare/Medicaid/workers' compensation. ERISA is regulated by the Department of Labor, and if the plan is an ERISA plan, the State Insurance Commissioners have no power to help with insurance carrier issues. Consequently, if the managed care organization is "related to" an employee benefit plan (EBP), the requirements of ERISA and its regulations are of overriding importance and severely restrict patient rights.

No employer is obligated to establish an EBP. To encourage them to do so, Congress has given them, their plans, their HMOs and insurers, and their administrators substantial immunities from liability. State regulation of HMOs administered by self-insured EBPs is preempted by ERISA; therefore employees cannot be protected by those state laws that limit the excesses of other HMOs not subject to ERISA.

Any case "relating to" an EBP falls under federal jurisdiction and is always removed from state to federal court when a lawsuit is initiated. There the patient and provider will find that the usual state law tort claims also are preempted by ERISA; therefore any claims against the HMO or EBP for medical malpractice, wrongful death, fraud, nonpayment or incorrect payment of claims, and so on will be summarily dismissed if filed in state courts. As of January 1, 2003, new changes were made to ERISA about time limitations on claims processing and the appeals process. Therefore know if the policy is paid for by the patient or employer. Refer to the resources at the end of this chapter for more information on ERISA.

RESOURCES ON THE INTERNET

American Association of Health Plans (AAHP) [formerly known as American Managed Care and Review Association and American Association of Foundations for Medical Care]
www.aahp.org
Employee Retirement Income Security Act (ERISA)
www.dol.gov
Then do a search and select "E." ERISA is listed as a selection.
Federal Register
www.gpo.gov

STUDENT ASSIGNMENT LIST

✔ Study Chapter 10.
✔ Answer the review questions in the *Workbook* to reinforce the theory learned in this chapter and to help prepare you for a future test.
✔ Complete the assignments in the *Workbook* to give you hands-on experience in abstracting information from a medical record to complete treatment authorization forms for prepaid health insurance cases.
✔ Turn to the Glossary at the end of this textbook for a further understanding of the Key Terms used in this chapter.

MEDICARE

Medicare

CHAPTER OUTLINE

Medicare Summary Notice

Beneficiary Representative/
Representative Payee

Posting Payments

Review and Appeal Process

OBJECTIVES*

After reading this chapter, you should be able to:

- Explain eligibility criteria for Medicare.
- Name important information to abstract from a patient's Medicare card.
- Identify the benefits and nonbenefits of Medicare.
- List the federal laws adopted to increase health benefits for employed workers and the elderly.
- Name the conditions when an HMO-Medicare patient can be seen by a nonmember HMO physician.
- Differentiate between an HMO Risk Plan and an HMO Cost Plan.
- Name the federal laws that relate to cost containment of health services and to reduction of fraud and abuse issues.
- Explain when to obtain a patient's signature on a waiver of liability agreement.
- Define a Medicare-mandated prepayment screen.
- State the benefits for a participating versus nonparticipating physician.
- Calculate a payment for a procedure using the current conversion factor.
- List situations for using a lifetime beneficiary claim authorization and information release document.

- Determine the time limit for submitting a Medicare claim.
- Explain claims submission for individuals who have Medicare with other insurance.
- List CMS-1500 block numbers that require Medigap information when submitting a Medicare/Medigap claim.
- Post information on the patient's financial accounting record after a Medicare payment has been received.

KEY TERMS

advance beneficiary notice (ABN)

approved charges

assignment

benefit period

Centers for Medicare and Medicaid Services (CMS)

Correct Coding Initiative (CCI)

crossover claim

diagnostic cost groups (DCGs)

disabled

end-stage renal disease (ESRD)

fiscal intermediary (FI)

hospice

hospital insurance

intermediate care facilities (ICFs)

limiting charge

medical necessity

Medicare Part A

Medicare Part B

Continued.

Provider Identification
  Numbers

Patient's Signature
  Authorization

Time Limit

Manual Claims

Electronic Claims

Medicare/Medicaid Claims

Medicare/Medigap Claims

Medicare/Supplemental and
  MSP Claims

Deceased Patients Claims

Physician Substitute Coverage

After Claim Submission

Remittance Advice

---

*Performance objectives and exercises for hands-on practical experience for this chapter
appear in the *Workbook*.

KEY TERMS—cont'd

Medicare Part C

Medicare/Medicaid (Medi-Medi)

Medicare Secondary Payer (MSP)

Medicare Summary Notice (MSN)

Medigap (MG)

national alphanumeric codes

nonparticipating physician (nonpar)

nursing facility (NF)

participating physician (par)

peer review organization (PRO)

premium

prospective payment system (PPS)

qui tam **action**

reasonable fee

relative value unit (RVU)

remittance advice (RA)

resource-based relative value scale (RBRVS)

respite care

Supplemental Security Income (SSI)

supplementary medical insurance (SMI)

volume performance standard (VPS)

Background

Although Social Security is one of the United States' most important domestic programs, this system is by no means the first. There were a number of social insurance programs throughout Europe and Latin America before the Social Security Act was signed into law in 1935. Before the United States had Social Security, 20 other nations already had similar systems in operation. Another 30 countries had different social insurance programs in place, such as workers' compensation.

Policies and Regulations

Medicare is run by the **Centers for Medicare and Medicaid Services (CMS),** formerly known as the Health Care Financing Administration (HCFA). CMS is subdivided into three divisions with the following responsibilities:

1. The Center for Medicare Management oversees traditional fee-for-service Medicare, including development of payment policy and management of fee-for-service contractors.
2. The Center for Beneficiary Choices provides beneficiaries with information on Medicare, Medicare Select, and Medicare Plus (+) Choice programs and Medigap options. It also manages the Medicare + Choice plans, consumer research, and grievance and appeals functions.
3. The Center for Medicaid and State Operations focuses on federal–state programs, such as Medicaid, the State Children's Health Insurance Program, insurance regulations, and the Clinical Laboratory Improvements Act (CLIA).

Eligibility Requirements

Local Social Security Administration (SSA) offices take applications for Medicare and provide information about the program. The eligible person must apply to receive the benefits. Eligible persons may apply at age 65 to receive full-time retirement benefits and Medicare Parts A or B. In the year 2000, the retirement age gradually increased for people born in the year 1938 or later. By 2027, full-time retirement age will be 67 for people born after 1959. Benefits may increase if retirement is delayed beyond full-retirement age. As of this edition, Medicare still may be applied for at age 65. Those who apply for Social Security early (at age 62 years) do not receive Medicare but receive monthly reduced Social Security benefits.

Medicare is a federal health insurance program for the following categories of people:

1. People 65 years of age or older who are retired on Social Security
2. People 65 years of age or older who are retired from the railroad or civil service
3. **Disabled** individuals who are eligible for Social Security disability benefits* and are in the following categories:
   a. Disabled workers of any age
   b. Disabled widows of workers who are fully or currently insured through the federal government, civil service, SSA,

---

*Note: In the disabled categories, a person must be disabled for not less than 12 months to apply for disability benefits. A disabled beneficiary must receive disability benefits for 24 months before Medicare benefits begin. See Chapter 15 for further information on this topic.

Supplemental Security Income (SSI), or the Railroad Retirement Act and whose husbands qualified for benefits under one of these programs

   c. Adults disabled before age 18 whose parents are eligible for or retired on Social Security benefits

4. Children and adults who have chronic kidney disease requiring dialysis or **end-stage renal disease (ESRD)** requiring kidney transplant

5. Kidney donors (all expenses related to the kidney transplantation are covered)

All persons who meet one of the previously stated eligibility requirements are eligible for **Medicare Part A** (hospital coverage). Those who qualify for full Medicare benefits may also elect to take **Medicare Part B** (outpatient coverage). Medicare Part B recipients pay annually increasing basic premiums to the SSA, and some pay a Medicare surtax on federal income tax payments. This premium may be deducted automatically from the patient's monthly Social Security check if he or she wishes. Those individuals not eligible for Medicare Part A (hospital insurance) at age 65 may purchase Part B from the SSA.

Aliens

An alien on Medicare may be eligible for Part A or B coverage. To be eligible, the applicant must have lived in the United States as a permanent resident for 5 consecutive years. It is usually not necessary to state on the CMS-1500 form that the patient is an alien when billing Medicare.

Health Insurance Card

The patient should present his or her Medicare health insurance card indicating the patient's insurance claim number (Figs. 11–1 and 11–2). The claim number is the Social Security number of the wage earner with an alpha suffix. The card indicates hospital and medical coverage, effective date, and patient status. When a husband and wife both have Medicare, they receive separate cards and claim numbers. Medicare cards are red, white, and blue, and cards issued after 1990 are plastic.

The letters after the Medicare number on the patient's identification card indicate the patient's status as follows (this is only a partial listing):

A = wage earner (shown in Fig. 11–1)

B = husband's number (wife 62 years or older)

D = widow

HAD = disabled adult

C = disabled child

J, Kl, or Jl = special monthly benefits, never worked under Social Security

M = Part B benefits only

T = uninsured and entitled only to health insurance benefits

A patient whose Medicare card claim number ends in "A" has the *same* Social Security and claim numbers. A patient whose Medicare card claim number ends in "B" or "D" has *different* Social Security and claim numbers. A quick check between Social Security and card claim numbers may identify a submission error and forestall a claims rejection.

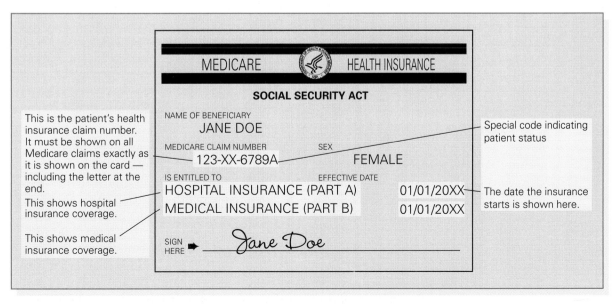

Figure 11–1. Medicare Health Insurance Identification Card.

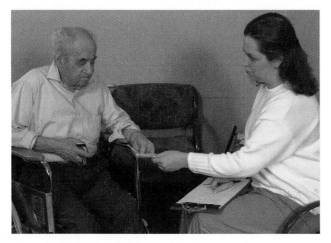

Figure 11–2. Insurance billing specialist obtaining the identification card from a disabled Medicare patient.

The letters preceding the Medicare number on the patient's identification card indicate *railroad retirees:*

A   retired railroad employee
                 Examples: A 000000 (6 digits);
                 A 000-00-0000 (9 digits)
MA   Spouse of a retired railroad employee
WA/WD   Widow or widower of deceased
                 employee (age or disability)
                 Examples: WA000000 (6 digits);
                 WA000-00-0000 (9 digits)
CA   Child or student
WCA/WCD   Widow of retiree with child in her
                 care or disabled child of deceased
                 employee
PA/PD   Parent of deceased employee (male or
                 female)
H   Railroad retirement board pensioner
                 before 1937
MH   Wife of railroad retirement board
                 pensioner before 1937
WH   Widowed wife of railroad retirement
                 board pensioner before 1937
WCH   Widow of railroad retirement board
                 pensioner with child in her care
PH   Parent of railroad retirement board
                 pensioner before 1937
JA   Widow receiving a joint and survivor
                 annuity
X   Divorced spouse's annuity, for use on
                 forms AA-3 and AA-7 only
                 Example: CA 123-45-6789C

Enrollment Status

An individual is eligible to enroll in Medicare 3 months before his or her 65th birthday, and the enrollment period ends 3 months after the month in which the person turns 65. If the enrollment period is missed, the individual must wait until the next general enrollment period, January 1 through March 31.

A telephone hotline or, in some states, a modem is available to verify the enrollment status. This is useful because patients can switch coverage to a senior managed care plan on a month-to-month basis. Most carriers also allow information on deductible status. The patient's numeric information (Medicare number and date of birth) is entered into the telephone system, and the digital response indicates how much of the deductible has been satisfied. Contact the Medicare local fiscal agent for information about this service.

Benefits and Nonbenefits

Medicare Part A: Hospital Benefits

Part A of Medicare is **hospital insurance** benefits for the aged, disabled, and blind. Funds for this health service come from special contributions from employees and self-employed persons, with employers matching contributions. These contributions are collected along with regular Social Security contributions from wages and self-employment income earned during a person's working years.

A **benefit period** begins the day a patient enters a hospital and ends when the patient has not been a bed patient in any hospital or **nursing facility (NF)** (formerly called skilled nursing facility) for 60 consecutive days. It also ends if a patient has been in a nursing facility but has not received skilled nursing care for 60 consecutive days. A nursing facility offers nursing or rehabilitation services that are medically necessary to a patient's recovery. Services provided are not custodial. Custodial services are those that assist the patient with personal needs (e.g., dressing, eating, bathing, and getting in and out of bed). Hospital insurance protection is renewed every time the patient begins a new benefit period. There is no limit to the number of benefit periods a patient can have for hospital or nursing facility care. However, special limited benefit periods apply to hospice care.

Medicare Part A provides benefits to applicants in any of the following situations:

1. A bed patient in a hospital (up to 90 hospital days for each benefit period)
2. A bed patient in a nursing facility (up to 100 extended-care days for each benefit period)
3. A patient receiving home health care services
4. A patient who needs care in a psychiatric hospital (up to 190 days in a lifetime)
5. A terminally ill patient diagnosed as having 6 months or less to live who needs hospice care. A **hospice** is a public agency or private organization that is primarily engaged in providing

pain relief, symptom management, and supportive services to terminally ill people and their families.

6. A terminally ill patient who needs respite care. **Respite care** is a short-term inpatient stay that may be necessary for the terminally ill patient to give temporary relief to the person who regularly assists with home care. Inpatient respite care is limited to stays of no more than 5 consecutive days for each respite period.

Figure 11–3 contains information on five major classifications of inpatient hospital cost-sharing benefits for Medicare Part A. Miscellaneous hospital services and supplies might consist of intensive care unit (ICU) costs, blood transfusions, drugs, x-ray and laboratory tests, medical supplies (casts, surgical dressings, splints), use of wheelchair, operating room (OR) and recovery room costs, and therapy (physical, occupational, and speech language). There are no benefits for personal convenience items (television, radio, and telephone), private duty nurses, or a private room unless it is determined medically necessary. Similar benefits also relate to nursing facilities.

Benefits for hospice and respite care consist of nursing and physicians' services, drugs, therapy (physical, occupational, and speech-language pathology), home health aide, homemaker services, medical social services, medical supplies and appliances, short-term inpatient care, and counseling.

Medicare Part B: Medical Benefits

Part B of Medicare is **supplementary medical insurance (SMI)** benefits for the aged and disabled. Funds for this program come equally from those who sign up for it and the federal government. A medical insurance **premium** is automatically deducted from monthly checks for those who receive Social Security benefits, railroad retirement benefits, or a civil service annuity. Others pay the premium directly to the SSA. In some states, when a person is

MEDICARE (PART A): HOSPITAL INSURANCE-COVERED SERVICES FOR 2003

Services	Benefit	Medicare Pays	Patient Pays
HOSPITALIZATION Semiprivate room and board, general nursing and miscellaneous hospital services and supplies. (Medicare payments based on benefit periods.)	First 60 days	All but $840	$840 deductible
	61st to 90th day 91st to 150th day[1]	All but $210 a day	$210 a day
	60-reserve-days benefit	All but $420 a day	$420 a day
	Beyond 150 days	Nothing	All costs
NURSING FACILITY CARE Patient must have been in a hospital for at least 3 days and enter a Medicare-approved facility generally within 30 days after hospital discharge.[2] (Medicare payments based on benefit periods.)	First 20 days	100% of approved amount	Nothing
	21st to 100th day	All but $105 a day	Up to $105 a day
	Beyond 100 days	Nothing	All costs
HOME HEALTH CARE Part-time or intermittent skilled care, home health aide services, durable medical equipment and supplies, and other services.	Unlimited as long as Medicare conditions are met and services are declared "medically necessary."	100% of approved amount; 80% of approved amount for durable medical equipment.	Nothing for services; 20% of approved amount for durable medical equipment.
HOSPICE CARE Pain relief, symptom management, and support services for the terminally ill.	If patient elects the hospice option and as long as doctor certifies need.	All but limited costs for outpatient drugs and inpatient respite care.	Limited cost sharing for outpatient drugs and inpatient respite care.
BLOOD	Unlimited if medically necessary.	All but first 3 pints per calendar year.	For first 3 pints.[3]

[1] This 60-reserve-days benefit may be used only once in a lifetime.
[2] Neither Medicare nor private Medigap insurance will pay for most long-term nursing home care.
[3] To the extent the blood deductible is met under Part B of Medicare during the calendar year, it does not have to be met under Part A.

Figure 11–3. Five major classifications of Medicare Part A benefits. (Updated from *Your Medicare Handbook for Railroad Retirement Beneficiaries*. U.S. Government Printing Office, 2003.)

eligible for Medicare Part B and Medicaid, Medicaid pays for the monthly Part B premiums.

Figure 11–4 contains information on six major classifications of medical benefits for Medicare Part B. In addition to medical and surgical services by a doctor of medicine (MD), doctor of osteopathy (DO or MD), or a doctor of dental medicine or dental surgery (DDS), certain services by a doctor of podiatric medicine (DPM), and limited services by a doctor of chiropractic (DC) are paid for. Dental care is covered only for fractures or surgery of the jaw. Optometric examinations are provided if a person has aphakia (absence of the natural lens of the eye).

Preventive care benefits that Medicare will pay for are the following:

▶ Annual mammograms for women age 40 and older, plus a one-time baseline mammogram for women aged 35 to 39
▶ Papanicolaou (Pap) tests every 2 years. Medicare will pay for an annual examination for women at high risk for cervical and vaginal cancer and those with a recent abnormal Pap test
▶ Colorectal cancer screening for people age 50 and older. The test covered is dependent on the patient's risk level and the time elapsed from his or her last screening

MEDICARE (PART B): MEDICAL INSURANCE-COVERED SERVICES FOR 2003

Services	Benefit	Medicare Pays	Patient Pays
MEDICAL EXPENSES Doctor's services (not routine physical exams), outpatient medical and surgical services and supplies, diagnostic tests, ambulatory surgery center facility fees for approved procedures, and durable medical equipment (such as wheelchairs, hospital beds, oxygen, and walkers). Also covers second surgical opinions, outpatient mental health care, and outpatient physical and occupational therapy, including speech-language therapy.	Unlimited if medically necessary.	80% of approved amount (after $100 deductible). Reduced to 50% for most outpatient mental health services.	$100 deductible,[1] plus 20% of approved amount or limited charges.[2]
CLINICAL LABORATORY SERVICES Blood tests, urinalyses, and more.	Unlimited if medically necessary.	100% of approved amount.	Nothing for services.
HOME HEALTH CARE Part-time skilled nursing care, physical therapy, occupational therapy, speech-language therapy, home health aide services, medical social services, durable medical equipment (such as wheelchairs, hospital beds, oxygen, and walkers), medical supplies, and other services.	Unlimited as long as patient meets conditions and benefits are declared medically necessary.	100% of approved amount; 80% of approved amount for durable medical equipment.	Nothing for services; 20% of approved amount for durable medical equipment.
OUTPATIENT HOSPITAL TREATMENT Services for the diagnosis or treatment of illness or injury.	Unlimited if medically necessary.	Medicare payment to hospital based on hospital cost.	$100 deductible, plus 20% of whatever the hospital charges.
BLOOD	Unlimited if medically	80% of approved amount	First 3 pints plus 20% of approved amounts for additional pints (after $100 deductible).[3]

[1]Once the patient has had $100 of expenses for covered services in the year, the Part B deductible does not apply to any further covered services received for the rest of the year.

[2]See Figure 11–8 for an explanation of approved amount for participating physicians and limited charges for nonparticipating physicians.

[3]To the extent the blood deductible is met under Part A of Medicare during the calendar year, it does not have to be met under Part B.

Figure 11–4. Five major classifications of Medicare Part B benefits. (Updated from *Your Medicare Handbook for Railroad Retirement Beneficiaries.* U.S. Government Printing Office, 2003.)

- Annual prostate cancer screening procedures, including digital rectal examinations and prostate-specific antigen (PSA) blood tests, for men older than age 50
- Purchase of home glucose monitors and testing strips for people with diabetes. A wider range of diabetes self-management training and therapeutic shoes for severe diabetic foot disease may also be covered
- Glaucoma screening once every 12 months
- Bone mass measurements for women 65 and older at high risk for osteoporosis
- Vaccines (influenza, pneumococcal pneumonia, and hepatitis B)
- Ambulance service meeting medical necessity requirements
- Rental or purchase of durable medical equipment for home use, prosthetic devices for internal body organs, artificial limbs and eyes, and braces or supports (leg, arm, back, and neck)

Nonbenefits consist of routine physical examination, routine foot care, eye or hearing examinations, and cosmetic surgery unless caused by injury or performed to improve functioning of a malformed part. A physician may bill a patient separately for noncovered services.

There are many other benefits and nonbenefits too numerous to list here. Refer to Medicare newsletters or contact the Medicare carrier to find out whether a particular procedure qualifies for payment.

Medicare Part C: Medicare Plus (+) Choice Program

The Balanced Budget Act of 1997 created **Medicare Part C** called Medicare + Choice. This program increased the number of health care options in addition to those that are available under Part A and Part B. Medicare + Choice plans receive a fixed amount of money from Medicare to spend on their Medicare members. Some plans may require members to pay a premium similar to the Medicare Part B premium.

Plans available under this program may include the following: health maintenance organization (HMO), point-of-service (POS) plan, preferred provider organization (PPO), private fee-for-service (PFFS) plan, provider sponsored organization (PSO), religious fraternal benefit society (RFBS), and a pilot program, medical savings account (MSA). Most of these are discussed in Chapters 2 and 10, except for PSO, RFBS, and MSA.

A PSO is a managed care plan that is owned and operated by a hospital and provider group instead of an insurance company. An RFBS is a managed care option that is associated with a church, group of churches, or convention. Membership is restricted to church members and is allowed regardless of the

person's health status. In an MSA plan, the patient chooses an insurance policy approved by Medicare that has a high annual deductible. Medicare pays the premiums for this policy and deposits the dollar amount difference between what it pays for the average beneficiary in the patient's area and the cost of the premium into the patient's MSA. The patient uses the MSA money to pay medical expenses until the high deductible is reached. If the MSA money becomes depleted, the patient pays out of pocket until the deductible is reached. Unused funds roll over to the next year.

Railroad Retirement Benefits

Railroad Retirement Board offices take applications for Medicare and provide information about the program for railroad workers and their beneficiaries. Medical insurance premiums are automatically deducted from the monthly checks of people who receive railroad retirement benefits. Those who do not receive a monthly check pay their premiums directly or, in some cases, have premiums paid on their behalf under a state assistance program. If the allowed fees differ from those allowed by the regular Medicare carrier, write or fax the Medicare railroad retiree carrier, asking that fees be based on fee data from the local carrier.

Railroad retirement beneficiaries generally are entitled to benefits for covered services received from a qualified American facility. However, under certain circumstances a Medicare beneficiary may receive care in Canada or Mexico. Benefits and deductibles under Parts A and B are the same as for other Medicare recipients.

Some railroad retirees are members of a railroad hospital association or a prepayment plan. These members pay regular premiums to the plan and then can receive health services the plan provides without additional charges. In some plans small charges are made for certain services, such as drugs or home visits. Many prepayment plans make arrangements with Medicare to receive direct payments for services they furnish that are covered under Medicare Part B. Some prepayment plans have contracts with Medicare as HMOs or competitive medical plans and can receive direct payment for services covered by either hospital or medical insurance. After a claim is submitted to the Medicare railroad retiree carrier, a Remittance Advice (RA) document is generated, explaining the decision made on the claim and what services Medicare paid.

Employed Elderly Benefits

To understand various types of scenarios that may be encountered when submitting claims for elderly individuals, one must know about several powerful federal laws that regulate health care coverage of those age 65 and older who are employed. Such individuals may have group insurance or a Medigap (MG) policy and may fall under billing categories of Medicare First Payer or Medicare Secondary Payer (all are presented in detail later in this chapter).

Omnibus Budget Reconciliation Act

The Omnibus Budget Reconciliation Act (OBRA) of 1981 required that, in the case of a current or former employee or dependent younger than age 65 and Medicare eligible solely because of ESRD, the employer's group coverage is primary for up to 12 months. This act applies to all employers regardless of the number of employees. OBRA of 1986, effective in 1987, required that if an employee or dependent younger than age 65 has Medicare coverage because of a disability other than ESRD, the group coverage is primary and Medicare is secondary. This act applies only to large group health plans having at least 100 full- or part-time employees.

Tax Equity and Fiscal Responsibility Act

The Tax Equity and Fiscal Responsibility Act (TEFRA) of 1982 established that an employee or spouse aged 65 to 69 years is entitled to the same health insurance benefits offered under the same conditions to younger employees and their spouses. The group insurance is primary and Medicare is secondary. TEFRA applies to employers with at least 20 full- or part-time employees.

Deficit Reduction Act

The Deficit Reduction Act (DEFRA) of 1984, effective 1985, was an amendment to TEFRA and stated that a spouse aged 65 to 69 years or an employee of any age is entitled to the same group health plan offered to younger employees and their spouses. The group's coverage is primary and Medicare is secondary. DEFRA applies to employers with at least 20 full- or part-time employees.

Consolidated Omnibus Budget Reconciliation Act

The Consolidated Omnibus Budget Reconciliation Act (COBRA) of 1985, effective 1986, is another amendment to TEFRA eliminating the age ceiling of 69 years. An employee or spouse age 65 or older is entitled to the same group health plan offered to younger employees and their spouses. COBRA requires that third-party payers reimburse for certain care rendered in government-run veteran and military hospitals. The group's coverage is primary and Medicare is secondary. COBRA applies to employers with at least 20 full- or part-time employees.

Tax Reform Act

The Tax Reform Act was passed in 1986; it clarified certain aspects of COBRA. A spouse and dependents may elect to receive continued coverage even if the employee does not wish insurance coverage and terminates the plan. However, the spouse and dependents must have been covered under the plan before the covered employee terminates it. Spouses who are widowed or divorced while receiving continued coverage must report such changes to the benefit plan administrator within 60 days of the employee's death to determine how many additional months of coverage are available.

Additional Insurance Programs

Many Medicare recipients have Medicare in combination with other insurance plans. This section explains various coverage combinations. Guidelines for processing claims for these plans are presented later in this chapter.

Medicare/Medicaid

Patients designated as **Medicare/Medicaid (Medi-Medi)** are on both Medicare and Medicaid (in California Medi-Cal) simultaneously and are those who qualify for Old Age Security (OAS) assistance benefits (older than age 65), the severely disabled, and the blind.

Medicare/Medigap

A specialized insurance policy devised for the Medicare beneficiary is called **Medigap** or *Medifill*. This type of policy is designed to supplement coverage under a fee-for-service Medicare plan. It may cover prescription costs and the deductible and copayment (e.g., 20% of the Medicare allowed amount) that are typically the patient's responsibility under Medicare. These plans are offered by private third-party payers to Medicare beneficiaries.

The federal government in, conjunction with the insurance industry, established predefined minimum benefits for 10 Medigap policies categorized by alpha letters A through J (Fig. 11–5). Basic benefits are found in policy A. Each subsequent letter represents basic benefits plus other coverage, with the most comprehensive benefits in Policy J. Sale of all policies are not available in all states, so individuals in some states have fewer options than others.

A slightly different variation of a Medigap policy is *Medicare Select*. This policy has the same coverage as regular Medigap policies, but there is a restriction in that the beneficiary must obtain medical care from a list of specified network doctors and providers.

TEN MEDIGAP STANDARDIZED POLICIES

(Not all may be available in all states.)

A	B	C	D	E	F	G	H	I	J
Basic Benefit	Basic Benefit	Basic Benefit	Basic Benefit	Basic Benefit	Basic Benefit	Basic Benefit	Basic Benefit	Basic Benefit	Basic Benefit
		Skilled Nursing Coinsurance	Skilled Nursing Coinsurance	Skilled Nursing Coinsurance	Skilled Nursing Coinsurance	Skilled Nursing Coinsurance	Skilled Nursing Coinsurance	Skilled Nursing Coinsurance	Skilled Nursing Coinsurance
	Part A Deductible	Part A Deductible	Part A Deductible	Part A Deductible	Part A Deductible	Part A Deductible	Part A Deductible	Part A Deductible	Part A Deductible
		Part B Deductible			Part B Deductible				Part B Deductible
					Part B Excess 100%	Part B Excess 100%		Part B Excess 100%	Part B Excess 100%
		Foreign Travel Emergency	Foreign Travel Emergency	Foreign Travel Emergency	Foreign Travel Emergency	Foreign Travel Emergency	Foreign Travel Emergency	Foreign Travel Emergency	Foreign Travel Emergency
			At-Home Recovery			At-Home Recovery		At-Home Recovery	At-Home Recovery
							Basic Drug Benefit ($1250 Limit)	Basic Drug Benefit ($1250 Limit)	Extended Drug Benefit ($3000 Limit)
				Preventive Care					Preventive Care

Figure 11–5. Ten Medigap standardized policies.

Medicare Secondary Payer

In some instances, Medicare is considered secondary and classifies the situation as **Medicare Secondary Payer (MSP).** Follow the suggested steps in the next procedure to identify whether Medicare is primary or secondary and know what additional benefits the patient might have.

> **PROCEDURE: Determining if Medicare Is Primary or Secondary and Determining Additional Benefits**

1. Inquire whether the patient is covered under one or more of the following plans or situations:
   ▶ *Automobile liability insurance, no-fault insurance, and self-insured liability insurance.* An individual injured or ill because of an automobile accident may be covered by liability insurance or no-fault insurance.
   ▶ *Disability insurance.* Disability insurance coverage offered through an employer-sponsored large group health plan (LGHP).
   ▶ *Employee group health plan (EGHP).* Insurance policies for individuals aged 65 years or older who are still employed. Employers with 20 or more employees are required to offer workers and their spouses aged 65 through 69 the same health benefits offered to younger workers. Workers may accept or reject the employer's health insurance plan. If they accept it, Medicare becomes the secondary insurance carrier.
   ▶ *Employer supplemental insurance.* A Medicare beneficiary has this plan through a former employer. Some people are covered by employment plans even after retirement, provided the plan allows it and the insured informs the insurance company he or she wishes to maintain coverage. Benefits can vary in these supplemental plans, and these policies are not considered "Medigap" as defined by federal law. *Note:* When an employee retires and Medicare becomes the primary coverage, the company's group health plan coordinates

benefits with Medicare. These are known as conversion policies.

▶ *Federal Black Lung Act.* An act was formed to cover employees or former coal miner employees who have illness related to black lung disorder and have acceptable diagnoses that occur on the Department of Labor's list.

▶ *Veterans Affairs (VA).* A Medicare beneficiary is also receiving benefits from the Department of Veterans Affairs. In this situation, there must be a decision made as to where to send the claim. Medicare is not secondary to the VA and the VA is not secondary to Medicare. The claim is sent where specified by the patient. The claim can be sent to Medicare, where, if the claim is processed, the patient must satisfy his or her contractual requirement to pay any deductible and copayment amounts. If the patient asks that the claim be sent to the VA instead of Medicare, the claim is processed and any payments issued are considered as payment in full. Many veterans want the claim sent to the VA.

▶ *Workers' compensation.* An individual suffers a disease or injury connected with employment.

▶ These plans are billed as **primary** (first) **payer** and Medicare second. Payments for these types of policies may not necessarily go to the physician but may go to the insured.

2. Ask to see the Medicare card, as well as any other insurance cards, and make photocopies of both sides of each card.

3. Inquire from the patient whether the supplemental coverage was carried over (conversion policy) from his or her employer.

4. Call the carrier if the type of plan is not clearly identified.

5. Bill the correct insurance plan.

▶ For Medigap cases, nonparticipating physicians may collect copayments and deductibles up to their limiting charge (unless the state forbids collection of more than the allowed amount) from patients at the time of service. Participating physicians may not collect copayments/deductibles from patients covered by Medigap if the patient requests the physician to submit the claim to the Medigap insurer. Collect copayments after receiving the Medicare/Medigap RA document.

▶ For other secondary insurance, write the patient's group and policy (or certificate) numbers on the Medicare RA, attach it to a copy of the original Health Insurance Claim Form CMS-1500, and submit it to the secondary carrier. Then copy the physician's billing statement showing date of treatment, description of service(s) rendered, fees, and diagnosis.

Managed Care and Medicare

When a patient's primary insurance is a managed care plan that requires fixed copayments, it is possible to obtain reimbursement from Medicare for those amounts. An assigned MSP claim must be filed with Medicare after the MCO has paid. When Medicare's copayment reimbursement has been received, the provider must refund to the patient the copayment amount previously collected.

The practice is paid a capitated amount, and there will be no Explanation of Benefits (EOB) document. Have the patient sign a statement that explains the situation. Attach the statement and the copayment receipts to the claim. The statement may read as shown in the following box:

Patient Name _____
Medicare Number _____
There is no Explanation of Benefits documentation available for the attached billed services. I am currently enrolled with _____ managed care plan for my health care. My physician, _____ MD, is paid on a capitated basis, and the copayment that I pay is $ _____, for each service or visit.
Patient's signature _____
Date _____

A nonparticipating physician must file an unassigned MSP claim. The patient is directly reimbursed by Medicare, and no refund is necessary.

Automobile or Liability Insurance Coverage

Liability insurance is not secondary to Medicare because there is no contractual relationship between the injured party and third-party payer. A physician who treats a Medicare patient who has filed a liability claim must bill the liability insurer first *unless* the insurer will not pay promptly (e.g., within 120 days after the liability insurance claim is filed). After 120 days have gone by without a payment from the liability insurer and if the services performed are covered Medicare benefits, a par or nonpar physician may seek conditional payment from Medicare. However, if a claim is filed with Medicare, the provider must drop the claim against the liability insurer.

If the payment made by the liability insurer is less than the physician's full charge, the physician may file an assigned claim and must accept as full payment the greater of either the Medicare-approved charge or sum of the liability insurance primary payment and the Medicare secondary payment.

A nonpar physician may file an unassigned claim for Medicare secondary payment only if the payment by the liability insurer is less than the Medicare limiting charge. If the payment equals or exceeds the limiting charge, the physician must accept the disbursement as full payment.

If Medicare payments have been made but should not have been because the services are excluded under this provision, or if the payments were made on a conditional basis, they are subject to recovery. A copy of the notice of payment or denial form from the other insurer should be included when sending in the CMS-1500 claim form. Medicare is secondary even if a state law or a private contract of insurance states that Medicare is primary. The physician must bill the other insurer first. A claim for secondary benefits may be submitted to Medicare only after payment or denial has been made by the primary coverage. Liability insurance is not considered a Medicare secondary payer.

Medicare Managed Care Plans

Health Maintenance Organizations

During the spring of 1984 the Department of Health and Human Services published regulations giving Medicare enrollees the right to join and assign their Medicare benefits to HMOs. HMOs had been in operation for nearly 50 years when they became available as an option for Medicare enrollees. With a Medicare HMO (also known as a senior HMO or senior plan), the patient does not need a Medicare supplemental insurance plan. Upon enrollment the Medicare beneficiary is sent an insurance card from the managed care plan (Fig. 11–6). However, Medicare cards are not forfeited and an elderly patient may show two cards, leading to confusion about what the coverage is and who to bill.

Medicare makes payments directly to the HMO on a monthly basis for Medicare enrollees who use the HMO option. Enrollees pay the HMO a monthly premium, which is an estimate of the coinsurance amounts for which the enrollee would be responsible plus the Medicare deductible. It appears that HMOs contracting to provide services for Medicare patients will be converted to a Medicare + Choice plan as their contract renewal dates come up.

Some HMOs provide services not usually covered by Medicare, such as eyeglasses, prescription drugs, and routine physical examinations. Once a person has converted from Medicare to an HMO, he or she cannot go back to a former physician of personal choice and expect Medicare to pay the bill. The patient should receive services from a physician and hospital facility that are contracted with the HMO plan.

If a Medicare patient has switched over to a managed care plan and wishes to disenroll, the patient must do the following:

1. Notify the plan in writing of disenrollment.
2. Complete Medicare form Medicare Managed Care Disenrollment CMS-566, attach a copy of the disenrollment letter, and take it to the Social Security office.

Many plans allow the patient to enroll and disenroll at any time during the year. It may take the plan 30 days for disenrollment, and Medicare may take as long as 60 days to reenroll a patient. Patients who disenroll may have to requalify for supplemental coverage at a higher cost.

There are two types of HMO plans that may have Medicare Part B contracts: HMO risk plans and HMO cost plans.

Risk Plan

As a condition of enrollment in an HMO risk plan, beneficiaries receive Medicare-covered services (except emergency, urgent need, and prior authorized services) only from providers who are contracted members of the HMO network. Enrollees of HMO risk plans are referred to as "restricted" beneficiaries. Usually services rendered by "out-of-plan" physicians are not covered when the same services are available through the organization unless a referral or prior authorization is obtained. The only exception is for emergency care. Claims for HMO risk plan beneficiaries must be sent directly to the organization.

A system of Medicare reimbursement for HMOs with risk contracts is called **diagnostic cost groups (DCGs).** The HMO enrollees are classified into various DCGs on the basis of each beneficiary's prior

---

Health America Senior
Offered by CarePlus

I.D. NUMBER   04865-01 LAC

MEMBER SINCE: 04/01/95

NAME: TOWNGATE, IRENE B.

MEDICAL   COLLEGE CLINIC
$3   (555) 486-9002

DENTAL   MASROUR-RAD, GUSTAVA
$5   (555) 884-4224

$20 ER
RX YES

BASIC

Figure 11–6. A senior managed care plan card.

12-month history of hospitalization, and payments are adjusted accordingly. This payment system does not apply to disabled and hospice patients, those on renal dialysis, or those enrolled only in Medicare Part B. Patients are reclassified each year according to their previous year's use of hospital service.

Cost Plan

Under an HMO cost plan, beneficiaries receive Medicare-covered services from sources in or outside of the HMO network. Enrollees are referred to as "unrestricted" beneficiaries. Claims for cost plan beneficiaries may be sent to the HMO plan or the regular Medicare carrier.

Noncontract Physician

If a noncontract physician treats a Medicare HMO patient, the services are considered "out-of-plan" services. The claim must be submitted to the managed care plan, which will determine whether it is responsible to pay for the services. Conditions that must be met follow:

1. The service was an emergency and the patient was not able to get to an HMO facility or member physician (patient was out of the HMO area).
2. The service was covered by Medicare.
3. The service was medically necessary.
4. The service was prior authorized or an approved referral.

The patient is responsible for the fee if the HMO determines there was no emergency and denies payment. The HMO reimburses according to the Medicare Fee Schedule Allowable Amount, so the physician cannot bill the patient for the balance. If the physician does not receive 100% of the allowable, steps must be taken through the HMO's appeals process. If this fails, contact the Medicare Managed Care Department at the Medicare Regional CMS Operations Office. Denied services can be billed to the patient (no more than the Medicare fee schedule or limiting charge) after the HMO EOB is received.

Carrier Dealing Prepayment Organization

A Carrier Dealing Prepayment Organization may be set up by a medical practice under contract to the government. Such plans are considered a service contract rather than insurance. In the past, such plans were run by HMOs, but now practices of 12 to 15 physicians are opting to run their own plans. These organizations must be incorporated and have their own Medicare provider number. The organization must furnish physicians' services through employees and partners or under formal arrangement with medical groups, independent practice

associations, or individual physicians. Part B services must be provided through qualified hospitals or physicians. When operating this type of organization, the physician accepts Medicare assignment and agrees to deal with the Medicare carrier instead of CMS. Patients sign a contract agreeing to pay a monthly fee (usually $20 to $25). This is supposed to cover all Medicare copayments, deductibles, and nonreimbursable expenses (annual physical examinations and preventive care). The patient is not responsible to pay for noncovered services.

Utilization and Quality Control

Peer Review Organization

A **peer review organization (PRO)** is a state-based group of physicians working under government guidelines reviewing cases for hospital admission and discharge, extended stay, or extended services. The PRO evaluates physicians on the quality and appropriateness of professional care and settles fee disputes. It is involved in implementing a quality of improvement plan using statistical data. Case reviews focus on admission and discharge, invasive procedures, documentation, extraordinarily high costs (outlier costs), and limitation of liability determinations.

CMS has assigned a point system for medical documentation as discussed in Chapter 3. If sufficient points are lacking, penalties can lead to fines or forfeiture of the physician's license. Therefore it is extremely important that each patient's care be well documented from the treatment standpoint, as well as for justifying maximum reimbursement. A physician who receives a letter from a PRO about quality of care should consult his or her attorney before responding by letter or personal appeal. A photocopy of the patient's medical record can be used to substantiate the claim if there is detailed clinical documentation.

Federal False Claims Amendment Act

Another federal law to prevent overuse of services and to spot Medicare fraud is the Federal Claims Amendment Act of 1986. This act offers financial incentives of 15% to 25% of any judgment to informants who report physicians suspected of defrauding the federal government. This is called a *qui tam* **action.** The laws are intended to help catch Medicare and Medicaid cheaters. The health insurance companies that process Medicare claims have a Medicare fraud unit whose job is to catch people who steal from Medicare. The Office of the Inspector General (OIG), Department of Health and Human Services, is the law enforcement agency that investigates and prosecutes people who steal from Medicare. The OIG works closely with Medicare insurance companies, the Federal Bureau of Investigation (FBI), the Postal Inspection Service, and other federal law enforcement agencies. If the physician is on an optical disk retrieval (ODR) A-1000 system, it is possible for the OIG to obtain procedure codes that show comparison billing with peers in the area. The Centers for Medicaid and Medicare Services alerts offices of whom to investigate.

For information on fraud and abuse, see Chapter 1, Box 1–1 and Box 1–2. See Chapter 14 for information about fraud in the workers' compensation program.

HIPAA Compliance Alert

Medicare Billing Compliance Issues

Because Medicare is a federal program, legislation sets down the policies that must be followed. Therefore whoever participates in the program must comply with all the regulations. The following four sections are marked for emphasis about billing issues about which medical practices should be aware. These may include but are not limited to:

▶ Release of medical information
▶ Reassignment of payment
▶ Limiting charges for nonparticipating providers
▶ Correct procedural code assignment and service utilization
▶ Accurate diagnostic code assignment
▶ Medical necessity of services performed
▶ Billing for ancillary employees (physician assistants and nurse practitioners) called "incident to" billing
▶ Documentation related to selection of procedural codes for services performed
▶ Ancillary orders and supervision requirements
▶ Teaching physician and resident billing
▶ Routine waiver of copayments, deductibles, or professional courtesy discounts
▶ Stark I and II antireferral and compensation regulations
▶ Credit balance refunds
▶ Correct coding initiative edits

Health Insurance Portability and Accountability Act

The Health Insurance Portability and Accountability Act of 1996 (HIPAA) has a section that deals with prevention of health care fraud and abuse of patients on Medicare and Medicaid. Insurance billing specialists, coders, physicians, and any individuals who knowingly and willfully break the law could suffer a penalty or fine, imprisonment, or both. Civil monetary penalties are assessed for the following:

▶ Intentional incorrect coding that will result in greater payment than appropriate
▶ A pattern of claims being submitted for a service or product that is not medically necessary
▶ Offering remuneration to induce an individual to order from a particular provider or supplier who receives Medicare or state health funds

The federal criminal sanctions of this act are established for those who

▶ Knowingly or willfully defraud a health care program
▶ Knowingly embezzle, steal, or misapply a health care benefit program

Civil Monetary Penalties Law

In 1983 the federal government passed the Civil Monetary Penalties Law (CMPL) to prosecute cases of Medicare and Medicaid fraud. The law carries three separate forms of sanction:

1. A penalty of up to $2000 for each item or service wrongfully listed in a payment request to Medicare or Medicaid
2. An assessment of up to twice the total amount improperly claimed
3. Suspension from the programs for whatever period the Department of Health and Human Services determines

A physician may be penalized when participating in the following violations:

▶ Billing more than once for the same service to obtain greater reimbursement
▶ Billing for services that were not provided
▶ Fragmenting billed services that could be described accurately by one procedural code
▶ Upgrading the reported level or complexity of services, more than those services actually furnished to obtain greater reimbursement

A physician who fails to practice due care to ensure the accuracy of Medicare and Medicaid claims prepared in his or her office risks enormous financial penalties. The CMPL makes no distinction between outright fraud and negligence in billing. Therefore if an employee submits billings that the physician knows nothing about, the physician may be held liable. Reckless disregard of federal and state regulations by the insurance billing specialist can affect the way claims are submitted and possibly cause a physician to incur a civil monetary penalty. Incorrectly coded procedures can affect the penalties imposed on a physician.

The insurance billing specialist should periodically attend Medicare and Medicaid training workshops to keep up-to-date and gain a better understanding of federal and state government claim requirements. Medicare and Medicaid manuals and bulletins should be kept up-to-date and accessible for quick reference. Keep documentation to support claims submission in the event of an audit. If a record is missing, make a written note that it has been lost or destroyed because it might be presumed that the physician deliberately destroyed the documents to conceal evidence. If a billing error is discovered after a claim submission or an overpayment is received, notify the fiscal agent or insurance carrier immediately.

Always document any meetings with representatives of the fiscal agent or state welfare department and include the advice given. If the advice later proves to be erroneous, such records can support the physician's good faith. The Office of the Inspector General of the Department of Health and Human Services and each state's Medicaid fraud control unit investigates violations. Notify the physician's attorney if the physician is advised that he or she is being investigated. Documents should be released only after the attorney's approval. Retain photocopies of all documents given to the investigator.

Stark I and II Regulations: Physician Self-Referrals

Stark I went into effect on January 1, 1992, but the regulations included in this federal legislation were not followed until they were published in 1995. This law prohibits a physician or a member of his or her family from referring patients to a laboratory if the physician has a financial relationship with that facility. Clinical laboratories must submit financial information to the CMS, including the names and identification numbers of physicians who hold a financial interest in the business. Stark II, an amendment, took effect on January 1, 1995, and expanded these regulations by prohibiting Medicare and Medicaid payments for treatment that results from the referral of a patient by a physician (or immediate family member of the physician) who has a financial relationship (ownership interest or compensatory arrangement) with providers of designated health services. It also prohibits the provider from billing for the designated health service. These services include the following:

▶ Clinical laboratory services
▶ Durable medical equipment and supplies
▶ Home health services

▶ Inpatient and outpatient hospital services
▶ Occupational therapy services
▶ Outpatient prescription drugs
▶ Parenteral and enteral nutrients, related equipment, and supplies
▶ Physical therapy services
▶ Prosthetics, orthotics, and prosthetic devices and supplies
▶ Radiation therapy services and supplies
▶ Radiology services, including magnetic resonance imaging, computed tomography, and ultrasound services

Many states have passed laws and administrative rules that may apply the same principles to other private payers. Uncovered self-referral deceits or failure of a laboratory to report financial information can lead to hefty fines, sanctions, payment denials, and exclusion from the Medicare/Medicaid programs by the Office of the Inspector General, Department of Health and Human Services. There are some general exceptions related to ownership or investment and compensation arrangements, so obtain a complete description of this legislation for proper compliance.

Clinical Laboratory Improvement Amendment

The CLIA of 1988 established federal standards, quality control, and safety measures for all freestanding laboratories, including physician laboratories. Various laboratory procedures fall within CLIA categories depending on the complexity of each test. Each category level requires a yearly licensing fee to be paid by the physician. A certificate is then issued and must be posted in the laboratory. Various levels of quality control measures are necessary for each CLIA level and must be performed in a timely manner (e.g., daily or weekly). Fines may be levied if federal standards are not maintained. This has had an impact on office laboratories; because of the strict requirements, many physicians send patients to independent laboratories for tests (e.g., blood cell counts, cytology specimens, and cultures). However, some physicians prefer to draw blood from a patient, particularly if the patient has a history of difficult venous access.

When claims to Medicare fiscal intermediaries are submitted for laboratory services performed in the physician's office, the 10-digit CLIA certificate number should be entered in Block 23 of the CMS-1500 claim form (Fig. 11–7). Physicians billing patients for outside laboratory work are not held to these standards but may charge the patient only what the laboratory charges (based on a fee schedule), plus any additional services the physician provides

Figure 11-7. Section of the CMS-1500 claim form with Block 23 emphasized indicating where to insert a certificate number for laboratory services (CLIA No.) or a prior authorization number for a procedure when permission has been granted.

(e.g., drawing, handling, shipping, and interpretation of the blood or office visit).

Payment Fundamentals

Provider

Participating Physician

In a **participating physician (par)** agreement, a physician agrees to accept payment from Medicare (80% of the **approved charges**) plus payment from the patient (20% of approved charge) after the $100 deductible has been met (Fig. 11-8). The Medicare annual deductible is based on the calendar year, January 1 through December 31. This agreement is referred to as accepting **assignment.** The physician must complete and submit the CMS-1500 claim form to the fiscal intermediary. The assignment of benefits, Block 12, is signed by the patient, the physician indicates that assignment is being accepted by checking "Yes" in Block 27, and the payment goes directly to the physician (Fig. 11-9). Physicians, practitioners, and suppliers who fail to submit claims are subject to civil monetary penalties up to $2500 for each claim.

Nonparticipating Physician

A **nonparticipating physician (nonpar)** does not have a signed agreement with Medicare and has an option about assignment. The physician may decline assignment for all services or accept assignment for some services and collect from the patient for other services performed at the same time and place. An exception to this policy is mandatory assignment for clinical laboratory tests and services by physician assistants.

Nonpar physicians receive only 95% of the Medicare-approved amount. Nonpar physicians may decide on a case-by-case basis whether to accept assignment. If the nonpar physician accepts assignment for a claim, Medicare pays 80% of the nonpar Medicare-approved amount directly to the physician and the physician collects the remaining 20% from the patient. If the nonpar physician does not take assignment on a particular claim, he or she may balance bill the patient 115% of the nonpar rate because Medicare will send the payment to the patient. For example, if the nonpar rate is $100, the provider can balance bill the patient for $115. However, in this case even though the physician is required to submit the claim to Medicare, the carrier pays the patient directly and the physician therefore must collect his or her entire fee from the patient; thus physicians must "chase the money." Consequently, physicians should evaluate whether the ability to balance bill and collect a higher fee from the patient is worth the potential extra billing and collection costs. Furthermore, some hospitals and states—including Minnesota, Pennsylvania, Vermont, and New York—prohibit or limit balance billing, so physicians must ascertain whether or not these restrictions apply before making a Medicare participation or nonparticipation decision.

Limiting charge is a percentage limit on fees, specified by legislation, that nonpar physicians may bill Medicare beneficiaries above the allowed amount. Nonpar physicians may submit usual and customary fees for assigned claims. Because of these two situations, nonpar physicians usually maintain two fee schedules, one with usual fees and one with

PAYMENT EXAMPLES

	Actual charge	Medicare approved amount*	Deductible	Medicare pays	Beneficiary responsible for	Medicare courtesy adjustment**
Doctor A accepts assignment	$480	$400	$100 already satisfied	$320 (80% of approved amount)	$80 (20% of approved amount)	$80 (difference between actual charge and approved amount)
Doctor B does not accept assignment and charges the limiting amount	$437	$380	$100 already satisfied	$304 (80% of approved amount)	$133 (20% of approved amount [$76] plus difference between limiting charge [actual charge] and approved amount [$57] = $133)	None
Doctor C accepts assignment; however, the patient has not met the deductible amount	$480	$300 ($400 minus the deductible)	$100 has not been met	$200 (80% of approved amount determined after subtracting the deductible)	$60 (20% of approved amount determined after subtracting the deductible)	$80 (difference between actual charge and approved amount)

* The Medicare approved amount is less for nonparticipating physicians than for participating physicians.
** The courtesy adjustment is the amount credited to the patient's account in the adjustment column. The word "courtesy" implies that Medicare patients are treated well and is preferred to phrases like "not allowed."

Figure 11–8. Payment examples for three physicians showing a physician accepting assignment versus not accepting assignment, and the amounts the patient is responsible for paying with deductible satisfied and not met.

limiting charges. Some states have set limiting charges that are more restrictive than Medicare policies. These states are Connecticut, Massachusetts, New York, Ohio, Pennsylvania, Rhode Island, and Vermont. Inquire from the fiscal intermediary of those states for guidelines.

Prior Authorization

Many insurance carrier group plans and MCO senior plans require prior authorization for surgical procedures, diagnostic testing, and referrals to specialists. Some of these procedures requiring authorization are on a mandatory list, whereas others are chosen by the regional carrier. The mandatory list is composed of such procedures as:

▶ Bunionectomy
▶ Carotid endarterectomy
▶ Cataract extractions
▶ Cholecystectomy
▶ Complex peripheral revascularization
▶ Coronary artery bypass graft surgery
▶ Hysterectomy
▶ Inguinal hernia repair
▶ Joint replacements (hip, shoulder, or knee)
▶ Transurethral prostatectomy

Carriers may have a toll-free line to call for authorization, require the completion of a preauthorization form, or require a letter only if there is a dispute over claims payment. Check with the local carrier on its policy for preauthorization.

The prior authorization number is used when billing the Medicare carrier and is entered on the CMS-1500 claim form in Block 23 (Fig. 11–7). If the procedure is not approved, the carrier sends a denial to the physician, patient, and hospital, if applicable. If the procedure is done as an emergency, notify the carrier within the time frame designated by the insurance plan so an authorization can be arranged.

Waiver of Liability Provision

Limited Liability

When a patient is to receive a service from a participating physician that might be denied for **medical necessity** or because of *limitation of liability* by Medicare, inform the patient and have him or her agree to pay for the denied service in advance. If the Medicare guidelines or parameters are not known for a certain procedure or service, refer to Medicare bulletins or call the Medicare carrier and ask. Instruct the patient to sign an **advance beneficiary notice (ABN),** also known as a waiver of liability agreement or responsibility statement, as shown in Figures 11–10 and 11–11. This form should not be given to someone who is in a medical emergency, confused, legally incompetent, or otherwise under great duress. It cannot be signed after a patient has

PLEASE
DO NOT
STAPLE
IN THIS
AREA

APPROVED OMB-0938-008

CARRIER

| | PICA | **HEALTH INSURANCE CLAIM FORM** | PICA | |

1. ☐ MEDICARE (Medicare #) ☐ MEDICAID (Medicaid #) ☐ CHAMPUS (Sponsor's SSN) ☐ CHAMPVA (VA File #) ☐ GROUP HEALTH PLAN (SSN or ID) ☐ FECA BLK LUNG (SSN) ☐ OTHER (ID)   1a. INSURED'S I.D. NUMBER   (FOR PROGRAM IN ITEM 1)

2. PATIENT'S NAME (Last Name, First Name, Middle Initial)

3. PATIENT'S BIRTH DATE MM DD YY   SEX M ☐ F ☐

4. INSURED'S NAME (Last Name, First Name, Middle Initial)

5. PATIENT'S ADDRESS (No., Street)

6. PATIENT RELATIONSHIP TO INSURED   Self ☐ Spouse ☐ Child ☐ Other ☐

7. INSURED'S ADDRESS (No., Street)

CITY   STATE

8. PATIENT STATUS   Single ☐ Married ☐ Other ☐   Employed ☐ Full-Time Student ☐ Part-Time Student ☐

CITY   STATE

ZIP CODE   TELEPHONE (Include Area Code) (   )

ZIP CODE   TELEPHONE (Include Area Code) (   )

9. OTHER INSURED'S NAME (Last Name, First Name, Middle Initial)

10. IS PATIENT'S CONDITION RELATED TO:

11. INSURED'S POLICY GROUP OR FECA NUMBER

a. OTHER INSURED'S POLICY OR GROUP NUMBER

a. EMPLOYMENT? (CURRENT OR PREVIOUS) ☐ YES ☐ NO

a. INSURED'S DATE OF BIRTH MM DD YY   SEX M ☐ F ☐

b. OTHER INSURED'S DATE OF BIRTH MM DD YY   SEX M ☐ F ☐

b. AUTO ACCIDENT?   PLACE (State) ☐ YES ☐ NO

b. EMPLOYER'S NAME OR SCHOOL NAME

c. EMPLOYER'S NAME OR SCHOOL NAME

c. OTHER ACCIDENT? ☐ YES ☐ NO

c. INSURANCE PLAN NAME OR PROGRAM NAME

d. INSURANCE PLAN NAME OR PROGRAM NAME

10d. RESERVED FOR LOCAL USE

d. IS THERE ANOTHER HEALTH BENEFIT PLAN? ☐ YES ☐ NO   If yes, return to and complete item 9 a-d.

PATIENT AND INSURED INFORMATION

READ BACK OF FORM BEFORE COMPLETING & SIGNING THIS FORM.

12. PATIENT'S OR AUTHORIZED PERSON'S SIGNATURE I authorize the release of any medical or other information necessary to process this claim. I also request payment of government benefits either to myself or to the party who accepts assignment below.

SIGNED *SOF*   DATE

13. INSURED'S OR AUTHORIZED PERSON'S SIGNATURE I authorize payment of medical benefits to the undersigned physician or supplier for services described below.

SIGNED

14. DATE OF CURRENT: ILLNESS (First symptom) OR INJURY (Accident) OR PREGNANCY (LMP) MM DD YY

15. IF PATIENT HAS HAD SAME OR SIMILAR ILLNESS. GIVE FIRST DATE MM DD YY

16. DATES PATIENT UNABLE TO WORK IN CURRENT OCCUPATION FROM MM DD YY TO MM DD YY

17. NAME OF REFERRING PHYSICIAN OR OTHER SOURCE

17a. I.D. NUMBER OF REFERRING PHYSICIAN

18. HOSPITALIZATION DATES RELATED TO CURRENT SERVICES FROM MM DD YY TO MM DD YY

19. RESERVED FOR LOCAL USE

20. OUTSIDE LAB? ☐ YES ☐ NO $ CHARGES

21. DIAGNOSIS OR NATURE OF ILLNESS OR INJURY. (RELATE ITEMS 1,2,3 OR 4 TO ITEM 24E BY LINE)

1. ___   3. ___   2. ___   4. ___

22. MEDICAID RESUBMISSION CODE   ORIGINAL REF. NO.

23. PRIOR AUTHORIZATION NUMBER

24. A DATE(S) OF SERVICE From MM DD YY To MM DD YY	B Place of Service	C Type of Service	D PROCEDURES, SERVICES, OR SUPPLIES (Explain Unusual Circumstances) CPT/HCPCS	MODIFIER	E DIAGNOSIS CODE	F $ CHARGES	G DAYS OR UNITS	H EPSDT Family Plan	I EMG	J COB	K RESERVED FOR LOCAL USE
1											
2											
3											
4											
5											
6											

PHYSICIAN OR SUPPLIER INFORMATION

25. FEDERAL TAX I.D. NUMBER   ☐ SSN ☐ EIN

26. PATIENT'S ACCOUNT NO.

27. ACCEPT ASSIGNMENT? (For govt. claims, see back) ☒ YES ☐ NO

28. TOTAL CHARGE $

29. AMOUNT PAID $

30. BALANCE DUE $

31. SIGNATURE OF PHYSICIAN OR SUPPLIER INCLUDING DEGREES OR CREDENTIALS (I certify that the statements on the reverse apply to this bill and are made a part thereof.)

SIGNED   DATE

32. NAME AND ADDRESS OF FACILITY WHERE SERVICES WERE RENDERED (If other than home or office)

33. PHYSICIAN'S, SUPPLIER'S BILLING NAME, ADDRESS, ZIP CODE & PHONE #

PIN#   GRP#

(APPROVED BY AMA COUNCIL ON MEDICAL SERVICE 8/88)

FORM HCFA-1500 (12-90)
FORM OWCP-1500   FORM RRB-1500

Figure 11–9. Block 12 of the CMS-1500 claim form where the patient signs authorizing payment to be sent to the physician and Block 27 marked with an X showing that the physician accepts Medicare assignment of benefits.

received the service and must specifically state what service or procedure is being waived.

Obtain guidance from the insurance carrier when in doubt about using an ABN form. An office policy should be in place for handling patients who refuse to sign an ABN. When sending in a claim, the HCPCS Level II modifier -GA (waiver of liability on file) must be added to pertinent codes to indicate a patient has signed the waiver. The Medicare carrier then informs the patient that he or she is responsible for the fee. Keep this signed waiver with other patient financial documents and not with the patient's medical record.

If the service was not reasonable because of Medicare guidelines but the patient thought it was covered and there is no advance notice given with signed waiver of liability agreement, then:

▶ Medicare or the patient cannot be collected from.

Patient Name: *Mary Judd*   Medicare # (HICN): 432XX1234

ADVANCE BENEFICIARY NOTICE (ABN)

Note: You need to make a choice about receiving these health care items or services.

We expect that Medicare will not pay for the item(s) or service(s) that are described below. Medicare does not pay for all of your health care costs. Medicare only pays for covered items and services when Medicare rules are met. The fact that Medicare may not pay for a particular item or service does not mean that you should not receive it. There may be a good reason your doctor recommended it. Right now, in your case, **Medicare probably will not pay for –**

Items or Services: *B12 injections*

Because: *Medicare does not usually pay for this injection or this many injections.*

The purpose of this form is to help you to make an informed choice about whether or not you want to receive these items or services, knowing that you might have to pay for them yourself.
Before you make a decision about your options, you should **read this entire notice carefully.**
● Ask us to explain, if you don't understand why Medicare probably won't pay.
● Ask us how much these items or services will cost you (**Estimated Cost**: $35.00   ),
   in case you have to pay for them yourself or through other insurance.

PLEASE CHOOSE **ONE** OPTION. CHECK **ONE** BOX. **SIGN & DATE** YOUR CHOICE.

☒ **Option 1. YES.   I want receive these items or services.**
I understand that Medicare will not decide whether to pay unless I receive these items or services. Please submit my claim to Medicare. I understand that you may bill me for items or services and that I may have to pay the bill while Medicare is making its decision.
If Medicare does pay, you will refund to me any payments I made to you that are due to me.
If Medicare denies payment, I agree to be personally and fully responsible for payment.
That is, I will pay personally, either out of pocket or through any other insurance that I have.
I understand I can appeal Medicare's decison.

☐ **Option 2. NO.   I have decided not to receive these items or services.**
I will not receive these items or services. I understand that you will not be able to submit a claim to Medicare and that I will not be able to appeal your opinion that Medicare will not pay.

March 20, 20XX   *Mary Judd*
Date   Signature of patient or person acting on patient's behalf

NOTE: Your health information will be kept confidential. Any information that we collect about you on this form will be kept confidential in our offices. If a claim is submitted to Medicare, your health information on this form may be shared with Medicare. Your health information, which Medicare sees, will be kept confidential by Medicare.

OMB Approval No. 0938-0566   Form No. CMS-R-131-G   (June 2002)

Figure 11–10. Advance Beneficiary Notice, which is also known as a responsibility statement or waiver of liability agreement.

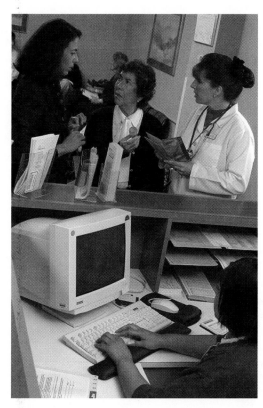

Figure 11-11. Insurance billing specialist instructing an elderly patient to sign an Advance Notice Medicare Beneficiary Waiver of Liability Agreement for services not covered.

▶ The patient does not have to pay the deductible or coinsurance.

▶ The patient is refunded any amount paid to the provider on the item or service.

If assignment is accepted and the physician and patient thought the service was covered under reasonable assumptions, then:

▶ Medicare is billed to pay for the service.

▶ The patient must pay the deductible and co-insurance.

▶ Medicare will not seek a refund of money already paid to the physician.

Nonparticipating providers must refund any amounts collected from the beneficiary when services are later found to be not reasonable and necessary.

Noncovered Services

Do not get confused with the issue of *noncovered* Medicare services because these may always be billed to the patient. Some physicians prefer to obtain a Waiver of Liability for noncovered services; however, it is not mandated. Services denied as inclusive of another service (a payment already made for the other service) are not considered a noncovered item and may not be billed to the patient. If a formal denial is necessary to bill the patient or another insurer, a claim should be sent with a letter attached stating the need for the denial to bill another payer; otherwise to bill for a non-covered service is inappropriate and may be viewed as fraud.

Elective Surgery Estimate

Effective October 1, 1987, under the Tax Reform Act, a nonparticipating physician who does not accept assignment for an *elective surgery* for which the actual charge will be $500 or more must provide the beneficiary with the following in writing: (1) the estimated fee for the procedure; (2) the estimated Medicare-approved allowance for the procedure; and (3) the difference in the physician's actual charge (limiting charge and the allowed amount) (Fig. 11-12). *Elective surgery* means a surgical procedure that can be scheduled in advance, is not an emergency, and is discretionary on the part of the physician and the patient. Failure to undergo elective surgery does not pose a mortality threat. Give a copy of the estimation letter to the Medicare patient and keep the original for the files. Document the patient's acknowledgment by obtaining his or her signature at the bottom of the letter.

Prepayment Screens

On some procedures, Medicare limits the number of times a given procedure can be billed during 1 year (e.g., four office visits per month or one treatment every 60 days for routine foot care). This is known as a Medicare Prepayment Screen. The screens or flags are computer triggers that suspend processing. These screens are used to identify and review claims for medical necessity and determine compliance with other appropriate criteria. The suspended claim is checked by a reviewer who decides if the services are medically necessary. If the patient previously submitted a claim for the procedure performed in the same year by another physician and has met the limit for the year, the claim will be downcoded or denied. Refer to the local Medicare fiscal agent's newsletters or bulletins or contact them for a complete list of the Medicare Prepayment Screens applicable locally.

To avoid problems, use good procedure code guidelines discussed in Chapter 5 and adhere to the following criteria.

▶ The level of service is appropriate to documentation.

▶ The procedure is accurate to the gender of the patient.

▶ The frequency is appropriate.

WORKSHEET FOR
ESTIMATED MEDICARE PAYMENT FOR ELECTIVE SURGERY

Worksheet

1. Physician's actual fee (limiting charge) $ 1248.03
2. Medicare approved or allowed amount $ 1085.24
3. Difference between physician's actual fee and
   Medicare approved or allowed amount   − 162.79
   (1 − 2 = 0)
4. Twenty percent coinsurance (0.20 × 2 = 0)   + 217.05
5. Beneficiary's out-of-pocket expense (3 + 4 + 0) $ 379.84
   Assume the $100 deductible has been met

Items 1, 2, and 5 must be included in the letter to the beneficiary

A

Beneficiary Letter

Dear Patient:

Because I do not accept assignment for elective surgery, Medicare requires that I give you certain information before surgery when my charges are $500 or more.

The following information concerns the surgery we have discussed. These estimates assume that you have already met the $100 deductible.

Type of surgery .....Osteotomy, proximal left tibia......

Limiting charge $ ....1248.03..........
Medicare estimated payment $ ....868.19...........
Patient's estimated payment $ ....379.84...........

This estimate is based upon our present expectations of what surgical procedure(s) will be required. Please remember that this is only an estimate of charges; we cannot be sure that additional procedures will or will not be necessary.

Sincerely,

John Doe, M.D.
Medicare Provider Number..........126XX5479..........

I understand the foregoing physician charges and my financial responsibility with respect to those estimated charges.

Patient's Signature.......... *Jane Doe*.......... Date.. 5-18-20XX..
                                                                    Jane Doe

B

Figure 11–12. A, Worksheet and, **B,** sample beneficiary letter for estimated Medicare payment for elective surgery.

▶ The diagnosis and procedure match.
▶ The provider has certification for performing services (e.g., laboratories).
▶ The fee is within the Medicare-approved charge.

Correct Coding Initiative

Medicare's **Correct Coding Initiative (CCI)** is implemented by CMS in an attempt to eliminate unbundling or other inappropriate reporting of Current Procedural Terminology (CPT) codes. Coding conflicts are picked up and claims are reviewed, suspended, or denied when conflicts occur. Software is available to give physicians, private insurance companies, and billing services access to the same government database used in auditing physicians for improper use of CPT codes.

Medicare Reimbursement

Chronology of Payment

For many years Medicare payments were based on reasonable fees (e.g., the amounts approved by the Medicare carrier [fiscal agents]). Medicare paid 80% of the approved charge. On October 1, 1983, an important development in the Medicare Part A program, the **prospective payment system (PPS),** became effective. Under the regulations enacted by the Social Security Amendments of 1983, hospitals treating Medicare patients are reimbursed according to preestablished rates for each type of illness treated based on diagnosis. Payments to hospitals for Medicare services are classified according to 503 diagnosis-related group (DRG) numbers. Beneficiaries (patients) cannot be billed beyond the preestablished DRG rate except for normal deductible and copayment amounts. (See Chapter 16 for an in-depth discussion of DRGs.)

In 1984 the Deficit Reduction Act established a participating physician program that offered incentives to participating physicians and froze the fees of nonparticipating physicians. The 1987 Omnibus Budget Reconciliation Act (OBRA) introduced the maximum allowable actual charge (MAAC) formula, which developed the maximum fee (limiting charge) a nonpar physician could charge Medicare patients for each service.

Reasonable Fee

Reasonable fee means the amount that Medicare participating providers agree to accept. It is listed on the RA, formerly known as the EOB, as an allowed (approved) charge for a procedure. This charge may be higher or lower than the fee the physician lists on the claim. When a physician accepts assignment, he or she may bill the patient only 20% of the Medicare-allowed charge. Charging for completion and submission of a claim form on an assignment claim violates the terms of the assignment. Interest fees cannot be assessed to Medicare patients. It is permissible to collect the deductible at the time of service, but the Medicare copayment should not be collected until Medicare pays.

Mandatory assignment laws have been adopted in several states, and legislation is under consideration and pending in many more states. These state laws would require physicians to accept the approved charge for their Medicare patients as a condition for being licensed to practice medicine in the state. Arkansas, Florida, Illinois, Maryland, Montana, and New Hampshire have rejected mandatory assignment proposals.

Resource-Based Relative Value Scale

A **resource-based relative value scale (RBRVS)** system was established as a means to redistribute Medicare dollars among physicians more equitably. This became the basis for physicians' payments nationwide for a 5-year phase-in that began on January 1, 1992. This system consists of a fee schedule based on relative values. The formula for obtaining relative value units is somewhat complex and involves a bit of mathematics in computing three components: a **relative value unit (RVU)** for the service, a geographic adjustment factor (GAF), and a monetary conversion factor (CF).

Relative value unit formula:
RVU × GAF × CF = Medicare $ per service

RVUs are based on the physician work RVU, the practice expense RVU, and the malpractice insurance RVU. To bring the fees in line for the region where the physician practices and to adjust for regional overhead and malpractice costs, each of the RVUs is adjusted for each Medicare local carrier by geographic practice cost indices (GPCIs), pronounced "gypsies."

A CF is used to convert a geographically adjusted relative value into a payment amount. This CF is updated to a new amount each year. Figure 11–13 provides an example of calculating payment for one procedure code.

The figures to work out this formula in the chart for each service are published annually in the Federal Register.

RVSs help when determining cost accounting because they take into account the practice expense,

Figure 11–13. Formula used to calculate the fee for a specific procedure using the Resource-Based Relative Value Scale system.

Code	Work	Overhead	Malpractice
RVUs	1.04	0.70	0.06
91000	× 1.028	× 1.258	× 1.370
GAF*	1.07 +	0.88 +	0.08 = Total adjusted RVUs, 2.03

For 2003, the Conversion Factor for nonsurgical care is $36.7856 × 2.03 = Allowed amount $74.67

* The medical practice location is Oakland, California.

TABLE 11–1	RBRVS Crosswalk						
A	**B**	**C**	**D**	**E**	**F**	**G**	**H**
Code	Code Description	RBRVS/RVUs	Conversion Factor	Fee	Contract Conversion Factor	Contract Fee	% Contract Payment
99212	Ofc Visit	0.68	72.06	$49	64.71	$44.00	90%

malpractice expense, work effort, and cost of living. They also are helpful when negotiating the best contract available with managed care plans; therefore office managers or individuals assisting physicians should know and understand RBRVS data. A crosswalk is an effective way to see how the practice may be affected by an RBRVS contract (Table 11–1). To develop one, make several columns using spreadsheet software. In column A, list common procedure codes used by the practice; column B, the code description; and column C, the RBRVS RVUs. Leave column D blank to insert a conversion factor. In column E, put in the present fee-for-service rate (rounded-out figure). Divide the fee in column E by column C to get the conversion factor. Leave a blank for column F to insert a conversion factor for the contract. List the managed care contract payment in column G. Divide column G by column C to get the conversion factor for column F. Then divide the plan's contract fee by the physician's fee for column H to work out the percentage being paid at the contract rate.

Medicare Fee Schedule

Beginning in 1996, each Medicare local carrier annually sends each physician a Medicare fee schedule for his or her area or region number listing three columns of figures: participating amount, nonparticipating amount, and limiting charge for each procedure code number. To see an example of this, refer to the Mock Fee Schedule shown in Appendix A of the *Student Workbook for the Insurance Handbook for the Medical Office.*

Healthcare Common Procedure Coding System (HCPCS)

As mentioned in Chapter 5, the federal government developed the Healthcare Common Procedure Coding System (HCPCS) for the Medicare program. To obtain correct payment for a procedure or service, a code number must be selected from Level I, II, or III of HCPCS coding system. When submitting a claim, be sure to use the Level II HCPCS **national alphanumeric codes** and modifiers rather than CPT procedure codes for certain appliances and procedures when

indicated. When billing CPT modifiers, a good reference is presented in Chapter 5, Table 5–4, as helpful hints in italics entitled "Medicare Payment Rule."

Claim Submission

Fiscal Intermediaries and Fiscal Agents

An organization handling claims from hospitals, NFs, **intermediate care facilities (ICFs),** long-term care facilities (LTCFs), and home health agencies is called a **fiscal intermediary (FI).** The National Blue Cross Association holds the fiscal intermediary contract for Medicare Part A; in turn it subcontracts it out to member agencies.

Organizations handling claims from physicians and other suppliers of services covered under Medicare Part B are called *carriers* or *fiscal agents.* Medicare Part B payments are handled by private insurance organizations under contract with the government. Since January 1, 1992, the rule for where to send a Medicare claim is to bill the carrier who covers the area where the service occurred or was furnished, *not* the carrier who services the physician's office.

See Appendix A for the name and address for claims submission in each state and to obtain further information about this program.

Provider Identification Numbers

Another requirement of the Tax Reform Act was the establishment of several types of identification numbers for each physician and nonphysician practitioner providing services paid by Medicare. Because there are so many numbers, they are easily confused and end up being the source of many errors when completing blocks on the CMS-1500 claim form. The numbers defined and shown in template examples with correct placement in Chapter 6 follow:

- Provider identification numbers (PINs); group and individual
- Unique physician identification numbers (UPINs)
- Performing physician identification number (PPINs)

College Clinic
4567 Broad Avenue
Woodland Hills, XY 12345-0001
Tel (555) 486-9002
Fax (555) 487-8976

LIFETIME BENEFICIARY CLAIM AUTHORIZATION AND INFORMATION RELEASE

Patient's
Name _____ Jane Doe _____ Medicare I.D. number _____ 540-XX-8755A _____

I request that payment of authorized Medicare benefits be made either to me or on my behalf to (name of physician/supplier) for any services furnished me by that physician/supplier. I authorize any holder of medical information about me to release to the Center for Medicare and Medicaid Services and its agents any information needed to determine these benefits or the benefits payable to related services.

I understand my signature requests that payment be made, and I consent to the release of medical information necessary to pay the claim. If other health insurance is indicated in Item 9 of the CMS-1500 claim form or elsewhere on other approved claim forms or electronically submitted claims, my signature authorizes release of the information to the insurer or agency shown. In Medicare assigned cases, the physician or supplier agrees to accept the allowed amount of the Medicare carrier as the full charge, and the patient is responsible only for the deductible, coinsurance, and noncovered services. Coinsurance is based upon the allowed amount of the Medicare carrier.

_____   _____
Patient's Signature   January 3, 20XX
                                                                                  Date

Figure 11–14. Lifetime Assignment of Benefits and Information Release.

▶ National provider identifier (NPI)
▶ Durable Medical Equipment (DME) supplier number

Patient's Signature Authorization

A Medicare patient's signature authorization for release of medical information and assignment of benefits to the insurance carrier is obtained in Block 12 of the CMS-1500 claim form. This block should be signed regardless of whether the physician is a participating or nonparticipating physician. The signed authorization should be kept on file in the patient's medical record for an episode of care or for a designated time frame (e.g., 1 year or lifetime). Subsequent claims may then indicate "Signature on file" or "SOF" in Block 12 of the claim form. The lifetime beneficiary claim authorization and information release form shown in Figure 11–14 is an example that can be used for assigned and nonassigned Medicare claims and kept in the patient's medical record. An original copy of a CMS-1500 claim form may be used to obtain a lifetime signature authorization. Write across the top of the form "Lifetime Signature Authorization" and file as just described. Further information on this topic may be found in Chapters 3 and 6.

Signature on file situations that may occur in a medical practice are the following:

▶ **Illiterate or physically handicapped.** When an illiterate or physically handicapped enrollee signs by mark (X), a witness should sign his or her name and address next to the mark. If the claim is filed for the patient by another person, that person should enter the patient's name and write "By," sign his or her own name and address, indicate relationship to the patient, and state why the patient cannot sign.

▶ **Confinement in a facility.** Sometimes it is not possible to obtain the signature of a Medicare patient because of confinement in a nursing facility, hospital, or home. In such cases, physicians should obtain a lifetime signature authorization from the patient.

▶ **Medigap claim.** When submitting a crossover claim to a Medigap carrier, obtain a lifetime signature authorization for the Medigap carrier.

▶ **Deceased patient.** Refer to section on "Deceased Patient Claims" later in this chapter for signature requirements.

▶ **Medicare/Medicaid (Medi-Medi) claim.** These crossover claims do not require the patient's signature.

Time Limit

The *time limit* for sending in claims is the end of the calendar year after the fiscal year in which services were furnished. The fiscal year for claims begins October 1 and ends September 30 (see the following box).

For services furnished on:	The time limit for filing is:
Oct. 1, 2003–Sept. 30, 2004	December 31, 2005
Oct. 1, 2004–Sept. 30, 2005	December 31, 2006

On assigned claims, the provider may file without penalty up to 27 months after providing service if reasonable cause for the delay is shown to the insurance carrier. Otherwise there is a 10% reduction in the reimbursement. On unassigned claims the provider may be fined for delinquent claim submission up to $2000 or dropped from Medicare. When submitting a late claim, ask the fiscal intermediary for the guidelines CMS considers reasonable cause for delay.

Manual Claims

The form that physicians use to submit paper claims to Medicare is the CMS-1500. Refer to Chapter 6 for instructions on how to complete the CMS-1500 claim form for the Medicare program. The reference templates for Medicare and supplemental coverage shown at the end of that chapter are:

Medicare, No secondary coverage	Figure 6–9
Medicare/Medicaid, Crossover	Figure 6–10
Medicare/Medigap, Crossover	Figure 6–11
Other insurance/Medicare MSP	Figure 6–12

Patients are not allowed to submit claims to Medicare (with four exceptions). Situations when a patient may file a claim are the following:

◗ Services covered by Medicare for which the patient has other insurance that should pay first; called MSP
◗ Services provided by a physician who refuses to submit the claim
◗ Services provided outside the United States
◗ Situations where durable medical equipment is purchased from a private source

Medicare claim status is also explained in detail in Chapter 6 (e.g., clean, incomplete, rejected, invalid, dirty, dingy, and other claims). Refer to Appendix A to obtain the mailing address for the Medicare claim form for the state or county. Go to the Internet Web site or contact the nearest Social Security office for further information and booklets, pamphlets, and the annual Medicare Handbook.

Electronic Claims

Medicare requests that all providers submit claims electronically. All electronic transmission formats are scheduled to be standardized by the use of ANSI ASC X12N (837) Version 4010. Refer to Chapter 7 on how to submit claims electronically to the Medicare carrier.

Medicare/Medicaid Claims

Medi-Medi patients qualify for the benefits of Medicare and Medicaid. Use the CMS-1500 claim form and check "Yes" for the assignment in Block 27.

If the physician does not accept assignment, then payment goes to the patient and Medicaid (in California Medi-Cal) will not pick up the residual. The CMS-1500 claim form will be crossed over and processed automatically by Medicaid after processing is completed by Medicare. The fiscal intermediary may refer to this as a **crossover claim,** or *claims transfer.* It is not necessary to submit another form. Claims should be sent according to the time limit designated by the Medicaid program in the state. Generally the Medicare payment exceeds the Medicaid fee schedule, and little or no payment is received except when the patient has not met his or her annual Medicare deductible.

In some states the fiscal intermediary for a crossover claim may have a different address from that used for the processing of a patient who is on Medicare only. Write or call the nearest Medicare fiscal intermediary for the guidelines pertinent to the state.

Medicare/Medigap Claims

Medicare has streamlined the processing of Medicare/Medigap claims in most states. Medicare carriers transmit Medigap claims electronically for participating physicians, thus eliminating the need to file an additional claim. This is also called a *crossover claim.* Medigap payments go directly to the participating physicians, and a Medicare Summary Notice is sent to the patient that states, "This claim has been referred to your supplemental carrier for any additional benefits."

To assure the crossover of the Medicare/Medigap claim, complete Blocks 9 through 9d of the CMS-1500 claim form and list the PAYRID number of the Medigap plan in Block 9d. The PAYRID for Medigap plans is referred to as the Other Carrier Name and Address (OCNA) number, and a list of all OCNAs is published in the Medicare newsletter.

If automatic crossover capabilities are not offered in one's state, attach the Medicare RA to the claim form and submit a claim to the Medigap plan separately.

Refer to Figure 6–11 for submitting claims when Medicare is primary and the patient has a Medigap (supplemental) policy.

Medicare/Supplemental and MSP Claims

Completing the CMS-1500 claim form for a Medicare patient who has supplemental insurance can be confusing. First, decide whether the case is Medicare primary or secondary payer. If Medicare is primary and the secondary payer is a Medigap policy, follow Medicare/Medigap processing guidelines. After determining who is primary, follow the directions on what should be entered in each block of the CMS-1500 claim form, depending on the primary payer, or follow MSP guidelines.

Templates shown at the end of Chapter 6 make it easier to learn which blocks to complete and which to ignore, depending on the primary and secondary payer. Figure 6–12 is for billing other insurance primary and Medicare secondary (MSP). A copy of the front and back sides of the primary insurance's EOB document must be attached to the claim when billing Medicare.

See Chapter 6 for general instructions for completing claims in Medicare and Medicare Secondary Payer cases.

Deceased Patients Claims

There are two ways in which to submit billing for a patient who has expired. They are the following:

1. Participating physician accepts assignment on the claim form. This results in the quickest payment. No signature by a family member is needed on the CMS-1500 claim form. Type "Patient died on (indicate date)" in Block 12 where the patient's signature is necessary.
2. The nonparticipating physician does not accept assignment, bills Medicare, and submits the following:
   a. A CMS-1500 claim form signed by the estate representative who is responsible for the bill
   b. A statement or claim for all services provided
   c. Name and address of the responsible party
   d. Provider's statement, signed and dated, refusing to accept assignment

Nothing can be done about the open balance on the account until the estate is settled, and then Medicare will pay.

Physician Substitute Coverage

Many times special substitute coverage arrangements are made between physicians (e.g., on-call, vacation, or unavailable because of another commitment). These arrangements are referred to as either reciprocal for on-call situations or *locum tenens* for a vacation situation. Specific modifiers are used to distinguish these situations, and special billing guidelines are stated as follows:

▶ *Reciprocal Arrangement.* When submitting Medicare claims, the *regular* physician must identify the service provided by the *substitute* doctor by listing the -Q5 modifier after the procedure code.
▶ *Locum Tenens Arrangement.* When submitting Medicare claims, the *regular* physician must identify the service provided by the *substitute* doctor by listing the -Q6 modifier after the procedure code.

After Claim Submission

Remittance Advice

Medicare sends a payment check and a nationally standardized document to participating physicians called a **Medicare remittance advice (RA),** formerly known as an explanation of Medicare benefits (EOMB). On the front side of the RA are status codes that are the same nationwide, representing the reason a claim may not have been paid in full, denied, and so forth. These codes are defined on the reverse side of the RA. If the patient has Medigap coverage, the "other payer" statement will say whether the claim has been transferred to the supplemental insurer.

Nonparticipating physicians also receive a remittance advice with payment information about unassigned claims. The remittance advice will separate payment information about assigned claims from unassigned claims to avoid posting errors by the practice. Check the payment against the fee schedule to determine whether the benefits are for the correct amount. On each claim form, note the date the payment is posted for reference. Optional items to document are amount of payment, RA processing data, and batch number.

Offices transmitting claims electronically receive an electronic remittance advice (ERA) showing payment data, and this may be automatically uploaded into the office computer system. The ERA electronically posts payments, and the provider does not have to manually post them. Paper and electronic remittance notices have the same format.

Medicare Summary Notice

A patient is mailed a similar document called a **Medicare Summary Notice (MSN).** This document is designed to be easier for the patient to understand, but because many patients do not know what is meant by *amount charged, Medicare approved, deductible, and coinsurance,* it often becomes necessary for the insurance billing specialist to educate the patient. First, photocopy an RA to be used as an example, deleting the patient's name to ensure confidentiality. Then use the RA to illustrate to future patients what various terms mean. This will increase patient understanding and save time.

Beneficiary Representative/Representative Payee

Medicare beneficiaries may have memory impairment or may be confined to a wheelchair or bed so they have a legal right to appoint an individual to serve as their representative.

Claims assistance professionals (CAPs) act as client representatives. They have some legal standing and are recognized by Medicare to act on the beneficiary's behalf if the beneficiary completes a Beneficiary Representative Form SSA-1696. This form is available from the Social Security District Office. Copies of the completed form should be sent to the Medicare intermediary or carrier when appropriate.

In contrast, a representative payee is an individual or organization chosen by the SSA to receive and administer SSA benefit funds on behalf of the beneficiary. Other duties consist of assisting the beneficiary with check writing for financial obligations, such as personal care and maintenance, housing, medical service expenses, and investing any surplus monies for the beneficiary's benefit. A representative payee is responsible for using payments received only for the benefit of the beneficiary, accounting for the benefits received on request, and contacting SSA when anything affects eligibility for SSA benefits or prevents the representative payee's ability to perform these responsibilities. Additional information on CAPs is found in Chapters 1 and 17.

Posting Payments

Usually a physician's charge is higher than the charge approved by the Medicare carrier or fiscal agent. This does not mean that his or her charges are unreasonable. As mentioned, payments are established using a fee schedule based on an RBRVS, a **volume performance standard (VPS)** for expenditure increases, and a *limiting charge* for nonparticipating physicians.

Because some services may be disallowed or the payments on them may be lower than those charged by the physician, know how to post payments to the patient's financial accounting record card or computerized account. Figure 11–15 illustrates how payments and courtesy adjustments are posted. The word "courtesy" implies that Medicare patients are treated well and is preferred to phrases like "not allowed" or "write off."

Medicare does not allow for the standardized waiving of copayments. Medicare regulations require that a patient be billed for the copayment at least three times before the balance is adjusted off as uncollectable. Document this as further justification if the patient is suffering financial hardship.

When an RA is received, it may list many patients (Fig. 11–16). Do not post the entire payment made in a lump sum to the daysheet. Individually post each line item paid to the patient's financial accounting record card or computerized account and to the daysheet (Fig. 11–17). To prevent funds from going astray, some offices prefer to post Medicare payments to a separate daysheet and deposit each multiple reimbursement check separately. The daysheet totals will then agree with the deposit slip totals and not get confused with other monies collected.

Figure 11–18, *A* illustrates an example of a Medicare/Medicaid case after payment by Medicare. Medicare applied the patient's full $100 deductible amount to the Medicare allowed amount, reducing payment to $4. The Medicaid RA (Fig. 11–18, *B*) shows reimbursement of the coinsurance and deductible amounts dual-billed to Medicaid.

Calculation are shown in the following box:

Medicare		Medicaid	
$105	Allowed amount	$105	Medicare allowed
−100	Deductible		amount
$ 5	Balance on which	−32	Medicaid cutback
	payment is	$ 73	Medicaid allowed
× .80	calculated		
$ 4	Medicare paid 80%	−4	Medicare paid
		$ 69	Medicaid payment

When referring to the Medicaid program, a *cutback* means a reduction and would require an adjustment entry on the patient's financial accounting record. Cutbacks are common on Medicaid claims.

Medicare overpayments can occur in the following situations:

▶ The carrier processes the charge more than once.
▶ The physician receives duplicate payments from Medicare and a secondary payer.
▶ The physician is paid directly on an unassigned claim.
▶ The item is not covered but is paid.
▶ The payment is made on erroneous information.

If an overpayment check is received, deposit the check and then write to Medicare notifying them of the overpayment. Include a copy of the check and the RA. This overpayment will be deducted from the next Medicare payment and will be shown on the RA. If the physician wishes to repay a Medicare overpayment on the installment plan, Financial Statement of Debtor CMS-379 form may be used. This form is sent to the physician when the carrier notifies the physician that money is due back.

Refer to Chapter 8 for additional information about Explanation of Benefits documents from private insurance carriers.

Review and Appeal Process

As you have read Chapter 8 outlines in detail the steps to take for having a claim reviewed and the process of appealing a claim in the Medicare program.

STATEMENT

College Clinic
4567 Broad Avenue
Woodland Hills, XY 12345-0001
Telephone: 555-486-9002
Fax: 555-487-8976

Account No. 946
John Smith
100 James Street
Woodland Hills, XY 12345-0001

DATE	PROFESSIONAL SERVICE DESCRIPTION	CHARGE		CREDITS		CURRENT BALANCE	
				PAYMENTS	ADJUSTMENTS		
2-15-xx	Surgery	800	00			800	00
2-17-xx	Medicare/Medigap billed (2-15-xx)					800	00
4-2-xx	Medicare payment voucher #12498 (2-15-xx)			440	00	360	00
4-12-xx	Medigap payment voucher #45500 (2-15-xx)			110	00	250	00
4-12-xx	Medicare courtesy (adjustment 2-15-xx)				250	00	-0-

Due and payable within 10 days

Pay last amount in balance column

Key: PF: Problem-focused	SF: Straightforward	CON: Consultation	HCD: House Call (Day)
EPF: Expanded problem-focused	LC: Low complexity	CPX: Complete Phys Exam	HCN: House Call (Night)
D: Detailed	MC: Moderate complexity	E: Emergency	HV: Hospital visit
C: Comprehensive	HC: High complexity	ER: Emergency Dept.	OV: Office Visit

Figure 11–15. Financial accounting record (ledger card) illustrating how payments and courtesy adjustments should be posted. The Medicare allowed amount is $550 in the case illustrated.

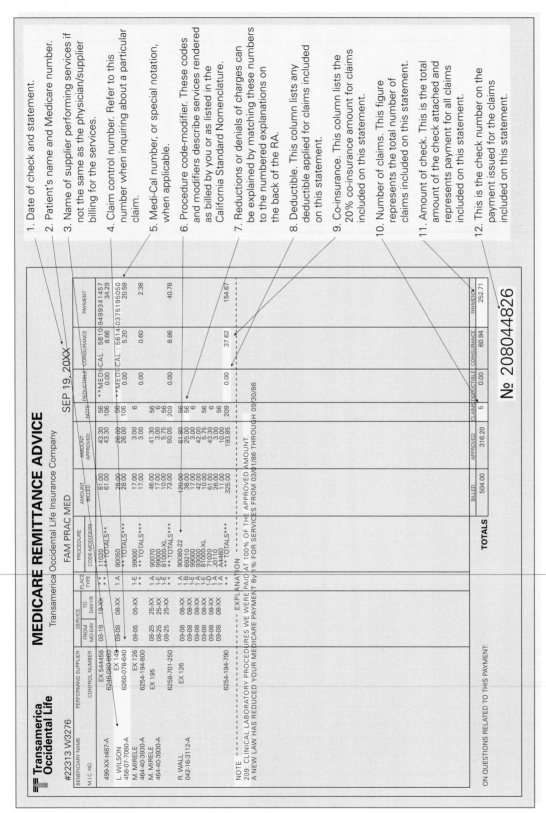

Figure 11-16. Medicare Remittance Advice (RA) document. **A,** Front. Insurance carriers are required to use Center for Medicare and Medicaid Services messages for Medicare RA, but each carrier has its own code numbers to denote the messages.

EXPLANATION OF NOTES   Additional notes may be listed on the front of this form.

1 – See enclosed letter.

2 – Claim was filed after the time limit.

4 – These bills are handled by a special intermediary.

5 – This payment is for an adjustment of a previous claim.

6 – Charges over the maximum Medicare allowance are not covered.

7 – Services before Medicare entitlement are not covered.

8 – Services after Medicare entitlement ended are not covered.

10 – Other charges submitted with this claim may be on a separate statement which you have received or will receive soon.

12 – Routine examinations and related services are not covered.

13 – Immunizations or other routine and preventative services are not covered.

16 – We need an itemization of this charge. Please resubmit your claim with this information.

17 – Prescription drugs are not covered.

18 – Charges for this physician/supplier are not covered.

19 – We need a full description of the service or supply to consider this charge. Please resubmit your claim with this information.

23 – We need a written report for this service. Please resubmit your claim with this information.

26 – More than $312.50 annual psychiatric expense is not covered.

27 – We need from the prescribing physician the specific length of time this medical equipment is needed. Please resubmit your claim with this information.

30 – This charge was previously considered.

37 – Claims for these services will be made by a home health agency or hospital.

39 – Equipment that is not medically necessary is not covered. (See Note 89)

42 – These supplies or services are not covered.

45 – Over 62½% of psychiatric expenses is not covered.

46 – Routine foot care is not covered.

47 – Routine eye examinations or eye refractions are not covered.

48 – Partial payment of this claim was made to the beneficiary.

49 – This service cannot be considered until the hospital makes the necessary arrangement with the carrier for its processing.

50 – The beneficiary is not responsible for this reduction/denial under the assignment agreement.

54 – Care before and/or after surgery is included in the surgery benefit. (See Note 50)

56 – This is the full charge allowed based upon the prevailing or usual and customary rate.

62 – Payment has been reduced because this test is commonly part of an automated test group. (See Note 50)

66 – This service is not covered when done by this laboratory.

70 – There were no charges or bills with your claim form. Please resubmit your claim with this information.

72 – We need a signed and dated prescription showing medical necessity and specific length of time needed. Please resubmit your claim with this information.

73 – Before another month's payment can be made, we need a new signed and dated prescription showing further necessity of the medical equipment and specific length of time needed.

80 – We need to know the place of service to consider this charge. Please resubmit your claim with this information.

83 – SSA advises us that they are unable to verify the patient's eligibility for Part B Medical Insurance Plan. For this reason, no payment can be made on this claim.

84 – The patient's HIC number shown on this claim was incorrect. Please use the correct HIC number on all future claims.

85 – The patient's name shown on this claim was incorrect. Please use the correct name on all future claims.

86 – Over 62⅓% of the allowable charges for psychiatric services is not covered.

89 – If you did not know that Medicare does not pay for this medical service, you may request a review of this decision. See below paragraph entitled "Your right to review of a case."

90 – This service by a chiropractor is not covered.

93 – Over $500.00 annual expense billed by a physical therapist is not covered.

95 – These specific services by this supplier are not covered.

96 – Please verify the date of this service. Resubmit your claim with this information.

99 – We need a complete diagnosis before the claim can be considered. Please resubmit your claim with this information.

106 – The Medicare covered services on this claim have been forwarded for additional processing under Medi-Cal.

107 – This claim was not forwarded for Medi-Cal processing. Please bill Medi-Cal directly and attach a copy of this statement.

108 – The bills for these services have been transferred to Blue Shield of California Medicare Claims, Chico, CA 95976. You will hear from them.

129 – Payment for services prior to July 1 is based on the previous year's payment rate.

131 – Payment for this physician service in a hospital department is reduced since this service is commonly performed in the physician's office. (See Note 50)

138 – This amount is more than Medicare pays for maintenance treatment of renal disease.

147 – This charge is not covered because an allowance for purchase of the same equipment was previously made.

151 – Your claim was transferred to a Health Maintenance Organization for processing.

153 – These are more visits (treatments) for this diagnosis than Medicare covers unless there were unusual circumstances. (See Note 89)

154 – This service is not covered for your patient's reported condition. (See Note 89)

155 – Only one visit per month to a nursing home is covered unless special need is indicated. (See Note 89)

156 – This laboratory test for the reported condition and/or illness is not covered. (See Note 89)

158 – Procedures whose effectiveness has not been proven are not covered. (See Note 89)

161 – The frequency of services for this condition are not covered. (See Note 89)

162 – More than one visit per day for this condition are not covered. (See Note 89)

172 – This type of services billed by a psychologist are not covered.

179 – The amount for this service is included in the approved amount for the consultation/office/hospital visit.

181 – Payment for this service is included in the major surgical fee.

187 – We need the name and address of the individual doctor who performed this service. Please resubmit your claim with this information.

192 – Medicare benefits have been reduced because the patient's employer group health plan has paid some of these expenses.

198 – A claim must be sent to the patient's employer group health plan first. After the claim has been processed by that plan, resubmit this claim with the bills and the notice the other insurance company sent you.

203 – Clinical laboratory services. Blood Gas Studies and Rhythm Strips (1–3 leads) furnished in a hospital setting are reimbursed through the hospital.

205 – The date of this service is after the patient's expiration date provided to us by SSA. If service was rendered to this patient on this date, have the patient's estate contact the local Social Security Office for assistance.

206 – For payment, these services must be billed by the performing laboratory with the assignment accepted.

213 – We did not send this claim to Medicaid. Please send this statement and a copy of the claim to the agency that handles Medicaid in your area.

216 – This service or item cannot be processed until your application for a Medicare provider identification number is received and approved.

218 – Since you are Medicare participating, we have processed this claim as assigned. Future claims must be billed on assignment. If the bill was paid in full, you must immediately refund the amount due to the beneficiary.

219 – We need this charge submitted on your letterhead bill. Please resubmit your claim with this information.

221 – The name and Medicare number submitted on this claim do not match. Please verify for whom these services were rendered and provide the correct name and number on the claim and resubmit.

223 – We did not consider this for payment because you did not send the extra information we asked for. Payment can be requested again by sending us another claim form and all the information.

226 – Medicare will pay rent for the prescribed number of months or until the equipment is no longer needed, whichever occurs first. This is the first monthly rental payment.

227 – You will receive a notice each month when additional rental payments are paid.

231 – Medicare will no longer pay for rental on this item since the purchase price has been paid.

237 – The amount of this payment is the difference between the approved purchase allowance and the rental payments you have received.

YOUR RIGHT TO REVIEW OF A CASE

If you have a problem or question about the way a claim was handled or about the amount paid, please write Transamerica Occidental Life, Box 54905, Terminal Annex, Los Angeles, California 90054, within 6 months of the date of this notice. We will give your request full consideration.

Your Social Security office will help you file a request for review of a claim if it is more convenient for you.

WHERE TO SEND REFUNDS

When refunding a payment you should send a check with a letter of explanation. The letter should include your Transamerica Occidental/Medicare check number, beneficiary name and Medicare identification number (HIC No.), control number to which the payment relates and any other information which may be pertinent to the refund. Send this information to:

Transamerica Occidental Life
C/O Check and Payment Control
Box 54905, Terminal Annex
Los Angeles, CA 90054-0905

KEY TO CODES FOR PLACE AND TYPE OF SERVICE

Place of service	Type of service
1. Office	A. Medical care
2. Home	B. Surgery (includes treatment of fractures)
3. Inpatient hospital	C. Consultation
4. Skilled nursing facility	D. Diagnostic X-ray
5. Outpatient hospital	E. Diagnostic laboratory
6. Independent laboratory	F. Radiation therapy
7. Other	G. Anesthesia
8. Independent kidney disease treatment center	H. Assistance at surgery
	I. Other medical service
	J. Whole blood or packed red cells

B

Figure 11–16, cont'd. B, Back of Medicare RA document.

Figure 11–17. Insurance billing specialist explaining a Medicare Remittance Advice document that the physician's office has received.

MEDICARE REMITTANCE ADVICE
XYZ Insurance Company

Physician or Supplier Name	Dates of service From To MMDD MMDDYY	See back serv typl	Sub code (alwcode)	Billed amount	Amount allowed	See ** act cde	Beneficiary obligation Deductible Co-ins		Medicare payment to Beneficiary Provider
BENEFICIARY: BILL HUTCH CONTROL NO.: 92106-30810-00	DE/MI: 2121D52			HIC NUMBER: 5432-112-34					
John Doe MD 0310 031094		D 03	120101	145.00	105.00	101	100.00	1.00 0.00	4.00
CLAIM TOTALS:				145.00	105.00	101	100.00	1.00 0.00	4.00

A

MEDICAID REMITTANCE ADVICE

RECIPIENT NAME	RECIPIENT MEDICAID ID NO.	CLAIM CONTROL NUMBER	SERVICE DATE MO DAY YR	PROCEDURE CODE	PATIENT ACCT. NO.	QTY.	MEDICARE ALLOWED	MEDICAID ALLOWED	PATIENT LIABILITY	COMPUTED MCR AMT.	MEDICAID PAID	EOB MESSAGE
BILL HUTCH	521345678	4006984891200	03 10 XX	49555–80		001	105.00	73.00		4.00	.00	
		4006984891200	00 00 XX			000	105.00	73.00		4.00	69.00	
BLOOD DEDUCT 00 DEDUCTIBLE 100.00 COINSUR 1.00 CUTBACK 32.00												CUTBACK 443

B

Figure 11–18. A, A Medicare/Medicaid case after payment by Medicare. **B,** The Medicaid Remittance Advice shows reimbursement of the coinsurance and deductible amounts dual billed to Medicaid.

STUDENT ASSIGNMENT LIST

✔ Study Chapter 11.

✔ Answer the review questions in the *Workbook* to reinforce the theory learned in this chapter and to help prepare you for a future test.

✔ Complete the assignments in the *Workbook* to give you experience in computing Medicare in mathematic calculations, selecting HCPCS code numbers, abstracting from patients' medical records, preparing financial accounting record cards, and completing forms pertinent to the Medicare program.

✔ Turn to the Glossary at the end of this textbook for a further understanding of the Key Terms used in this chapter.

COMPUTER ASSIGNMENT

Do the exercises for cases 8, 9, and 10 on the CD ROM to review concepts you have learned for this chapter.

Medicaid and Other
State Programs

MEDICAID

12

- State eligibility requirements and claims procedures for the Maternal and Child Health Program.
- Identify those eligible for the Medicaid Qualified Medicare Beneficiaries program.
- Explain basic operations of a Medicaid-managed care system.
- Describe basic Medicaid claim procedure guidelines.
- File claims for patients who have Medicaid and other coverage.
- Minimize the number of insurance forms rejected because of improper completion.

KEY TERMS

categorically needy

covered services

Early and Periodic Screening, Diagnosis, and Treatment (EPSDT)

fiscal agent

Maternal and Child Health Program (MCHP)

Medicaid (MCD)

Medi-Cal

medically needy (MN)

prior approval

recipient

share of cost

Supplemental Security Income (SSI)

OBJECTIVES*

After reading this chapter, you should be able to:

- Understand the benefits and nonbenefits of Medicaid.
- Define terminology inherent to Medicaid.
- Interpret Medicaid abbreviations.
- Name the two Medicaid eligibility classifications.
- List important information to abstract from the patient's Medicaid card.

---

*Performance objectives and exercises for hands-on practical experience for this chapter appear in the *Workbook*.

History

Federal participation in providing medical care to needy persons began between 1933 and 1935 when the Federal Emergency Relief Administration made funds available to pay the medical expenses of the needy unemployed. The Social Security Act of 1935 set up the public assistance programs; and although no special provision was made for medical assistance, the federal government paid a share of the monthly assistance payments, which could be used to meet the costs of medical care. However, the payment was made to the assistance recipient rather than the provider of medical care.

In 1950 Congress passed a law mandating that all states set up a health care program of assistance, which meant that the states had to meet minimum requirements. As a result of this mandate, the states set up **Medicaid (MCD)** programs. Congress authorized *vendor payments* for medical care—payments from the welfare agency directly to physicians, health care institutions, and other providers of medical services. By 1960 four fifths of the states made provisions for medical vendor payments.

A new category of assistance recipient was established for the medically needy aged population. The incomes of these individuals were too high to qualify them for cash assistance payments, but they needed help in meeting the costs of medical care. The federal government financially supports the minimum assistance level, and the states must wholly support any part of the program that goes beyond the federal minimum. This is referred to as *state share.*

In 1965 Title XIX of the Social Security Act became federal law, and Medicaid legally came into being. To a large extent it was the result of various attempts during the previous 30 years to provide medical care to the needy. The program has always had somewhat of a split personality. On one hand it is viewed as an attempt on the part of the government to provide comprehensive quality health care to those unable to afford it. On the other hand Medicaid has been seen as merely a bill-paying mechanism that uses the most efficient and economic system possible to administer the provision of health care.

Since 1983 the trend in many states has been to expand Medicaid eligibility requirements and services. Changes in Medicaid eligibility allowing more people into the program were made by many states after the passage by the federal government of the Deficit Reduction Act of 1984 (DEFRA) and the Child Health Assurance Program (CHAP).

In 1982 the Tax Equity and Fiscal Responsibility Act (TEFRA) set down laws affecting those under the Medicare program, as well as Medicaid medically needy recipients and those in certain other categories. See Chapter 11 for information about how this act affects Medicare recipients.

Medicaid Programs

Title XIX of the Social Security Act provides for a program of medical assistance for certain low-income individuals and families. The program is known as Medicaid in 48 states and **Medi-Cal** in California. Arizona is the only state without a Medicaid program similar to those existing in other states. Since 1982 it has received federal funds under a demonstration waiver for an alternative medical assistance program (prepaid care) for low-income persons called the Arizona Health Care Cost Containment System (AHCCCS).

Medicaid is administered by state governments with partial federal funding. Coverage and benefits vary widely from state to state because the federal government sets minimum requirements and the states are free to enact more benefits. Thus each state designs its own Medicaid program within federal guidelines. The Centers for Medicaid and Medicare Services (CMS) of the Bureau of Program Operations of the United States Department of Health and Human Services is responsible for the federal aspects of Medicaid. Medicaid is not so much an insurance as an assistance program.

Maternal and Child Health Program

Each state and certain other jurisdictions, including territories and the District of Columbia (56 programs total), operate a **Maternal and Child Health Program (MCHP)** with federal grant support under Title V of the Social Security Act. Although Title V has been amended on a number of occasions, notably between 1981 and 1987, no changes have been as sweeping as those in the Omnibus Budget Reconciliation Act (OBRA) of 1989. Federal funds are granted to states, enabling them to:

▶ Provide low-income mothers and children access to quality maternal and child health services.
▶ Reduce infant mortality and the incidence of preventable diseases and handicapping conditions among children.
▶ Increase the number of children immunized against disease and the number of low-income children receiving health assessments and follow-up diagnostic and treatment services.
▶ Promote the health of mothers and infants by providing prenatal, delivery, and postpartum care for low-income, at-risk pregnant women.
▶ Provide preventive and primary care services for low-income children.
▶ Provide rehabilitation services for the blind and disabled younger than age 16 years.
▶ Provide, promote, and develop family-centered, community-based, coordinated care for children with special health care needs.

The state agency tries to locate mothers, infants, and children younger than 21 years of age who may have conditions eligible for treatment under the MCHP. The conditions are diagnosed, and the necessary medical and other health-related care, any hospitalization, and any continuing follow-up care are given.

After a child is examined at an MCHP clinic and a diagnosis is made, the parents are advised about the treatment that will benefit the child. The state agency then helps them locate this care. If the parents cannot afford this care, the agency assists them with financial planning and may assume part or all of the cost of treatment, depending on the child's condition and the family's resources.

Low-Income Medicare Recipients

There are three aid programs for Medicare patients who have low incomes and have difficulty paying Medicare premiums, copayments, and deductibles. Each program addresses a different financial category, and the monthly income figures are adjusted each year. The titles of the three programs follow:

◗ Medicaid Qualified Medicare Beneficiary Program
◗ Specified Low-Income Medicare Beneficiary Program
◗ Qualifying Individuals Program

The programs usually are administered through county social services departments, the same ones that administer Medicaid. One application is completed that pertains to all three programs, and an individual is placed in one of the programs depending on how he or she qualifies financially.

Medicaid Qualified Medicare Beneficiary Program

The Medicaid Qualified Medicare Beneficiary (MQMB) program was introduced in the Medicare Catastrophic Act of 1988 as an amendment to the Social Security Act. In 1990 the Omnibus Budget Reconciliation Act allowed for assistance to qualified Medicare beneficiaries (QMBs, pronounced "kwim-bees") who are aged and disabled and are receiving Medicare and have annual incomes *below the federal poverty level*. Eligibility also depends on what other financial resources an individual might have.

Under this act, states must provide limited Medicaid coverage for QMBs. They must pay Medicare Part B premiums (and Part A premiums if applicable), along with necessary Medicare deductibles and coinsurance amounts. Coverage is restricted to Medicare cost sharing unless the beneficiary qualifies for Medicaid in some other way. Medicaid will not pay for the service if Medicare does not cover the service to the patient.

States also are required to pay Part A premiums, but no other expenses, for qualified disabled and working individuals. It is optional for states to provide full Medicaid benefits to QMBs who meet a state-established income standard.

Specified Low-Income Medicare Beneficiary Program

The Specified Low-Income Medicare Beneficiary (SLMB, pronounced "slim-bee") program was established in 1993 for elderly individuals who are *20% above the federal poverty level*. It pays the entire Medicare Part B premium. The patient must pay the deductible, copay, and for noncovered items.

Qualifying Individuals Program

The Qualifying Individuals (QI) program was created in 1997 for qualifying individuals who are *135% above the poverty standard*. It also pays for the Medicare Part B premium.

Medicaid Eligibility

Medicaid is available to certain needy and low-income people, such as the aged (65 years or older), blind, disabled, and members of families with dependent children deprived of the support of at least one parent and financially eligible on the basis of income and resources. If a person is eligible for Medicaid, he or she goes to the local welfare office and applies for benefits.

Verifying Eligibility

After acceptance into the program, the patient brings a form or card to the physician's office that verifies acceptance into the program (Fig. 12–1), but this does not indicate proof of eligibility. It is the provider's

Figure 12–1. Medicaid patient checking in with the receptionist.

GROUPS ELIGIBLE FOR MEDICAID BENEFITS

CLASSIFICATIONS	GROUPS

CATEGORICALLY NEEDY	1. Families, pregnant women, and children
	   a) Aid to Families with Dependent Children (AFDC)-related groups
	   b) Non-ADFC pregnant women and children
	
	2. Aged and disabled persons
	   a) Supplemental Security Income (SSI)-related groups
	   b) Qualified Medicare Beneficiaries (QMBs)
	
	3. Persons receiving institutional or other long-term care
	   in nursing facilities (NFs) and intermediate care facilities (ICFs)
	   a) Medicaid beneficiaries
	   b) Medi/Medi beneficiaries

MEDICALLY NEEDY	4. Medically indigent low-income individuals and families 5. Low-income persons losing employer health insurance coverage (Medicaid purchase of COBRA coverage)

Figure 12–2. Classifications and basic groups eligible for Medicaid benefits.

responsibility to verify that the person to receive care is eligible on the date the service is rendered and is the individual to whom the card was issued.

Each state decides which services are covered and what the payments are for each service. There are two classifications that contain several basic groups of needy and low-income individuals.

Categorically Needy

The first classification, the **categorically needy** group, includes all cash recipients of the Aid to Families with Dependent Children (AFDC) program, certain other AFDC–related groups, most cash recipients of the **Supplemental Security Income (SSI)** program, other SSI–related groups, QMBs, and institutional and long-term care and intermediate-care facility patients (Fig. 12–2).

Medically Needy

The second classification involves state general assistance programs for low-income people, the medically indigent, and individuals losing employer health insurance. This classification is sometimes referred to as the **medically needy (MN)** class. A Medicaid **recipient** in this category may or may not pay coinsurance or a deductible, which must be met within the eligibility month or other specified time frame before he or she can receive state benefits (also known as **share of cost**). Emergency care and pregnancy services are exempt by law from copayment requirements. This may be a component of a state's general assistance program for low-income people. For those individuals who may become

medically indigent as a result of high medical care expenses and inadequate health insurance coverage, a number of states have adopted a State Program of Assistance for the Medically Indigent. See Figure 12–2 for a clear, simple explanation of the classes and basic groups for Medicaid eligibility.

Maternal and Child Health Program Eligibility

Specific conditions qualify a child for benefits under the MCHP. The state law under which each agency operates either defines the conditions to be included or directs the children's agency to define them. All state laws include children who have some kind of handicap that requires orthopedic treatment or plastic surgery; a few states add other conditions. A list of both types of conditions that qualify children for MCHP follows:

‣ Cerebral palsy
‣ Chronic conditions affecting bones and joints
‣ Cleft lip
‣ Cleft palate
‣ Clubfoot
‣ Cystic fibrosis*
‣ Epilepsy*
‣ Hearing problems*
‣ Mental retardation*
‣ Multiple handicaps*
‣ Paralyzed muscles
‣ Rheumatic and congenital heart disease*
‣ Vision problems requiring surgery*

---

*Only some states include this item in their Maternal and Child Health Program.

Accepting Medicaid Patients

Individual physicians have their own office procedures for handling Medicaid patients. A patient can be on Medicaid 1 month and off the following month or on the program for several months or years; therefore each case is different. The physician may accept or refuse to treat Medicaid patients but must make the decision on the basis of the entire Medicaid program, not an individual patient's personality, medical situation, or other discriminating factor. The patient must receive quality care and be treated the same as the paying patient. If the physician decides to take Medicaid patients, he or she must accept the Medicaid allowance as payment in full (Fig. 12–3).

When obtaining personal information from the patient at the time of the first visit or a follow-up visit, check the patient's name, address, and telephone number in a reverse address directory to verify that it is correct. Another type of directory available is one that lists everyone on a given block or even in an apartment building who has a telephone. These easy reference guides cut verification time in half. Some Medicaid individuals are homeless and may list fake addresses, which makes locating them difficult.

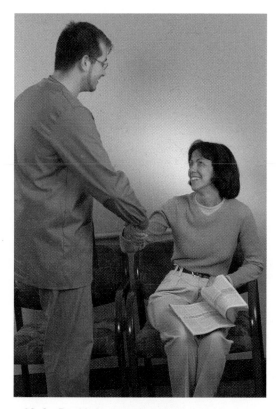

Figure 12–3. Disabled patient being welcomed by an insurance biller who is asking for her Medicaid card.

Identification Card

A plastic or paper Medicaid identification card (or coupons in some states) usually is issued monthly (Fig. 12–4). Under certain classifications of eligibility, identification cards are issued in some states on the 1st and 15th of each month, every 2 months, every 3 months, or every 6 months. Sometimes an unborn child can be issued an identification card that is used for services promoting the life and health of the fetus.

Obtain a photocopy of the front and back of the card. Carefully check the expiration date of the card each time the patient visits the physician's office to see whether eligibility is indicated for the month of service. Note whether the patient has other insurance, copayment requirements, or restrictions, such as being eligible for only certain types of medical services.

Point-of-Service Machine

When professional services are rendered, eligibility for that month must be verified, which may be done in a number of ways. The Potomac Group, Inc., in Nashville, TN, has developed MediFAX for some states. This is a machine that allows the user to verify coverage in seconds and is available for several states. There are some states that provide their own electronic system for Medicaid verification via touch-tone telephone, modem, or specialized Medicaid terminal equipment such as a point-of-service (POS) machine (Fig. 12–5). Some states issue cards that contain adhesive labels listing the month of eligibility that must be used on the billing claim form.

Retroactive Eligibility

Retroactive eligibility may be granted to a patient in some cases. When patients are seeking medical care who are in hope of qualifying for Medicaid but have not done so at the time of service, the account must be set up as a cash account until retroactive eligibility has been established. If the patient has documentation or a retroactive card confirming this and has paid for any services during the retroactive period, a refund must be made and Medicaid billed. As described and shown in the previous chapter, a waiver of liability agreement rewritten to the Medicaid program and signed by the patient might be used in such cases.

Medicaid Benefits

Covered Services

Under Federal guidelines the state Medicaid basic benefits offered to eligible recipients include the types of **covered services** shown in Box 12–1; consult state regulations for additional benefits.

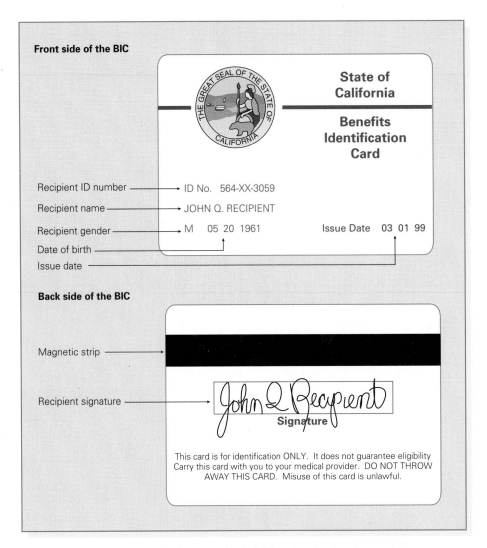

Front side of the BIC

THE GREAT SEAL OF THE STATE OF CALIFORNIA

State of California

Benefits Identification Card

Recipient ID number ⟶ ID No. 564-XX-3059

Recipient name ⟶ JOHN Q. RECIPIENT

Recipient gender ⟶ M   05 20 1961   Issue Date   03 01 99

Date of birth

Issue date

Back side of the BIC

Magnetic strip ⟶

Recipient signature ⟶ *John Q Recipient*
Signature

This card is for identification ONLY. It does not guarantee eligibility
Carry this card with you to your medical provider. DO NOT THROW
AWAY THIS CARD. Misuse of this card is unlawful.

Figure 12–4. Plastic Medi-Cal benefits identification card.

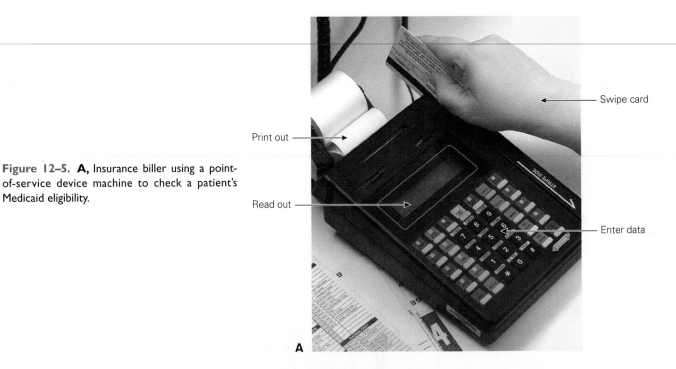

Figure 12–5. A, Insurance biller using a point-of-service device machine to check a patient's Medicaid eligibility.

Swipe card

Print out

Read out

Enter data

A

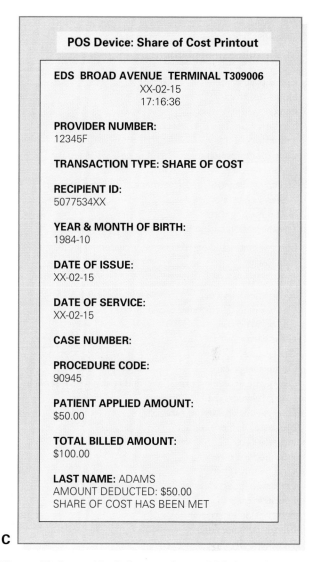

POS Device: Medi-Service Printout

EDS BROAD AVENUE TERMINAL T309006
XX-02-15
17:16:36

PROVIDER NUMBER:
12345F

TRANSACTION TYPE: MEDI-SERVICES

RECIPIENT ID:
5077534XX

YEAR & MONTH OF BIRTH:
1975-12

DATE OF ISSUE:
XX-02-15

DATE OF SERVICE:
XX-02-15

PROCEDURE CODE:
45339

LAST NAME: MORRISON MEDI SVC
RESERVATION APPLIED

B

Figure 12–5, cont'd. **B,** Printout from a POS device for Medi-Service.

POS Device: Share of Cost Printout

EDS BROAD AVENUE TERMINAL T309006
XX-02-15
17:16:36

PROVIDER NUMBER:
12345F

TRANSACTION TYPE: SHARE OF COST

RECIPIENT ID:
5077534XX

YEAR & MONTH OF BIRTH:
1984-10

DATE OF ISSUE:
XX-02-15

DATE OF SERVICE:
XX-02-15

CASE NUMBER:

PROCEDURE CODE:
90945

PATIENT APPLIED AMOUNT:
$50.00

TOTAL BILLED AMOUNT:
$100.00

LAST NAME: ADAMS
AMOUNT DEDUCTED: $50.00
SHARE OF COST HAS BEEN MET

C

Figure 12–5, cont'd. **C,** Printout from a POS device for share of cost.

Early and Periodic Screening, Diagnosis, and Treatment

Another benefit of the Medicaid program is the **Early and Periodic Screening, Diagnosis, and Treatment (EPSDT)** service. This is a program of prevention, early detection, and treatment of welfare children (younger than age 21). In California (Medi-Cal), it is known as the Child Health and Disability Prevention (CHDP) program. Because many states are changing the name of EPSDT and the services offered under the program, check with the state Medicaid vendor.

The EPSDT guidelines include a medical history and physical examination; immunization status assessment; dental, hearing, and vision screening; developmental assessment; and screening for anemia and lead absorption, tuberculosis, bacteriuria, and sickle cell disease and trait. States are required to provide necessary health care, diagnostic services, treatment, and other services to correct physical or mental defects found.

Disallowed Services

If a service is totally disallowed by Medicaid (denied claim), a physician is within legal rights in many states to bill the patient; consult state regulations before deciding to bill. However, it is wise to have the patient sign a waiver of liability agreement if the service to be provided may be a denied service from known past claim submission experience. An example of a waiver of liability agreement is shown in Chapter 11, Figure 11–10. Write or telephone the state agency (see Appendix A) to obtain up-to-date information and details on the Medicaid program in a particular state.

Medicaid Managed Care

As early as 1967, some states began bringing managed care to their Medicaid programs. In the past decade many states have adopted pilot projects to see whether a managed care system will work and what benefits might be received. Mainly this has been done as an effort to control escalating health care costs by curbing unnecessary emergency department visits and emphasizing preventive care.

Medicaid Basic Benefits

Family planning
Home health care
Immunizations
Inpatient hospital care
Laboratory and x-ray
Outpatient hospital care
Physicians' care
Screening, diagnosis, and treatment of children younger
     than 21 years of age
Skilled nursing care
Transportation to and from health care providers

In some states additional services included might be the
     following:

Allergy care
Ambulance services
Certain medical cosmetic procedures
Chiropractic care
Clinic care
Dental care
Dermatologic care
Diagnostic, screening, preventive, and rehabilitative services
     (e.g., physical therapy)
Emergency department care
Eyeglasses and eye refractions
Hospice care
Intermediate care
Occupational therapy
Optometric services
Podiatric care
Prescription drugs
Private duty nursing
Prosthetic devices
Psychiatric care
Respiratory care
Speech therapy

When the last state, Arizona, joined Medicaid, it began with prepaid care rather than adhering to the way most states have structured their programs. By then most states had been struggling with Medicaid for nearly 20 years. In these systems the Medicaid recipient enrolls either in an existing or specifically formed plan similar to a health maintenance organization (HMO). Some plans are run by independent commissions appointed by county boards of supervisors. Usually the patient can either choose or be assigned a gatekeeper (primary care physician) who must approve all specialty care and inpatient or outpatient hospital treatment. Patients must use physicians, clinics, and hospitals participating in their assigned plan.

Patients can be cared for side by side with private-paying patients. Some states have adopted capitated (a flat fee per patient) rather than fee-for-service reimbursement. There may be a small copayment for

services. In programs run for a number of years, it has been found that there is better access to primary health care and savings of monies in delivering the care if the programs are well managed.

Claim Procedure

Medicaid policies and claim procedures about identification cards, prior approval regulations, claim forms, and time limits vary from state to state. General guidelines for submitting claims are stated here.

For specific state guidelines consult the current Medicaid Handbook or state fiscal agent. See Appendix A for the name and address in a region.

Claim procedures and information on the Medi-Cal program are presented in Appendix C to assist those working as an insurance billing specialist for a clinic or physician's practice in California.

Copayment

There are two types of copayment requirements that may apply to a state. Some states require a small fixed copayment paid to the provider at the time services are rendered. This policy was instituted to help pay some of the administrative costs of physicians participating in the Medicaid program.

Another requirement is the *share of cost* copayment. Some Medicaid recipients must meet this copayment requirement each month before Medicaid benefits can be claimed. The amount may change from month to month so be sure to verify the copayment each time it is collected. Obtain this copay amount when the patient comes in for medical care and report on the claim form that it has been collected.

Prior Approval

Many times **prior approval** is necessary for various services, except in a bona fide emergency. Some of these services are the following:

▶ Durable medical equipment
▶ Hearing aids
▶ Hemodialysis
▶ Home health care
▶ Inpatient hospital care
▶ Long-term care facility services
▶ Medical supplies
▶ Medications
▶ Prosthetic or orthotic appliances
▶ Surgical procedures
▶ Transportation
▶ Some vision care

Usually prior authorization forms are completed to obtain permission for a specific service or hospitalization (Fig. 12–6) and mailed or faxed to the

STATE USE ONLY

SERVICE CATEGORY

TYPEWRITER ALIGNMENT
Elite   Pica

CONFIDENTIAL PATIENT INFORMATION
FOR F.I. USE ONLY

CCN

TREATMENT AUTHORIZATION REQUEST
STATE OF CALIFORNIA DEPARTMENT OF HEALTH SERVICES

F.I. USE ONLY
40 □   41 □
42 □   43 □

TYPEWRITER ALIGNMENT
Elite   Pica

(PLEASE TYPE)   FOR PROVIDER USE   (PLEASE TYPE)

VERBAL CONTROL NO.

TYPE OF SERVICE REQUESTED	REQUEST IS RETROACTIVATE?	IS PATIENT MEDICARE ELIGIBLE?	PROVIDER PHONE NO.
□ DRUG ☒ OTHER	□ YES ☒ NO	□ YES ☒ NO	(555) 555-1111 AREA

PATIENT'S AUTHORIZED REPRESENTATIVE (IF ANY)
ENTER NAME AND ADDRESS
•
•
•
•

PROVIDER NAME AND ADDRESS

PLEASE TYPE YOUR NAME AND ADDRESS HERE

SMITH, SUSAN MD
727 ELM BLVD
ANYTOWN, CA 90101

PROVIDER NO.
HSC12345F

30   83

FOR STATE USE

33   PROVIDER; YOUR REQUEST IS:

1 ☒ APPROVED AS REQUESTED   □   □ DEFERRED

2 □ APPROVED AS MODIFIED (ITEMS MARKED BELOW AS AUTHORIZED MAY BE CLAIMED)   □ JACKSON VS RANK PARAGRAPH CODE

BY   *John Doe*
MEDICAL CONSULTANT

NAME AND ADDRESS OF PATIENT

PATIENT NAME (LAST, FIRST, M. I.)
APPLEGATE, NANCY

MEDICAL IDENTIFICATION NO.
253971060

STREET ADDRESS
1515 RIVER ROAD

SEX	AGE	DATE OF BIRTH
F	32	06 18 70

CITY, STATE, ZIP CODE
SACRAMENTO, CA 95822

☒ HOME   □ BOARD AND CARE

PHONE NUMBER
(555) 545-1123

PATIENT STATUS: □ SNF/ICF   □ ACUTE HOSPITAL

34 I.D. # 0 1   35 DATE 0 8 20 X X   44 □ REVIEW COMMENTS INDICATOR

DIAGNOSIS DESCRIPTION:
ENDOMETRIOSIS

ICD-9-CM DIAGNOSIS CODE
617.9

MEDICAL JUSTIFICATION:
VISTA HOSPITAL - 1200 MAPLE ST., ANYTOWN, CA

UNCONTROLLABLE ENDOMETRIOSIS

COMMENTS/ EXPLANATION

RETROACTIVE AUTHORIZATION GRANTED IN ACCORDANCE WITH SECTION 51003 (B)
36 □1 □2 □3 □4 □5 □6

	AUTHORIZED YES / NO	APPROVED UNITS	SPECIFIC SERVICES REQUESTED	UNITS OF SERVICE	PROCEDURE OR DRUG CODE	QUANTITY	CHARGES
1	9 ☒ □	10 *3*	DAYS: 3 HOSPITAL DAYS REQUESTED		11	12	$
2	13 ☒ □	14 *1*	HYSTERECTOMY	1	15 5815070	16 1	$ $1300.00
3	17 □ □	18			19	20	$
4	21 □ □	22			23	24	$
5	25 □ □	26			27	28	$
6	29 □ □	30			31	32	$

TO THE BEST OF MY KNOWLEDGE, THE ABOVE INFORMATION IS TRUE, ACCURATE AND COMPLETE AND THE REQUESTED SERVICES ARE MEDICALLY INDICATED AND NECESSARY TO THE HEALTH OF THE PATIENT.

Susan Smith   MD   8-10-XX
SIGNATURE OF PHYSICIAN OR PROVIDER   TITLE   DATE

AUTHORIZATION IS VALID FOR SERVICES PROVIDED

37 FROM DATE	38 TO DATE
0 9 01 X X	0 9 3 0 X X

TAR CONTROL NUMBER

36 OFFICE	SEQUENCE NUMBER	PI
12	61240229	0

NOTE: AUTHORIZATION DOES NOT GUARANTEE PAYMENT. PAYMENT IS SUBJECT TO PATIENT'S ELIGIBILITY. BE SURE THE IDENTIFICATION CARD IS CURRENT BEFORE RENDERING SERVICE.   SEND TO FIELD SERVICES (F.I. COPY)

SEE YOUR PROVIDER MANUAL FOR ASSISTANCE REGARDING THE COMPLETION OF THIS FORM.   50-1 12/87

Figure 12–6. Completed prior authorization form.

Department of Health or a certain office in a region for approval. In some cases time does not allow for a written request to be sent for prior approval, so an immediate authorization can be obtained via a telephone call to the proper department in any locale. Note the date and time the authorization was given, the name of the person who gave authorization, and any verbal number given by the field office. Usually a treatment authorization form indicating that the service was already authorized must be sent in as follow up to the telephone call.

Time Limit

Each state has its own time limit for the submission of a claim. The time limit can vary from 2 months to 1 year or year and a half from the date that the service was rendered. A bill can be rejected if it is submitted after the time limit unless there is some valid justification that the state recognizes. Some states have separate procedures for billing Over One Year (OOY) claims. A percent of the claim may be reduced according to the date of a delinquent submission. Prescription drugs and dental services are often billed to a different intermediary than are services performed by a physician, depending on the state guidelines.

Reciprocity

Most states have reciprocity for Medicaid payments if a patient requires medical care while out of state. Contact the Medicaid intermediary in the patient's home state and ask for the appropriate forms. If the case was an emergency, state this on the form. File the papers with Medicaid in the patient's home state. Reimbursement will be at that state's rate.

Claim Form

As of October 1, 1986, federal law has mandated that the CMS-1500 Insurance Claim Form be adopted for the processing of Medicaid claims in all states that do not optically scan their claims for payment. States that use optical scanners must adopt a form that is as similar as possible to the format of Form CMS-1500.

Physicians either submit a claim form to a **fiscal agent,** which might be an insurance company, or the bill is sent directly to the local Department of Social Services (Fig. 12–7). Refer to Appendix A for the Medicaid fiscal agent's address for each state.

In Chapter 6 there are general instructions for block-by-block entries on how to complete the CMS-1500 claim form for the Medicaid program. Because guidelines for completing the form vary among all Medicaid intermediaries, refer to the local Medicaid intermediary for their directions. Figure 6–8

Figure 12–7. Physician holding a child and interacting with an insurance biller.

is a template emphasizing placement of basic elements on the claim form and shaded blocks that do not require completion.

To keep up-to-date, always read the current bulletins or newsletters on the Medicaid or Medi-Cal program published by the state fiscal agent. Obtain the state-published handbook with updates of its Medicaid rules. Read and implement the rule changes and updates to avoid rejected claims.

Medicaid Managed Care

When filing a claim for a Medicaid managed care patient, send the bill to the managed care organization (MCO) and not the Medicaid fiscal agent. The MCO receives payment for services rendered to eligible members via the capitation method.

Maternal and Child Health Program

Each jurisdiction operates its own MCHP with its own unique administrative characteristics. Thus each has its own system and forms for billing and related procedures. The official plans and documents are retained in the individual state offices and are not available on either a regional or national office basis. For specific information about a state's policies, write to the MCHP state agency listed in Appendix A.

Medicaid and Other Plans

When Medicaid and a third-party payer cover the patient, Medicaid is always considered the payer of last resort. The third-party payer is billed first.

Government Programs and Medicaid

When a Medicaid patient has Medicare (referred to as a crossover case), TRICARE, or CHAMPVA, always send the insurance claim first to the federal program fiscal agent servicing the region. Then bill Medicaid second and attach to the claim form the remittance advice/explanation of benefits (RA/EOB) that has been received from the federal program. Only send in a claim if the other coverage denies payment or pays less than the Medicaid fee schedule, or if Medicaid covers services not covered by the other policy.

Electronic claims may be automatically crossed over from primary government programs. Chapter 11 gives additional information on crossover claim submission. In Chapter 6, Figure 6–10 is a template emphasizing placement of basic elements on the claim form and shaded blocks that do not require completion for a crossover claim. Chapter 13 gives further information on patients who receive benefits from TRICARE and CHAMPVA.

Group Health Insurance and Medicaid

It is possible that a person can be eligible for Medicaid and also have group health insurance coverage through an employer. Third-party liability occurs if any entity is liable to pay all or part of the medical cost of injury, disease, or disability. In these cases, the primary carrier is the other program or insurance carrier, and it is sent the claim first. After an RA/EOB is received from the primary carrier, Medicaid (the secondary carrier) is billed; a copy of the RA/EOB is enclosed.

Medicaid and Aliens

Some aliens may have Medicare Part A or Part B or both (see chapter 11). If an alien is older than 65 years and on Medicaid (Medi-Cal in California) and not eligible for Medicare benefits, bill the Medicaid processing agent and use the proper Medicaid claim form for the region. On the CMS-1500 claim form in Block 19 indicate, "Alien is older than 65 years and not eligible for Medicare benefits."

After Claim Submission

Remittance Advice

A remittance advice (RA), formerly known as an explanation of benefits (EOB) form, accompanies all Medicaid payment checks sent to the physician. Sometimes five categories of adjudicated claims appear on an RA—adjustments, approvals, denials, suspends, and audit/refund (A/R) transactions— although this terminology may vary from one fiscal agent to another (Fig. 12–8).

Adjustments occur from overpayments or underpayments. Approval is when an original claim or a previously denied claim is approved for payment. Denied claims are listed with a reason code on the RA. Claims in suspense for a certain period of time may be listed on the RA. A/R transactions are miscellaneous transactions as a result of cost settlements, state audits, or refund checks received. An RA for a Medicare or Medicaid case may be found in Chapter 11, Figure 11–18, A and B.

Appeals

The time limit to appeal a claim varies from state to state, but it is usually 30 to 60 days. Most Medicaid offices consider an appeal filed when they receive it, not when it is sent. Usually appeals are sent on a special form or with a cover letter along with photocopies of documents applicable to the appeal (e.g., claim form, remittance advice, and preauthorization forms). Appeals go first to the regional fiscal agent or Medicaid bureau, next to the Department of Welfare, and then to an appellate court that evaluates decisions by local and government agencies. At each level an examiner looks at the case and makes a decision. If not satisfied, the physician may ask for further review at the next level.

HIPAA Compliance Alert
Medicaid Fraud Control

Each state has a Medicaid Fraud Control Unit (MFCU), which is a federally funded state law enforcement entity usually located in the state Attorney General's office. The MFCU investigates and prosecutes cases of fraud and other violations, including complaints of mistreatment in long-term care facilities. The state Medicaid agency must cooperate and ensure access to records by the MFCU and agree to refer suspected cases of provider fraud to this division of the Attorney General's office for investigation.

RESOURCES ON THE INTERNET

Many states have Medicaid Web sites. Get the Internet address for the state by contacting the local Medicaid office. To compare state-to-state Medicaid programs and obtain general data, contact the Centers for Medicaid and Medicare Services's Web site at *http://www.CMS.gov/Medicaid.*

MEDICAID REMITTANCE ADVICE				TO: ANYBODY, FERNANDO G. 1000 ELM STREET ANYTOWN, XY 12345-0001						

REFER TO PROVIDER MANUAL FOR DEFINITION OF RAD CODES

PROVIDER NUMBER 00AX65800		CLAIM TYPE MEDICAL	WARRANT NO 39248026		EDS SEQ NO 20000617		DATE 06/01/20XX		PAGE 1 of 1 pages	

RECIPIENT NAME	RECIPIENT MEDICAID I.D. NO.	CLAIM CONTROL NUMBER	SERVICE DATES FROM MMDDYY	TO MMDDYY	PROCED CODE MODIFIER	PATIENT ACCOUNT NUMBER	QTY	BILLED AMT	PAYABLE AMT			PAID AMT	RAD CODE
APPROVES (RECONCILE TO FINANCIAL SUMMARY)													
TORRES R	559978557	5079350917901	030720XX	030720XX	Z4802		0001	20.00	16.22			16.22	0401
		5079350917901	030720XX	030720XX	Z4802		0001	20.00	16.22			16.22	0401
						TOTAL		40.00	32.44			32.44	
CHAN B	561198435	5044351314501	020320XX	020320XX	Z4800		0001	30.00	27.03			27.03	0401
		5044351314501	020320XX	020320XX	Z4800		0001	20.00	16.22			16.22	0401
						TOTAL		50.00	43.25			43.25	
	TOTALS FOR APPROVES							90.00	75.69			75.69	
												75.69	AMT PAID
DENIES (DO NOT RECONCILE TO FINANCIAL SUMMARY)													
GOMEZ M	624163192	501134031900	122720XX	122720XX	Z4800		0001	30.00					0036
	TOTAL NUMBER OF DENIES						0001						
SUSPENDS (DO NOT RECONCILE TO FINANCIAL SUMMARY)													
HERN D	562416373	5034270703001	010520XX	010520XX	Z4800		0001	20.00					0602
MART E	623105478	5034270712305	010520XX	010520XX	Z4800		0001	20.00					0602
		5034270712305	010520XX	010520XX	Z4800		0001	20.00					0602
						TOTAL		40.00					0602
LOPEZ C	560291467	5034270712502	012420XX	012420XX	Z4800		0001	20.00					0602
	PAT LIAB 932.00 OTH COVG			0.00		SALES TX		0.00					
	TOTAL NUMBER OF SUSPENDS						0004	80.00					

EXPLANATION OF DENIAL/ADJUSTMENT CODES
0401 PAYMENT ADJUSTED TO MAXIMUM ALLOWABLE
0036 RESUBMISSION TURNAROUND DOCUMENT WAS EITHER NOT RETURNED OR WAS RETURNED UNCORRECTED, THEREFOR YOUR CLAIM IS FORMALLY DENIED
0602 PENDING ADJUDICATION
            OHC CARRIER NAME AND ADDRESS
N049 NORTHWESTERN NATIONAL LIFE   111 WASHINGTON AVE. FL 3   MINNEAPOLIS MN 55401

Figure 12–8. Medicaid Remittance Advice form showing adjustments, cutbacks, denied claims, and claims in suspense.

STUDENT ASSIGNMENT LIST

✔ Study Chapter 12.
✔ Answer the review questions in the *Workbook* to reinforce the theory learned in this chapter and to help prepare you for a future test.
✔ Complete the assignments in the *Workbook* to give you hands-on experience in abstracting from case histories, posting to financial accounting record cards, and completing forms pertinent to the Medicaid program in your state. *Note:* For students in California, study Appendix C, Medi-Cal. Complete the assignments in the *Workbook* for Chapter 12 and apply the knowledge learned from Appendix C.
✔ Turn to the Glossary at the end of this textbook for a further understanding of the Key Terms used in this chapter.

TRICARE

CHAMPVA

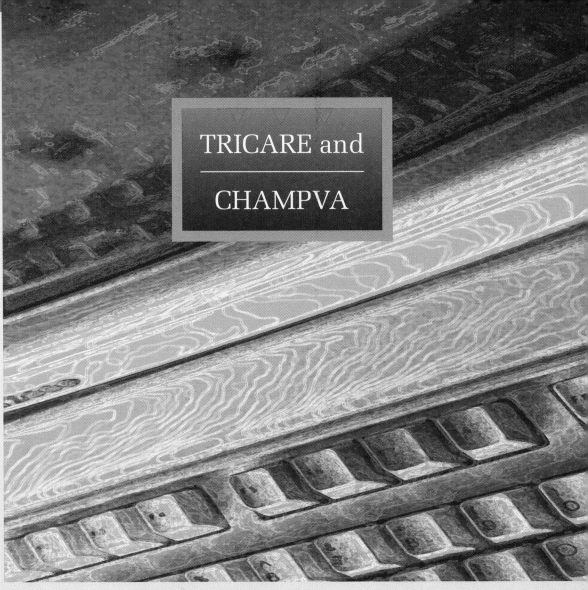

TRICARE and

CHAMPVA

13

TRICARE Hospice Program

TRICARE and HMO Coverage

CHAMPVA Program

Eligibility

Enrollment

Identification Card

Benefits

Provider

Preauthorization

Medical Record Access

Privacy Act of 1974

Computer Matching and
  Privacy Protection Act of 1988

Claims Procedure

Fiscal Intermediary

TRICARE Standard and
  CHAMPVA

TRICARE Extra and TRICARE
  Prime

TRICARE Prime Remote and
  Supplemental Health Care
  Program

TRICARE for Life

TRICARE/CHAMPVA and
  Other Insurance

Medicaid and
  TRICARE/CHAMPVA

Medicare and TRICARE

Medicare and CHAMPVA

Dual or Double Coverage

Third Party Liability

Workers' Compensation

*Procedure: Completing a
CHAMPVA Claim Form*

After Claim Submission

TRICARE Summary Payment
  Voucher

CHAMPVA Explanation of
  Benefits Document

Quality Assurance

Claims Inquiries and Appeals

OBJECTIVES*

**After reading this chapter
you should be able to:**

- State who is eligible for
  TRICARE and CHAMPVA.
- Define pertinent TRICARE
  and CHAMPVA terminology
  and abbreviations.
- Enumerate the differences
  between TRICARE Prime
  and Extra and the TRICARE
  Standard programs.
- Identify the difference
  between the TRICARE
  program and CHAMPVA.
- Explain the benefits and
  nonbenefits of these
  government programs.
- Name various forms used
  with these federal health
  care programs.

- List the circumstances
  when a nonavailability
  statement is necessary.
- Describe how to process
  claims for individuals who
  are covered by TRICARE
  and CHAMPVA.

KEY TERMS

**active duty service member
(ADSM)**

allowable charge

authorized provider

beneficiaries

catastrophic cap

catchment area

CHAMPVA

cooperative care

coordination of benefits

cost-share

**Defense Enrollment
Eligibility Reporting
System (DEERS)**

emergency

fiscal intermediary (FI)

**health benefits advisor
(HBA)**

Health Care Finder (HCF)

**medically (or psychologi-
cally) necessary**

**military treatment facility
(MTF)**

**Nonavailability Statement
(NAS)**

**nonparticipating provider
(nonpar)**

**other health insurance
(OHI)**

participating provider (par)

partnership program

**point-of-service (POS)
option**

Continued.

*Performance objectives and exercises for hands-on practical experience for this chapter appear in the *Workbook*.

KEY TERMS—cont'd

preauthorization

primary care manager (PCM)

quality assurance program

service benefit program

service-connected injury

service retiree (military retiree)

sponsor

summary payment voucher

total, permanent service-connected disability

TRICARE Extra

TRICARE for Life (TFL)

TRICARE Prime

TRICARE Service Center (TSC)

urgent care

veteran

History of TRICARE

The U.S. Congress created CHAMPUS in 1966 under Public Law 89-614 because individuals in the military were finding it increasingly difficult to pay for the medical care required by their families. CHAMPUS (Civilian Health and Medical Program of the Uniformed Services) is a congressionally funded comprehensive health benefits program. Beginning in 1988 CHAMPUS beneficiaries had a choice of retaining their benefits under CHAMPUS or enrolling in a managed care plan called CHAMPUS Prime, a plan to control escalating medical costs and standardize benefits for active duty families, military retirees, and their dependents. In January 1994 TRICARE became the new title for CHAMPUS. Individuals have three choices to obtain health care under TRICARE:

⬧ TRICARE Standard (fee-for-service cost-sharing type of option)
⬧ TRICARE Extra (preferred provider organization type of option)
⬧ TRICARE Prime (health maintenance organization type of option)

TRICARE Programs

Eligibility

The following individuals are entitled to medical benefits under TRICARE:

⬧ Active duty service members in a program called TRICARE Prime Remote
⬧ Eligible family members of active duty service members
⬧ Military retirees and their eligible family members
⬧ Surviving eligible family members of deceased active or retired service members
⬧ Wards and preadoptive children
⬧ Former spouses of active or retired service members who meet certain length-of-marriage rules and other requirements
⬧ Family members of active duty service members who were court-martialed and separated for spouse or child abuse
⬧ Abused spouses, former spouses, or dependent children of service members who were retirement-eligible but lost that eligibility as a result of abuse of the spouse or child
⬧ Spouses and children of North Atlantic Treaty Organization (NATO) nation representatives, under certain circumstances
⬧ Families of activated reservists and National Guard members if military sponsor's active duty orders are for 30 consecutive days or an indefinite period
⬧ Disabled beneficiaries younger than 65 years of age who have Medicare parts A and B and qualify under one of the aforementioned categories
⬧ Medicare-eligible beneficiaries in a program called TRICARE for Life

An individual who qualifies for TRICARE is known as a **beneficiary**; the active duty service member is called the **sponsor.** A person who is retired from a career in the armed forces is known as a **service retiree** or **military retiree** and remains in a TRICARE program until age 65, at which time the individual becomes eligible for the Medicare program. No further family benefits are provided in the event that an active duty military person served from 4 to 6 years and then chose to leave the armed services, thereby giving up a military career. CHAMPVA beneficiaries are not eligible for TRICARE.

Defense Enrollment Eligibility Reporting System

All TRICARE–eligible persons must be enrolled in the **Defense Enrollment Eligibility Reporting System (DEERS)** computerized database. TRICARE claims processors check DEERS before processing claims to verify beneficiary eligibility. A TRICARE beneficiary may check his or her status by contacting the nearest personnel office of any branch of the service or by calling the toll-free number of the DEERS center.

Nonavailability Statement

A **Nonavailability Statement (NAS)** is a certification from a military hospital stating that it cannot provide the care needed (Fig. 13–1). This type of certification is necessary for all TRICARE and CHAMPVA beneficiaries who wish to receive treatment as inpatients at a civilian hospital and who live within a catchment area surrounding a **military treatment facility (MTF)**. An MTF is a uniformed services hospital sometimes referred to as a military hospital, formerly called a U.S. Public Health Service (USPHS) hospital. TRICARE may not pay if this certification is not obtained. An NAS is no longer required for an outpatient procedure.

An NAS is not needed for inpatient care in the following situations:

1. In a medical emergency when delay could cause death or serious threat to health
2. When the patient has other non–TRICARE major medical insurance that pays first on the bills for TRICARE covered care (e.g., when TRICARE is second pay)
3. When the person is a TRICARE beneficiary and lives within the service area of a uniformed hospital
4. When maternity care and birthing services are at a TRICARE Standard–authorized birthing center or a hospital-based birthing room
5. When inpatient services are needed in substance use disorder rehabilitation facilities, skilled nursing facilities, student infirmaries, and residential treatment centers

Catchment Area

The **catchment area** is defined by ZIP codes and is based on an area of approximately 40 miles in radius surrounding each U.S. MTF. Individuals whose home address ZIP code falls outside the local military hospital's service area do not need an NAS before they seek civilian health care under TRICARE.

Automated NAS System

The NAS system has been automated since October 1, 1991. This means that instead of a paper copy of the NAS being sent in with the TRICARE or CHAMPVA claim, the uniformed service medical facility enters the NAS electronically into the DEERS computer files. The patient should always be asked if he or she is enrolled in DEERS. Electronically filed statements are the only ones accepted for processing claims. A hard (paper) copy of DD Form 1251 may be printed if the patient needs one to show the hospital or physician.

TRICARE Standard

Enrollment

Those entitled to medical benefits under TRICARE are automatically enrolled in the TRICARE Standard program.

Identification Card

All dependents 10 years of age or older are required to have a Uniformed Services (military) identification and privilege card for TRICARE Standard. Dependents and survivors of active duty personnel and retirees carry a military identification card DD Form 1173 (Fig. 13–2). Dependents younger than 10 years of age are not normally issued Uniformed Services identification cards; information for their claims should be provided from either parent's card. Refer to the back of the card under "medical" to ensure that the card authorizes civilian medical benefits. Essential information must be abstracted from the front and back of the card; therefore photocopy both sides to retain in the patient's medical record.

Benefits

In the TRICARE Standard program, beneficiaries may receive a wide range of civilian health care services, with a significant portion of the cost paid by the federal government. Patients are not limited to using network providers, and benefits include medical or psychological services or supplies that are considered appropriate care. Such services generally are accepted by qualified professionals to be reasonable and adequate for the diagnosis and treatment of illness, injury, pregnancy, and mental disorders, or are reasonable and adequate for well-baby care. These services are referred to as **medically (or psychologically) necessary.**

Beneficiaries also may receive urgent care and emergency care services. **Urgent care** is medically necessary treatment needed for an immediate illness or injury that would not result in further disability or death if not treated immediately. Treatment should not be delayed but should occur within 24 hours to avoid development of further complications.

NONAVAILABILITY STATEMENT DEPENDENTS MEDICAL CARE PROGRAM

(AR 40-121, SECNAV INST 6320.8A, AFR 160-41, PHS GEN CIR NO 6)

(This Statement is Issued for your Immediate use)

THE ISSUANCE OF THIS STATEMENT MEANS:

1. The medical care requested is not available to you at a Uniformed Services facility in this area.
2. If you receive medical care from civilian sources and such care is determined to be authorized care under the Medicare Program, it will be paid for by the Government to the extent that the program permits.
3. If you receive medical care from civilian sources and it is determined that all or part of the care is not authorized under the Medicare Program, THE GOVERNMENT WILL NOT PAY for the unauthorized care.

The determination of whether medical care you may receive from civilian sources is authorized for payment cannot be made at this time because this determination depends, among other things, upon the care you actually receive. Further, no statement regarding your condition or diagnosis made hereon will be considered in any way determinative as to whether care rendered for such condition is payable under the Medicare Program.

The use of this statement is subject to the conditions and limitations set forth in the regulation issued under the Dependents' Medical Care Act as codified in 10 U.S.C. 1071-1085.

This form must be presented with your Uniformed Services Identification and Privilege Card (DD Form 1173), identified below, when you obtain civilian medical care.

DEPENDENT, SPOUSE OR CHILD, RESIDING WITH SPONSOR				
DEPENDENT'S LAST NAME - FIRST NAME - MIDDLE INITIAL	UNIFORMED SERVICES IDENTIFICATION AND PRIVILEGE CARD (DD FORM 1173)			
	CARD NUMBER			EXPIRATION DATE
	PREFIX	NUMERICAL	SUFFIX	
DOE, MARY B.	EU	18352	A	20XX JUNE 15

DEPENDENT'S ADDRESS (Complete mailing address)

503 CORN DRIVE, WOODLAND HILLS, XY 12345-0002

SPONSOR MEMBER OF UNIFORMED SERVICES ON ACTIVE DUTY	
SPONSOR'S LAST NAME - FIRST NAME - MIDDLE INITIAL DOE, JOHN B.	BRANCH OF SERVICE [ ] ARMY [X] NAVY [ ] AIR FORCE
SERVICE NUMBER GRADE OR RANK 000-00-0001 LT/03	[ ] MARINE CORPS [ ] PUBLIC HEALTH [ ] COAST GUARD [ ] COAST & GEODETIC SURVEY

ORGANIZATION AND OFFICIAL DUTY STATION

POINT MUGU NAVAL STATION, POINT MUGU, CALIFORNIA

REMARKS

STATION AT WHICH PERMIT ISSUED POINT MUGU NAVAL STATION, POINT MUGU, CALIFORNIA	DATE ISSUED 20XX MAY 12
GRADE OR RANK AND POSITION OF ISSUING OFFICER COMMANDING OFFICER LT CMDR	SIGNATURE OF ISSUING OFFICER *George M. Plates*

DISTRIBUTION (Three signed copies of this statement will be furnished the dependent for distribution as follows):

DEPENDENT (Original Copy)   ATTENDING PHYSICIAN (Duplicate copy)   CIVILIAN MEDICAL FACILITY (Triplicate copy)

Figure 13–1. TRICARE Nonavailability Statement DD Form 1251 for inpatient care rendered in a nonmilitary hospital.

Figure 13–2. A, TRICARE Standard active duty dependent's identification card (DD Form 1173) from which essential information must be abstracted. **B,** Sample identification card (DD Form 1173) for a retiree's widowed spouse. Cards indicate: *1*, sponsor's status and rank; *2*, authorization status for treatment by a civilian provider; and *3*, expiration date.

An **emergency** is a sudden and unexpected medical condition, or the worsening of a condition, which poses a threat to life, losing a limb, or sight and requires immediate treatment to alleviate suffering (e.g., shortness of breath, chest pain, and drug overdose). Usually it is obtained at a hospital emergency department.

TRICARE Standard patients usually seek care from a military hospital near their home. The military physician may refer the patient to a civilian source if the service hospital that is managing the TRICARE Standard patient cannot provide a particular service or medical supplies. **Cooperative care** consists of services or supplies that may be cost-shared by TRICARE Standard under certain conditions.

A **partnership program** is another option that lets TRICARE Standard–eligible persons receive inpatient or outpatient treatment from civilian providers of care in a military hospital, or from uniformed services providers of care in civilian facilities. Whether a partnership program is instituted at a particular military hospital is up to the facility's commander, who makes the decision based on economics.

In addition, there are times when there is no service hospital in the area and a TRICARE Standard beneficiary may seek care through a private physician's office or hospital. Delivery of care through the private physician is emphasized in this chapter.

Read carefully through Figures 13–3 and 13–4 to see the overall picture of TRICARE benefits, which includes cost-sharing (deductibles and copayments).

Fiscal Year

The TRICARE fiscal year begins October 1 and ends September 30. It is different from most programs; therefore office staff should be alert when collecting deductibles.

ADFM = active duty family members RFMS = retirees, family members, and survivors	**Benefit and Coverage Chart**					
Inpatient Services	**Programs and Beneficiary Costs**					
Program and Classification	**Tricare Prime**		**Tricare Extra**		**Tricare Standard**	
	ADFM	**RFMS**	**ADFM**	**RFMS**	**ADFM**	**RFMS**
Hospitalization* including **Maternity Benefits***	No copayment	$11.45/day; civilian care $11/day or $25 min charge per/admission, whichever is greater	$11.45/day; civilian care $11/day or $25 min charge per/admission, whichever is greater	$11.45/day; civilian care $250/day or 25% cost-share (contracted fee) whichever is less, plus 20% cost-share for separately billed professional charges	$11.45/day; civilian care $11/day or $25 min charge per/admission, whichever is greater	$11.45/day; civilian care $401/day or 25% cost-share (contracted fee) whichever is less, plus 25% cost-share (maximum allowable charge) for separately billed professional charges
Skilled Nursing Care					$25/admission, or $11.45/day, whichever is greater	25% cost-share (billed charges), plus 25% cost-share (maximum allowable charge) for separately billed professional charges
Mental Ilness Hospitalization* and **Substance Use Treatment*** (inpatient, partial hospital program)	None	$40/day (no copayment or cost-share for separately billed professional charges)	$20/day	20% cost-share (contracted fee), plus 20% cost-share (contracted fee) for separately billed professional charges	$20/day	25% cost-share (max allowable charge), for separately billed professional charges plus: 25% of (1) per diem, (2) fixed daily amount or billed charges, or (3) 25% of allowed amount (RTC & partial hospitalization)
Partial Hospitalization* (mental illness)	None	$40/day or $25/admission, whichever is greater	$20/day	20% cost-share (contracted fee), plus 20% cost-share for separately billed professional charges	$20/day	25% of allowed amount, plus 25% maximum allowable charge for separately billed professional charges
Hospice Care	Available in lieu of other TRICARE benefits (provided by Medicare approved program).					
*Preauthorization required						

Figure 13–3. TRICARE Prime, Extra, and Standard Inpatient Services Benefits and Coverage Chart.

Authorized Providers of Health Care

An **authorized provider** may treat a TRICARE Standard patient. This means the provider can be reimbursed by TRICARE for its share of costs for medical benefits and the provider is qualified to provide certain health benefits to TRICARE beneficiaries. Only "certified" providers, those who have passed a credentialing process, can be authorized by TRICARE. Beneficiaries who use *nonauthorized* providers may be responsible for their entire bill, and

there are no legal limits on the amounts these providers can bill beneficiaries. Examples of non-authorized providers are most chiropractors and acupuncturists and those physicians who do not meet state licensing or training requirements or were rejected for authorization by TRICARE. Authorized providers include:

◗ Doctor of medicine (MD)
◗ Doctor of osteopathy (DO or MD)
◗ Doctor of dental surgery (DDS)
◗ Doctor of dental medicine (DDM)

ADFM = active duty family members RFMS = retirees, family members and survivors	**Benefit and Coverage Chart**					

Outpatient Services	Programs and Beneficiary Costs					
Program and Classification	**Tricare Prime**		**Tricare Extra**		**Tricare Standard**	
	ADFM	**RFMS**	**ADFM**	**RFMS**	**ADFM**	**RFMS**
Annual Enrollment Fee* (per fiscal year)	None	$230/person $460/family	None ⟶		None ⟶	
Annual Deductible (per fiscal year 10/1 to 9/30) (applied to outpatient services before cost-share is determined)	None (except when using Point-of-Service option)		E-4 and below $50/person $100/family E-5 and above $150/person $300/family	$150/person $300/family	E-4 and below $50/person $100/family E-5 and above $150/person $300/family	$150/person $300/family
Physician Services	None	$12	15% of contracted fee	20% of contracted fee	20% of maximum allowable charge	25% of maximum allowable charge
Ancillary Services (certain radiology, laboratory, & cardiac services)	None ⟶ (RFMS may have $12 copay if test provided independent of office visit)					
Ambulance Services	None	$20				
Home Health Services	None	$12				
Family Health Services	None	$12				
Durable Medical Equipment (greater than $100)	None	20% cost-share				
Emergency Services (network and non-network)	None	$30 copayment				
Outpatient Behavioral Health (limitations apply)	None	$25 copayment $17 group visits				
Immunizations (for required overseas travel)	None	Not covered		Not covered		Not covered
Ambulatory Surgery (same day)	None	$25 copayment (applied to facility charges only)	$25 copayment for hospital charges	20% of contracted fee	$25 copayment for hospital charges	*Professional:* 25% of maximum allowable charge *Facility:* 25% of maximum allowable charge OR billed charges, whichever is less
Eye Examinations (limitations apply)	None	Clinical Preventive Service	15% of contracted fee	Not covered	20% of maximum allowable charge	Not covered
Prescription Drugs– Network Pharmacy	$3 copayment for each 30-day supply of **generic** medication $9 copayment for each 30-day supply of **brand name** medication					
Prescription Drugs– National Mail Order Pharmacy	$3 copayment for each 90-day supply of **generic** medication $9 copayment for each 90-day supply of **brand name** medication (Note: if the beneficiary has primary insurance that covers presciption medication, the beneficiary is not eligible for the mail order pharmacy benefit)					
Prescription Drugs– Non-network Pharmacy	$9 or 20% of total cost (whichever is greater) plus deductible					

*No enrollment fee for those who are eligible for Medicare (enrolled in Part B) on the basis of disability or end-stage renal disease

NOTE: TRICARE Prime Remote–benefits are similar to TRICARE Prime program; however, ADSMs have no copayment costs-share or deductible

Program for Persons with Disabilities–no deductible; monthly cost-share varies from $25 to $250, depending on sponsor's rank

Figure 13–4. TRICARE Prime, Extra, and Standard Outpatient Services Benefits and Coverage Chart.

▶ Doctor of podiatric medicine or surgical chiropody (DPM or DSC)

▶ Doctor of optometry (DO)

▶ Psychologist (PhD)

Other authorized nonphysician providers include audiologists, certified nurse midwives, clinical social workers, licensed practical nurses, licensed vocational nurses, psychiatric social workers, registered nurses, registered physical therapists, and speech therapists.

Preauthorization

There are certain referral and **preauthorization** requirements for TRICARE Standard patients. When specialty care or hospitalization is necessary, the military treatment facility must be used if services are available. If services are not available, the **Health Care Finder (HCF)** will assist with the referral or preauthorization process. An HCF is a health care professional, usually a registered nurse, who helps the patient work with his or her primary care physician to locate a specialist or obtain a preauthorization for care. HCFs are found at a **TRICARE Service Center (TSC),** which is an office staffed by HCFs and beneficiary service representatives. All admissions, ambulatory surgical procedures, and other selected procedures require preauthorization. Certain types of health care services requiring prior approval from the TRICARE health contractor follow:

▶ Arthroscopy

▶ Breast mass or tumor removal

▶ Cardiac catheterization

▶ Cataract removal

▶ Cystoscopy

▶ Dental care

▶ Dilatation and curettage

▶ Durable medical equipment purchases

▶ Gastrointestinal endoscopy

▶ Gynecologic laparoscopy

▶ Hernia repairs

▶ Laparoscopic cholecystectomy

▶ Ligation or transection of fallopian tubes

▶ Magnetic resonance imaging (MRI)

▶ Mental health care

▶ Myringotomy or tympanostomy

▶ Neuroplasty

▶ Nose repair (rhinoplasty and septoplasty)

▶ Strabismus repair

▶ Tonsillectomy or adenoidectomy

Payment

Deductible and Copayment

Deductibles and copayments are determined according to two groups: (1) active duty family members; and (2) retirees, their family members, and survivors.

Spouses and Children of Active Duty Members

For inpatient (hospitalized) care, the beneficiary pays the first $25 of the hospital charge or a small fee for each day, whichever is greater, and TRICARE pays the remainder of the allowable charges for authorized care.

For outpatient (nonhospitalized) care, the beneficiary pays the first $150 (deductible) plus 20% of the charges more than the $150 deductible. A family with two or more eligible beneficiaries pays a maximum of $300 (deductible) plus 20% of the charges in excess of $300. TRICARE pays the remainder of the allowable charges, which is 80%.

All Other Eligible Beneficiaries

This category includes retired members, dependents of retired members, dependents of deceased members who died in active duty, and so forth.

For inpatient (hospitalized) care, the beneficiary pays 25% of the hospital charges and fees of professional personnel. TRICARE pays the remaining allowable charges for authorized care, or 75%.

For outpatient (nonhospitalized) care, the beneficiary pays $150 (deductible) plus 25% of the charges more than the $150 deductible. A family with two or more eligible beneficiaries pays a maximum of $300 plus 25% of the charges in excess of $300. TRICARE pays the remainder of the allowable charges for authorized care, which is 75%.

Refer to Figures 13–3 and 13–4 for further clarification and to see the differences in benefits between the three TRICARE program options.

Participating Provider

If the physician agrees to accept assignment a TRICARE Standard case, the **participating provider (par)** agrees to accept the TRICARE–determined **allowable charge** as payment in full. Providers may choose to accept TRICARE assignment on a case-by-case basis. Assignment should always be accepted when the service member is transferring within 6 months because this will avoid collection problems. The provider may bill the patient for his or her **cost-share** or coinsurance (20% to 25% of the allowable charge after the deductible has been met) and for any noncovered services or supplies. The provider may not bill for the difference between the provider's usual charge and the allowable charge.

Beneficiaries pay only a certain amount each year for the cost-share and annual deductible. This amount is known as the **catastrophic cap.** After this cap is reached, TRICARE pays 100% of the allowable charges for the rest of the year. A note should be attached to the claim when the patient has met the catastrophic cap; this may help expedite claims processing and payment. After the claim is completed and sent to the fiscal intermediary, the payment goes directly to the physician.

Nonparticipating Provider

A health care provider who chooses not to participate in TRICARE is called a **nonparticipating provider (nonpar)** and, as of November 1, 1993, may not bill the patient more than 115% of the TRICARE allowable charge. For example, if the TRICARE allowable charge for a procedure is $100, providers who decide not to participate in TRICARE may charge TRICARE patients no more than $115 for that procedure. The patient pays the deductible (20% or 25% of the charges determined to be allowable) and any amount more than the allowable charge up to 115% when the physician does not accept assignment.

TRICARE Extra

Enrollment

TRICARE Extra is a preferred provider organization type of option in which the individual does not have to enroll or pay an annual fee. On a visit-by-visit basis, the individual may seek care from an authorized network provider and receive a discount on services and reduced cost-share (copayment). A nonenrolled beneficiary automatically becomes a TRICARE Extra beneficiary when care is rendered by a network provider. If a nonenrolled beneficiary receives care from a non-network provider, the services received are covered under TRICARE Standard. Providers receive a contract rate for giving care.

Identification Card

A TRICARE Extra beneficiary must present the military identification card when receiving care as proof of eligibility. The military identification card indicates a "Yes" in Box 15B (back of card) if the beneficiary is eligible. Children younger than 10 years of age may use the sponsor's identification card (attach a copy of the child's card to the claim). Individuals older than 10 years must have their own identification card. Contact the local HCF to verify eligibility. Active duty and retiree dependents and survivors carry an orange or brown military identification card (Fig. 13–2). Retirees carry a blue-gray military identification card.

Benefits

See Figures 13–3 and 13–4 for outpatient and inpatient benefits and deductible and copayment amounts.

Network Provider

The network provider is the physician who provides medical care to TRICARE beneficiaries under the TRICARE Extra program at contracted rates. They have discount agreements with the TRICARE program.

Preauthorization

Referrals from other network providers are coordinated through the HCF. The network provider refers the beneficiary for additional services, when necessary, after precertification requirements and completing a referral form.

Payments

Deductible and Copayment

Deductibles and copayments are determined by group: (1) active duty family members; and (2) retirees, their family members, and survivors.

Spouses and Children of Active Duty Members

No copayment is required for inpatient (hospitalized) care.

For outpatient (nonhospitalized) care, the beneficiary pays the first $150 (deductible) plus 15% of the charges more than the $150 deductible. A family with two or more eligible beneficiaries pays a maximum of $300 (deductible) plus 15% of the charges in excess of $300. TRICARE pays the remainder of the allowable charges (85%).

All Other Eligible Beneficiaries

For inpatient (hospitalized) care, the copayment is $250 per day or 25% of the plan's allowable charges, whichever is less, plus 20% of separately billed professional charges at the plan's allowable rate.

For outpatient (nonhospitalized) care, the beneficiary pays $150 (deductible) plus 20% of the charges more than the $150 deductible. A family with two or more eligible beneficiaries pays a maximum of $300 plus 20% of the charges in excess of $300. TRICARE pays the remainder of the allowable charges for authorized care (80%).

See Figures 13–3 and 13–4 for further clarification of deductibles and copayments.

TRICARE Prime

TRICARE Prime is a voluntary health maintenance organization (HMO)–type option. Participation in TRICARE Prime is optional. Beneficiaries who are not enrolled as members in TRICARE Prime may continue to receive services through TRICARE Extra from network providers or through TRICARE Standard using non-network providers. The beneficiary may no longer use the TRICARE Standard program once enrolled in TRICARE Prime.

Enrollment

An individual must complete an application and enroll for a minimum of 12 months to become a TRICARE Prime member. There is an annual enrollment fee charged per person or family except for active duty families, who may enroll free. Active duty service members are enrolled automatically in TRICARE Prime and are not eligible for benefits under TRICARE Standard or TRICARE Extra. These members are able to use the local military and civilian provider network with necessary authorization.

Enrollees normally receive care from within the Prime network of civilian and military providers. The beneficiary has the option of choosing or being assigned a **primary care manager (PCM)** for each family member. The PCM manages all aspects of the patient's health care (except emergencies) including referrals to specialists. Enrolled beneficiaries may not use a non-network provider, except in emergencies or for pharmaceuticals, without a specific referral from an HCF.

Identification Card

Individuals who enroll are issued a TRICARE Prime identification card, as shown in Figure 13–5. This card does not guarantee TRICARE eligibility; therefore providers must check the TRICARE Uniformed Services military identification card for the effective

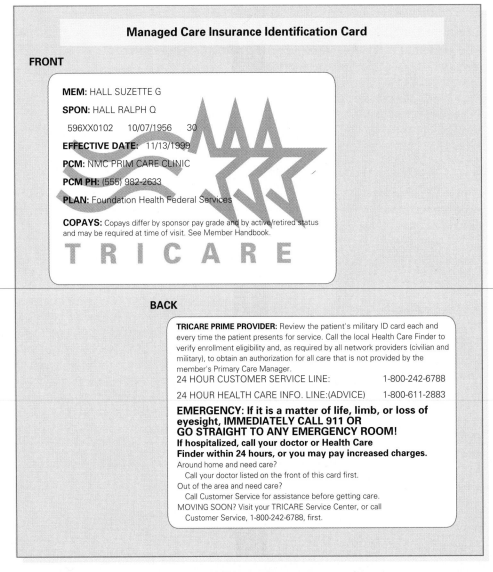

Figure 13–5. TRICARE Prime identification card. A new TRICARE Prime identification card has been redesigned to incorporate essential contact information to help enrollees access health care. This card will be introduced gradually.

and expiration dates or call the local HCF. Copies of the military identification card and the TRICARE Prime card should always be made and retained in the patient's file. For TRICARE Prime patients, both cards should be checked at every visit.

Benefits

Covered services are the same as those for TRICARE Standard patients plus additional preventive and primary care services. For example, periodic physical examinations are covered at no charge under TRICARE Prime but are not covered under TRICARE Extra or TRICARE Standard. Prime also covers certain immunizations and annual eye examinations for dependent children of retirees that are not a benefit under Extra or Standard. A dental plan is available for an additional monthly premium. An NAS is necessary for certain inpatient services if the beneficiary resides within the designated military treatment facility catchment area. See Figures 13–3 and 13–4 for outpatient and inpatient benefits and deductible and copayment amounts.

Primary Care Manager

The **PCM** is a physician who is responsible for coordinating and managing the entire beneficiary's health care unless there is an emergency. A provider who decides to participate in a managed care program goes through a credentialing process. This is done approximately every 2 years for all physicians who participate as providers. The PCM may refer the beneficiary for additional services, when necessary, but specific referral and preauthorization requirements must be carried out. Referral patterns are evaluated to determine excessive or inappropriate referrals to specialists. A pattern of such referrals could result in termination of participation in TRICARE Prime.

Preauthorization

All admissions, ambulatory surgical procedures, and other selected procedures require preauthorization. Outpatient or ambulatory surgery must be on the approved procedure list before it is performed. The list is in the TRICARE Policy Manual available on the Web site: *www.tricare-on@csd-mail.med com.amedd.army.mil.*

An NAS may be needed for some types of surgery performed in approved ambulatory surgery centers or hospitals.

The **health benefits advisor (HBA)** at the nearest military medical facility should be called to find out if an NAS statement is needed for the procedure before the surgery is scheduled in the approved facility. An HBA is a person at a military hospital or clinic who is there to help beneficiaries obtain medical care needed through the military and TRICARE. A **point-of-service (POS) option** is available if no authorization is obtained. This means that the individual can choose to get TRICARE–covered nonemergency services outside the Prime network of providers without a referral from the PCM and without authorization from the HCF. There is an annual deductible and 50% cost-share if the POS option is used.

Payments

Copayment

TRICARE Prime copayments for inpatient hospital services vary for active duty family members and for retirees and their family members and survivors. For outpatient services, copayments are the same for active duty family members and for retirees and their family members and survivors but vary in amounts depending on the type of service received. They always should be collected at the time services are rendered. Refer to Figures 13–3 and 13–4 for further clarification of copayments.

TRICARE for Life

In October 2001 **TRICARE for Life (TFL)** was enacted and offered additional TRICARE benefits as a supplementary payer to Medicare for uniformed service retirees, their spouses, and survivors age 65 or older. When beneficiaries become entitled to receive Medicare Part A and to purchase Medicare Part B upon attaining the age of 65, they experience no break in TRICARE coverage. The only change is that TRICARE will pay secondary to Medicare beginning on the first day of the month they turn 65.

TRICARE for Life is provided to the following beneficiaries:

▶ Medicare–eligible uniformed service retirees, including retired guard and reservists
▶ Medicare–eligible family members, including widows and widowers
▶ Certain former spouses if they were eligible for TRICARE before age 65

Note: Dependent parents and parents-in-law are not eligible for TRICARE benefits. They may continue to receive services within a military treatment facility on a space-available basis.

Enrollment

Most beneficiaries must be eligible for Medicare Part A and enrolled in Medicare Part B to qualify for TFL. An exception is Uniformed Services Family Health Plan (USFHP) members. Prospective TFL beneficiaries do not have to sign up or enroll for the program; however, they should be enrolled in DEERS. There are no enrollment fees for TRICARE for Life. The member is required to enroll in Medicare Part B and must pay Medicare Part B monthly fees.

The DEERS notifies a beneficiary within 90 days before his or her 65th birthday that the medical benefits are about to change. They ask the beneficiary to contact the nearest Social Security Administration office about enrollment in Medicare. Remember that the beneficiary must elect to enroll in Medicare Part B to be eligible for TRICARE for Life benefits. If the beneficiary is age 65 or older and only has Medicare Part A, he or she can enroll in Medicare Part B during the annual general enrollment period, which runs from January 1st to March 31st every year. Medicare Part B coverage then begins on July 1st of the year in which the beneficiary enrolls.

Refer to Resources on the Internet at the end of this chapter for more information about enrolling in Medicare Part B and monthly fees that apply.

Identification Card

Beneficiaries who qualify for TFL do not need a TRICARE enrollment card.

Benefits

Each beneficiary receives a matrix comparing Medicare benefits to TRICARE benefits. Refer to Resources at the end of this chapter for the TRICARE Management Activity Web site address to download this information. Certain benefits (e.g., prescription medications) are covered under the TRICARE Senior Pharmacy Program. Pharmacy benefits provide Medicare–eligible retirees of the Uniformed Service, their family members, and survivors the same pharmacy benefit as retirees who are under age 65. This includes access to prescription drugs at MTFs, retail pharmacies, and through the National Mail Order Pharmacy. Medicare Part B enrollment is not mandatory to receive TRICARE Senior Pharmacy Program benefits.

Referral and Preauthorization

There are no preauthorization requirements for the TFL program. All services and supplies must be benefits of the Medicare or TRICARE programs to be covered.

Payment

The following four scenarios represent most cases and explain the payment mechanism:
1. Services covered under both Medicare and TRICARE. Medicare pays first at the Medicare rate and the remaining is paid by TRICARE, which covers the beneficiary's cost-share and deductible. No copayment, cost-share, or deductible is paid by the TFL beneficiary.
2. Services covered under Medicare but not TRICARE. Medicare pays the Medicare rate and the beneficiary pays the Medicare cost-share and deductible amounts. TRICARE pays nothing.
3. Services covered under TRICARE but not Medicare. TRICARE pays the allowed amount and Medicare pays nothing. The beneficiary is responsible for the TRICARE cost-share and the deductible amounts.
4. Services not payable by TRICARE or Medicare. The beneficiary is entirely responsible for the medical bill.

TRICARE Plus

Enrollment

TRICARE Plus is open to persons eligible for care in military facilities and not enrolled in TRICARE Prime or a commercial HMO. TRICARE Plus allows some Military Health System (MHS) beneficiaries to enroll with a military primary care provider. There is no enrollment fee.

Identification Card

Persons enrolled in TRICARE Plus are issued an identification card and identified in the DEERS.

Benefits

The TRICARE Plus program is designed to function in the following ways:
- Enrollees use the military treatment facility as their source of primary care; it is not a comprehensive health plan.
- Enrollees may seek care from a civilian provider but are discouraged from obtaining nonemergency primary care from sources outside the MTF.
- Enrollees are not guaranteed access to specialty providers at the MTF.
- Enrollees may not use their enrollment at another facility.

The military treatment facility's commander determines the enrollment capacity at each MTF.

Payment

TRICARE Plus offers the same benefits as TRICARE Prime when using an MTF. It has no effect on the enrollees' use or payment of civilian health care benefits; therefore TRICARE Standard, TRICARE Extra, or Medicare may pay for civilian health care services obtained by a TRICARE Plus enrollee.

TRICARE Prime Remote Program

Enrollment

TRICARE Prime Remote (TPR) is a program designed for **active duty service members (ADSMs)** who work and live more than 50 miles or 1 hour from military treatment facilities (military hospitals and clinics). ADSMs must enroll for this program, which enables them to receive care from any civilian provider.

Family members of active duty service members in the TPR program are not eligible for TPR. They may enroll in TRICARE Prime or receive care through the TRICARE Standard and TRICARE Extra options.

Identification Card

Active duty service members must present their military identification card to receive care from providers (Fig. 13–6). Photocopy front and reverse sides of the card so information is available for reference when completing the insurance claim form.

Benefits

TPR program benefits are similar to TRICARE Prime. Services may be received from an MTF when available or from any civilian provider. Primary routine care does not require prior authorization (e.g., office visits and preventive health care). The HCF must be contacted to receive authorization for referrals, inpatient admissions, maternity, physical therapy, orthotics, hearing appliances, family planning (tubal ligation or vasectomy), outpatient and inpatient behavioral health services, and transplants. See Figure 13–7 for a summary of the unique aspects of TPR.

Referral and Preauthorization

Routine primary care does *not* require prior authorization (e.g., office visits and preventive health care). The PCM must initiate all specialty referrals and coordinate requests through the HBA for certain outpatient services, all inpatient surgical or medical services, maternity services, physical therapy, orthotics, hearing appliances, family planning, transplants, and inpatient or outpatient behavioral health services. The HBA is a government employee who is responsible for helping all MHS beneficiaries to obtain medical care.

Payments

Those covered and receiving benefits under TPR are not responsible for any out-of-pocket costs. Active duty service member claims for services provided by a TRICARE network provider are paid at the same contracted rate as other TRICARE beneficiary claims.

Supplemental Health Care Program

Enrollment

The Supplemental Health Care Program (SHCP) covers both military treatment facility–referred care as well as civilian health care provided to active duty service members. The military treatment facility always administers routine care (e.g., routine office visits and preventive health care).

Identification Card

Active duty service members must present their military identification card to receive care from providers (Fig. 13–6). The front and reverse sides of

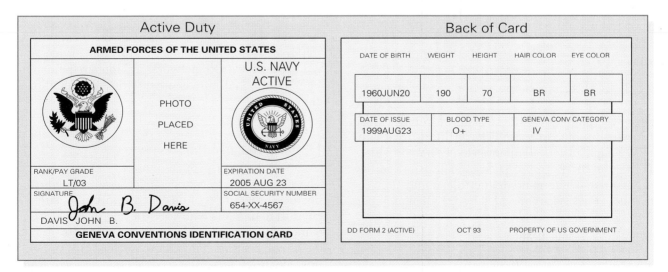

Figure 13–6. Military identification card for an active duty individual in the Armed Forces. It is used as the identification card for the TRICARE Prime Remote Program and is considered a sponsor identification card.

	TRICARE Prime Remote (TPR)	Supplemental Health Care Program (SHCP)
Plan description	TPR is a program for Active Duty Service Members (ADSMs) who live and work more than 50 miles or one hour from a military treatment facility. ADSMs must enroll.	SHCP is a program for • Active Duty Service Members (ADSMs) • Inpatients at military treatment facilities who are not TRICARE eligible (e.g., eligible parents, parents-in-law) referred by an MTF to a civilian provider for care (usually for a specific test, procedure or consultation). • Non-MTF referred ADSMs (e.g., ROTC students, cadets/midshipmen, eligible foreign military).
Provider type	Any civilian provider.	Any civilian provider.
Beneficiary access to care	TPR ADSMs receive from any civilian provider, or from a military treatment facility when available. Under TPR, ADSMs will have the same priority to care as other ADSMs at the MTF.	The beneficiary may receive services from any civilian provider, in accordance with referral and preauthorization requirements, below.
Beneficiary responsibility	TPR ADSMs have no annual deductible, cost-shares or copayments. The TPR ADSM must present his/her Military ID card at the time care is received.	ADSMs and others, eligible for SHCP referred to civilian providers have no copayment, deductible, or cost share. Beneficiary must present his/her Military ID card at the time care is recieved.
Point-of-Service (POS)	Point-of-Service does not apply. If the ADSM receives care without a referral or preauthorization, the claim will be processed if it meets all other TRICARE requirements on a case-by-case basis.	The Point-of-Service option does not apply.
Program benefits	Offers benefits similar to TRICARE Prime. Some benefits (including all behavioral health care) require preauthorization.	Offers benefits similar to TRICARE Prime. Some benefits (including all behavioral health care) require preauthorization.
Referrals and preauthorizations	Primary care – ADSMs can receive primary care from a provider without a referral or preauthorization. ADSMs with an assigned PCM will receive primary care from their PCM. ADSMs with no PCM can use any TRICARE-certified provider. Or, he/she can contact a HCF for assistance in locating a provider. Specialty and inpatient care – The SPOC will review requests for specialty and inpatient care.	Specialty and inpatient care – The MTF will review all requests for specialty and inpatient care for ADSMs. **The MTF Commander or designee signature on a DD Form 2161** is required for designated patients **referred** for civilian care. Preauthorization for **non-referred** Active Duty Service Members for specialty, inpatient, and behavioral health care must be **obtained from the SPOC or the Health Care Finder.**

Figure 13–7. Summary of unique aspects of TRICARE Prime Remote Program and Supplemental Health Care Program.

the card should be photocopied so information is available for reference when the insurance claim form is completed.

Benefits

See Figure 13–7 for a summary of the unique aspects of SHCP.

SHCP enables beneficiaries to be referred to a civilian provider for care. The military treatment facility must initiate all referrals to civilian providers and use a DD Form 2161 signed by the facility commander. There is no deductible, copayment, or cost-share for services provided by a civilian provider.

Referral and Preauthorization

The MTF initiates all referrals for ADSMs and other designated patients to civilian specialists when needed.

Payments

Those covered and receiving benefits under SHCP are not responsible for any out-of-pocket costs. Active duty service member claims for services provided by a TRICARE network provider are paid at the same contracted rate as other TRICARE beneficiary claims.

TRICARE Hospice Program

The TRICARE hospice program is based on Medicare's hospice program. It is designed to provide care and comfort to patients who are expected to live less than 6 months if the terminal illness runs its normal course. Those persons who receive care under the hospice program cannot receive other services under the TRICARE basic programs (treatments aimed at a cure) unless the hospice care has been formally revoked. There are a number of additional rules and limits to the hospice program; therefore HBA at the nearest military medical facility should be called and a copy of the guidelines requested.

TRICARE and HMO Coverage

TRICARE considers HMO coverage to be the same as any other primary health insurance coverage. TRICARE shares the cost of covered care received from an HMO (including the HMO's user fees), after the HMO has paid all it is going to pay, under the following conditions:

▶ The provider must meet TRICARE provider certification standards.
▶ The type of care must be a TRICARE benefit and medically necessary.
▶ TRICARE does not pay for emergency services received outside the HMO's normal service area.

TRICARE does not cost-share services an individual obtains outside the HMO if the services are available through the HMO. For example, if an HMO provides psychiatric services but the patient does not like the HMO's psychiatrist and obtains services outside the HMO, TRICARE will not pay anything on the claim.

CHAMPVA Program

The Veterans Health Care Expansion Act of 1973 (PL93-82) authorized a CHAMPUS–like program called **CHAMPVA** (Civilian Health and Medical Program of the Veterans Administration; now known as the Department of Veterans Affairs), which became effective on September 1, 1973. CHAMPVA is not an insurance program in that it does not involve a contract guaranteeing the indemnification of an insured party against a specified loss in return for a premium paid. It is considered a **service benefit program;** therefore there are no premiums.

This program is for the spouse and children of a veteran with a **total, permanent service-connected disability** or for the surviving spouse and children of a veteran who died as a result of a service-connected disability. A **veteran** is any person who has served in the armed forces of the United States, is no longer in the service, and has received an honorable discharge. Just as in the TRICARE program, individuals who qualify for CHAMPVA are known as beneficiaries and the active duty service member is called the sponsor.

Examples of service-connected total, permanent disabilities include: an injury with paraplegic results, a bullet wound with neurologic damage, and loss of a limb. This contrasts with a chronic or temporary service-connected disability, which might exist if an individual improperly lifts a heavy object while in the Navy, suffers a back injury with ongoing sporadic symptoms, and requires continuing medical care after leaving the service. Both scenarios present service-connected disabilities; however, the first example illustrates a person permanently disabled, whereas the second illustrates what may be a chronic or temporary disability.

Eligibility

The following persons are eligible for CHAMPVA benefits as long as they are not eligible for TRICARE Standard and not eligible for Medicare Part A as a result of reaching age 65:

▶ The husband, wife, or unmarried child of a veteran with a total disability, permanent in nature, resulting from a service-connected injury
▶ The husband, wife, or unmarried child of a veteran who died as the result of a service-connected disability or who, at the time of death, had a total disability, permanent in nature, resulting from a **service-connected injury**
▶ The husband, wife, or unmarried child of an individual who died in the line of duty while in active service

Qualifying children are those unmarried and younger than the age of 18, regardless of whether dependent or not, or those up to age 23 who are enrolled in a course of instruction at an approved educational institution.

Determination of eligibility is the responsibility of the Department of Veterans Affairs. The prospective beneficiary visits the nearest VA medical center and receives a VA identification card if eligible.

Enrollment

Dependents of veterans must have a Social Security number and have contacted the local VA regional office to establish dependency on the veteran sponsor. The individual obtains and completes an application by phone, fax, or downloading from the VA's Web site (see Resources on the Internet at the end of this chapter).

Identification Card

The issuing station's number appears on the identification card to identify the home station where the beneficiary's case file is kept. The identification card number is the veteran's VA file number with an alpha suffix. The suffix is different for each beneficiary of a sponsor. All dependents 10 years of age or older are required to have a Uniformed Services (military) identification and privilege card for CHAMPVA, as shown in Figure 13–8.

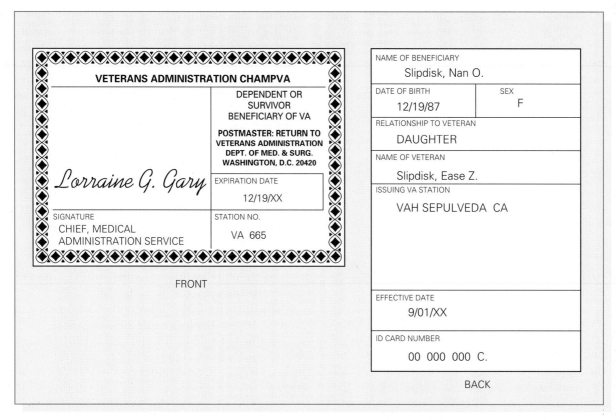

Figure 13–8. CHAMPVA card.

Benefits

The Department of Veterans Affairs (VA) elected to provide these beneficiaries with benefits and cost-sharing plans similar to those received by dependents of retired and deceased uniformed services personnel under TRICARE Standard. An overall picture of CHAMPVA benefits, which includes cost-sharing (deductibles and copayments), can be seen in Figure 13–9.

Provider

The beneficiaries of the CHAMPVA program have complete freedom of choice in selecting their civilian health care providers.

Preauthorization

Preauthorization is necessary for organ and bone marrow transplants, hospice services, most mental health or substance abuse services, all dental care, and all durable medical equipment with a purchase price or total rental cost of $300 or more. Preauthorization for mental health and substance abuse care must be requested from Health Management Strategies (HMS) International, Inc., at 800-240-4068 or mailed to CVAC-MHP, P.O. Box 26128, Alexandria, VA 22313. All other preauthorization requests are made directly to CHAMPVA at 303-331-7599, by fax at 303-331-7804, or by mail to VA Health Administration Center, CHAMPVA, Attn: Preauthorization, P.O. Box 65023, Denver, CO 80206-9023.

HIPAA Compliance Alert
Medical Record Access

Privacy Act of 1974

The Privacy Act of 1974 became effective on September 27, 1975, and establishes an individual's right to review his or her medical records maintained by a federal medical care facility, such as a VA medical center or U.S. Public Health Service facility, and to contest inaccuracies in such records. The Act directs each agency to make its own rules establishing access procedures. Agencies are allowed to adopt special procedures when it is believed that direct access could be harmful to a person. The Act requires that an individual from whom personal information is requested be informed of: (1) the authority for the request; (2) the principal purpose of the information requested; (3) routine use of the information; and (4) the effect on an individual who does not provide the information.

Computer Matching and Privacy Protection Act of 1988

The Computer Matching and Privacy Protection Act of 1988 was established and permits the government to verify information by way of computer matches.

Both of these acts are mentioned on the back of the CMS-1500 claim form. TRICARE patients must be made aware of this information by physicians who treat them, so that they are knowledgeable about routine use and disclosure of medical data.

Patients may make a Privacy Protection Act request in writing, in person, or by telephone. Individuals should call the facility to determine the required procedures to obtain access to the records and what to include in making a written request.

Claims Procedure

Fiscal Intermediary

TRICARE Standard is governed by the Department of Defense (DoD). As such, it is not subject to those state regulatory bodies or agencies that control the insurance business. The DoD and the VA have agreed to use the Office of the Assistant Secretary of Defense and the TRICARE Standard system of fiscal

Benefit (Covered Services)	Beneficiary Pays [1,2]		CHAMPVA Pays
	Deductible ($50/individual or $100/family per calendar year)	**Cost Share**	
CHAMPVA Cost Share Summary			
Outpatient services			
Ambulatory surgery *Family services*	No	25% of allowable	75% of allowable
Professional services	Yes	25% of allowable	75% of allowable
Pharmacy services	Yes	25% of allowable	75% of allowable
Durable Medical Equipment (DME)			
Non–VA source VA source	Yes No	25% of allowable NONE	75% of allowable 100% of VA cost
Inpatient services			
Facility services DRG based	No	Lesser of: 1) per day amt x number of inpatient days; 2) 25% of billed amount; or 3) DRG rate	DRG rate less beneficiary cost share
Non–DRG based	No	25% of allowable	75% of allowable
Mental health High volume/RTC	No	25% of allowable	75% of allowable
Low volume	No	Lesser of: 1) per day amt x number of inpatient days; 2) 25% of billed amount.	Balance of allowable AFTER beneficiary cost share
Professional services	No	25% of allowable	75% of allowable

[1] Services received at VA health care facilities under the CHAMPVA Inhouse treatment Intiative (CITI) program are exempt from beneficiary cost sharing.
[2] Under catastrophic protection plan (Cat Cap), annual beneficiary cost sharing is limited to $7500.

Figure 13–9. CHAMPVA Service Benefits and Cost Share Summary Chart.

intermediaries and hospital contractors to receive, process, and pay CHAMPVA claims, following the same procedures currently used for TRICARE Standard.

A **fiscal intermediary (FI)** (also known as a contractor or claims processor) is an organization under contract to the government that handles insurance claims for care received under the TRICARE Standard or CHAMPVA program.

TRICARE Standard and CHAMPVA

TRICARE Standard and CHAMPVA claims must be billed on the CMS-1500 claim form and submitted to the claims processor (fiscal intermediary). Remember to abstract the correct information from front and back sides of the patient's identification card. Refer to Chapter 6 and follow the TRICARE or CHAMPVA instructions for completing the CMS-1500 claim form. Refer to Figure 6–13 for an example of a completed TRICARE case with no other insurance and Figure 6–14 for an example of a completed CHAMPVA case. If electing to complete the VA Form 10-1759A for a CHAMPVA case, refer to the instructions presented later in this chapter.

If the physician is nonparticipating and does not accept assignment, the patient completes the top portion of the CMS-1500 claim form, attaches the physician's itemized statement, and submits the claim. Alternatively, the patient may submit on the white TRICARE claim DD Form 2642 Patient's Request for Medical Payment. Patients and providers of care for health services in foreign countries must use DD Form 2520. The Uniform Bill (UB-92) form is used for inpatient hospital billing.

Time Limit

Effective January 1, 1993, claims must be filed within 1 year from the date a service is provided or (for inpatient care) within 1 year from the patient's date of discharge from the inpatient facility.

Claims Office

The TRICARE program is administered by the Department of Defense, TRICARE Management Activity, 16401 East Centretech Parkway, Aurora, CO 80011-9043, but claims are not processed in Colorado. The medical biller must understand that when sending the claim to TRICARE, the claim is sent to the TRICARE claims office nearest to the residence of the military sponsor. For example, if the patient is a child that was treated in California, but the sponsor is an active duty service member stationed in Florida, the claim should be sent to the TRICARE claims office in Camden, SC, and not to the claims office in Surfside Beach, SC. Refer to

Appendix A for the address for submitting a TRICARE Standard claim in each state. Write to the TRICARE Support Office or contact the HBA at the nearest MTF to obtain a current TRICARE Standard Handbook or for answers to any questions about the name of the regional claims processor, benefits, nonbenefits, when an NAS is necessary, and so on.

Because of the September 11, 2001, attack and the activation of the United States National Guard and Reserve components to the Middle East, the provider's office may come into contact with members of the National Guard or Reserve Component. The members of these two organizations normally join a unit located near their place of residence. The Guard and Reserve are only called to active duty in certain circumstances. Otherwise they are required to perform their duties once a month with what is called "Drill Status" and to participate in what is called "Annual Training." Drill status occurs on a Saturday and a Sunday. Annual Training occurs for 2 weeks, normally during the summer months. While these service members are on drill status or in annual training, they are entitled to medical care at government expense. The government will pay for an illness or injury incurred while on the way to drill status, during drill status, and on the way home from drill status. If they stop anywhere on the way to or from drill (e.g., to put gas in their car), any injury they receive is not paid for by the government. Sometimes when a service member is injured or becomes ill, he or she may have medical personnel available within the unit to provide medical care. If not, the service member is sent to a clinic or hospital near the drill center. This injury or illness is not covered by workers' compensation. The military unit must be contacted to be compensated for the medical care. Each unit has a staff member called a Full Time Manager (FTM). This person is assigned to the unit and works full-time during the week and attends drills with the unit on weekends. He or she processes all medical claims for unit members. Medical records must accompany the claim for it to be paid. The unit also may require the physician to prepare additional forms that must accompany the claim. The payment is not paid by the unit. The claim is sent to a higher command where the illness or injury is investigated. This is a very time-consuming procedure, and it could take months for the claim to be paid. It is better to bill the service member for payment if payment is not received with 60 to 90 days.

The CHAMPVA program is administered by the Department of Veterans Affairs, Health Administration Center, P.O. Box 65023, Denver, CO 80206-9023.

TRICARE Extra and TRICARE Prime

The beneficiary does not file any claim forms under TRICARE Extra or TRICARE Prime programs when using network providers. Providers must submit claims on CMS-1500 claim forms to TRICARE subcontractors listed in Appendix A for services given to beneficiaries. Referral and preauthorization numbers are required on claim forms when applicable.

Time Limit

For outpatient care a claim must be received by the state's or region's TRICARE contractor within 1 year of the date the provider rendered the service to the patient. For inpatient care a claim must be received by the contractor within 1 year from the date the patient was discharged from the facility. If a claim covers several different medical services or supplies that were provided at different times, the 1-year deadline applies to each item on the claim.

When a claim is submitted on time but the contractor returns it for more information, the claim should be resubmitted with the requested information so it is received by the contractor no later than 1 year after the medical services or supplies were provided or 90 days from the date the claim was returned to the provider, whichever is later.

A contractor may grant exemptions from the filing deadlines for several reasons. A request that includes a complete explanation of the circumstances of the late filing, all available documentation supporting the request, and the claim denied for late filing should be submitted to the contractor.

Claims Office

See Appendix A for the name and address that claims should be submited to and to obtain further information about this program.

TRICARE Prime Remote and Supplemental Health Care Program

Outpatient professional services are submitted using a CMS-1500 claim form. Primary care service claims are processed and paid without a referral or preauthorization from a network or non-network provider. A referral number provided by the HCF must be included on the claim form for specialty medical or surgical care and for behavioral health counseling and therapy sessions. The POS option and NAS requirements do not apply to TPR and SHCP claims.

Time Limit

A claim must be filed within 1 year from the date a service is provided or (for inpatient care) within 1 year from the patient's date of discharge from the inpatient facility.

Claims Office

Do not file claims of active duty armed service patients to TRICARE. Claims for patients on active duty must be sent to the specific branch of service (e.g., Army, Navy, Air Force, or Marines). Claims are submitted to Palmetto Government Benefits Administrators (PGBAs) for processing and payment (see Appendix A for the address).

TRICARE for Life

If the beneficiary receives care from a civilian provider, the provider submits claims to Medicare. Medicare pays its portion and then automatically forwards the claim to TRICARE for the remaining amount. TRICARE sends its payment directly to the provider. The beneficiary receives a TRICARE summary payment voucher that indicates the amount paid to the provider.

TRICARE/CHAMPVA and Other Insurance

By law TRICARE/CHAMPVA is usually the second payer when a beneficiary is enrolled in **other health insurance (OHI),** a civilian health plan, or belongs to an HMO or preferred provider organization (PPO). However, there are two exceptions:

▶ When a plan is administered under Title XIX of the Social Security Act (Medicaid)
▶ When coverage is specifically designed to supplement TRICARE benefits (e.g., Medigap health plan)

When the patient has other health insurance that is primary (meaning that it pays before TRICARE Standard or CHAMPVA does), submit the claim using the CMS-1500 insurance claim form. Attach the explanation of benefits from the primary carrier. If the patient is submitting his or her claim to the other insurance, take these steps:

1. Bill the other insurance carrier with the form it has supplied.
2. Bill TRICARE or CHAMPVA by completing the top section of the CMS-1500 after receiving payment and an explanation of benefits from the other insurance company. Submit the physician's itemized statement, which must contain the following:
   a. Provider's name
   b. Date the services or supplies were provided
   c. Description of each service or supply
   d. Place of treatment
   e. Number or frequency of each service
   f. Fee for each item of service or supply
   g. Procedure code numbers
   h. Diagnostic code number or description of condition for which treatment is being received
   i. Billing statements showing only total charges, canceled checks, or cash register receipts

(or similar-type receipts) are not acceptable as itemized statements.

3. Attach a photocopy of the explanation of benefits from the other insurance company.
4. Send the TRICARE or CHAMPVA claim to the local claims processor (fiscal intermediary).

Medicaid and TRICARE/CHAMPVA

File TRICARE or CHAMPVA claims first if the beneficiary is a recipient of the Medicaid program.

Medicare and TRICARE

TRICARE is considered secondary to Medicare for persons younger than age 65 who have Medicare Part A as a result of a disability and who have enrolled in Medicare Part B. Those eligible for Medicare Part A are not covered by TRICARE unless disabled. Claims should be submitted to Medicare, then to TRICARE with a copy of the Medicare remittance advice. Services covered by TRICARE but not covered by Medicare (e.g., prescriptions) are paid by TRICARE. Participating providers may obtain a TRICARE fee schedule by contacting their fiscal intermediary.

Medicare and CHAMPVA

Effective December 5, 1991, CHAMPVA became secondary payer to Medicare for persons younger than age 65 who are enrolled in Medicare Parts A and B and who are otherwise eligible for CHAMPVA. Claims first must be submitted to Medicare because CHAMPVA is a secondary payer.

Dual or Double Coverage

A claim must be filed if a patient has additional insurance that provides double coverage. Refusal by the beneficiary to claim benefits from other health insurance coverage results in a denial of TRICARE benefits. In double coverage situations, TRICARE pays the lower of:

1. The amount of TRICARE allowable charges remaining after the double coverage plan has paid its benefits
2. The amount TRICARE would have paid as primary payer

There must be **coordination of benefits** so that there is no duplication of benefits paid between the double coverage plan and TRICARE.

Third-Party Liability

If the patient is in an automobile accident or receives an injury that may have third-party involvement, the following two options are available for reimbursement:

Option 1: TRICARE Form DD 2527 (Statement of Personal Injury, Possible Third-Party Liability) must be sent in with the regular claim form for cost-sharing of the civilian medical care. All five sections of the form should be completed by the patient. This form allows TRICARE to evaluate the circumstances of the accident and the possibility that the government may recover money for the medical care from the person who injured the patient. If a CMS-1500 claim form is submitted without TRICARE Form DD 2527, a request is made to complete it. This form must be returned within 35 days of the request, or the claims processor will deny the original and all related claims. Then the fiscal intermediary submits a claim to the third party for reimbursement or files a lien for reimbursement with the liability insurance carrier, the liable party, or the attorneys or court involved.

Option 2: The provider can submit claims exclusively to the third-party liability carrier for reimbursement. Claims submitted with ICD-9-CM diagnostic codes between 800 and 999 (Injury and Poisoning) trigger the fact that there might be third-party litigation, and the claims processor may request the completion of DD Form 2527.

Workers' Compensation

If a TRICARE or CHAMPVA beneficiary is injured on the job or becomes ill because of his or her work, a workers' compensation claim must be filed with the compensation insurance carrier. TRICARE or CHAMPVA can be billed when all workers' compensation benefits have been exhausted.

In some situations it must be decided whether a case that involves an accident or illness is work-related, and the claim might be sent to the TRICARE or CHAMPVA claims fiscal intermediary. In those instances the claims processor files a lien with the workers' compensation carrier for recovery when the case is settled.

> **PROCEDURE: Completing a CHAMPVA Claim Form**

An example of a completed CHAMPVA claim form is provided in Figure 13-10.

1. Enter the patient's last name, first name, and middle initial (do not use nicknames or abbreviations).
2. Enter the patient's Social Security number exactly as it appears on the Social Security card. If the patient does not have a Social Security number, print "None."

OMB NC: 2900-
Estimated burden: 30 min

VA Department of Veterans Affairs	**CHAMPVA CLAIM FORM**

CHAMPVA CENTER, 4500 Cherry Creek Drive South, Box 300, Denver CO 80222

WARNING: IF YOU KNOWINGLY MAKE A FALSE STATEMENT OF ANY MATERIAL FACT IN OR IN
CONNECTION WITH THIS CLAIM, YOU ARE SUBJECT TO PROSECUTION IN A U.S. COURT

PART 1 - PATIENT INFORMATION (To be completed by the beneficiary, patient or sponsor)

1. PATIENT'S NAME CHIEU, MARION W.	2. PATIENT'S SOCIAL SECURITY NUMBER 742-XX-0491

3. PATIENT'S ADDRESS (Street, City, State, ZIP)   (Check if new address)
321 OAK STREET,   WOODLAND HILLS, XY 12345

4. TELEPHONE NUMBER (Include area code) (555)492-7800	5B. EFFECTIVE DATE			5C. EXPIRATION DATE		
	MONTH	DAY	YEAR	MONTH	DAY	YEAR
5A. CHAMPVA IDENTIFICATION CARD/AUTHORIZATION NUMBER 49-467-081C	09	01	XX	12	19	XX

6. PATIENT'S DATE OF BIRTH (Month, day, year) 12-01-77	7. PATIENT'S RELATIONSHIP TO SPONSOR (Check one) ☒ SPOUSE ☐ CHILD	8. PATIENT'S SEX (Check one) ☐ MALE ☒ FEMALE

PART II - SPONSOR INFORMATION (To be completed by the beneficiary, patient or sponsor)

9. SPONSOR'S NAME (Last, first, middle initial) CHIEU, FRANK T.	10. VA CLAIM/FILE NUMBER 421-05-0129

11. SPONSOR'S ADDRESS IF DIFFERENT FROM PATIENT'S (Street, City, State, Zip)

PART III - PATIENT INSURANCE INFORMATION (To be completed by the beneficiary, patient or sponsor)

12A. IS PATIENT'S TREATMENT COVERED BY OTHER HEALTH INSURANCE
☐ YES   ☒ NO   IF YES, PLEASE COMPLETE ITEMS 12B THROUGH 12G BELOW

12B. TYPE OF COVERAGE ☐ GROUP HEALTH ☐ PRIVATE (NON–GROUP) ☐ MEDICARE ☐ CHAMPVA SUPPLEMENTAL ☐ MEDICAID ☐ WORKERS COMPENSATION ☐ OTHER ☐ NONE	12C. NAME AND ADDRESS OF INSURANCE CARRIER	12D. IF COVERAGE IS THROUGH WORK, NAME AND ADDRESS OF EMPLOYER
12E. POLICY IDENTIFICATION NUMBER	12F. INSURANCE AGENT'S NAME	12G. AGENT'S TELEPHONE NUMBER

PART IV - TREATMENT INFORMATION (To be completed by the beneficiary, patient or sponsor)

13. TYPE OF CLAIM (Check one) ☐ INPATIENT ☐ DENTAL ☒ OUTPATIENT ☐ DME ☐ PHARMACY ☐ OTHER ☐ TRAVEL	14. WAS NEED OF TREATMENT DUE TO A PHYSICAL INJURY? YES ☐ NO ☒ (If "Yes", briefly describe injuries and give a statement of circumstances)

15. I authorize the identified provider of service to disclose to CHAMPVA medical record information that pertains to the medical services described on this form. Unless limitations are shown below, this consent pertains to all of my medical records, including records related to treatment for medical or dental conditions, psychological or psychiatric impairments, drug or alcohol abuse, acquired immune deficiency syndrome (AIDS) or infection with the human immunodeficiency virus (HIV), and sickle cell disease.

The information will be used to process my CHAMPVA claim and determine my (or the patient identified above) eligibility for medical benefits. I also authorize the release of or obtaining of medical and/or other coverage information to and from another organization with which I have other medical benefits plan or health insurance coverage. I understand that I may revoke this authorization at any time, except to the extent that action has already been taken to comply with it. Without my express revocation, this consent will automatically expire: (1) upon satisfaction of the need for disclosure; (2) on February 2, 20XX (date supplied by the beneficiary); or (3) under the following conditions:

LIMITATIONS:

16. I assign payment to the provider(s) of these claim services   ☐ YES   ☒ NO

17. I CERTIFY THAT THE ABOVE STATEMENTS AND ATTACHMENTS ARE CORRECT AND REPRESENT ACTUAL SERVICES, DATES AND FEES CHARGED TO ME OR MY ELIGIBLE DEPENDENTS.

17A. CLAIMANT'S SIGNATURE	17B. DATE 2–2–XX	17C. RELATIONSHIP TO SPONSOR WIFE

Figure 13–10. Completed CHAMPVA Claim Form VA Form 10-7959A, used when billing for professional services.

Continued.

PATIENT'S NAME (Last, first, middle initial)	SPONSOR'S NAME (Last, first, middle initial)
CHIEU, MARION W.	CHIEU, FRANK T.

PART V - PHYSICIAN/OTHER PROVIDER (To be completed by physician or other provider)

18. PROVIDER'S NAME	19. PROVIDER'S TAX I.D. NUMBER	20. NAME OF REFERRING PHYSICIAN OR OTHER SOURCE (e.g. public health agency)
DOE, JOHN M.D.	93-4267890	

21. WHEN SERVICES ARE RELATED TO A PERIOD OF HOSPITALIZATION, GIVE DATES	22. NAME AND ADDRESS OF FACILITY WHERE SERVICES RENDERED (if other than home office)

ADMITTED	DISCHARGED	

23. DIAGNOSIS OR NATURE OF ILLNESS OR INJURY. RELATE DIAGNOSIS TO PROCEDURE BY USING PROCEDURE NUMBER IN COLUMN 24E BELOW.

A. Dysfunctional uterine bleeding.

B.

C.

24A DATE OF SERVICE	24B * PLACE OF SERVICE	24C PROCEDURE CODE	24D DESCRIBE UNUSUAL SERVICE OR CIRCUMSTANCES	24E DIAGNOSIS CODE	24F CHARGES	24G DAYS OR UNITS	24H TYPE OF SERVICE
02-02-XX	0	99213	Ofc visit Eval & Mgmt Level 3	626.8	45 00	1	1

25. I certify that the statements on the reverse of this bill apply and are made a part hereto.	26. PROVIDER'S SOCIAL SECURITY NO 272-XX-5731	27. TOTAL CHARGES 45.00	
John Doe, MD 02-02-XX SIGNATURE OF PROVIDER DATE	28. PROVIDER'S ADDRESS, ZIP CODE AND TELEPHONE NUMBER 123 MAIN STREET, WOODLAND HILLS, XY 12345 013/486-9002		

* PLACE OF SERVICE CODE FOR ITEM 24B
  IN -INPATIENT HOSPITAL
  OH -OUTPATIENT HOSPITAL
  O -DOCTOR'S OFFICE
  H -PATIENT'S HOME
  DCF -DAY CARE FACILITY (PSY)

NCF -NIGHT CARE FACILITY (PSY)
NH -NURSING HOME
SNF -SKILLD NURSING FACILITY
AMB -AMBULANCE
OL -OTHER LOCATIONS

IL -INDEPENDENT LABORATORY
OF -OTHER MEDICAL/SURGICAL FACILITY
RTC -RESIDENTIAL TREATMENT CENTER
STF - SPECIALIZED TREATMENT FACILITY

PART VI- PHARMACY INFORMATION (To be completed by pharmacist)	PATIENT'S NAME

29A. NATIONAL DRUG CODE	29B. RX NUMBER	29C. PHARMACY NAME	29D. FILL DATE (Month, day, year)	29E. PHYSICIAN NAME	29F. CHARGES

30. TOTAL CHARGES – $

VA FORM 10-7959A
DEC 1990

Pg II

reference initials

Figure 13–10, cont'd.

3. Enter the patient's complete address. If the patient's address has changed, place an "X" in the box.

4. Enter the patient's home telephone number. Include the area code.

5A. Enter the number from Item 6 of the patient's current CHAMPVA Authorization Card.

5B. Enter the date from Item 4 of the patient's current CHAMPVA Authorization Card.

5C. Enter the date from Item 5 of the patient's current CHAMPVA Authorization Card.

6. Enter the patient's date of birth.

7. Enter the patient's relationship to the sponsor.

8. Enter the patient's gender.

9. Enter the sponsor's last name, first name, and middle initial (do not use nicknames or abbreviations).

10. Enter the sponsor's VA Claim or File Number.

11. Enter the sponsor's complete address (if different from the patient's).

12A. Place an "X" in the appropriate box if the patient is covered under any other medical benefits plan or health insurance coverage. CHAMPVA does not duplicate benefits of any other health insurance plan or program.

12B. Place an "X" beside all applicable types of medical plans or other health insurance to which the patient is entitled.

12C. Enter the name and address of the other insurance carrier.

12D. Enter the name and address of the employer if other health insurance is provided by the patient's employer.

12E. Enter the policy identification number of the other health insurance carrier.

12F. Enter the insurance agent's name. If this information is not known, enter "Unknown."

12G. Enter the insurance agent's telephone number. If this information is not known, enter "Unknown."

13. Check the appropriate box according to the type of medical care the patient received.

   ▶ Inpatient: Check the Inpatient box for admission to a civilian hospital.

   ▶ Outpatient: Check the Outpatient box for all eligible CHAMPVA beneficiaries provided medical care from civilian facilities unless otherwise authorized by the VA.

   ▶ Pharmacy: Check the Pharmacy box for claims for payment of drugs and medicines requiring a prescription by law.

   ▶ Travel: Check the Travel box for claims for ambulance travel to, from, or between hospitals for inpatient care.

   ▶ Dental: Check the Dental box for dental care for which the patient has an approved preauthorization.

   ▶ Durable Medical Equipment (DME): Check the DME box for payment of durable medical equipment costing more than $100.

   ▶ College Infirmary: Check the Other box for College Infirmary.

   ▶ Other Inpatient Care: Check the Inpatient box for admissions to an approved nursing facility (including a Christian Science sanatorium).

14. If the patient needs treatment for any kind of an injury (e.g., broken toe, sprained knee, lacerated forehead, or back injury), check "YES" and briefly describe the injury and circumstances of how the patient was injured.

15. Be sure to read the release of medical record information contained in this item and complete the blanks, if appropriate.

16. CHAMPVA is a benefit program. As such the patient (or sponsor) *must* assign the benefit to the provider of care if he or she wishes the payment to be made to the provider. Otherwise payment will be made to the patient.

17A. Every CHAMPVA claim must be signed by a patient 18 years of age or older. If the beneficiary is unable to sign on his or her own behalf, the sponsor (or other parent) may sign. In the absence of either parent, a guardian or fiduciary may sign. (*Note:* For privacy reasons a patient younger than 18 years of age may sign his or her own claim form.)

17B. Insert date of signature.

17C. Enter the claimant's relationship to sponsor.
Part V: To be completed by physician or other provider.
Top of page II: Enter patient and sponsor's last name, first name, and middle initial.

18. Enter provider's (physician's) name and title.

19. Enter provider's tax identification number.

20. Enter the name of the referring physician or agency.

21. Enter the admission and discharge dates if the patient is hospitalized.

22. Enter the name and address of the facility where services were rendered if other than home or office.

23. Enter diagnostic description or nature of illness or injury.

24A. Enter the date of service.

24B. Enter the place of service using one of the codes shown midway down on this page of the form.

24C. Enter the CPT procedure code number with modifier.

24D. Insert a description of the service or procedure.

24E. Enter the ICD-9-CM diagnostic code number for each diagnosis as described in Item 23.

24F. Enter the fee for each service, procedure, or test described in 24D.

24G. Enter the number of days or units. This block is commonly used for multiple visits, number of miles, units of supplies including drugs, anesthesia minutes, or oxygen volume.

24H. Enter the type of service code from the following list:

    1 Medical care
    2 Surgery
    3 Consultation
    4 Diagnostic x-ray
    5 Diagnostic laboratory dialysis
    6 Radiation therapy
    7 Anesthesia
    8 Assistance at surgery
    9 Other medical service
    0 Blood or packed red cells
    A Used DME
    F Ambulatory surgical center
    H Hospice
    L Renal supply in home
    M Alternate payment for maintenance
    N Kidney donor
    V Pneumococcal vaccine
    Y Second opinion on elective surgery
    Z Third opinion on elective surgery

25. Show the signature of the physician, or his or her representative, and the date the form was signed.

26. Enter the provider's Social Security number.

27. Enter the total of all charges.

28. Enter the provider's street address, city, state, ZIP code, and telephone number, including area code.

Items 29A through 30 may be completed if the patient is receiving prescription drugs.

After Claim Submission

TRICARE Summary Payment Voucher

For each TRICARE claim the claims processor issues a **summary payment voucher** (Fig. 13–11) that details the payment of the claim. When the provider participates (accepts assignment), the voucher is sent to him or her with the check. The patient always receives a copy of the voucher, even if the provider receives payment directly from the fiscal intermediary.

CHAMPVA Explanation of Benefits Document

Upon completion of the processing of a claim, a payment check is generated and an explanation of benefits document is sent to the beneficiary (including the provider if the claim is filed by the provider). The explanation of benefits summarizes the action taken on the claim and contains information as graphically illustrated and explained in Figure 13–12. Beneficiaries who receive durable medical equipment or VA services from a CHAMPVA In-house Treatment Initiative (CITI, pronounced "city") do not receive an explanation of benefits.

Quality Assurance

A **quality assurance program** continually assesses the effectiveness of inpatient and outpatient care. The quality assurance department reviews providers' outpatient records on a random basis for clinical and administrative quality. Grievance procedures have been established for members and providers if any complaint arises from an administrative process, a service provided by a physician, or an issue involving quality of care.

TRICARE–managed care programs have a quality assurance program to continually assess the effectiveness of care and services rendered by providers. This includes inpatient and outpatient hospital care, mental health services, long-term care, home health care, and programs for the handicapped. Providers are notified in writing when a potential quality issue has been confirmed as a breach of quality standards. Recommended corrective action plans are given, and noncompliance may lead to suspension or termination of a provider.

Claims Inquiries and Appeals

Through the appeal process, providers may request reconsideration of a denial of certification for coverage or of the amount paid for a submitted claim. See Chapter 8 for inquiring about the status of a claim and to learn the procedures on how to file reviews and appeals.

┌───┐
│ RESOURCES ON THE INTERNET │
└───┘

CHAMPVA
http://www.va.gov/hac/champva
Medicare
http://www.medicare.gov
Social Security Administration (for information about enrolling in Medicare Part B)
http://www.ssa.gov
TRICARE (for download of a TRICARE manual)
http://www.tricare.osd.mil/tricaremanuals/
TRICARE military health care beneficiary
http://www.TRICAREOnline.com
TRICARE University (basic student course)
http://199.211.83.208/public
VA government forms
http:// www.va.gov/forms/medical

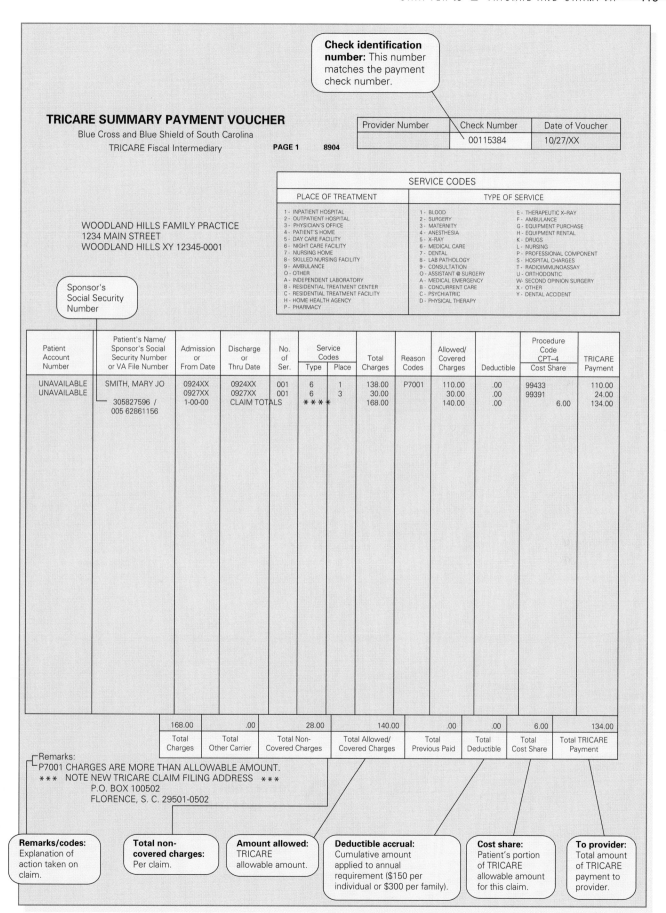

Check identification number: This number matches the payment check number.

TRICARE SUMMARY PAYMENT VOUCHER

Blue Cross and Blue Shield of South Carolina

TRICARE Fiscal Intermediary   PAGE 1   8904

Provider Number	Check Number	Date of Voucher
	00115384	10/27/XX

WOODLAND HILLS FAMILY PRACTICE
1234 MAIN STREET
WOODLAND HILLS XY 12345-0001

Sponsor's Social Security Number

SERVICE CODES

PLACE OF TREATMENT	TYPE OF SERVICE	
1 - INPATIENT HOSPITAL	1 - BLOOD	E - THERAPEUTIC X-RAY
2 - OUTPATIENT HOSPITAL	2 - SURGERY	F - AMBULANCE
3 - PHYSICIAN'S OFFICE	3 - MATERNITY	G - EQUIPMENT PURCHASE
4 - PATIENT'S HOME	4 - ANESTHESIA	H - EQUIPMENT RENTAL
5 - DAY CARE FACILITY	5 - X-RAY	K - DRUGS
6 - NIGHT CARE FACILITY	6 - MEDICAL CARE	L - NURSING
7 - NURSING HOME	7 - DENTAL	P - PROFESSIONAL COMPONENT
8 - SKILLED NURSING FACILITY	8 - LAB PATHOLOGY	S - HOSPITAL CHARGES
9 - AMBULANCE	9 - CONSULTATION	T - RADIOIMMUNOASSAY
O - OTHER	O - ASSISTANT @ SURGERY	U - ORTHODONTIC
A - INDEPENDENT LABORATORY	A - MEDICAL EMERGENCY	W - SECOND OPINION SURGERY
B - RESIDENTIAL TREATMENT CENTER	B - CONCURRENT CARE	X - OTHER
C - RESIDENTIAL TREATMENT FACILITY	C - PSYCHIATRIC	Y - DENTAL ACCIDENT
H - HOME HEALTH AGENCY	D - PHYSICAL THERAPY	
P - PHARMACY		

Patient Account Number	Patient's Name/ Sponsor's Social Security Number or VA File Number	Admission or From Date	Discharge or Thru Date	No. of Ser.	Service Codes Type	Service Codes Place	Total Charges	Reason Codes	Allowed/ Covered Charges	Deductible	Procedure Code CPT-4 Cost Share	TRICARE Payment
UNAVAILABLE UNAVAILABLE	SMITH, MARY JO	0924XX 0927XX	0924XX 0927XX	001 001	6 6	1 3	138.00 30.00	P7001	110.00 30.00	.00 .00	99433 99391	110.00 24.00
	305827596 / 005 62861156	1-00-00	CLAIM TOTALS	****			168.00		140.00	.00	6.00	134.00

168.00	.00	28.00	140.00	.00	.00	6.00	134.00
Total Charges	Total Other Carrier	Total Non-Covered Charges	Total Allowed/ Covered Charges	Total Previous Paid	Total Deductible	Total Cost Share	Total TRICARE Payment

Remarks:
P7001 CHARGES ARE MORE THAN ALLOWABLE AMOUNT.
*** NOTE NEW TRICARE CLAIM FILING ADDRESS ***
    P.O. BOX 100502
    FLORENCE, S. C. 29501-0502

Remarks/codes: Explanation of action taken on claim.

Total non-covered charges: Per claim.

Amount allowed: TRICARE allowable amount.

Deductible accrual: Cumulative amount applied to annual requirement ($150 per individual or $300 per family).

Cost share: Patient's portion of TRICARE allowable amount for this claim.

To provider: Total amount of TRICARE payment to provider.

Figure 13–11. TRICARE Summary Payment Voucher.

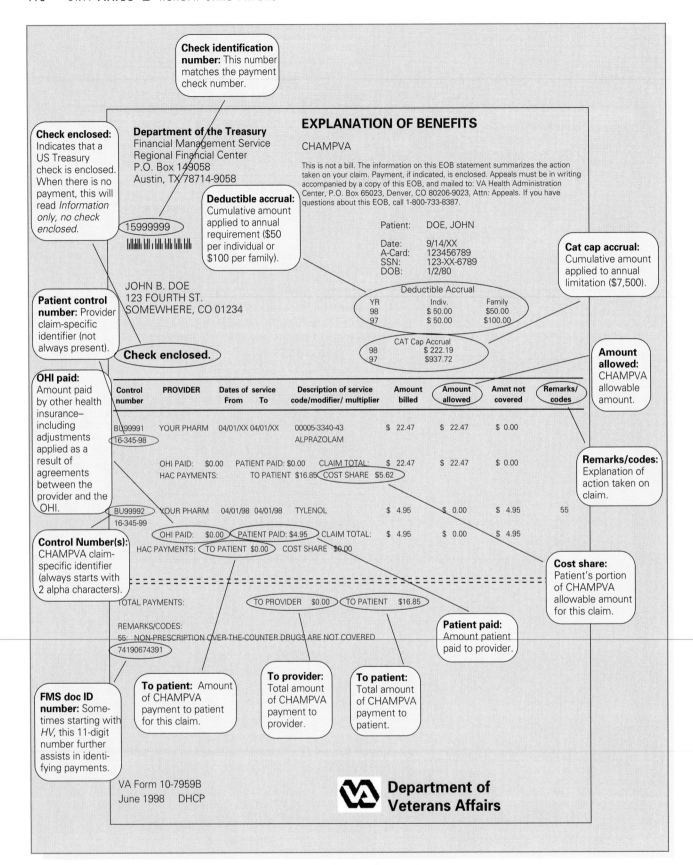

Figure 13–12. CHAMPVA Explanation of Benefits document.

STUDENT ASSIGNMENT LIST

✔ Study Chapter 13.

✔ Answer the review questions in the *Workbook* to reinforce the theory learned in this chapter and help prepare you for a future test.

✔ Complete the assignments in the *Workbook* for computing mathematical calculations and giving you hands-on experience in completing TRICARE and CHAMPVA insurance claim forms and proficiency in procedural and diagnostic coding.

✔ Turn to the Glossary at the end of this textbook for a further understanding of the Key Terms used in this chapter.

COMPUTER ASSIGNMENT

 Complete Case 7 on the CD-ROM to review concepts you have learned for this chapter.

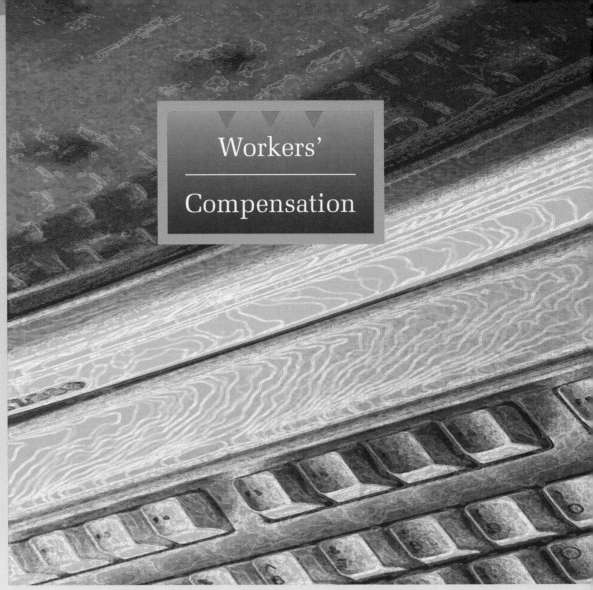

Workers' Compensation

WORKERS' COMP

14

Procedure: Completing the Doctor's First Report of Occupational Injury or Illness

Progress or Supplemental Report

Final Report

Claim Submission

Financial Responsibility

Fee Schedules

Helpful Billing Tips

Billing Claims

Out-of-State Claims

Delinquent or Slow Pay Claims

KEY TERMS

accident

adjudication

by report (BR)

claims examiner

compromise and release (C and R)

deposition

ergonomic

extraterritorial

Federal Employees' Compensation Act (FECA)

fee schedule

independent medical evaluator (IME)

injury

insurance adjuster

lien

medical service order

nondisability (ND) claim

occupational illness (or disease)

Occupational Safety and Health Administration (OSHA)

permanent and stationary (P and S)

permanent disability (PD)

petition

second injury fund

sequelae

sub rosa films

Continued.

KEY TERMS—cont'd

subsequent-injury fund (SIF)

temporary disability (TD)

third-party liability

third-party subrogation

waiting period (WP)

work hardening

Workers' Compensation Appeals Board (WCAB)

workers' compensation (WC) insurance

History

Before the establishment of a workers' compensation program in the United States, the employer was responsible for any injury or death to his or her employees resulting from administrative negligence. *Employees* are individuals employed by another, generally for wages, in exchange for labor or services. A physician who is incorporated also is considered an employee under workers' compensation laws.

Originally the worker had to prove legally that injury was caused by negligence on the part of the employer. By the close of the nineteenth century the number of accidents had increased and legal processes were uncertain; therefore federal and state legal provisions were required. As an outcome in the early 1900s employers' liability laws were adopted by many states, but there was still a great need for improvement. In 1911 the first workers' compensation laws were enacted that allowed injured employees to receive medical care without first taking employers to court. All states have workers' compensation laws today.

Workers' compensation insurance is the most important coverage written to insure industrial accidents. Previously this form of insurance was known as workmen's compensation. The term *workmen* was changed to *workers* for a more generic title and to avoid sexual bias in language. Employers use employers' liability coverage occasionally to protect themselves when their employees do not come within the scope of a compensation law.

Workers' Compensation Statutes

There are two kinds of statutes under workers' compensation: federal compensation laws and state compensation laws. Federal laws apply to miners, maritime workers, and those who work for the government; they do not apply to state and private business employees. State compensation laws apply to employers and employees within each state, but the laws vary for each state.

The workers' compensation statutes relieve the employer of liability for injury received or illness contracted by an employee in a work situation, except in gross negligence cases. They also enable the employee to be more easily and quickly compensated for loss of wages, medical expenses, and permanent disability. Before these statutes were passed the employer could be found legally responsible for his or her employees' injuries or illnesses, and frequently there were delays in the employee's attempt to recover damages.

Workers' Compensation Reform

By 1994 dysfunctional workers' compensation systems were costing companies more than $65 billion annually in many U.S. cities, driving insurers to deny insurance to businesses and causing companies to close their doors. Some employers began moving their businesses to states requiring lower premiums. Widespread legal and medical corruption and abuse had evolved throughout the system in the form of record-high medical treatment and legal expenses. Reforms of the compensation of health care workers became necessary because of these problems. Reform laws have been introduced in a number of states that deal with the following issues:

◗ Antifraud legislation and increased penalties for workers' compensation fraud

▶ Antireferral provisions (e.g., restrictions of physicians referring patients for diagnostic studies to sites where the physician has a financial interest)

▶ Proof of the medical necessity for treatment (or tests), as well as appropriate documentation. If not adhered to, the carrier may refuse to pay the entire fee (e.g., utilization review of inpatient and outpatient claims and treatment plans)

▶ Preauthorization for major operations and expensive tests (e.g., computed tomography and magnetic resonance imaging)

▶ Caps on vocational rehabilitation

▶ Utilization of a disabled worker in another division of the company he or she was employed in so that the person may be gainfully employed while not using the injured part of the body

▶ Increase in occupational safety measures

▶ Employers offering a variety of managed care plans from which employees can choose, with some of these restricting their choice of provider (e.g., health maintenance organizations [HMOs] and preferred provider organizations [PPOs])

▶ Development of fee schedules

▶ Medical bill review (mandatory review by law or payers' voluntary review identifying duplicate claims and billing errors)

▶ Use of mediators instead of lawyers to reach agreement between employers and the injured employee

▶ Prosecuting physicians, lawyers, and employees who abuse the system

Although the system is far from perfect or complete, much progress has been made toward reducing high costs by trimming reimbursement for medical services and minimizing abuses of the system.

Workers' Compensation Laws and Insurance

Purposes of Workers' Compensation Laws

Workers' compensation laws have been developed for a variety of reasons and accomplish much:

1. Provide the best available medical care necessary to ensure a prompt return to work of any injured or ill employee, as well as the achievement of maximum recovery.

2. Provide income to the injured or ill worker or to his or her dependents, regardless of fault.

3. Provide a single remedy and reduce court delays, costs, and workloads arising out of personal injury litigation.

4. Relieve public and private charities of financial drains resulting from uncompensated industrial accidents.

5. Eliminate payment of fees to attorneys and witnesses, as well as time-consuming trials and appeals.

6. Encourage maximum employer interest in safety and rehabilitation through an appropriate experience-rating mechanism.

7. Promote the study of causes of accidents and reduce preventable accidents and human suffering rather than concealing fault.

Self-Insurance

Self-insurance is another way that employers can fight high medical costs after an accident. A very large employer can save money by self-insuring employees for a predetermined amount of money and then purchasing policies with large deductibles to cover catastrophic problems. A self-insuring company pays for medical expenses instead of insurance premiums. Benefits are variable from plan to plan, and precertification for certain services may be required.

Self-insured employers are covered by the Employee Retirement Income Security Act (ERISA). This federal law mandates reporting and disclosure requirements for group life and health plans, with guidelines for administration, servicing of plans, some claims processing, and appeals; therefore the state insurance commissioner does not have jurisdiction over such plans. Because they are not state regulated, they often overlook timely payment. ERISA regulations state that a claim must be paid or denied within 90 days of receipt or submission; however, this regulation is not helpful because there is no penalty for violation of the 90-day deadline. Thus physicians who care for individuals under such plans may wish to negotiate payment terms to be 60 days or less.

Sometimes a self-insured plan may have stop-loss or reinsurance that becomes active on large claims, or a set dollar limit per policy year or employee, depending on how it is structured. Such provisions give them an excuse to delay claims until the reinsurer decides to fund the claim. In such cases it may be necessary to become aggressive and ask for the name, address, and telephone number of the reinsurer to learn the claim status. Prompt processing and payment should be demanded because delaying claims is a violation of federal laws and ERISA regulations. Read the Conclusion at the end of Chapter 10 for additional information on ERISA.

A form of self-insurance designed to serve a small manufacturing company is known as *captive insurance.* This is best for companies that have good safety records and those willing to implement worker safety programs to keep claims to a minimum. Members of captive self-insurance programs may hire an outside firm to process claims and purchase extra insurance for major claims. They share overhead expenses and investment income if any remains after paying expenses and claims. Most captive programs are based in Bermuda or the Cayman Islands to take advantage of favorable tax benefits.

Managed Care

Increasing numbers of employers are seeking managed care contracts with PPOs and HMOs. Some states have adopted laws authorizing managed care programs, and other states are conducting pilot programs to test the effectiveness of managed care networks. Managed care contracts are not uniform and may limit the choice of providers, use fee schedule-based payments, require precertification for certain procedures, implement hospital and medical bill review, and incorporate utilization review of medical services.

Eligibility

Individuals entitled to workers' compensation insurance coverage are private business employees, state employees, and federal employees (e.g., postal workers, Internal Revenue Service [IRS] employees, coal miners, and maritime workers). **Workers' compensation (WC) insurance** coverage provides benefits to employees and their dependents if employees suffer work-related injury, illness, or death.

Industrial Accident

An **accident** is an unplanned and unexpected happening traceable to a definite time and place and causing **injury** (damage or loss).

Workers' compensation (industrial) accidents do not necessarily occur at the customary work site. For example, an individual may be asked to obtain cash for the petty cash reserve during the lunch hour. He or she may misstep off the curb while walking to the bank and suffer a fractured ankle. This person is considered to be working, although not at the customary work site, and the injury is covered under workers' compensation insurance.

Occupational Illness

Occupational illness or disease is any abnormal condition or disorder caused by exposure to environmental factors associated with employment, including acute and chronic illnesses or diseases that may be caused by inhalation, absorption, ingestion, or direct contact. Occupational diseases usually become apparent soon after exposure. However, some diseases may be latent for a considerable amount of time. Therefore some states have extended periods during which claims may be filed for certain slowly developing occupational diseases. These diseases include

silicosis, asbestosis, pneumoconiosis, berylliosis, anthracosilicosis, radiation disability, loss of hearing, cumulative trauma, or repetitive motion illnesses (e.g., carpal tunnel syndrome).

Coverage

Federal Laws

Employees who work for federal agencies are covered by a number of federal workers' compensation laws:

▶ *Workmen's Compensation Law of the District of Columbia.* This law became effective on May 17, 1928, and provides benefits for those working in Washington, DC.
▶ *Federal Coal Mine Health and Safety Act.* This act, also referred to as the Black Lung Benefits Act, became effective on May 7, 1941. The act provides benefits to coal miners and is administered through the national headquarters in Washington, DC.
▶ *Federal Employees' Compensation Act.* The **Federal Employees' Compensation Act (FECA)** was instituted on May 30, 1908, to provide benefits for on-the-job injuries to all federal employees. The insurance is provided through an exclusive fund system. Many different claim forms are used depending on the type of injury. Payment is based on a schedule of maximum allowable charges. The time limit for submitting a bill is by December 31 of the year after the year in which services were rendered (or by December 31 of the year after the year the condition was accepted as work compensable, whichever is later). For further information contact the Office of the FECA by writing to the nearest office as listed in Appendix A.
▶ *Longshoremen's and Harbor Workers' Compensation Act (LHWCA).* This act became effective on March 4, 1927, and provides benefits for private or public employees engaged in maritime work nationwide. It is administered through regional offices in Boston, Chicago, Cleveland, Denver, Honolulu, Jacksonville, Kansas City, New Orleans, New York City, Philadelphia, San Francisco, Seattle, and Washington, DC. This type of insurance corresponds to that available through the private insurance system. Contact the nearest district office as listed in Appendix A for further information.

State Laws

State compensation laws cover those workers not protected by the previously mentioned federal statutes. Federal law mandates that states set up laws to meet minimum requirements. If an employer does not purchase workers' compensation insurance from a private insurance company, the employer must self-insure and have enough cash in reserve to cover the cost of medical care for all workers who suffer work-related injuries. An employer may be reluctant to file a workers' compensation report with the state in some instances, preferring to pay medical expenses out of pocket rather than have premium rates increase. It is illegal for an employer to fail to report a work-related accident when reporting is required by state law, and some states consider it a misdemeanor. Different penalties can be imposed, depending on state law, such as imprisonment or assessment of fines of from $50 to $2500 or more.

Statutes require that employers have employers' liability insurance in addition to workers' compensation protection. The difference between workers' compensation insurance and employers' liability insurance is that the latter is coverage that protects against claims arising out of bodily injury to others (nonemployees) or damage to their property when someone is on business premises. It is not considered insurance coverage for someone who is working at a business site.

State compensation laws are compulsory or elective, which may be defined as follows:

1. *Compulsory law.* Each employer is required to accept its provisions and provide for specified benefits.
2. *Elective law.* The employer may accept or reject the law. If the statute of the law is rejected, the employer loses the three common-law defenses, which are the following:
   a. Assumption of risk
   b. Negligence of fellow employees
   c. Contributory negligence

Coverage is elective in only two states, New Jersey and Texas. This means that in effect all laws are "compulsory."

Minors

Minors are covered by workers' compensation; in some states, double compensation or added penalties are provided. Minors also receive special legal benefit provisions in many states.

Interstate Laws

Questions may arise as to which state's law determines payment of compensation benefits if a worker's occupation takes him or her into another state. Most compensation laws are **extraterritorial** (effective outside of the state) by either specific provisions or court decision.

Volunteer Workers

Several states have laws to compensate civil defense and other volunteer workers, such as firemen who are injured in the line of duty.

Funding

Six states (Nevada, North Dakota, Ohio, Washington, West Virginia, and Wyoming), two U.S. territories, and most provinces require employers to insure through a *monopolistic state* or *provincial fund.* Puerto Rico and the Virgin Islands require employers to insure through a *territorial fund.* Employers may qualify as self-insurers in 48 states and territories. A number of states permit employers to purchase insurance from either a competitive state fund or a private insurance company.

The employer pays the premiums for workers' compensation insurance, the amount depending on the employee's job and the risk involved in job performance. The physician usually must supply comprehensive information, and the reporting requirements vary from state to state (Table 14–1). The state bureau or individual insurance carrier should be contacted to obtain instructions and proper forms. State bureaus are listed in Appendix A.

Second-Injury Fund (Subsequent-Injury Fund)

The **second-injury fund**, also known as the **subsequent-injury fund (SIF)**, was established to meet problems arising when an employee has a preexisting injury or condition and is subsequently injured at work. The preexisting injury combines with the second injury to produce disability that is greater than that caused by the latter alone.

Two functions of the fund are: (1) to encourage hiring of the physically handicapped and (2) to allocate more equitably the costs of providing benefits to such employees. Second-injury employers pay compensation related primarily to the disability caused by the second injury, even though the employee receives benefits relating to the combined disability. The difference is made up from the subsequent-injury fund.

Scenario: Second-Injury Fund

Bob Evans loses his left thumb while working a lathe. Two years later Bob loses his left index finger in a second work-related accident. A question could arise of whether the second injury added to a preexisting condition or was related to the prior injury. This case illustrates that the existence of the former injury or disability substantially increased (added to) the disability caused by the latter injury. The employer pays compensation related to the second injury, and funds come from a second-injury fund to pay for the difference between the first and second injuries.

TABLE 14–1	**Employers' or Physicians' Report of Accident**[1]	
Jurisdiction	**Time Limit**	**Injuries Covered**
Alabama	Within 15 days	Death or disability exceeding 3 days
Alaska	Within 10 days	Death, injury, disease, or infection
Arizona	Within 10 days	All injuries
Arkansas	10 days from notice of injury	Indemnity, injuries, or death. Medical claims reported monthly[2]
California	Immediately[3] (employer)	Death or serious injuries
	As prescribed	1-day disability or more than first aid
	Within 5 days	Occupational diseases or pesticide poisoning
Colorado	Immediately[4a]	Death
	Within 10 days[4a]	Injuries causing lost time of 3 days or more[4b]
	Immediately	Any accident in which three or more employees are injured
	10 days[4a]	Occupational disease cases
	10 days[4a]	Cases of permanent physical impairment
Connecticut	7 days or as directed	Disability of 1 day or more
Delaware	Within 48 hours[5]	Death or injuries requiring hospitalization
	Within 10 days	Other injuries
District of Columbia	Within 10 days	All injuries
Florida	Within 24 hours[6]	Death
	Within 7 days of carrier receipt of notice	All injuries
Georgia	Within 21 days[7]	All injuries requiring medical or surgical treatment or causing over 7 days of absence
Guam	Within 10 days[8]	Injury, illness, or death
Hawaii	Within 48 hours	Death
	Within 7 working days	All injuries
Idaho	As soon as practicable but not later than 10 days after the accident[9]	All injuries requiring medical treatment or causing 1 day's absence
Illinois	Within 2 working days	Death or serious injuries
	Between 15th and 25th of month	Disability of more than 3 days
	As soon as determinable	Permanent disability
Indiana	Within 7 working days[10]	Disability of more than 1 day
Iowa	Within 4 days	Disability of more than 3 days, permanent partial disability, death
Kansas	Within 28 days[11]	Death
	Within 28 days	Disability of more than remainder of day or shift
Kentucky	Within 7 days[12]	Disability of more than 1 day
Louisiana	Within 10 days of employer's actual knowledge of injury[13]	Lost time more than 1 week or death
Maine	Within 7 days[14]	Only injuries causing 1 day or more of lost time[14]
Maryland	Within 10 days	Disability of more than 3 days
Massachusetts	Within 7 days, except Sundays and holidays	Disability of 5 or more calendar days
Michigan	Immediately	Death disability of 7 days or more, and specific losses
Minnesota	Within 48 hours	Death or serious injury
	Within 14 days	Disability of 3 days or more
Mississippi	Within 10 days	Death or disability of more than 5 days[15]
Missouri	Within 10 days[16]	Death or injury
Montana	Within 6 days	All injuries
Nebraska	Within 48 hours[17]	Death
	Within 7 days	All injuries
Nevada	Within 6 working days after report from physician[18]	All injuries requiring medical treatment
New Hampshire	Within 5 calendar days	All injuries involving lost time or medical expenses
New Jersey	Immediately[19]	All injuries
New Mexico	Within 10 days of employer notification	Any injury or illness resulting in 7 or more days of lost time

TABLE 14–1	**Employers' or Physicians' Report of Accident[1]—cont'd**	
Jurisdiction	**Time Limit**	**Injuries Covered**
New York	Within 10 days	Disability of 1 day beyond working day or shift on which accident occurred or requiring medical care beyond 2 first aid treatments
North Carolina	Within 5 days[20]	Disability of more than 1 day
North Dakota	Within 7 days	All injuries
Ohio	Within 1 week	Injuries causing total disability of 7 days or more
Oklahoma	Within 10 days or a reasonable time	All injuries causing lost time or requiring treatment away from worksite
Oregon	Within 5 days[21]	All injuries requiring medical treatment[21]
Pennsylvania	Within 48 hours	Death
	After 7 days but not later than 10 days	Disability of 1 day or more
Puerto Rico	Within 5 days	All injuries
Rhode Island	Within 48 hours	Death
	Within 10 days	Disability of 3 days or more and all injuries requiring medical treatment
	Within 2 years of injury	Any claim resulting in medical expense to be reported within 10 days
South Carolina	Within 10 days[22]	All injuries requiring medical attention costing more than $500, more than 1 day disability or permanency
South Dakota	Within 7 days	All injuries[23]
Tennessee	Within 14 days	All injuries requiring medical attention
Texas	Within 8 days[22]	Disability of more than 1 day, or occupational disease
Utah	Within 7 days	All injuries requiring medical attention
Vermont	Within 72 hours[22]	Disability of 1 day or more requiring medical care
Virgin Islands	Within 8 days	Injury or disease
Virginia	Within 10 days[22]	All injuries
Washington	Within 8 hours	Death and accidents resulting in workers' hospitalizations or inability to work
West Virginia	Within 5 days	All injuries
Wisconsin	Within 14 days	Disability beyond 3-day waiting period
Wyoming	Within 10 days	Compensable injuries
FECA	Immediately	All injuries involving medical expenses, disability, or death
LHWCA	10 days	Injuries that cause loss of 1 or more shifts of work or death

[1]Federal Occupational Safety and Health Act of 1970 established uniform requirements and forms to meet its criteria for all businesses affecting interstate commerce to be used for statistical purposes and compliance with the Act. 12 U.S.C. §651.

[2]Arkansas. Medical only claims reported monthly.

[3]California. To Division of Occupational Safety and Health. Within 5 days of employer's notice or knowledge of employee death, employer must report death to the Department of Industrial Relations.

[4]Colorado. (a) Failure to report tolls time limit for claims. (b) Disability of less than 3 days must be reported to insurer.

[5]Delaware. Supplemental report upon termination of disability.

[6]Florida. Report to carrier within 7 days, if injury caused employee to lose 7 or more work days. Supplemental report within 30 days after final payment.

[7]Georgia. Supplemental report on first payment and suspension of payment and within 30 days after final payment.

[8]Guam. Failure to report tolls limits for claims.

[9]Supplemental report required after 60 days (for Rhode Island and South Carolina every 6 months), or upon termination of disability.

[10]Indiana. Supplemental report within 10 days after termination of compensation period.

[11]Kansas. Failure to report tolls time limit for claims. *Childress v. Childress Painting Co.,* 1979.

[12]Kentucky. Supplemental report required after 80 days or upon termination of disability

[13]Louisiana. Employers with more than 10 employees must also report, within 90 days, death, any nonfatal occupational illness or injury causing loss of consciousness, restriction of work or motion, job transfer, or medical treatment other than first aid. Violation of confidentiality of any record, subject to $500 fine.

[14]Maine. Must report asbestosis, mesothelioma, silicosis, and exposure to heavy metals no later than 30 days from date of diagnosis.

[15]Mississippi. Permanent disability, serious head or facial disfigurement also covered. $100 may be added to any award and $100 may be ordered payable to the Commission.

Continued.

| TABLE 14–1 | **Employers' or Physicians' Report of Accident[1]—cont'd** |

[16]Missouri. Supplemental report within 1 month after original notice to Division.

[17]Nebraska. Report may be made by insurance carrier or employer. Failure to report tolls time limits.

[18]Nevada. For minor injuries not requiring medical treatment, the employee may file a "Notice of Injury," which must be retained by the employer for 3 years.

[19]New Jersey. Uninsured employers are required to report compensable injuries only. If insured, carrier is also required to make report.

[20]North Carolina. Supplemental report required after 60 days or upon termination of disability.

[21]Oregon. Insurers to send disabling claims to Workers' Compensation Department within 21 days of employer knowledge.

[22]South Carolina, Texas, Vermont, and Virginia. Supplemental report required after 60 days or upon termination of disability.

[23]South Dakota. Any injury that requires treatment other than first aid or that incapacitates employee for at least 7 calendar days.

Minimum Number of Employees

Table 14–2 shows the minimum number of employees required by each state before the state workers' compensation law comes into effect. There are exemptions in many states for certain occupations such as domestic or casual employees, laborers, babysitters, newspaper vendors or distributors, charity workers, and gardeners. Some states do not require compensation insurance for farm laborers or may specify a larger number of farm employees than the number shown in the table.

Waiting Periods

The laws state that a **waiting period (WP)** must elapse before income benefits are payable. This waiting period affects only wage compensation because medical and hospital care are provided immediately. See Table 14–3 to find the waiting period of each state.

State Disability and Workers' Compensation

Five states and one U.S. territory have state disability insurance (also known as unemployment compensation disability insurance): California, Hawaii, New Jersey, New York, Rhode Island, and Puerto Rico. If a recipient is collecting benefits from a workers' compensation insurance carrier and the amount that the compensation carrie pays is less than that allowed by the state disability insurance program, then the latter pays the balance. See Chapter 15 for further information on state disability insurance.

| TABLE 14–2 | **Minimum Number of Employees for State Workers' Compensation Laws** |

Number of Employees						
1		**3**		**4**		**5**
Alaska	Nebraska	American Samoa		Florida		Alabama
Arizona	Nevada	Arkansas		South Carolina		Mississippi
California	New Hampshire	Georgia				Missouri
Colorado	New Jersey	Michigan				Tennessee
Connecticut	New York	New Mexico				
Delaware	North Dakota	North Carolina				
District of Columbia	Ohio	Virginia				
Guam	Oklahoma					
Hawaii	Oregon					
Idaho	Pennsylvania					
Illinois	Puerto Rico					
Indiana	Rhode Island					
Iowa	South Dakota					
Kansas	Texas					
Kentucky	Utah					
Louisiana	Vermont					
Maine	Virgin Islands					
Maryland	Washington					
Massachusetts	West Virginia					
Minnesota	Wisconsin					
Montana	Wyoming					

TABLE 14-3	**Waiting Period for Income and Medical Benefits***			
Jurisdiction	**Waiting Period (Days)**		**Jurisdiction**	**Waiting Period (Days)**
Alabama	3		Nebraska	7
Alaska	3		Nevada	5
Arizona	7		New Hampshire	3
Arkansas	7		New Jersey	7
California	3		New Mexico	7
Colorado	3		New York	7
Connecticut	3		North Carolina	7
Delaware	3		North Dakota	5
District of Columbia	3		Ohio	7
Florida	7		Oklahoma	3
Georgia	7		Oregon	3
Guam	3		Pennsylvania	7
Hawaii	3		Puerto Rico	3
Idaho	5		Rhode Island	3
Indiana	7		South Dakota	7
Illinois	3		South Carolina	7
Iowa	3		Tennessee	7
Kansas	0		Texas	7
Kentucky	7		Utah	3
Louisiana	7		Vermont	3
Maine	7		Virgin Islands	0
Maryland	3		Virginia	7
Massachusetts	5		Washington	3
Michigan	7		West Virginia	3
Minnesota	3		Wisconsin	3
Mississippi	5		Wyoming	3
Missouri	3		FECA	3
Montana	6		LHWCA	3

*These are statutory provisions for waiting periods. Statutes provide that a waiting period must elapse during which income benefits are not payable. This waiting period affects only compensation, because medical and hospital care are provided immediately. FECA, Federal Employees Compensation Act; LHWCA, Longshoremen's and Harbor Workers' Compensation Act.

Benefits

Five principal types of state compensation benefits that may apply in ordinary cases are the following:

1. *Medical treatment.* This includes hospital, medical and surgical services, medications, and prosthetic devices. Treatment may be rendered by a licensed physician, osteopath, dentist, or chiropractor.
2. *Temporary disability indemnity.* This is in the form of weekly cash payments made directly to the injured or ill person.
3. *Permanent disability indemnity.* This may consist of either weekly or monthly cash payments based on a rating system that determines the percentage of permanent disability or a lump sum award. California has a unique system of permanent disability evaluation that requires a separate determination by the disability rating bureau in San Francisco. No other state has this system.
4. *Death benefits for survivors.* This consists of cash payments to dependents of employees who are

fatally injured. A burial allowance also is given in some states.
5. *Rehabilitation benefits.* This can be medical or vocational rehabilitation in cases of severe disabilities.

Types of State Claims

There are three types of state workers' compensation claims: nondisability (ND) claims, temporary disability claims, and permanent disability claims. Each type is discussed in detail for a clear definition and understanding of the determination process.

Nondisability Claim

This is the simplest type of claim. Generally an **ND claim** involves a minor injury in which the patient is seen by the doctor but is able to continue working (Fig. 14–1). This type of case does not require weekly temporary disability payments.

Temporary Disability Claim

Temporary disability (TD) occurs when a worker has a work-related injury or illness and is unable to perform the duties of his or her occupation for a specific time or range of time. The time period of temporary disability can extend from the date of injury until the worker either returns to full duty without residual ratable disability (discussed later), returns to modified work, or has ratable residual disability that the physician states is permanent and stationary.

An **insurance adjuster** is the person at the workers' compensation insurance carrier who oversees the industrial case. He or she is responsible for keeping in contact with the physician's office about the patient's ongoing progress. The insurance adjuster's most important function is *adjusting an industrial claim*. This means that the insurance adjuster must evaluate the injury or illness, predict in advance the amount of money reserves needed to cover medical expenses, and calculate as accurate a reserve as possible for weekly TD payments to the injured. This is frequently a difficult task because a seemingly minor back strain ultimately may require fusion, or a

Figure 14–1. Physician interacting with an injured worker in the examination room.

small cut may become gangrenous and lead to an amputation. The insurance carrier wants to provide the best possible medical care for the patient. The patient is immediately referred to the specialist if a specialist is necessary.

Usually workers' compensation weekly TD payments are based on the employee's earnings at the time of the injury. Compensation benefits are not subject to income tax.

Sometimes a patient is released to modified work to effect a transition between the period of inactivity caused by disability and a return to full duty, especially when heavy work is involved. Other times an employee is returned to the company and placed in a different department or division so that he or she is gainfully employed while not using the injured body part. This topic is further detailed in the next section.

Vocational Rehabilitation

Many states provide rehabilitation in the form of retraining, education, job guidance, and placement, to assist an injured individual in finding work before temporary disability compensation benefits expire. In any successful rehabilitation program, insurance carrier, physician, physical therapist, employer supervisor, and personnel department must act as a team with the common goal of getting an injured employee back to light duty or regular work as soon as possible. It is believed that the longer a person remains out of work, the less chance there is that he or she will return to the workplace. The employer and insurance adjuster must keep in communication with rehabilitation center therapists to determine when the injured person will be able to resume some form of work. The physician may suggest a rehabilitation center that provides good care, or the employer may have an in-house program.

Work Hardening

Sports medicine therapy and physical medicine rehabilitation often are used to strengthen the injured worker. Physical medicine/therapy CPT codes 97001 to 97542 are used to report these services. Another type of therapy, called **work hardening,** is an individualized program using simulated or real work tasks to build up strength and improve the worker's endurance toward a full day's work. CPT codes 97545 and 97546 are used to report work hardening conditioning.

Ergonomics

In some cases an **ergonomic** evaluation of the work site is performed and modifications may be instituted to the job or work site to lessen the possibility of future injury and to get the employee back to gainful employment. CPT code 97537 may be used to report a work site modification analysis. Injured individuals also may be retrained into another career field if their disability prevents them from returning to their former occupation.

Permanent Disability Claim

In this type of claim the patient or injured party is usually on TD benefits for a time and then concludes that he or she is unable to return to his or her former occupation. The physician states in the report that the patient has residual disability that will hamper his or her opportunity to compete in the open job market. Examples of residual disability include loss of a hand, eye, or leg or neurologic problems. Each patient who has **permanent disability (PD)** is rated according to the severity of the injury, the age of the injured person, and the patient's occupation at the time of the injury. The older the person, the greater the PD benefit. One might think that a younger person deserves higher compensation because he or she will be disabled for a longer portion of his or her working career. However, the workers' compensation laws assume that a young person has a better chance of being rehabilitated into another occupation.

In a PD claim the physician's final report must include the words "**permanent and stationary**" **(P and S).** This phrase means that damage from the injury or illness is permanent, the patient has recovered to the fullest extent possible, the physician is unable to do anything more for the patient, and the patient will be hampered by the disability to some extent for the rest of his or her life. The P and S examination usually is comprehensive, and a level 5 CPT code may be appropriate. Depending on the fee schedule, a modifier indicating that the Evaluation and Management service is a P and S examination also may be used. The case is rated for PD, and a settlement is made called a **compromise and release (C and R).** This is an agreement between the injured party and insurance company on a total sum. The case can then be closed.

Reasons that may delay closing a workers' compensation case include the following:

1. Unanswered questions or incomplete answers to data required on workers' compensation forms by the employee, employer, or physician
2. Vague terminology used by the physician in medical reports
3. Omitted signatures on forms or written reports by the employee, employer, or physician
4. Incorrect billing by the physician's office
5. Inadequate progress reports (e.g., the physician fails to send in a medical report routinely to update the insurance carrier when the injured employee is seen in subsequent visits)

Rating

Final determination of the issues involving settlement of an industrial accident is known as **adjudication,** or the rating of a case. A physician does not rate disability but renders a professional opinion on whether the injured individual has temporary or permanent disability that prevents him or her from gainful employment. Rating itself is carried out by the state's industrial accident commission or workers' compensation board. Wage loss, earning capacity, and physical impairment are three categories that may be taken into consideration to rate temporary partial, permanent partial, or total disabilities.

In addition, permanent partial disabilities may be rated by using a scheduled or nonscheduled injury award system. This system is based on a set number of weeks of compensation for a specific loss, such as 288 weeks for the loss of a leg. Scheduled injuries may include loss of a body part, disfigurement, permanent hearing loss, and so on. Nonscheduled injuries are more general, such as disability caused by injury to the back or neck.

If an injured person is dissatisfied with the rating after the case has been declared P and S, he or she may appeal the case (by **petition**—formal written request) to the **Workers' Compensation Appeals Board (WCAB)** or the Industrial Accident Commission.

Surveillance

Sub rosa films sometimes are provided when rating a case to document the extent of a patient's permanent disability. *Sub rosa* means under the rose. In ancient times the rose was a symbol of silence or secrecy. Videotapes are made over a period of 2 to 3 days without the patient's knowledge. This surveillance is expensive and is used as a last resort, especially in a case in which a person receiving workers' compensation benefits is suspected of making exaggerated complaints. It is also used in cases when a worker has been off work for a long period of time and supposedly is unable to perform any work activity, even light duty.

Investigators have been known to carry a camera in a gym bag and videotape a supposedly disabled claimant bench pressing at the gym. Patients also have been videotaped going into the physician's office for an appointment wearing a neck brace and removing the brace after returning to their car.

Fraud and Abuse

Increases for fraudulent workers' compensation claims were noted throughout many large metropolitan cities in the 1990s. These problems involved employers, employees, insurers, medical providers, and lawyers. An increasing number of states have enacted some kind of antifraud legislation and stiffened penalties for workers' compensation fraud, making it a felony. Some states require reporting suspected insurance fraud and have forms to incorporate wording in regard to fraudulent statements. An example is shown in Figure 14–2.

Physicians are responsible for determining the legitimacy of work injuries and reporting findings accurately. If a report is prepared with the intent to use it in support of a fraudulent claim, or if a fraudulent claim is knowingly submitted for payment under an insurance contract, the physician may be subject to fines or imprisonment and the revocation or suspension of his or her medical license. Some physicians sign and send a disclosure statement with the medical report certifying that they personally performed an evaluation. The physician may list the total time spent in reviewing records, face-to-face time with the patient, preparation of a report, and other relevant activities.

It is the responsibility of all individuals who deal with workers' compensation cases to notify the insurance carrier of any suspicious situation. By doing so, action can be taken to have the case investigated further by personnel from the fraud divisions or referred to the district attorney's office. Perpetrators and signs of workers' compensation fraud and abuse are listed in Box 14–1.

See Chapters 1, 11, and 12 for further information on fraud and abuse in the medical setting.

Occupational Safety and Health Administration Act of 1970

Background

Congress has established an office known as the **Occupational Safety and Health Administration (OSHA)** to protect employees against on-the-job health and safety hazards. This program includes strict health and safety standards and a sensible complaint procedure enabling individual workers to trigger enforcement measures.

Work standards are designed to minimize exposure to on-the-job hazards such as faulty machinery, noise, dust, and toxic chemical fumes. Employers are required by law to meet these health and safety standards. Failure to do so can result in fines against the employer that could run into thousands of dollars.

Coverage

The Act provides that if a state submits an OSHA plan and it is approved by the government, the state may assume responsibility for carrying out OSHA policies and procedures and is excluded from federal jurisdiction.

The Act applies to almost all businesses, large or small. It applies to heavy, light, and service industries, nonprofit and charitable institutions, churches' secular activities in hospitals, farmers, and retailers. Employees of state and local governments are also covered. Federal employees, a farmer's immediate family, church employees engaged in religious activities, independent contractors, and household domestic workers are *not* covered.

Regulations

Specific regulations that affect the medical setting are those aimed at minimizing exposure to hepatitis B virus (HBV), human immunodeficiency virus (HIV), and other blood-borne pathogens. Any worker who comes in contact with human blood and infectious materials must receive proper information and training and use universal precautions to avoid infection. Vaccinations must be provided for those who are at risk for exposure to hepatitis B, and comprehensive records must be maintained. For fact sheets, booklets, and guidelines on blood-borne pathogens, contact the nearest OSHA office or write to OSHA Publications Office, 200 Constitution Avenue, NW, Room N3101, Washington, DC 20210.

Chemicals and hazardous substances are used that impose dangers in many work settings. Businesses are required to obtain material safety data sheets (MSDS) for each hazardous chemical used on site. Employers that produce a hazardous chemical must develop material safety data sheets. A compliance kit is available from the Superintendent of Documents, U.S. Government Printing Office, Washington, DC 20402.

Filing a Complaint

To file a complaint, the proper form is obtained from the federal Division of Industrial Safety or a state OSHA office and completed by the employee. It is against the law for an employer to take any adverse action against an employee who files such a complaint.

Inspection

A compliance officer (inspector) may call for an appointment or may be sent unannounced to the place of employment. If an officer arrives unannounced, the office manager must be notified so an appointment may be arranged for the inspection to take place. A court warrant may be required to search a company's premises if the employer does not consent to OSHA entry. A business may be cited and, depending on the violation, fines or criminal penalties may be imposed.

State of California
Department of Industrial Relations
DIVISION OF WORKERS' COMPENSATION

Estado de California
Departmento de Relaciones Industriales
DIVISION DE COMPENSACIÓN AL TRABAJADOR

EMPLOYEE'S CLAIM FOR WORKERS' COMPENSATION BENEFITS

PETICION DEL EMPLEADO PARA BENEFICIOS DE COMPENSACIÓN DEL TRABAJADOR

If you are injured or become ill because of your job, you may be entitled to workers' compensation benefits.

Complete the **"Employee"** section and give the form to your employer. Keep the copy marked **"Employee's Temporary Receipt"** until you receive the dated copy from your employer. You may call the Division of Workers' Compensation at **1-800-736-7401** if you need help in filling out this form or in obtaining your benefits. An explanation of workers' compensation benefits is included on the back of this form.

You should also have received a pamphlet from your employer describing workers' compensation benefits and the procedures to obtain them.

Si Ud. se ha lesionado o se ha enfermado a causa de su trabajo, Ud. tiene derecho a recibir beneficios de compensación al trabajador.
Complete la sección "Empleado" y entregue la forma a su empleador. Quédese con la copia designada "Recibo Temporal del Empleado" hasta que Ud. reciba la copia fechada de su empleador. Si Ud. necesita ayuda para completar esta forma o para obtener sus beneficios, Ud. puede hablar con la Division de Compensación al Trabajador llamando al 1-800-736-7401. En la parte de atrás de esta forma se encuentra una explicación de los beneficios de la compensación al trabajador.

Ud. también debería haber recibido de su empleador un folleto describiendo los beneficios de compensación al trabajador lesionado y los procedimientos para obtenerlos.

Any person who makes or causes to be made any knowingly false or fraudulent material statement or material representation for the purpose of obtaining or denying workers' compensation benefits or payments is guilty of a felony.

Toda aquella persona que a propósito haga o cause que se produzca cualquier declaración o representación material falsa o fraudulenta con el fin de obtener o negar beneficios o pagos de compensación a trabajadores lesionados es culpable de un crimen mayor "felonía".

Employee: *Empleado*

1. Name. *Nombre.* Ima B. Hurt Today's date. *Fecha de hoy.* 4-3-20XX
2. Home address. *Dirección residencial.* 300 East Central Avenue
3. City. *Ciudad.* Woodland Hills State. *Estado.* XY Zip. *Código postal* 12345-0001
4. Date of injury. *Fecha de la lesión (accidente).* 4-3-XX Time of injury. *Hora en que ocurrió.* ____ a.m. 2:00 p.m.
5. Address and description of where injury happened. *Dirección/lugar dónde occurió el accidente.* The Conk Out Company 45 South Gorman Street, Woodland Hills, XY 12345 injured in stock room
6. Describe injury and part of body affected. *Describa la lesión y parte dél cuerpo afectada.* Fell off ladder in stock room. Injured left ankle.
7. Social Security Number. *Número de Seguro Social del Empleado.* 120 XX 6542
8. Signature of employees. *Firma del empleado.* *Ima B. Hurt*

Employer–complete this section and give the employee a copy immediately as a receipt.
Empleador–complete esta sección y déle inmediatamente una copia al empleado como recibo.

9. Name of employer. *Nombre del empleador.* The Conk Out Company
10. Address. *Dirección.* 45 South Gorman Street, Woodland Hills, XY 12345
11. Date employer first knew of injury. *Fecha en que el empleador supo por primera vez de la lesión o accidente.* 4-3-20XX
12. Date claim form was provided to employee. *Fecha en que se le entregó al empleado la petición.* 4-3-20XX
13. Date employer received claim form. *Fecha en que el empleado devolvió la petición al empleador.* 4-3-20XX
14. Name and address of insurance carrier or adjusting agency. *Nombre y dirección de la compañía de seguros o agencia administradora de seguros.* XYZ Insurance Company, P.O. Box 5, Woodland Hills, XY 12345
15. Insurance policy number. *El número de la poliza del Seguro.* B 12345
16. Signature of employer representative. *Firma del representante del empleador.* *J. D. Hawkins*
17. Title. *Título.* Owner 18. Telephone. *Teléfono.* 555-430-3488

Employer: You are required to date this form and provide copies to your insurer or claims administrator and to the employee, dependent or representative who filed the claim within **one working day** of receipt of the form from the employee.

SIGNING THIS FORM IS NOT AN ADMISSION OF LIABILITY

Empleador: Se requiere que Ud. feche esta forma y que provéa copias a su compañía de seguros, administrador de reclamos, o dependiente/répresentante de reclamos y al empleado que hayan presentado esta peticíon dentro del plazo de **un día hábil** desde el momento de haber sido recibida la forma del empleado.

EL FIRMAR ESTA FORMA NO SIGNIFICA ADMISION DE RESPONSABILIDAD

Original (Employer's Copy)
DWC Form 1 (REV. 1/94)

ORIGINAL (Copia del Empleador)
DWC Forma 1 (REV. 1/94)

Figure 14–2. Employee's Claim for Workers' Compensation Benefits. Notice the insert about fraudulent material.

Perpetrators and Signs of Workers' Compensation Fraud and Abuse

Employee

- Misses the first physician's visit
- Cannot describe the pain or is overly dramatic (comes into the physician's office limping on the left leg, suddenly starts limping on the right leg, and then goes back to limping on the left leg)
- Delays in reporting the injury
- Does not report Friday's injury until Monday morning
- First reports an injury to a legal or regulatory agency
- Reports an injury after missing several days of work
- Changes physicians frequently
- Is a short-term worker
- Has a curious claim history
- Fabricates an injury
- Exaggerates a work-related injury to obtain larger benefits (A worker complains of back pain and an inability to bend over or lift. Surveillance cameras capture the individual at home repairing cars, a task he is supposedly unable to perform.)
- Blames the employer for an injury that occurred off the job

Employer

- Misrepresents the annual payroll to get lower premium rates
- Misrepresents the number of workers employed
- Gives a false address with the least expensive premium rates
- Falsely classifies the job duties of workers (The employer states the job title as clerical worker and defines it as nonhazardous when the employee is using a lathe every day.)

Insurer

- Refuses to pay valid medical claims
- Forces the injured worker to settle by using unethical tactics (An insurance agent tells an employee that he has a back sprain so the worker will settle the case. The worker later has a myelogram that reveals a herniated intervertebral disk that leaves the worker with a permanent partial disability.)

Medical Provider

- Orders or performs unnecessary tests
- Renders unnecessary treatment
- Charges the insurance carrier for services never rendered
- Participates in a provider mill scheme (see explanation under "Lawyer")
- Makes multiple referrals from a clinic practice regardless of type of injury
- Sends medical reports that look photocopied with the same information typed in (e.g., employer's address, description of injury) or that read almost identical to other reports
- Sends in many claims in which injuries are of a subjective nature, such as stress, emotional distress, headaches, or inability to sleep
- Sends in claims from one employer showing several employees with similar injuries, verified by the same physicians or attorneys

Lawyer

- Overbills clients
- Participates in a medical provider mill scheme. (An individual is solicited while in the unemployment line by a recruiter known as a "capper." The capper tells the worker it is possible to obtain more money on disability than through unemployment. The worker is referred to an attorney and a "provider mill" clinic, which help the individual fabricate a claim by claiming stress or an on-the-job injury. In some states such acts may be considered a public offense and punishable as a misdemeanor or felony.)

Recordkeeping and Reporting

Employers must keep records of their employees' work-related injuries and illnesses on OSHA Form No. 200. Forms may be obtained from the OSHA office or from any office of the U.S. Department of Labor. This document must be on file at the workplace and available to employees and OSHA compliance officers on request. Form 200 must be retained in the file for 5 years. After 6 days a case recorded on Form 200 must have a supplementary record (OSHA Form 101) completed and kept in the files. Some states have modified their workers' compensation forms so they may be used as substitutes for Form 101. Certain low-hazard industries are exempt from having to complete and retain Forms 200 and 101.

Companies with fewer than 11 employees must complete safety survey OSHA Form 200-S. Companies also are required to display OSHA posters to inform employees of their job safety rights. Federal law states that an accident that results in the death or hospitalization of five or more employees must be reported to OSHA.

Legal Situations

Medical Evaluator

Physicians who conduct medicolegal evaluations of injured workers must pass a complex medical examination. They are then certified by the Industrial Medical Council (IMC) and may be referred to under one of the following titles:

▶ Agreed Medical Evaluator (AME)
▶ Independent Medical Evaluator (IME)
▶ Qualified Medical Evaluator (QME)

The medical evaluator is hired by the insurance company or appointed by the referee or appeals board to examine an individual, independent from the attending physician, and render an unbiased opinion about the degree of disability of an injured worker. When the physician performs an evaluation on an injured worker, the workers' compensation fee schedule may have specific procedure codes to bill for the examination. Evaluation and Management consultation codes or the CPT code for work-related evaluation by "other" physician, 99456, may be used. Some state fee schedules may have specific medical legal (ML) procedure codes to bill for various levels of examination. When a case involves a medical evaluation, a deposition may be taken of his or her testimony.

Depositions

A **deposition** is a proceeding in which an attorney asks a witness questions about a case, and the witness answers under oath but not in open court. It may take place in the attorney's office or often in the physician's office. In permanent disability workers' compensation cases, depositions usually are taken from the physician and the injured party by the attorney representing the workers' compensation insurance company. The injured party's attorney is also present if the witness is the defendant. Direct questioning and cross-examination may be done by both attorneys.

The session may be recorded on a stenotype machine, in shorthand, or by audiotape or videotape. Video depositions are used in several instances. For example, if a plaintiff in a case is terminally ill and the plaintiff's attorney wishes to preserve the plaintiff's testimony, a video deposition may be used as substantive (essential) evidence. A video deposition also may be taken if a witness cannot be present at the trial. In a case in which a witness may be in Arizona and cannot appear in Pennsylvania, the attorney takes the deposition in Arizona and proves to the court that the witness is beyond its jurisdiction. The same is true for a physician defendant who is not available for some reason.

Exhibits may be entered into evidence. The witness is allowed to read the transcript and make corrections or changes. The witness may be asked to sign the transcript but can waive signature if his or her attorney recommends against signing it. The deposition is used when the case comes to trial.

Depositions may be taken to find out additional information, the physician's version of the facts, the patient's version of the facts, what kind of witnesses the physician and patient will be, and so on. Another use for a deposition is to impeach (challenge the credibility or validity of) a witness on cross-examination. If the witness takes the stand and the testimony is inconsistent with the deposition, the attorney will make this known to the jury.

Medical Testimony

In the instance of an accident case with third-party liability, the physician may have to testify as an expert witness, take time to give a deposition, or attend a pretrial conference. There should be a clear understanding of the terms of testimony and payment to eliminate future misunderstandings. A written agreement from the patient's lawyer should be obtained stating exactly what compensation the physician will receive for research (preparation), time spent waiting to testify (if appointments must be canceled), and actual testimony time (Fig. 14–3). In some cases the physician may want to ask for partial payment in advance. If the physician is subpoenaed he or she must appear in court regardless of whether an agreement exists. The correct CPT code for medical testimony is 99075. This agreement should be signed by the physician and sent to the attorney. The attorney should return the original to the physician, retaining a copy for his or her files.

Liens

The word **lien** derives from the same origin as the word *liable*, and the right of lien expresses legal claim on the property of another for the payment of a debt (Fig. 14–4). Liens sometimes are called encumbrances and may be filed for a number of reasons.

The advantages of filing a lien are as follows:

❭ It is a written agreement and is recognized in court.
❭ It is a source of protection in the event of litigation.
❭ It ensures that payment for previously rendered medical services will be received when the attorney and patient have reached a settlement with the insurance company in an accident case.
❭ It is an inexpensive method of collecting the fee. The physician can file suit and try to get a judgment against the patient, but this is relatively expensive in comparison with filing a lien.
❭ The physician will collect the full fee. If the physician assigns such a delinquent account to a collection agency, he or she may lose as much as 50% of the fee when it is collected.
❭ If the physician wishes to bill more than what is allowed for a given service or services, a lien can be filed and the judge will determine whether it is reasonable.
❭ It avoids harassment in trying to collect the bill.

The chief disadvantage of not filing a lien is that there is no legal documentation should the case go to court as far as collecting monies owed to the physician. A case could be settled, the attorney would get his or her fee, and the physician's fee may be placed last on the list for payment or remain unpaid.

MEDICAL TESTIMONY AGREEMENT

AGREEMENT made this _____ day of _____ 20XX, between _____
herein referred to as attorney, and _____ ,
of _____ , _____ , _____ _____ , a licensed _____ .
    (street address)   (city)   (state)   (ZIP code)

In consideration of their mutual covenants set forth herein, the parties agree as follows:

1. The doctor will give medical testimony in the case of:
_____

as a treating physician or as an expert witness (delete the unwanted phrase).

2. The doctor agrees to appear promptly when called and to present his or her medical testimony in a well-prepared professional manner.

3. The doctor will be compensated for time away from the practice of his or her medical duties in accordance with the following:
    (a) $_____ per hour for reports and preparation of medical testimony.
    (b) $_____ per hour for pretrial conferences.
    (c) $_____ per hour for court appearance, including travel time to and from the office.
    (d) $_____ per hour for deposition.
    (e) $_____ per hour for being on call with cancellation of appointments but not appearing in court.

4. The doctor will appear in court on _____ hour's notice from the attorney, unless prior arrangements have been made for the exact time of appearance.

5. The doctor will be compensated on completion of his or her medical testimony, and payment will not be contingent upon the outcome of the case. However, if the case is settled before reaching the court, the doctor will be compensated for being on call as noted above.

This contract shall be binding upon the parties.

IN WITNESS WHEREOF, the said parties hereto have subscribed their respective signatures.

_____
    (physician)
_____
    (attorney)

Date: _____

Figure 14–3. Example of a medical testimony agreement between physician and attorney. This is signed by the physician and sent to the attorney for signature. A copy is retained by the attorney and the original is kept by the physician.

Scenario: Filing a Lien

Problem 1: Suppose Attorney Blake advises a client Roger Reed not to pay the physician until after the trial or payment is not made for Dr. Practon's courtroom testimony and the case is lost? Suppose medical reports are ordered and Attorney Blake neglects to pay for them. What happens if Roger Reed forgets about the physician's bill?
Solution: If a lien had been signed, the money will be paid to the physician when the case has been settled. Otherwise the settlement belongs to the patient, Roger Reed, and he determines what he wants to do with the money.
Problem 2: Suppose Dr. Practon had an oral agreement covering his fee. The patient, Katie Crest, was unable to pay for medical treatment except on legal monetary recovery. When Katie Crest settled her case, the proceeds went almost entirely to welfare agencies because she received retroactive Medicaid. Dr. Practon sued the patient's attorney and lost.
Solution: If Dr. Practon had gotten a written assignment of the proceeds, the lawyer could have been held liable for the fee.

A time limit should be specified when a lien form is completed; reaching a settlement may involve several years of litigation. Some patients may be persuaded to pay before a legal settlement is made or at least make payments until a settlement is reached. The lien becomes null and void at the end of the time limit. If the patient's financial status has changed, one might be able to collect because the patient can now be billed. If not, an amended or subsequent lien should be filed that states the actual balance of the patient's account. The word "amended" should be typed on the new lien below the Workers' Compensation Appeals Board case number.

The physician's fee should be protected by having the attorney sign the lien, thereby indicating that he or she will pay the physician directly from any money received in a settlement. This makes the attorney responsible for the fee. The patient's file must be placed in a Hold for Settlement category until the case comes up in court. In some states the physician's fee owed by the patient constitutes a first lien against any such money settlement, and the

**REQUEST FOR ALLOWANCE OF LIEN
ASSIGNMENT AND AUTHORIZATION**

WHEREAS, I have a right or cause of action arising out of personal injury, to wit:

I, _____ hereby authorize _____ ,
    patient's name   physician's name

to furnish, upon request, to my attorney_____ ,
any and all medical records, or reports of examination, diagnosis, treatment, or prognosis but not necessarily limited to those items as set forth herein, in addition to an itemized statement of account for services rendered therefore or in connection therewith, which my attorney may from time to time request in connection with the injuries described above and sustained by me on the _____ day of _____ , 20XX.

I, hereby irrevocably authorize and direct my said attorney set forth herein to pay to_____ all charges for attendance in court,
                     physician's name

if required as an expert witness whether he testifies or not; reports or other data supplied by him; depositions given by said doctor; medical services rendered or drugs supplied; and any other reasonable and customary charges incurred by my attorney as submitted by_____ and in
                                   physician's name

connection with said injury. Said payment or payments are to be made from any money or monies received by my attorney whether by judgment, decree, or settlement of this case, prior to disbursement to me and payment of the amount as herein directed shall be the same as if paid by me. This authorization to pay the aforementioned doctor shall constitute and be deemed as assignment of so much of my recovery I receive. It is agreed that nothing herein relieves me of the primary responsibility and obligation of paying my doctor for services rendered, and I shall at all times remain personally liable for such indebtedness unless released by the aforementioned doctor or by payment disbursed by my attorney.
I accept the above assignment:
Dated: _____ Patient:_____

As the attorney of record for the above-named patient, I hereby agree to observe the terms of this agreement, and to withhold from any award in this case such sums as are required for the adequate protection of Dr._____
_____ .

Date: _____ Attorney:_____

Figure 14–4. Patient's authorization to release information to an attorney and grant lien to the physician against proceeds of settlement in connection with accident, industrial, or third-party litigation cases.

attorney must first satisfy the lien of the physician before the patient or attorney receives any money from the settlement. State laws should be checked. The office of the patient's attorney should be called at least quarterly for an update.

If there is a third-party litigation involved in an industrial case or a decision has not been reached as to whether an accident is caused by industrial or nonindustrial causes, both a regular lien and a workers' compensation lien should be filed. In most states a special lien form for workers' compensation filing is available and should be used. A copy of the lien should be completed and sent to all concerned parties:

▶ Appeals board
▶ Employer of the patient
▶ Employee (the patient)
▶ Insurance carrier
▶ Physician's files (lien claimant or one who is filing for the lien)

The patient/employee consents to the lien by his or her signature. Do not accept a lien form unless it is also signed by the patient's attorney. Check with the local Division of Industrial Accidents for forms pertinent to filing a lien and instructions on the formalities, number of copies required, and where they are to be sent.

Third-Party Subrogation

The legal term *subrogation* is the process of initiating a legal claim against another individual, an individual's insurer, or, in the case of a car accident, one's own automobile insurance company to pay health insurance bills. **Third-party subrogation** means "to substitute" one person for another. When applied to workers' compensation cases, it means a transfer of the claims and rights from the original creditor (workers' compensation insurance carrier) to the **third-party liability** carrier. In a compensation case the insurance carrier that is "subrogated" to the legal claims has a right to reimbursement of all of the moneys paid for the injuries. That reimbursement is obtained from any money the injured collects from a legal claim, directly from the individual who caused the injury, or from another insurer.

Scenario: **Third-Party Subrogation**

Problem: Monica Valdez, a secretary, goes to the bank to deposit some money for her employer. Monica's car is struck from behind by another automobile, and she is injured while on the errand.

Solution: In such a case there is no question of fault and no question of cause. Monica was hurt during the performance of her work, and the workers' compensation insurance carrier is liable. The carrier must adjust the claim, provide all medical treatment, and pay all TD and PD benefits.

However, the insurance carrier does have legal recourse. It may send a representative to visit with Monica, explain to her that she has a good subrogation case, encourage her to seek the advice of an attorney, and suggest that she sue the third party (other automobile driver) in civil court. This is sometimes referred to as litigation, which is the process of carrying on a lawsuit. If Monica agrees to sue, the insurance carrier files a demand with the court for repayment of all the money that it has paid out. This is called a lien, as discussed earlier in the chapter. If an award is made to Monica when the case is settled, the insurance carrier is reimbursed for all it has paid and Monica receives the balance. The patient is legally prevented from collecting twice in some states (e.g., California).

If the patient's attorney should call the physician's office for information, it is only ethical and legal to get a signed authorization from the patient and also to ask permission from the insurance carrier before giving out any medical information. The contract exists between the physician and insurance carrier, not the physician and patient.

Medical Reports

HIPAA Compliance Alert

Privacy and Confidentiality

Because there is a difference in the treatment of confidentiality for certain records in industrial cases, several aspects of the Health Insurance Portability and Accountability Act (HIPAA) covered by the Privacy Rule have been tailored to meet unique concerns of workers' compensation entities. The HIPAA Privacy Rule allows for the disclosure of Personal Health Information (PHI)

to workers' compensation insurers, state administrators, and employers to the extent necessary to comply with laws relating to workers' compensation. The Privacy Rule recognizes the legitimate need of insurers and other entities involved in the workers' compensation systems to have access to individuals' health information as authorized by state or other law. Because of the significant variability among such laws, the Privacy Rule permits disclosures of health information for workers' compensation purposes in a number of different ways.

1. *Disclosures Without Individual Authorization.* The Privacy Rule permits covered entities to disclose protected health information to workers' compensation insurers, State administrators, employers, and other persons or entities involved in workers' compensation systems, without the individual's authorization. This relates to workers' compensation injuries or illnesses and federal programs such as Black Lung Benefits Act, Federal Employees' Compensation Act, the Longshore and Harbor Workers' Compensation Act, and Energy Employees' Occupational Illness Compensation Program Act. The disclosure must comply with and be limited to what the state law requires. Disclosure is allowed for purposes of obtaining payment for any health care provided to the injured or ill worker.

2. *Disclosures With Individual Authorization.* Covered entities may disclose protected health information to workers' compensation insurers and others involved in workers' compensation systems where the individual has provided his or her authorization for the release of the information to the entity.

3. *Minimum Necessary.* Covered entities are required to limit the amount of protected health information disclosed to the minimum necessary to accomplish the workers' compensation purpose. Under this requirement, protected health information may be shared for such purposes to the full extent authorized by state or other law.

Documentation

Documentation always must show the necessity for the procedures performed. If there is not an accurate diagnostic code to explain the patient's condition, a report should be sent describing the details of the diagnosis. CPT code 99080 may be used to bill for workers' compensation reports. The monetary value assigned to the code usually is determined by the number of pages in the report. If medical records are reviewed before consulting or treating a workers' compensation patient, a bill should be submitted for this service. Refer to Chapter 3 for comprehensive information on this topic.

Medical Recordkeeping

If a private patient comes to the office with an industrial injury, a separate medical record (chart) and financial record (ledger) should be set up for the work-related injury. A private medical record should never be combined with an industrial case record because separate disclosure laws apply to each, and the workers' compensation case may go to court. Some medical practices use a colored file folder or tabs for the industrial medical record, which makes filing of all private and workers' compensation documents easier for the insurance billing specialist. If two charts are maintained, it is easy to pull the industrial medical record and financial accounting record quickly without having to go through the patients' previously unrelated private medical records.

It is preferable that a patient not be scheduled to see a physician for a workers' compensation follow-up examination and an unrelated complaint during the same appointment time. Separate appointments (back to back, if necessary) should be arranged. This allows for separate dictation without intermixing the required documentation for each chart.

Terminology

A majority of workers' compensation cases involve accidents causing bodily injuries. Therefore one should become familiar with anatomic terms, directional and range of motion words, types of fractures, body activity terms, and words that describe pain and symptoms. This terminology appears in progress chart notes and industrial injury reports. The more knowledgeable one becomes about the meaning of the documentation, the more proficient he or she will be in knowing if the procedure and diagnostic codes assigned are substantiated or if code selection is deficient and should be enhanced for better payment. Figures 14–5 through 14–9, Table 14–4, and Box 14–2 should be studied carefully. One should learn how to spell the words and find the definitions of the words in the dictionary.

Directional Terms

Directional terms are commonly used in workers' compensation reports. Figure 14–5 illustrates positional and directional terms referring to movements and planes of the body. The subject is standing upright, facing forward, arms at the sides with palms forward, and feet parallel. Imaginary lines divide the body in half, forming body planes (e.g., frontal plane dividing right and left sides and coronal plane dividing front and back).

The positional and directional terms indicate the location or direction of the body part with respect to each other (e.g., medial, toward the midline of the body, and lateral, toward the sides of the body).

Range of Motion of Upper and Lower Extremities

Figure 14–6 shows commonly dictated terms for range of motion (ROM) of upper and lower extremities. ROM tests determine if the body part is able to move to the full extent possible. Often after an injury to an extremity or joint there is restriction of motion and loss of strength (e.g., grip). ROM can be improved with activity and therapy and is measured with special measurement devices and documented each time a patient is examined.

Types of Fractures

A fracture is a break in the continuity of a bone. Figures 14–7 and 14–8 illustrate the many bones of the body and Figure 14–9 explains each type of fracture. Such injuries can occur from falling, blows, impact hits, a disease process, or direct violence, such as in an automobile accident. Healing may take months and depends on the location and severity of the injured part, associated injury, and complications or infections.

Reporting Requirements

Employer's Report

The laws clearly state that the injured person must promptly report the industrial injury or illness to his or her employer or immediate supervisor, which may be a safety officer in some businesses. The first report of an industrial injury submitted by the employer and the physician is required by law in most states. The employer sends in an Employer's Report of Occupational Injury or Illness Form (Fig. 14–10) to the insurance company. The time limit on submission of this form varies from immediately to as long as 30 days in different states (Table 14–1). Many states have adopted the form shown in Figure 14–10 to meet the requirements of the Federal Occupational Safety and Health Act of 1970 and for state statistical purposes.

Medical Service Order

In addition to the employer's report, the employer may complete and sign a **medical service order,** giving this to the injured employee to take to the

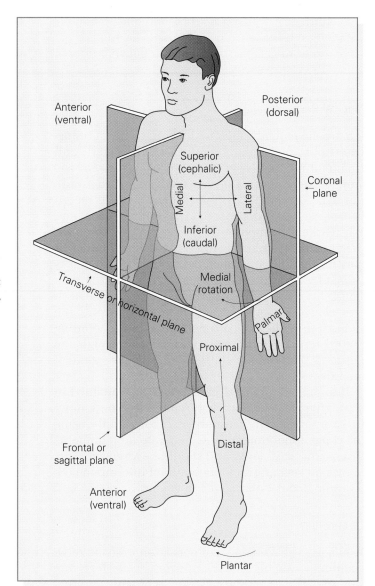

Figure 14–5. Directional terminology. (From Chabner DE: *Medical Terminology: A Short Course.* Philadelphia, Saunders, 1999.)

physician's office (Fig. 14–11). This authorizes the physician to treat the injured employee. The form should be photocopied and the copy retained for the physician's files. The original should be attached to the Doctor's First Report of Occupational Injury or Illness (preliminary report). An employer may prefer to write the service order on his or her business letterhead, billhead, or simply a piece of scratch paper.

Authorizations also may be obtained over the telephone. However, if a patient arrives for an appointment without written authorization, some offices prefer that the employer be telephoned and asked to have the authorized person fax the permission for treatment. Subsequently, if payment is not received or the claim is disputed, it may be easier to collect if a copy of the written authorization is included when sending collection follow-up correspondence.

The copayment should be collected when the patient has a managed care plan and neglects to bring in an authorization. It is the patient's responsibility to get the authorization if injured on the job (Fig. 14–12).

A charge can be made if an appointment was arranged by the employer or insurance company for a workers' compensation patient and was not canceled 72 hours before the appointment time. Check with the insurance company because this policy may vary, depending on state laws.

If outside testing or treatment is necessary, authorization should be obtained from the employer or the adjuster for the insurance company. When this is done by telephone, the name of the procedure or test and the medical necessity for it should be stated. The name and title of the person giving authorization should be obtained and written in the patient's chart and on the order form along with the date. No authorization numbers are issued in workers' compensation cases.

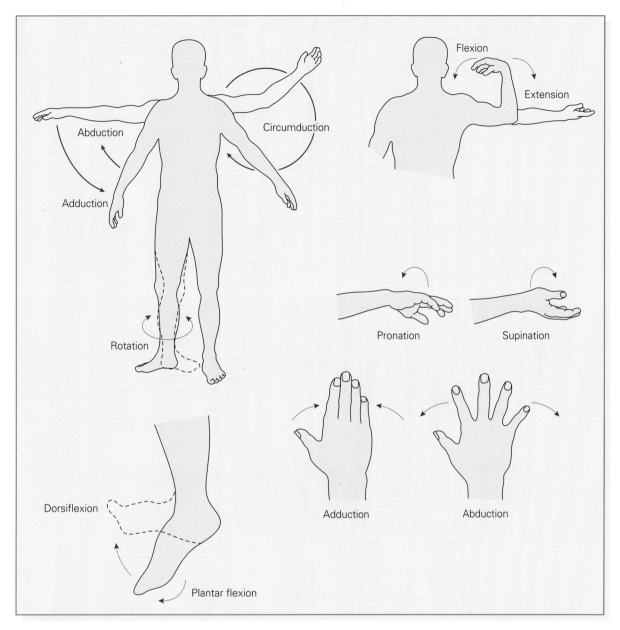

Figure 14–6. Range of motion for upper and lower extremities. (From Sloane S, Fordney MT: *Saunders Manual of Medical Transcription.* Philadelphia, Saunders, 1994.)

The insurance adjuster handling the case should be contacted if a translator is needed for a workers' compensation patient. He or she should make arrangements for an official translator to be present for all appointments. A member of the patient's family or the patient's friend should not be allowed to serve as a translator because there may be no legal recourse for the physician if miscommunicated information leads to a bad outcome.

Physician's First Report

After the physician sees the injured person, he or she sends in a completed First Treatment Medical Report (Fig. 14–13) or a Doctor's First Report of Occupational Injury or Illness form (used in California; see Fig. 14–14) as soon as possible.

If the physician prefers to submit a narrative letter, the medical report should include the components, if relevant, shown in Table 14–5. The time limit for filing this report varies; state requirements are provided in Table 14–1. Failure to file the report can be a misdemeanor. Copies of the report form go to the insurance carrier and the state. Some physicians also send a copy to the employer.

Because the report is a legal document, each copy *must be signed in ink* by the physician. The insurance company waits for the physician's report and bill, then issues payment to the physician. The case can be closed if there is no further treatment or disability.

THE SKELETON (ANTERIOR VIEW)

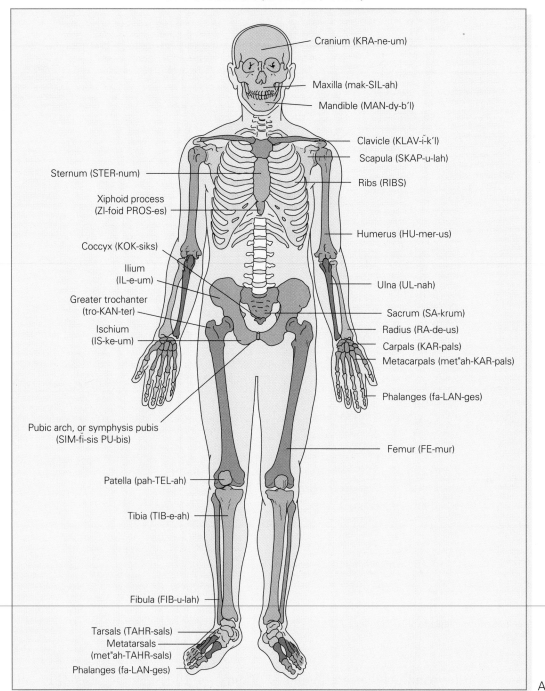

Figure 14–7. A and **B,** Terminology pertinent to the skeletal anatomy commonly used in reports on injury cases. (From Chabner DE: *The Language of Medicine,* 6th ed. Philadelphia, Saunders, 1999.)

PROCEDURE: Completing the Doctor's First Report of Occupational Injury or Illness

The submission of this form (Fig. 14–14) has a deadline, from immediately to within 5 days after the patient has been seen by the physician, depending on each state's law. An original and three or four copies should be distributed as follows:

▶ Original to the insurance carrier (unless more copies are required)
▶ One copy to the state agency
▶ One copy to the patient's employer
▶ One copy retained for the physician's files in the patient's workers' compensation file folder

THE SKELETON (POSTERIOR VIEW)

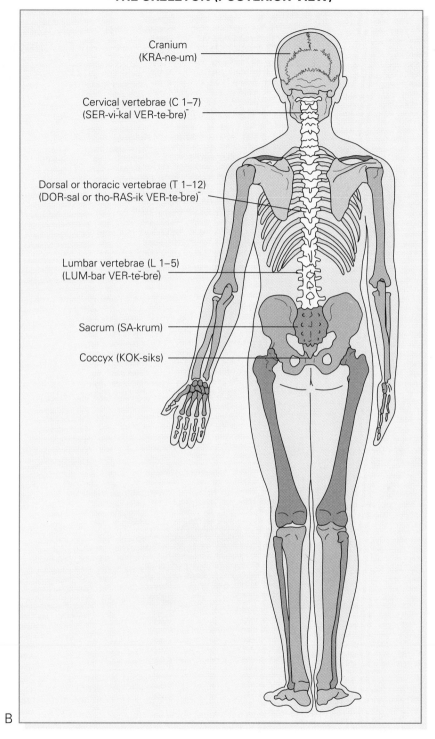

Cranium
(KRA-ne-um)

Cervical vertebrae (C 1–7)
(SER-vi-kal VER-te-bre)

Dorsal or thoracic vertebrae (T 1–12)
(DOR-sal or tho-RAS-ik VER-te-bre)

Lumbar vertebrae (L 1–5)
(LUM-bar VER-te-bre)

Sacrum (SA-krum)

Coccyx (KOK-siks)

B

Figure 14–7, cont'd.

In some states, attending physicians may file a single report directly to the insurer or self-insured employer within a specified number of days from initial treatment. The insurer or self-insured employer, in turn, is required to send a report to the state agency. This reduces paperwork and postage. Table 14–1 provides the time limit in each state during which the physician must submit the initial report.

1. Enter the insurance carrier's complete name, street address, city, state, and ZIP code.
2. Enter the employer's full name and policy number if known. Some insurance carriers file by employer and then by policy number. Sometimes

BONES OF THE HAND AND FOOT

Figure 14–8. Terminology pertinent to the, **A,** hand and, **B,** foot, indicating the common medical terms seen in reports on injury cases. (**A,** Redrawn from Marble HC: *The Hand: A Manual and Atlas for the General Surgeon.* Philadelphia, Saunders, 1960. **B,** Redrawn from Chabner DE: *The Language of Medicine,* 6th ed. Philadelphia, Saunders, 1999.)

the employer's telephone number is necessary on this line.

3. Enter the employer's street address, city, state, and ZIP code.

4. Enter the type of business (e.g., repairing shoes, building construction, and retailing men's clothes).

5. Enter the patient's complete first name, middle initial, and last name.

6. Enter a check mark in the appropriate box to indicate the patient's gender.

7. Enter the patient's birth date and list the year as four digits.

8. Enter the patient's street address, city, state, and ZIP code.

9. Enter the patient's home telephone number.

10. Enter the patient's specific job title. Be accurate in listing the occupation with the job title so that

Fracture	Definition		Fracture	Definition	
Closed or simple	Broken bone is contained within intact skin.		Pathologic	Results from weakening of bone by disease	
Open or compound	Skin is broken above the fracture, which is thus open to the external environment, resulting in potential for infection.		Nondisplaced	Bone ends remain in alignment	
Longitudinal	Fracture extends along the length of the bone.		Displaced	Bone ends are out of alignment	
Transverse	Produced by direct force applied perpendicularly to a bone		Spiral	Have long, sharp, pointed bone ends; produced by twisting or rotary forces	
Oblique	Produced by a twisting force with an upward thrust; fracture ends are short and run at an oblique angle across the bone		Compression	Produced by transmitted forces that drive bones together	
Greenstick	Produced by compression or angulation forces in long bones of children younger than 10. Bone is cracked on one side and intact on the other due to softness.		Avulsion	Produced by forceful contraction of a muscle against resistance, with a bone fragment tearing at the site of muscle insertion	
Comminuted	Has multiple fragments and is produced by severe direct violence		Depression	Bone fragments of the skull are driven inward	
Impacted	Produced by strong forces that drive bone fragments firmly together				

Figure 14–9. Terminology and illustration of different types of fractures. (From Chester GA: *Modern Medical Assisting.* Philadelphia, Saunders, 1998.)

TABLE 14–4	Body Activity Terms

Body activity terms are used when the physician describes activities the patient is capable of performing and restrictions when a patient returns to work before full recovery.

Balancing	Maintaining body equilibrium to prevent falling when walking, standing, crouching, or running on narrow, slippery, or erratically moving surfaces, or maintaining body equilibrium when performing gymnastic feats.
Bending	Angulation from neutral-straight position about joint (e.g., elbow) or spine (e.g., forward or lateral spine flexion).
Carrying	Transporting an object usually holding it in the hands or arms or on the shoulder.
Climbing	Ascending or descending ladders, stairs, scaffolding, ramps, and poles using feet and legs or hands or arms. For climbing, the emphasis is placed on body agility; for balancing, it is placed on body equilibrium.
Crawling	Moving about on hands and knees or hands and feet.
Crouching	Bending body downward and forward by bending legs and spine.
Feeling	Perceiving attributes of objects such as size, shape, temperature, or texture by means of receptors in skin like those of fingertips.
Fingering	Picking, pinching, or working with fingers primarily.
Handling	Seizing, holding, grasping, turning with hands, fingering not involved.
Kneeling	Bending legs at knees to come to rest on knees.
Lifting	Raising or lowering an object from one level to another.
Pulling	Exerting force on an object so the object moves toward the force (includes jerking).
Pushing	Exerting force on an object so the object moves away from the force (includes slapping, striking, kicking, and treadle action).
Reaching	Extending the arm(s) in any direction.
Sitting	Remaining in the normal seated position.
Standing	Remaining on one's feet in the upright position at a work station without moving about.
Stooping	Bending body downward and forward by bending spine and waist.

BOX 14–2	

Terms That Describe Intensity of Occurrence of Symptoms

Definitions that describe intensity of pain and frequency of symptoms were developed to assist the physician when documenting subjective complaints.

A **severe** pain precludes the activity causing the pain.

A **moderate** pain can be tolerated but causes marked handicap in the performance of the activity precipitating the pain.

A **slight** pain can be tolerated but causes some handicap in the performance of the activity precipitating the pain.

A **minimal** (mild) pain constitutes an annoyance but causes no handicap in the performance of the particular activity. It is considered a nonratable permanent disability.

Occasional means approximately 25% of the time.

Intermittent means approximately 50% of the time.

Frequent means approximately 75% of the time.

Constant means 90% to 100% of the time.

the insurance carrier may be certain the patient was doing the job for which he or she was insured.

11. Enter the patient's Social Security number. Some insurance carriers use the Social Security number as the industrial case number.

12. Enter the exact location where the patient was injured. Many times the injury may occur off the premises of the company or factory, depending on the type of job on which the employee was working. List the county where the patient was injured.

13. Enter the date the patient was injured and time of the injury. List the year as four digits.

14. Enter the date the patient last worked. This date should coincide with the date the patient reported to work and worked any portion of his or her shift (work day). This may be the same date of injury. This item is important because it informs the insurance carrier of the working status of the patient or whether the patient has been disabled and cannot return to work. List the year as four digits.

15. Enter the date and hour of the physician's first examination. The insurance carrier should know how soon after the accident the patient sought medical attention. List the year as four digits.

16. Enter a check mark in the appropriate box indicating whether the physician or an associate treated the patient previously.

17. Have the patient complete this section if possible in his or her own words, stating how the illness or injury occurred. The physician also may dictate this information after obtaining it from the patient.

18. Enter the answers to these questions about the patient's complaints and medical findings, which

State of California	Please complete in triplicate (type, if possible). Mail two copies to:		OSHA Case No.
EMPLOYER'S REPORT OF OCCUPATIONAL INJURY OR ILLNESS	**XYZ Insurance Company** PO Box 5 Woodland Hills, XY 12345		**# 18** ☐ Fatality

Any person who makes or causes to be made any knowingly false or fraudulent material statement or material representation for the purpose of obtaining or denying workers' compensation benefits or payments is guilty of a felony.

NOTICE: California law requires employers to report within **five days** of knowledge every occupational injury or illness which results in lost time beyond the date of the incident **OR** requires medical treatment beyond first aid. If an employee subsequently dies as a result of a previously reported injury or illness, the employer must file within **five days** of knowledge an amended report indicating death. In addition, every serious injury/illness, or death must be reported **immediately** by telephone or telegraph to the nearest office of the California Division of Occupational Safety and Health.

EMPLOYER

1. FIRM NAME *The Conk Out Company*	1A. POLICY NUMBER *B12345*	DO NOT USE THIS COLUMN
2. MAILING ADDRESS (Number and Street, City, ZIP) *45 South Gorman St. Woodland Hills, XY 12345*	2A. PHONE NUMBER *555-430-3488*	Case No.
3. LOCATION, IF DIFFERENT FROM MAILING ADDRESS (Number and Street, City, ZIP)	3A. LOCATION CODE	Ownership
4. NATURE OF BUSINESS, e.g., painting contractor, wholesale grocer, sawmill, hotel, etc. *Plumbing Repair*	5. STATE UNEMPLOYMENT INSURANCE ACCT. NO.	Industry
6. TYPE OF EMPLOYER [X] PRIVATE ☐ STATE ☐ CITY ☐ COUNTY ☐ SCHOOL DIST. ☐ OTHER GOVERNMENT - SPECIFY ___		Occupation

EMPLOYEE

7. EMPLOYEE NAME *Ima B. Hurt*	8. SOCIAL SECURITY NUMBER *120-XX-6542*	9. DATE OF BIRTH (mm/dd/yy) *3-4-66*	Sex
10. HOME ADDRESS (Number and Street, City, ZIP) *300 E.Central Ave. Woodland Hills, XY 12345*		10A. PHONE NUMBER *555-476-9899*	Age
11. SEX ☐ MALE [X] FEMALE	12. OCCUPATION (Regular job title — NO initials, abbreviations or numbers) *Clerk Typist*	13. DATE OF HIRE (mm/dd/yy) *1-20-86*	Daily Hours
14. EMPLOYEE USUALLY WORKS *8* hours per day *5* days per week *40* total weekly hours	14A. EMPLOYMENT STATUS (check applicable status at time of injury) [X] regular full-time ___ part-time ___ temporary ___ seasonal	14B. Under what class code of your policy were wages assigned? *7219*	Days per week
15. GROSS WAGES/SALARY $ *700.00* per *week*	16. OTHER PAYMENTS NOT REPORTED AS WAGES/SALARY (e.g. tips, meals, lodging, overtime, bonuses, etc.)? ☐ YES $ ___ [X] NO		Weekly hours

INJURY OR ILLNESS

17. DATE OF INJURY OR ONSET OF ILLNESS (mm/dd/yy) *4-3-XX*	18. TIME INJURY/ILLNESS OCCURRED ___ A.M. *2:00* P.M.	19. TIME EMPLOYEE BEGAN WORK *8:00* A.M. ___ P.M.	20. IF EMPLOYEE DIED, DATE OF DEATH (mm/dd/yy)	Weekly wage
21. UNABLE TO WORK AT LEAST ONE FULL DAY AFTER DATE OF INJURY? [X] YES ☐ NO	22. DATE LAST WORKED (mm/dd/yy) *4-3-XX*	23. DATE RETURNED TO WORK (mm/dd/yy)	24. IF STILL OFF WORK, CHECK THIS BOX [X]	County
25. PAID FULL WAGES FOR DAY OF INJURY OR LAST DAY WORKED? [X] YES ☐ NO	26. SALARY BEING CONTINUED? ☐ YES [X] NO	27. DATE OF EMPLOYER'S KNOWLEDGE/NOTICE OF INJURY/ILLNESS (mm/dd/yy) *4-3-XX*	28. DATE EMPLOYEE WAS PROVIDED *4-3-XX*	Nature of injury

29. SPECIFIC INJURY/ILLNESS AND PART OF BODY AFFECTED, MEDICAL DIAGNOSIS, if available, e.g., second degree burns on right arm, tendonitis of left elbow, lead poisoning.
ankle injury swelling, possible fracture — Part of body

30. LOCATION WHERE EVENT OR EXPOSURE OCCURRED (Number, Street, City) *45 South Gorman St. Woodland Hills, XY 12345*	30B. ON EMPLOYERS PREMISES? [X] YES ☐ NO	Source
31. DEPARTMENT WHERE EVENT OR EXPOSURE OCCURRED, e.g., shipping department, machine shop. *stock room*	32. OTHER WORKERS INJURED/ILL IN THIS EVENT? ☐ YES [X] NO	Event

33. EQUIPMENT, MATERIALS AND CHEMICALS THE EMPLOYEE WAS USING WHEN EVENT OR EXPOSURE OCCURRED, e.g., acetylene, welding torch, farm tractor, scaffold.
6 foot ladder — Sec. Source

34. SPECIFY ACTIVITY THE EMPLOYEE WAS PERFORMING WHEN EVENT OR EXPOSURE OCCURRED, e.g., welding seams of metal forms, loading boxes onto truck.
climbed ladder to remove a ream of paper from shelf; fell — Extent of injury

35. HOW INJURY/ILLNESS OCCURRED. DESCRIBE SEQUENCE OF EVENTS. SPECIFY OBJECT OR EXPOSURE WHICH DIRECTLY PRODUCED THE INJURY/ILLNESS, e.g., worker stepped back to inspect work and slipped on scrap material. As he fell, he brushed against fresh weld, and burned right hand. USE SEPARATE SHEET IF NECESSARY.
worker climbed ladder to remove a ream of paper from top shelf in stock room. She was descending and mis-stepped falling to the floor. She tried to land upright, and her left leg took the brunt of the fall.

36. NAME AND ADDRESS OF PHYSICIAN (Number and Street, City, ZIP) *Raymond Skeleton, MD 4567 Broad Ave., Woodland Hills, XY 12345*	36A. PHONE NUMBER *555-486-9002*
37. IF HOSPITALIZED AS AN INPATIENT, NAME AND ADDRESS OF HOSPITAL (Number and Street, City, ZIP)	37A. PHONE NUMBER

Completed by (type or print) J.D. Hawkins	Signature *J. D. Hawkins*	Title *owner*	Date *4-3-XX*

FILING THIS REPORT IS NOT AN ADMISSION OF LIABILITY

Figure 14–10. Employer's Report of Occupational Injury or Illness. This form complies with OSHA requirements as well as California State Workers' Compensation laws.

may be found in the patient's medical record. List all of the patient's subjective complaints.

19. *A.* Enter all objective findings from physical examination. *B.* Enter all x-ray and laboratory results; or if none, state "none" or "pending."

20. Enter a check mark in "yes" or "no" to indicate if chemical or toxic compounds are involved. Enter the diagnosis and diagnostic code number. Specify etiologic agent and duration of exposure if occupational illness.

**WORKERS' COMPENSATION
MEDICAL SERVICE ORDER**

To:　Dr./Clinic _____ Martin Feelgood, MD _____

Address　_____ 4567 Broad Avenue, Woodland Hills, XY 12345 _____

We are sending_____ Mrs. Ima Hurt _____

Address　_____ 300 East Central Ave. Woodland Hills, XY 12345 _____

Social Security No. ___ 120-XX-6542 ___ Date of birth 3-4-1966 ___
to you for treatment in accordance with the terms of the Workers'
Compensation Laws.　Please submit your report to the
_____ XYZ Insurance Company _____
at once.　Compensation cannot be paid without complete medical
information.

Insurance carrier___ XYZ Insurance Company _____

Address _P.O. Box 5, Woodland Hills, XY 12345_ Telephone _555-271-0562_

Employer　_____ The Conk Out Company _____

Address _45 S. Gorman St. Woodland Hills, XY 12345_ Telephone _555-430-3488_

Signature_____ *J.A. HAWKINS* _____Date___ 4-3-20XX ___
If patient is able to return to work today or tomorrow, please
show date and time below — sign and give to patient to return to
employer.　If there are any work restrictions indicate on the back
of this form.　Please submit your usual first report in any case.

Date/Time_____ By_____

Figure 14–11. Medical Service Order.

21. Enter a check mark in "yes" or "no" to indicate if the findings and diagnosis are consistent with the history of injury or onset of illness. Insert an explanation if "yes."

22. Enter a check mark in "yes" or "no" to indicate if there is any other current condition that will impede or delay the patient's recovery. Insert an explanation if "yes."

23. Enter a full description of what treatment was rendered.

24. Enter an explanation if further treatment is necessary and, if so, specify the treatment plan. Indicate if physical therapy is necessary and its frequency and duration.

25. Enter the name and location of the hospital, admission date, and estimated stay if the patient is to be hospitalized.

26. Enter a check mark in "yes" or "no" to indicate whether the patient is able to work as usual. If the answer is "no," give the date when it is estimated that the patient will be able to return to regular or modified work. List the year as four digits. Specify any work restrictions. It is very important for the insurance company to anticipate how long the patient will be off work so that money may be set aside for temporary disability benefits, medical benefits, and, if necessary, permanent disability benefits. If the estimated date of return to work should change after the form is submitted, a supplemental report or progress note should be sent to the insurance carrier to change the date of the disability.

Bottom of Form: If not preprinted, enter the physician's name and degree (e.g., MD, DC), complete

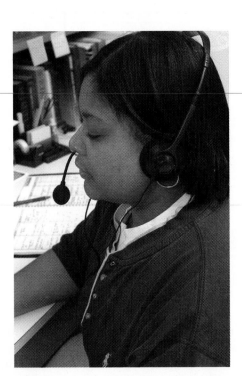

Figure 14–12. Receptionist receiving a medical service order via telephone for the worker to receive medical services.

NEBRASKA WORKERS' COMPENSATION COURT
First Treatment Medical Report
(Must be filed with Compensation Court & Employer within 7 days of first treatment)
(Shaded sections are not required)

TYPE OR PRINT

PATIENT & INSURED (SUBSCRIBER) INFORMATION

1. PATIENT'S NAME (First, name, middle initial, last name)	2. PATIENT'S DATE OF BIRTH	3. INSURED'S NAME (Employer)
Lester M. Task	05 | 06 | 60	Jonas Construction Company

4. PATIENT'S ADDRESS (Street, City, State, ZIP Code)	5. PATIENT'S SEX	6. INSURED'S I.D. NO. (Include any letters)
5400 Holly Street Woodland Hills, XY 12345	[X] MALE [ ] FEMALE	B 785700

	7. PATIENT'S RELATIONSHIP TO INSURED	8. INSURED'S GROUP NO. (Or Group Name)
	[ ] SELF [ ] SPOUSE [ ] CHILD [X] OTHER	5601

9. OTHER HEALTH INSURANCE COVERAGE - Enter Name of Policyholder and Plan Name and Address and Policy or Medical Assistance Number	10. WAS CONDITION RELATED TO: A. PATIENT'S EMPLOYMENT [X] YES [ ] NO B. AN AUTO ACCIDENT [ ] YES [ ] NO	11. INSURED'S ADDRESS (Street, City State, ZIP Code) 300 Main Street Woodland Hills, XY 12345

12. PATIENT'S OR AUTHORIZED PERSON'S SIGNATURE I Authorize the Release of any Medical Information Necessary to Process this Claim SIGNED	12A. PATIENT'S SOCIAL SECURITY NO 578 | XX | 1921 DATE 11-8-XX	13. I AUTHORIZE PAYMENT OF MEDICAL BENEFITS TO UNDERSIGNED PHYSICIAN OR SUPPLIER FOR SERVICE DESCRIBED BELOW SIGNED (Insured or Authorized Person)

PHYSICIAN OR SUPPLIER INFORMATION

14. DATE OF: 11-8-XX ILLNESS (FIRST SYMPTOM OR INJURY (ACCIDENT)	15. DATE FIRST CONSULTED YOU FOR THIS CONDITION 11-8-XX	16. HAS PATIENT EVER HAD SAME OR SIMILAR SYMPTOMS? [ ] YES [X] NO

17. DATE PATIENT ABLE TO RETURN TO WORK	18. DATES OF TOTAL DISABILITY FROM 11-8-XX THROUGH 12-8-XX	DATES OF PARTIAL DISABILITY FROM THROUGH

19. NAME OF REFERRING PHYSICIAN	20. FOR SERVICES RELATED TO HOSPITALIZATION GIVE HOSPITALIZATION DATES ADMITTED 11-8-XX DISCHARGED 11-10-XX

21. NAME & ADDRESS OF FACILITY WHERE SERVICES RENDERED (If other than home or office) Community Hospital, 400 Oak St., Woodland Hills, XY 12345	22. WAS LABORATORY WORK PERFORMED OUTSIDE YOUR OFFICE? [ ] YES [X] NO CHARGES:

23. DIAGNOSIS OR NATURE OF ILLNESS OR INJURY, RELATE DIAGNOSIS TO PROCEDURE IN COLUMN D BY REFERENCE TO NUMBERS 1,2,3, ETC. OR DX CODE

1. fracture of right patella   822.1 ▼
2.
3.
4.

24. A DATE OF SERVICE	B* PLACE OF SERVICE	C FULLY DESCRIBE PROCEDURES, MEDICAL SERVICE OR SUPPLIES FURNISHED FOR EACH DATE GIVEN PROCEDURE CODE (IDENTIFY:) (EXPLAIN UNUSUAL SERVICES OR CIRCUMSTANCES)	D DIAGNOSIS CODE	E CHARGES	F
11-8-XX	1	99222 Initial hospital care	1	125 00	
11-8-XX	1	27524 Open TX patellar fracture with internal fixation	1	600 00	

24A. HISTORY. GIVE BRIEF DESCRIPTION OF WHAT OCCURRED. PATIENT'S ACCOUNT OF ACCIDENT.

Patient was up on a scaffold at a construction site and fell off of it about

8 feet hitting the ground with his right knee.

25. SIGNATURE OF PHYSICIAN OR SUPPLIER SIGNED *Gregory T. Getwell, MD* DATE 11-8-XX	26. ACCEPT ASSIGNMENT (GOVERNMENT CLAIMS ONLY) [ ] YES [ ] NO PHYSICIAN'S SOCIAL SECURITY NO.	27. TOTAL CHARGE 725.00	28. AMOUNT PAID	29. BALANCE DUE 725 | 00
32. YOUR PATIENT'S ACCOUNT NO.	33. YOUR EMPLOYER I.D. NO. 95-32089XX	31. PHYSICIAN'S OR SUPPLIER'S NAME, ADDRESS, ZIP CODE & TELEPHONE NO Gregory T. Getwell, MD 60 North State Street Woodland Hills, XY 12345 I.D. NO. A123456 555-459-0087		

*PLACE OF SERVICE CODES

1—(IH) - INPATIENT HOSPITAL	4—(H) PATIENT'S HOME	7—(NH) NURSING HOME	O—(OL) OTHER LOCATIONS
2—(OH) - OUTPATIENT HOSPITAL	5— DAY CARE FACILITY (PSY)	8—(SNF) SKILLED NURSING FACILITY	A—(IL) INDEPENDENT LABORATORY
3—(O) - DOCTOR'S OFFICE	6— NIGHT CARE FACILITY(PSY)	9— AMBULANCE	B— OTHER MEDICAL/SURGICAL FACILITY

NWCC FORM 45 (Rev. 86)

reference initials

Figure 14–13. First Treatment Medical Report form used in Nebraska. This form follows the format of the Health Insurance Claim Form CMS-1500 developed by the American Medical Association Council on Medical Service (see Chapter 6).

STATE OF CALIFORNIA	**DOCTOR'S FIRST REPORT OF OCCUPATIONAL INJURY OR ILLNESS**

Within 5 days of your initial examination, for every occupational injury or illness, send two copies of this report to the **employer's workers' compensation insurance carrier** or the **self-insured employer.** Failure to file a timely doctor's report may result in assessment of a civil penalty. **In the case of diagnosed or suspected pesticide poisoning,** send a copy of this report to Division of Labor Statistics and Research, P.O. Box 420603, San Francisco, CA 94142-0603, and notify your local health officer by telephone within 24 hours.

	PLEASE DO NOT USE THIS COLUMN
1. **INSURER NAME AND ADDRESS** XYZ Insurance Company, P.O. Box 5, Woodland Hills, XY 12345	
2. **EMPLOYER NAME** The Conk Out Company Policy# B12345	Case No.
3. Address No. and Street City Zip 45 So. Gorman St. Woodland Hills, XY 12345	Industry
4. Nature of business (e.g., food manufacturing, building construction, retailer of women's clothes) plumbing repair	County
5. **PATIENT NAME** (first name, middle initial, last name) 6. Sex 7. Date of Mo. Day Yr. Ima B. Hurt ☐ Male ☒ Female birth 3-4-1966	Age
8. Address: No. and Street City Zip 9. Telephone number 300 East Central Ave., Woodland Hills, XY 12345 (555) 476-9899	Hazard
10. Occupation (Specific job title) 11. Social Security Number clerk typist 120-XX-6542	Disease
12. Injured at: No. and street City County 45 So. Gorman St., Woodland Hills, XY 12345 Humboldt	Hospitalization
13. Date and hour of injury Mo. Day Yr. Hour 14. Date last worked Mo. Day Yr. or onset of illness 4-3-20XX ____ a.m. 2:00 p.m. 4-3-20XX	Occupation
15. Date and hour of first Mo. Day Yr. Hour 16. Have you (or your office) previously examination or treatment 4-3-20XX ____ a.m. 4:00 p.m. treated patient? ☐ Yes ☒ NO	Return date/Code

Patient please complete this portion, if able to do so. Otherwise, doctor please complete immediately. Inability or failure of a patient to complete this portion shall not affect his/her rights to workers' compensation under the California Labor Code.

17. **DESCRIBE HOW THE ACCIDENT OR EXPOSURE HAPPENED** (Give specific object, machinery or chemical. Use reverse side if more space is required.)

I climbed a ladder in the stock room and while I was coming down I missed a step, lost my balance, and fell hurting my left ankle.

18. **SUBJECTIVE COMPLAINTS** (Describe fully. Use reverse side if more space is required.)

Pain in left ankle.

19. **OBJECTIVE FINDINGS** (Use reverse side if more space is required.)

A. Physical examination

Pain, swelling and discoloration of l. ankle

B. X-ray and laboratory results (state if none or pending.)   Ankle x-ray (left) 3 views

20. **DIAGNOSIS** (if occupational illness specify etiologic agent and duration of exposure.) Chemical or toxic compounds involved? ☐Yes   ☒ No

Trimalleolar ankle fracture (left)   ICD-9 Code ___ 824.6

21. Are your findings and diagnosis consistent with patient's account of injury or onset of illness?   ☒Yes   ☐ No if "no", please explain.

22. Is there any other current condition that will impede or delay the patient's recovery?   ☐Yes   ☒ No if "yes", please explain.

23. **TREATMENT RENDERED** (Use reverse side if more space is required.)

Examination, x-rays, closed treatment of trimalleolar ankle fracture (left) without manipulation. Return in one week for recheck.

24. If further treatment required, specify treatment plan/estimated duration.

25. If hospitalized as inpatient, give hospital name and location   Date admitted   Mo. Day Yr.   Estimated stay

26. WORK STATUS–Is patient able to perform usual work?   ☐Yes ☒ No
 If "no", date when patient can return to: Regular work _5_ / _17_ /20XX
 Modified work __ / __ /   Specify restrictions ___

Doctor's signature _Martin Feelgood, MD_   4-3-20XX   CA license number _A 12345_
 Doctor name and degree (please type) _Martin Feelgood, MD_   IRS number _95-36640XX_
 Address ___ 4567 Broad Avenue, Woodland Hills, XY 12345   Telephone number _(555) 486-9002_

FORM 5021 (REV. 4) 1992

Any person who makes or causes to be made any knowingly false or fraudulent material statement or material representation for the purpose of obtaining or denying workers' compensation benefits or payments is guilty of a felony.

reference initials

Figure 14–14. Doctor's First Report of Occupational Injury or Illness form, used in California.

TABLE 14–5	**Narrative Medical Report Issues, if Relevant**
History	Outline all specific details of accident, injury, or illness. Physician should state whether there is a causal connection between the accident and conditions that may appear subsequently but are not obvious **sequelae** (diseased conditions after, and usually resulting from, a previous disease). If facts were obtained by reviewing prior records or x-ray films, the source should be mentioned. When a history is obtained through an interpreter, include that person's name.
Present Complaints	Usually given as subjective complaints. *Subjective* refers to statements made by the patient about symptoms and how he or she feels. Subjective disability is evaluated by ▶ A description of the activity that produces the disability. ▶ The duration of the disability. ▶ The activities that are precluded by, and those that can be performed with, the disability. ▶ The means necessary for relief.
Past History	Describe any previous, current, subsequent medical information relevant to this injury or illness and state whether there is a preexisting defect that might entitle the injured person to benefits from the subsequent injury fund or represent the actual cause of the present condition.
Examination Findings	Usually given as *objective findings*. State all significant physical or psychiatric examination, testing, laboratory, or imaging findings.
Diagnostic Impression	State all diagnostic findings and opinion as to *relationship*, if any, between the injury or disease and the condition diagnosed. Use diagnostic terminology that corresponds to the diagnostic code book.
Disability/Prognosis	A. Period during which the patient has been unable to work because of the injury or illness. B. Opinion as to probable further temporary disability and a statement as to when the patient will be able to return to work or has returned to work. C. Statement indicating whether the condition is currently permanent and stationary, as well as the probability of future permanent disability. D. Statement indicating "All objective tests for organic pathology are negative. There is obviously a strong functional or emotional overlay," when a patient has multiple complaints but no clinical objective findings.
Work Limitations	Description of any limitations to all activities.
Causation	Description of how the permanent disability is related to the patient's occupation and the specific injury or cumulative events causing the illness.

address, state license number, federal tax identification number, and telephone number. Indicate the date the report is submitted. The insurance billing specialist should type reference initials in the lower left-hand corner of the form. This form *must be signed in ink* by the physician. Any carbon copies or photocopies also must be signed in ink. A stamped signature will *not* be accepted because sometimes these cases go into litigation or are presented for a permanent disability rating. Only those documents considered original medical records are acceptable; this means a handwritten signature by the attending physician is necessary.

Progress or Supplemental Report

In a TD case, a *supplemental report* is sent to the insurance carrier after 2 to 4 weeks of treatment to give information on the current status of the patient. If there is a significant change in the prognosis, a detailed progress report (sometimes called a *reexamination report*) is sent to the insurance carrier.

Subsequent progress or supplemental reports should be sent to the insurance carrier after each hospitalization and office visit to update the progress of a case. They may be narrative and are not necessarily completed on the special forms available in most states (Fig. 14–15). If the disability is ongoing over a period of time, monthly progress reports should be submitted. A follow-up report must contain the following information:

1. Date of most recent examination
2. Present condition and progress since last report
3. Measurements of function
4. X-ray or laboratory report since last examination
5. Treatment (give type and duration)
6. Work status (patient working or estimated date of return to work if patient is still temporarily disabled)
7. Permanent disability to be anticipated

The insurance carrier authorizing the examination should be furnished with the report in triplicate or quadruplicate, depending on its needs. A copy should be retained for the physician's files.

ATTENDING PHYSICIAN'S REPORT

Employee: Mrs. Ima B. Hurt   Claim number: 120 XX 6542

Employer: The Conk Out Company   Date of injury(ies): 4-3-20XX   Date of next exam: 4-24-20XX

Date of this exam: 4-10-XX   Patient Social Security No: 120 XX 6542

Current diagnosis: 824.6 closed fracture; L. trimalleolar ankle
(include ICD•9 code)

PATIENT STATUS

Since the last exam, this patient's condition has:

☒ improved as expected.   ☐ improved, but slower than expected.   ☐ not improved significantly.

☐ worsened.   ☐ plateaued, no further improvement is expected.   ☐ has been determined to be non-work related.

Briefly, describe any change in objective or subjective complaint:

TREATMENT

Treatment plan: (only list changes from prior status)   ☐ No change   ☐ Patient is/was discharged from care on

Est. discharge date: 5-18-20XX   Medications: Tylenol for pain

Therapy: Type   Times per week   Estimated date of completion

Diagnostic studies: X-ray, L. ankle 3 views

Hospitalization/surgery:

Consult/other service:

WORK STATUS

The patient has been instructed to:

☐ return to full duty with no limitations or restrictions.

☐ remain off the rest of the day and return to work tomorrow:

_____ with no limits or restrictions._____ with limits listed below.

☐ return to work on

work limitations:

☒ remain off work until 5-17-20XX — discharge exam scheduled

Estimated date patient can return full duty: 5-18-20XX

DISABILITY STATUS

☐ Patient discharged as cured.

Please supply a brief narrative report if any of the below apply:

☐ Patient will be permanently precluded from engaging in his/her usual and customary occupation.

☐ Patient's condition is permanent and stationary.

☐ Patient will have permanent residuals   ☐ Patient will require future medical care.

Physician name: Martin Feelgood, MD   Address: 4567 Broad Avenue, Woodland Hills, XY 12345

Date: April 10, 20XX   Telephone: (555) 482-9002

Signature: Martin Feelgood, MD

reference initials

Figure 14–15. Physician's Supplemental Report form.

Final Report

TD ends when the physician tells the insurance carrier that the patient is able to return to work. Sometimes a physician submits a final report at the time of discharge. When the patient resumes work, the insurance carrier closes the case, and the TD benefits cease.

A physician's final report indicating any impairment or permanent disability should be sent, accompanied by a statement listing total expenses incurred (Fig. 14–16).

XYZ INSURANCE COMPANY

DOCTOR'S FINAL (OR MONTHLY) REPORT AND BILL

Monthly itemized bills required on all cases under continuing treatment.
Services beginning late in month and extending into succeeding month may be itemized on one statement.

CASE No. __120 XX 6542__

EMPLOYEE _____Mrs. Ima B. Hurt_____
DATE OF INJURY _____April 3, 20XX_____
EMPLOYER _____The Conk Out Company_____

SERVICES FOR MONTH OF_____May_____ 20 _XX_

Patient refused treatment _____ 20 ____
Patient stopped treatment
    without orders _____ 20 ____
Patient entered hospital _____ 20 ____
Further treatment anticipated? ____X____
                 (Yes) _____ (No)
P.T L. Ankle 2 x wk 3 wks
Any other charges authorized such as Drugs? _____ Hospital? _____
                             (Check)   (Check)

Patient able to return to work _____May 18,_____ 20 _XX_
Patient discharged as cured _____ 20 ____
Condition at time of last visit ___fracture healed___

Code: O—Office: V—Home Visit: H—Hospital Visit: N—Night Visit: S—Operation: X—X-ray.

Month	1	2	3	4	5	6	7	8	9	10	11	12	13	14	15	16	17	18	19	20	21	22	23	24	25	26	27	28	29	30	31
May							O										O														

		RVS CODE		TOTALS
First aid treatment *(describe)* _____	# _____		$ _____
Office Visits ___5/7/XX and 5/17/XX___	# ___99213___		$	40.20
Home Visits _____	# ___99213___		$	40.20
Hospital Visits _____	# _____		$ _____
Operations _____	# _____		$ _____
MATERIAL *(Itemize at cost)* ___Left ankle films; complete 5/7/xx___	# ___73610___		$	34.26
5/17/xx	# ___73610___		$	34.26
	# _____		$ _____

Any charges shown above which are in excess of the scheduled fee must
be explained regarding nature of such services, indicating the date rendered.   TOTAL $ ___148.92___

Make check payable to:

Doctor _____Martin Feelgood, MD_____

Address _____4567 Broad Avenue_____
                        (Street)
_____Woodland Hills, XY 12345_____
      (City)   (Zip)

Internal Revenue Code Section 6109
requires you to furnish your Internal
Revenue Service Employer Identification
Number or Social Security Number.
Please enter the Identification Number
here ___95-36640XX___

Signature   *Martin Feelgood, MD*

Date _____May 18, 20XX_____

LEAVE BLANK	
APPROVED	
BY _____	
(Dollars) (Cents)	DATE _____

IMPORTANT—
Bills Must Be Submitted in Duplicate
MAIL ADDRESS: P.O. BOX S, WOODLAND HILLS, XY 12345

SCIF FORM 60 REV 5 78

Figure 14–16. Doctor's Final (or Monthly) Report and Bill form.

Claim Submission

Financial Responsibility

As discussed in Chapter 2, the contract for treatment in a personal illness or injury case is between the physician and patient, who is responsible for the entire bill. However, when a business is self-insured, a person is under a state program for care, or an individual is being treated as a workers' compensation case, the financial responsibility exists between the physician and insurance company or state program. As long as treatment is authorized by the insurance carrier, the insurance company is responsible for payment. A physician who agrees to treat a workers' compensation case must agree to accept payment in full according to the workers' compensation fee schedule. A copayment amount cannot be collected or the balance billed to the patient for any amount not covered.

If an injured worker refuses to accept the physician retained by the insurance company for the employer, the patient may be responsible for the cost of medical treatment. The employee should first contact the employer, then the insurance company, to find out if there are any provisions for a change of physicians.

Some states have a medical program where employers can reduce their workers' compensation rates by paying the first $1000 in medical bills. This is similar to a deductible for the employer's policy. The statement should be sent to the employer for payment in this situation.

Health insurance information should always be obtained in case services are provided that are not work related or should be billed for, or the injury or illness is declared nonindustrial. To assist in informing patients of financial responsibility for nonrelated illness, the worker should sign an agreement for nonrelated medical expenses, as shown in Figure 14–17.

Sometimes a physician discovers a problem unrelated to the industrial injury or illness (e.g., high blood pressure) while examining an injured worker. The physician may bill the workers' compensation carrier for the examination but should code the claim carefully with regard to treatment of the injury. If

Figure 14–17. Patient agreement to pay the physician's fees if the case is declared not work related or an illness is discovered and treated that is not work related.

PATIENT AGREEMENT

Patient's Name ___James Doland___ Soc. Sec. # _431-XX-1942_

Address_ 67 Blyth Dr., Woodland Hills, XY 12345 ___Tel. No. _555-372-0101_

WC Insurance Carrier ___Industrial Indemnity Company___

Address___ 30 North Dr., Woodland Hills ___ Telephone No. _555-731-7707_

Date of illness _2-13-20XX_ ___Date of first visit_ _2-13-20XX_

Emergency Yes __X__ No_____

Is this condition related to employment Yes _X_ No_____

If accident: Auto_____Other_____

Where did injury occur?___ Construction site ___

How did injury happen?___ fell 8 ft from scaffold suffering fractured right tibia ___

Employee/employer who verified this information ___Scott McPherson___

Employer's name and address___ Willow Construction Company ___

Employer's telephone No._ 555-526-0611 ___

In the event the claim for worker's compensation is declared fraudulent for this illness or condition or it is determined by the Workers' Compensation Board that the illness or injury is not a compensable workers' compensation case, I _James Doland_ , hereby agree to pay the physician's fee for services rendered.

I have been informed that I am responsible to pay any services rendered by Dr. _Raymond Skeleton_ with regard to the discovery and treatment of any condition not related to the workers' compensation injury or illness. I agree to pay for all services not covered by workers' compensation and all charges for treatment and personal items unrelated to my workers' compensation illness or injury.

Signed ___*James Doland*___ Date _2-13-20XX_

treatment is initiated for the patient's high blood pressure, that portion of the examination becomes the financial obligation of the patient and not the workers' compensation carrier.

Fee Schedules

Some states have developed and adopted a workers' compensation **fee schedule,** whereas other states pay medical claims based on the Medicare fee schedule plus a certain percentage. Fee schedules assist with the following:

1. They limit the fees providers can charge for standard medical procedures paid by workers' compensation companies.
2. They limit the amount that providers will be paid.
3. They make the allowable charges and procedures more consistent.
4. They provide follow-up procedures in case of a fee dispute.

Some workers' compensation fee schedules list maximum reimbursement levels for physicians and other nonhospital providers. However, the physician generally is expected to accept payment by the insurance company as payment in full when reimbursement is based on a fee schedule. If the fee charged is more than the amount listed, the following factors may be considered:

▶ Provider's medical training, qualifications, and time in practice
▶ Nature of services provided
▶ Fees usually charged by the provider
▶ Fees usually charged by others in the region where services were given
▶ Other relevant economic factors of the provider's practice
▶ Any unusual circumstances in the case

The insurance carrier may pay the additional amount if documentation is sent validating the fee and noting the aforementioned facts.

Types of Fee Schedules

Types of fee schedules include the following:

▶ *Percentile of charge schedule,* which is designed to set fees at a percentile of the providers' usual and customary fee.
▶ *Relative value scale schedule,* which takes into account the time, skills, and extent of the service provided by the physician. Each procedure is rated on how difficult it is, how long it takes, the training a physician must have to perform it, and expenses the physician incurs, including the cost of malpractice insurance. Many of the fee schedules are similar to the CPT format in regard to sections (e.g., Evaluation and Management; Anesthesia; Surgery; Radiology, Nuclear Medicine, and

Diagnostic Ultrasound; Pathology and Laboratory; and Medicine).

A *conversion factor* that uses a specific dollar amount is used for each of the sections of the fee schedule. Conversion factors may be adjusted to reflect regional differences and in some states are recalculated on an annual basis.

1999 Conversion Factors for Workers' Compensation in California

$8.50/unit	Evaluation and Management section
$34.50/unit	Anesthesia section
$153.00/unit	Surgery section
$12.50/unit	Radiology section (total unit value column)
$1.95/unit	Radiology section (professional component)
$1.50/unit	Radiology section (technical component)
$1.50/unit	Pathology section (technical component)
$6.15/unit	Medicine section

Actual covered procedures, descriptions, modifiers, global periods, and other elements of a fee guideline may significantly differ from those used for other plans or programs. Sometimes a schedule includes modifiers and code numbers not listed in the CPT code book. The workers' compensation codes should be used regardless of what is done for other insurance plans.

Reviews or audits may be performed by the following entities to enforce fee schedules:

▶ The state agency or state fund responsible for overseeing workers' compensation (bill review)
▶ The payer, employer, or insurance carrier (bill review)
▶ The payer (bill review) and state agency (compliance audit)

Helpful Billing Tips

The following are helpful hints for billing workers' compensation claims.

1. Ask whether the injury occurred within the scope of employment and verify insurance information with the benefits coordinator at the employer. This will promote filing initial claims with the correct insurance carrier.
2. Either ask the employer the name of the claims adjuster or request that the patient obtain the claim number of his or her case when he or she comes in for the initial visit.

3. Ask the workers' compensation carrier who is going to review the claim. Sometimes there are independent third-party billing vendors that work for the insurance carriers. Get the name and contact information.

4. Educate the patient with regard to the medical practice's billing policies for workers' compensation cases by having him or her complete the patient agreement form shown in Figure 14–17.

5. Verify if prior authorization is necessary before a surgical procedure is performed.

6. Document in a telephone log or patient's record all data for authorization of examination, diagnostic studies, or surgery (e.g., date, name of individual who authorizes, and response).

7. Obtain the workers' compensation fee schedule for the relevant state.

8. Use appropriate five-digit code numbers and modifiers to ensure prompt and accurate payment for services rendered.

9. Complete the Doctor's First Report of Occupational Injury or Illness form for the relevant state and submit it within the time limit shown in Table 14–1. Some states (e.g., California) allow a late fee if payment is not received within 30 to 45 days.

10. Ask if there is a state-specific insurance form or if the CMS-1500 form is acceptable.

11. Ask what year CPT and ICD-9-CM code books the insurance carrier uses. Some carriers use 2002 or earlier books, which means they do not reflect the deletion or addition of some procedure and diagnostic codes.

12. Submit a monthly itemized statement or bill on the termination of treatment for nondisability claims.

13. Clearly define any charges in excess of the fee schedule. Attach any x-ray reports, operative reports, discharge summaries, pathology reports, and so forth to clarify such excess charges or when **by report (BR)** is shown for a code selected from the workers' compensation procedure code book.

14. Itemize in detail and send invoices for drugs and dressings furnished by the physician. Bill medical supplies on a separate claim or statement and do not bill with services because this may be routed to a different claims processing department.

15. Call the insurance carrier and talk with the **claims examiner** who is familiar with the patient's case, if there is a question about the fee.

16. Search the Internet for a Web site or write to the workers' compensation state plan office in each state for booklets, bulletins, forms, and legislation information. See Appendix A for the workers' compensation address in each state.

17. Find out if the insurance carrier uses "usual and customary" payments tied to the physician's ZIP code. Most carriers use fee schedules.

18. Follow up and track the date the claim was filed. If no payment has been received or payment has been received beyond the 30 to 45 day deadline, see if it meets eligibility requirements for interest.

Billing Claims

For efficiency in processing industrial claims, many insurance carriers have developed their own forms for workers' compensation cases, whereas others allow use of the CMS-1500 claim form. Some carriers have made slight modifications to the CMS-1500 claim form as depicted in Figure 14–13.

Figure 6–15 is an illustration of a completed workers' compensation case on a nonmodified CMS-1500 claim form.

Electronic Claims Submission and Reports

Uniform data processing codes and universal electronic injury report forms have been developed by the American National Standards Institute (ANSI) and the International Association of Industrial Accident Boards and Commissions (IAIABC). ANSI is a national organization founded in 1918 to coordinate the development of voluntary business standards in the United States. Texas is one of the first states to establish an insurance regulation requiring workers' compensation carriers to use universal electronic transmission for first report of injury forms and subsequent reports developed by IAIABC.

Electronic Data Systems, Inc. (EDS) in Dallas, Texas, and Insurance Value-Added Network Services (IVANS) in Greenwich, CT, introduced the nation's first coast-to-coast electronic claims processing and report-filing network, called Workers' Compensation Reporting Service. EDS processes all claims and follow-up reports. IVANS provides the network service and marketing of software to employers. This system is operational in many states.

Some workers' compensation insurance companies are using telephone reporting of claims. Employers report injuries occurring on the job by calling a toll-free number. Calls go to a regional center where service representatives document the first report of injury and electronically transmit it to the local claim office handling workers' compensation insurance. Employers avoid tardiness of reporting when using this system. Employers neglecting prompt report of injuries could delay payments to physicians.

Because workers' compensation is operated under state laws, each state is required to report financial data, statistics on injuries and illnesses, and other information to state insurance regulators. In the states that use telephone reporting service, workers' compensation payers use the system to reduce the paper processing costs that have escalated out of proportion and to improve administrative efficiency.

Out-of-State Claims

When billing for an out-of-state claim, insurance billing specialists must follow all workers' compensation regulations from the jurisdiction (state) in which the injured was hired and not the state where the injury occurred.

Companies that have employees who travel to other states are required to obtain workers' compensation insurance in those states. Sometimes a patient may seek care from a physician in an adjacent state because he or she feels the physician provides a higher quality of care or the patient needs a specialized type of surgery, expensive diagnostic tests, or treatment. Referral requirements should be met before the patient is seen (e.g., letter of referral or preauthorization from the managing doctor with a copy to the workers' compensation carrier). Nine states hold the injured employee responsible for unauthorized care (Alabama, Alaska, Arkansas, New Jersey, North Dakota, Ohio, Washington, West Virginia, and Wisconsin). When a patient crosses a state line for treatment, he or she may be liable for some balance billing, and the patient should be informed of this fact. The date the employer subcontracts with another company to have to work performed must be researched. Many times the injured employee states that he or she works for ABC Company. The claim is denied because the employee is actually working for XYZ Company, which has subcontracted with ABC Company. This also happens with hospitals. One may think a hospital employee is being treated when an employee working for a company hired by the hospital actually is being treated. In these cases, extra time is spent identifying the subcontractor, and it may be discovered that the subcontractor does not have workers' compensation insurance and expected the hiring company to provide the coverage. In another scenario, a cruise ship employee injured at sea does not fall under state workers' compensation laws and is not required to have insurance in the state. Many cruise ships have maritime companies that settle these types of claims. Normally the claim should be paid in full, but many of these companies try to negotiate a much lower rate. This rate can be accepted in lieu of futile attempts to collect from the patient.

When the claim is billed, the out-of-state fee schedule should be obtained to determine the proper procedure codes, modifiers, and amounts. It should be determined whether the claimant's jurisdiction accepts electronic submission of the CMS-1500 claim form or another form and whether other documents (e.g., the operative report) are required to be submitted with the bill.

Delinquent or Slow Pay Claims

If payment of a workers' compensation claim is slow or the claim becomes delinquent, the insurance billing specialist should use an organized standard follow-up procedure:

1. Telephone the patient's employer. Note the name of the person talked to, name, address, and telephone number of the workers' compensation carrier, and the claim number. Verify the employer's address.
2. Send a copy of the claim form and an itemized copy of the financial account statement to the carrier. Send a letter and include details of the accident if necessary (Fig. 14–18). For problem claims it may be wise to obtain and complete a *Certificate of Mailing* form from the U.S. Postal Service. The form is initialed and postmarked at the post office and returned to the insurance biller for the office file. Because the post office does not keep a record

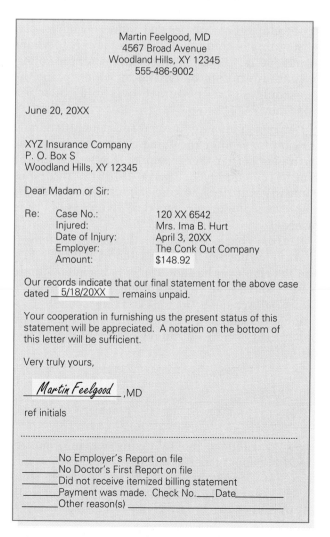

Figure 14–18. Letter sent to the insurance carrier when a workers' compensation claim becomes 45 days delinquent.

of the mailing, this certificate costs less than certified mail. It shows proof that a special communication was mailed or sent on a certain date if a deadline is in question.

3. Telephone the insurance carrier after 45 working days and request the expected date of payment.
4. Be reminded of that payment date by using a computer automated reminder or a note on the desk calendar. If payment is not received on or before that day, call the carrier again and ask for payment on a day determined by the facility's expectations.
5. Telephone the patient's employer and explain that there is difficulty with the carrier. Ask the employer to contact the carrier and have the carrier send payment immediately.
6. Send the employer a copy of the financial account statement showing the outstanding balance. If the carrier is not paying, ask the employer for payment. An employer's legal obligation to pay may vary from case to case.
7. Contact the patient only if given information by the carrier or employer that the injury is not work related.
8. Develop office policies that address when an outstanding account should be reviewed (perhaps after 90 or 120 days), whether to continue collection efforts internally, and at which point the account should be turned over to a collection agency.

It may be necessary to send subsequent letters to the employer after receiving a response from the insurance carrier. For example, a letter should be sent to the employer (Fig. 14–19) if the insurance company notifies the physician's office that the employer's preliminary report of injury has not been received.

If 30 days have elapsed from the date the letter was sent requesting the Employer's Report of Work Injury and the employer has not responded, a letter should be sent to the state Workers' Compensation Board or Industrial Accidents Commission (Fig. 14–20).

Refer to Chapter 8 for additional information and helpful suggestions on following up on delinquent claims.

Martin Feelgood, MD
4567 Broad Avenue
Woodland Hills, XY 12345
555-486-9002

June 20, 20XX

The Conk Out Company
45 South Gorman Street
Woodland Hills, XY 12345

Dear Madam or Sir:

Re: Case No.:   120 XX 6542
      Injured: Mrs. Ima B. Hurt
      Date of Injury: April 3, 20XX

I have been informed by your workers' compensation insurance carrier that they have not as yet received the employer's report in regard to the above injured person.

Unless you have already done so, may I ask your cooperation in completing and sending this report so that the case may be closed.

Should you have any questions or if I can be of assistance to you in any way, please do not hesitate to call on me.

Very truly yours,

Martin Feelgood , MD

ref initials

Figure 14–19. Letter sent to the employer when the insurance company notifies the physician's office that the employer's preliminary report of injury has not been received.

http://www.dol.gov/dol/esa/welcome.html
Inquiry can be directed to one of these departments:
Division of Coal Mine Workers' Compensation
Division of Federal Employees' Compensation
Division Longshoremen's and Harbor Workers' Compensation
Medicare Carriers Manual Sections 2370, 3330.6, and 330.8 (black lung and asbestos)
http://www.cms.gov
Contact the following for information about state benefits: Forms, statutes, news bulletins, links to all states
http://www.workerscompensation.com

RESOURCES ON THE INTERNET

Contact the following for information about federal benefits:
Department of Labor, Employment Standards Administration, Washington, DC 20210

STUDENT ASSIGNMENT LIST

✔ Study Chapter 14.
✔ Answer the review questions in the *Workbook* to reinforce the theory learned in this chapter and to help prepare you for a future test.

Martin Feelgood, MD
4567 Broad Avenue
Woodland Hills, XY 12345
555-486-9002

July 15, 20XX

Division of Industrial Accidents
State Office Building
107 South Broadway, Room 4107
Woodland Hills, XY 12345

Dear Madam or Sir:

Re: Failure of employer to follow Section No. 3760

Your office is being solicited to help secure an Employer's
Report of Work Injury from the employer listed below.

Case No.:	120 XX 6542
Name of Employer:	The Conk Out Company
Address:	45 South Gorman Street
	Woodland Hills, XY 12345
Name of Injured:	Mrs. Ima B. Hurt
Address:	300 East Central Avenue
	Woodland Hills, XY 12345
Date of Injury:	April 3, 20XX
Name of Insurance Carrier:	XYZ Insurance Company
Amount of Unpaid Bill:	$148.92

Your cooperation in this matter will be greatly appreciated. If you
need further information, please feel free to contact my office.

Sincerely yours,

Martin Feelgood , MD

ref initials

Figure 14–20. Letter sent to the Workers' Compensation Board or Industrial Accident Commission in your state if the employer does not respond to your letter requesting the Employer's Report of Work Injury after 30 days have elapsed from the date of the letter.

✔ Complete the assignments in the *Workbook* for hands-on experience in completing workers' compensation insurance claim forms and reports, as well as enhanced proficiency in procedural and diagnostic coding.

✔ Turn to the Glossary at the end of this textbook for a further understanding of the Key Terms used in this chapter.

DISABILITY

15

Disability Income Insurance
and Disability Benefit Programs

■ Name federal disability
benefit programs
■ Differentiate between SSDI
and SSI
■ State eligibility
requirements, benefits, and
limitations of SSDI and SSI
■ Explain disability benefit
programs for disabled active
military personnel, veterans,
and their dependents
■ Name states that have state
disability insurance plans
■ State eligibility
requirements, benefits, and
limitations of state disability
plans
■ Explain voluntary disability
insurance plans
■ Recognize forms used for
processing state disability
plans
■ Describe topics and contents
of a medical history report
■ List guidelines for federal,
state, individual, and group
disability claim procedures

OBJECTIVES*

After reading this chapter you should be able to:

■ Define terminology and
abbreviations pertinent to
disability insurance and
disability benefit programs
■ Describe benefits and
exclusions contained in
individual and group
disability income insurance
■ Define the words temporary
disability and permanent
disability, as related to each
type of disability program

---

*Performance objectives and exercises for hands-on practical experience for this chapter appear in the *Workbook*.

---

*Some of the insurance terms presented in this chapter are shown marked with an asterisk and may seem familiar from previous chapters. However, their meanings may or may not have a slightly different connotation when referring to disability income insurance.

459

Disability Claims

Not everyone has disability insurance, but when working with patients who have it, one may encounter some interesting and unique accidents, injuries, or illnesses. After reading these extracts or direct quotations from disability insurance claim applications, one may ask, "How in the world could something like this happen?" The following gems show just how funny some situations can appear.

Describe How Your Disability Occurred

"A hernia from pulling cork out of bottle."

"Put tire patch on Playtex girdle and it caused infection on right thigh."

"Fell out a two-story window while waving goodnight to friends."

"Back injury received from jumping off a ladder to escape being hit by a train."

One victim graphically described an experience most of us have had: "Getting on a bus, the driver started before I was all on." Can you hear them asking at the hospital, "Was this your assigned seat?"

Another victim stated, "I dislocated my shoulder swatting a fly." When asked, "Have you ever dislocated a shoulder at this sport?" he stated, "I have. I knocked over two table lamps, several high-balls, and skinned an elbow."

Because this is the end of the course on insurance billing and a great deal of information has been covered, one may feel a bit overwhelmed by the many rules and regulations and their ever-changing nature. The introduction to this chapter was intended to add a bit of levity before one delves into the world of disability insurance.

This chapter introduces various types of disability income insurance plans as well as a number of disability benefit programs. The first topic, **disability income insurance,** is a form of health insurance providing periodic payments under certain conditions when the insured is unable to work because of illness, disease, or injury—not as a result of a work-related accident or condition.

The second section describes major programs administered by the U.S. government related to industrial accidents and other disability benefit programs unrelated to work injuries.

The third part of the chapter deals with nonindustrial state disability programs administered in five states and Puerto Rico, as well as voluntary disability insurance plans.

Guidelines for federal, state, individual, and group disability claim procedures are presented at the end of the chapter.

History

Before the late 1800s, disability income insurance provided only accident protection. Some life insurance contracts had disability income riders attached to them that offered limited benefits. In the early 1880s insurance companies began selling disability income policies that offered coverage for accident and illness. The Paul Revere Life Insurance Company introduced the first noncancelable disability income policy in the early 1900s. The "noncancelable" clause guaranteed that the contract would be in force for a certain period of time and the premium would not be increased. By 1956 Congress had enacted legislation under the Social Security program that provided disability income protection to disabled individuals older than 50 years of age. This program was expanded in 1965 to cover workers without regard to age as long as certain eligibility standards were met.

Today disability income insurance is available from private insurance companies (individual policies) and employer-sponsored plans (group policies). Government-funded and state benefit programs are also available for disabled persons. All of these plans and programs are discussed in this chapter, along with the role of the insurance billing specialist in dealing with this type of insurance.

Disability Income Insurance

Individual

Individual disability income insurance is coverage that provides a specific monthly or weekly income when a person becomes unable to work, temporarily or totally, because of an illness or injury. Disability income policies do not provide medical expense benefits. The disability cannot be work related. As explained in the previous chapter, the illness or accident must be work related to be covered by workers' compensation insurance.

For individuals who are self-employed, this insurance is particularly important because a business could not meet its financial obligations if the owner became injured or too ill to work. For example, if an individual is self-employed with a home-based business, repetitive stress injuries (RSIs) would not allow that individual to use the computer for several months. The main purpose of these policies is to provide some benefits while the person is not able to work. To collect benefits, the individual must meet the policy's criteria of what constitutes partial, temporary, or total disability. These policies terminate when the individual retires or reaches a certain age, usually 65 years.

Waiting Period

The time period from the beginning of disability to receiving the first payment of benefits is called an elimination period or **waiting period.** During this initial period, a disabled individual is not eligible to receive benefits even though he or she is unable to work.

Benefit Period

A **benefit period** is the maximum amount of time that benefits will be paid to the injured or ill person for the disability (e.g., 2-year, 5-year, to age 65, or lifetime).

Benefits

Benefits paid to the insured disabled person are called indemnity and can be received daily, weekly, monthly, or semiannually, depending on the policy. Premiums and benefits depend on several risk factors, such as age, gender, health history and physical state, income, and occupational duties. Some policies include residual or partial disability income benefits. Benefits are not taxable if premiums are paid by the individual.

Residual benefits pay a partial benefit when the insured is not totally disabled. If one becomes partially disabled or can work only part-time or in a limited capacity, the residual benefits make up the difference between what an individual can earn at present and what he or she would have earned working full time.

Supplemental benefits may consist of insurance provisions that will increase monthly indemnity, such as a **future purchase option** or a **cost-of-living adjustment.** Provisions also distribute a percentage of the policy premiums if an individual keeps a policy in force for 5 or 10 years or does not file any claims.

An **accidental death and dismemberment** benefit is written into some contracts. This offers the insured person protection when loss of sight or loss of limb(s) occurs. In some policies (e.g., life insurance) a special provision known as **double indemnity** applies if an unintended, unexpected, and unforeseeable accident occurs resulting in death. This feature provides for twice the face amount of the policy to be paid if death results from accidental causes.

Types of Disability

A disability may be partial, temporary, or total. The definition of **total disability** that is stated in each disability income policy varies from one to the other because there is no standard definition. An example of a liberal definition might read, "The insured must be unable to perform the major duties of his or her specific occupation." Social Security has a restrictive definition presented later in this chapter.

The terms **residual disability** and **partial disability** are defined as occurring "when an illness or injury prevents an insured person from performing one or more of the functions of his or her regular job"—in other words, when a person cannot perform all of his or her job duties.

Temporary disability exists when a person cannot perform all the functions of his or her regular job for a limited period of time.

Clauses

With a **guaranteed renewable** policy, the insurer is required to renew the policy as long as premium payments are made for a specified number of years or to a specified age, such as 60, 65, or 70 years, or for life. However, the premium may be increased when it is renewed. When the policy has a **noncancelable clause,** the premium cannot be increased.

If a **waiver of premium** is included in the insurance contract, the policy pays all premiums while the employee is disabled; the employee does not have to pay. Usually this provision is used as a total and permanent disability benefit and may be available in certain other cases.

Exclusions

Exclusions are provisions written into the insurance contract denying coverage or limiting the scope of coverage. Examples are preexisting conditions; disability because of war, riot, self-inflicted injury, or attempted suicide; mental or nervous conditions; disability while legally intoxicated or under the influence of narcotics (unless prescribed by a licensed physician); conditions arising from normal pregnancy or during the act of committing a felony; or if benefits are being received under workers' compensation or a government program. The phrase "legally intoxicated" means intoxication in an individual who has a certain amount of alcohol in the blood that, when tested, exceeds limits set by state law.

Acquired Immunodeficiency Syndrome and Human Immunodeficiency Virus Infection

States have statutes governing questions that can and cannot be asked on insurance application forms about acquired immunodeficiency syndrome (AIDS) and human immunodeficiency virus (HIV) testing; therefore each state has developed its own forms. If a private insurance company wishes to test an applicant, a consent or notice form including acceptance of pretest and posttest counseling must be signed.

Group

Some employers elect to offer group disability income insurance as a fringe benefit. These contracts are drawn up between the insurer and employer. Premiums may be paid by the employer with or without contributions from the employee. Employees hold certificates of insurance and are covered under the employer's policy; therefore they are not called policyholders. When the employee leaves the company, the insurance terminates unless the employee is disabled. A few group policies allow conversion to a limited benefit individual policy.

Benefits

Benefits vary from one plan to another but are usually for **short-term disability insurance** (13 weeks to 24 months) or **long-term disability insurance** (to age 65). To qualify for benefits an individual must be unable to perform the major duties of his or her occupation during the initial period of disability (e.g., the first 2 years). Benefits cease when the employee returns to work, even part time. These policies offer the worker partial disability income benefits to motivate a disabled individual to return to work on a part-time basis. Monthly benefits usually are paid directly to the employee and are taxable if the employee is not making any contribution toward the premiums.

Exclusions

Disabilities commonly excluded from coverage include those seen in individual disability income insurance policies, as previously described.

Federal Disability Programs

Workers' Compensation

The federal government has a number of programs that cover workers from loss of income because of work-related disability. These programs were mentioned in Chapter 14 because work-related disabilities fall under workers' compensation laws. When an individual is eligible under more than one program, coordination of benefits is used so that a worker cannot receive benefits that result in an amount greater than what the person receives when working. Coordination of benefits is a provision preventing double payment for expenses by making one of the programs the primary payer and ensuring that no more than 100% of the costs are covered.

Disability Benefit Programs

The government's major disability programs are:

▶ **Social Security Disability Insurance (SSDI) program**
▶ Supplemental Security Income (SSI)
▶ **Civil Service Retirement System (CSRS)**
▶ **Federal Employees Retirement System (FERS)**
▶ **Armed Services Disability**
▶ **Veterans Affairs (VA) disability program**

The **Social Security Administration (SSA)** manages two programs that pay monthly disability benefits to people younger than age 65 who cannot work for at least a year because of a severe disability: SSDI and SSI. Medical requirements are the same for both programs.

Social Security Disability Insurance Program

Background

In 1935 the Social Security Act, the Old-Age, Survivors, Disability, and Health Insurance (OASDHI) Program, was enacted. It provided benefits for death, retirement, disability, and medical care. In 1956 Congress established a program for long-term disability known as Social Security Disability Insurance (SSDI) under Title II of the Social Security Act. This is an entitlement (not welfare) program that provides monthly benefits to workers and those self-employed who meet certain conditions.

Disability Definition

Disability under Social Security has a strict definition: "Inability to engage in any substantial gainful activity by reason of any medically determinable physical or mental impairment which can be expected to result in death or which has lasted or can be expected to last for a continuous period of not less than 12 months."

Eligibility

The following is a list of individuals who meet eligibility requirements for SSDI:

▶ Disabled workers younger than age 65 years and their families
▶ Individuals who become disabled before age 22 years, if a parent (or in certain cases, a grandparent) who is covered under Social Security retires, becomes disabled, or dies
▶ Disabled widows or widowers, age 50 years or older, if the deceased spouse worked at least 10 years under Social Security
▶ Disabled surviving divorced spouses older than age 50 years, if the ex-spouse was married to the disabled person for at least 10 years
▶ Blind workers whose vision in the better eye cannot be corrected to better than 20/200 or whose visual field in the better eye, even with corrective lenses, is 20 degrees or less

Workers must be fully insured in accordance with standards set by the Social Security Administration in terms of age, number of quarters worked, and amount of wages earned per quarter. The processing of eligibility application forms may take up to 2 months.

Benefits

Monthly benefits are paid to qualified individuals. After 24 months of disability payments, the disabled individual also becomes eligible for Medicare. The benefits convert to retirement benefits when an individual reaches age 65.

Supplemental Security Income

Eligibility

The SSI program is under Title XVI of the Social Security Act and provides disability payments to people (adults and children) with limited income and few resources. No prior employment is needed. Many SSI recipients also qualify for Medicaid, a state assistance program. The following individuals may qualify for SSI disability payments:

▶ Disabled persons younger than 65 years old who have very limited income and resources
▶ Disabled children younger than age 18 years, if the disability compares in severity with one that would keep an adult from working and has lasted or is expected to last at least 12 months or result in death
▶ Blind adults or children who have a visual acuity no better than 20/100 or have a visual field of 20 degrees or less in the better eye, with the use of corrective lenses

Disability Determination Process

To establish disability under SSDI or SSI, an individual calls or visits any Social Security office and completes application forms with the help of a social worker. This triggers a determination process. A physician may be involved in the determination process in one of three ways: (1) as a treating source who provides medical evidence on behalf of his or her patient; (2) as a **consultative examiner (CE)** who is paid a fee and examines or tests the applicant; or (3) as a full- or part-time medical or psychologic consultant reviewing claims for a state or **regional office (RO).**

In addition to a medical report from one of these sources, other criteria taken into consideration are the individual's age and vocational and educational factors that may contribute to the person's ability to work. It is possible that a person may be eligible for disability payments under one government program and not eligible under Social Security because the rules differ. The Social Security Administration may use reports that an applicant has from another agency to determine whether the person is eligible for Social Security disability payments. Many SSA state agencies have a division known as **Disability Determination Services (DDS).** Determination of disability is made by a DDS team composed of a physician or psychologist and disability examiner (DE), not by the applicant's physician.

Appeals Evaluation Process

If a claimant does not agree with the determination of disability, a four-level appeals process is available.

1. A **reconsideration,** which is a complete review of the claim by a medical or psychologic consultant or disability examiner team that did not take part in the original disability determination.
2. A **hearing** before an administrative law judge who had no part in the initial or reconsideration determinations of the claim. The hearing is held within 75 miles of the claimant's home. The claimant and his or her representative are permitted to present their case in person and present a written statement. They also are permitted to review information the judge will use to make a decision and question any witnesses.
3. A review by the Appeals Council, which considers all requests for review but may deny a request if it believes the decision by the administrative law judge was correct. If the Appeals Council decides the case should be reviewed, it will make a decision on the case or return it to an administrative law judge for further review.
4. A review by the federal court for which the claimant may file an action where he or she resides.

Disability cases are reviewed from time to time to be sure the individuals are still disabled. The frequency depends on the nature and severity of the impairment, the likelihood of improvement, rehabilitation, ability to work, and so on.

Benefits

Social Security disability programs are designed to give long-term protection and benefits to individuals totally disabled who are unable to do any type of work in the national economy. In contrast, short-term disability may be provided through workers' compensation, insurance, savings, and investments.

Work Incentives

Special rules allow disabled or blind people presently receiving Social Security or SSI to work and still receive monthly benefits as well as Medicare or Medicaid. There is a limit to how much the person can earn in a calendar year. These are referred to as "work incentives"; the rules are different for Social Security beneficiaries and SSI recipients.

Civil Service and Federal Employees Retirement System Disability

Eligibility

Federal employees who work in civil service fall under the CSRS. This system has provisions for those who become totally disabled. This program is a combination of federal disability and Social Security disability. Both portions of the program must be applied for by the worker. The disability cannot be work related, and 5 years of service are necessary before benefits are payable. Eighteen months of service are necessary under the FERS.

Benefits

Those who qualify are entitled to benefits that are payable for life.

An example is an individual who works for the Internal Revenue Service performing clerical and filing job duties and has an automobile accident on the weekend. The head injuries are so severe that the person is unable to return to gainful employment at any job. He or she could apply for benefits either under the CSRS or FERS, depending on his or her eligibility status.

Armed Services Disability

Eligibility

Individuals covered under this program must be members of the armed services on active duty.

Benefits

Monthly benefits are payable for life if a disability occurs or is aggravated while the individual is serving in the military service. Benefit amounts are based on years of service, base pay, and severity of disability. This also is subject to review.

Veterans Affairs Disability

Eligibility

The VA is authorized by law to provide a wide range of benefits to both those who have served their country in the armed forces and their dependents. If a veteran who is honorably discharged files a claim for a service-connected disability within 1 year of sustaining that injury, he or she is eligible for outpatient treatment. Veterans with non–service-connected disabilities who are in receipt of housebound or aid-in-attendance benefits are eligible for treatment from a private physician if they are unable to travel to a VA facility because of geographic inaccessibility. Their identification card, benefits, and claims procedures are identical to those of veterans with service-connected disabilities who receive out-patient medical care.

Benefits

The following is a general list of veterans' medical benefits. Each benefit requires that certain criteria be met. These criteria are ever-changing and are not mentioned here. A complete up-to-date booklet listing all the benefits is available.

▶ Federal Benefits for Veterans and Dependents. Department of Veterans Affairs, Washington, DC 20420. The booklet is published annually and is available for a small fee from the Superintendent of Documents, U.S. Government Printing Office, Mail Stop: SSOP, Washington, DC 20402-9328.
▶ Hospital care in a VA hospital
▶ Nursing home care in a VA facility
▶ Domiciliary care
▶ Outpatient medical treatment at a VA facility or by a private physician
▶ Emergency treatment in a hospital for a service-connected condition
▶ Prescription drugs and medication issued by a VA pharmacy or other participating pharmacy. Only bona fide emergency prescriptions can be filled by a private pharmacy.
▶ Certain medical equipment, such as oxygen, prosthetics, and so on
▶ Travel expenses when receiving VA medical care
▶ Outpatient dental treatment (if the veteran files a claim within 90 days from the date that he or she was discharged from the service)
▶ Treatment for Agent Orange or nuclear radiation exposure
▶ Alcohol and drug dependence outpatient care
▶ Readjustment counseling services

The physician must accept what the VA pays as payment in full for treatment of a service-connected disability and cannot bill the patient for any additional charges, even if there is a balance after the VA pays the claim. If the treatment is likely to cost more than $40 per month, the physician must obtain prior authorization from the nearest VA facility. A separate financial accounting record card must be prepared for VA benefits if the physician is also treating the patient for ailments other than a service-connected disability. Any professional service that is not related to a service-connected disability must be paid for by the veteran out of his or her own pocket.

Veterans with non–service-connected disabilities may have copayments when they seek treatment. For example, individuals on Medicare may be responsible for the deductible for the first 90 days of care during any 365-day period. For each additional 90 days of hospital care, the patient is charged one half of the Medicare deductible, $10 a day of hospital care, and $5 a day for VA nursing home care. For outpatient care the copayment is 20% of the cost of an average outpatient visit.

Outpatient Treatment

Veterans eligible for outpatient treatment may obtain outpatient medical care only for the disability as listed on the **VA outpatient clinic** card (Fig. 15–1). Usually a veteran seeks care at the nearest VA outpatient clinic. However, when a VA facility is not within reasonable distance, when the veteran is too ill to travel to the nearest location, or when the condition needs prompt attention, the veteran can apply for and be granted medical care by a private physician through the Home Town Care Program. The VA outpatient clinic must be notified within 15 days of the treatment rendered. In such cases the treating physician must submit evidence of medical necessity (e.g., detailed justification on the invoice) to the VA outpatient clinic. Form 10-583, Claim for Payment of Cost of Unauthorized Medical Services (Fig. 15–2), generally used for hospital emergency care, also can be used for professional care if the doctor is billing after the 15-day period has elapsed. There are patients who have both Medicare and medical coverage from the Veterans Affairs. In such cases Medicare is not secondary to the VA and the VA is not secondary to Medicare. The claim is to be sent where specified by the patient. The claim can be sent to Medicare, where, if the claim is processed, the patient must satisfy his or her contractual requirement to pay any deductible and copayment amounts. If the patient asks that the claim be sent to the VA instead of Medicare, the claim is processed and any payments issued are considered as payment in full. Many veterans prefer to have the claim sent to the VA.

Veterans Affairs Installations

For information on veterans' benefits or assistance in locating Veterans Affairs Installations, write or call one of the regional offices listed in Appendix A. Many states have toll-free telephone services to the Department of Veterans Affairs from communities in the state. Consult the local telephone directory or information assistance operator for the latest listing of these numbers.

State Disability Insurance

Background

In 1944 Rhode Island began a **State Disability Insurance (SDI)** program that proved successful. This form of insurance is part of an employment

BILLING AND REPORTS. Bill the Station of Jurisdiction monthly. Please itemize your usual statement to include (1) patient's name; (2) identification number; (3) condition treated; (4) treatment and dates rendered; and (5) your usual and customary fee. Bills for auxiliary medical services must reflect the name of the prescribing doctor of medicine or osteopathy. Submit a brief treatment report only when the cost of urgent treatment causes the $30.00 limitation to be exceeded, or when a significant clinical change in a disability occurs.

PAYMENT. Payment by the VA for services rendered is payment in full.

IMPORTANT: Direct inquiries and any change of address to the Station of Jurisdiction.

Station of Jurisdiction:

FOLD

```
┌                                              ┐
    VETERANS ADMINISTRATION
    OUTPATIENT C 9044/136A6
    428 SOUTH HILL ST.
    LOS ANGELES CA 90013
└                                              ┘
```

VA OUTPATIENT MEDICAL TREATMENT INFORMATION CARD

E. Z. Slipdisk   012-XX-5678
Beneficiary's name   Identification No.

DISABILITY FOR WHICH TREATMENT IS AUTHORIZED–VALID UNTIL CANCELLED BY VA

X P. O. HERNIATED NUC. PULPOSUS

VA FORM 10-1174, FEB 1971

Front

PLEASE READ CAREFULLY

TO VETERAN — You are authorized to obtain treatment within a reasonable distance from your permanent or temporary residence for the disability shown. When treatment is required, select a doctor of medicine or osteopathy who is licensed in the State in which treatment will be rendered. This card constitutes an agreement to provide care to you as a VA beneficiary within the limitations stated. Please alert the doctor to the instructions printed on the card and be sure he has your NAME, IDENTIFICATION NO. and the ADDRESS OF THE STATION OF JURISDICTION. If a specific therapy is authorized in lieu of listing disabilities, this card authorizes ONLY that therapy. IT MAY NOT BE USED TO OBTAIN OTHER MEDICAL SERVICES, SURGICAL PROCEDURES, NON-VA HOSPITALIZATION, OR PROSTHETIC APPLIANCES. Prescriptions of a recurring nature and others not needed at once should be brought or mailed to the VA station of jurisdiction. They will be filled promptly. When it is necessary to obtain medication immediately, PLEASE REQUEST THE PRIVATE PHARMACIST TO BILL THE STATION OF JURISDICTION SHOWN ON THIS CARD.

The VA may reimburse local, round trip, travel expenses between your permanent or temporary residence and the place treatment is obtained. A mileage allowance will be paid in lieu of actual and necessary expenses of travel (including lodging and subsistence).

Your one-time, written request for travel expenses, when received within 30 days from the date you first obtain medical services, will be approved to be effective with the first visit. A claim received after that 30-day-period will be effective from the date received. Generally, travel expenses are paid for a 3-month period.

TO PHYSICIAN — The beneficiary named on this card is authorized OUT-PATIENT TREATMENT for the disabilities shown by a doctor of medicine or osteopathy licensed in the state in which medical services are rendered. When treatment of these conditions requires eyeglasses, hearing aids, other prostheses, home nursing services, and/or dental services, notify the station of Jurisdiction. Items or services of this nature will be provided by the Veterans Administration. Please request additional medical or other information from the station of jurisdiction, if required.

MEDICAL SERVICES includes prescription and referral for auxiliary medical services when required. All routine treatment may not exceed a total cost of $30.00 per month without prior VA approval.

PHARMACY SERVICES: Please have Rxs filled by VA unless needed at once. Veteran may obtain stat Rx from private pharmacy if you certify Rx, "The VA has authorized me to treat the disability for which this prescription is written."

Back

Figure 15–1. Veterans Affairs outpatient clinic card.

---

security program that provides temporary cash benefits for workers suffering a wage loss because of off-the-job illness or injury. It can be referred to as **unemployment compensation disability (UCD)** or **temporary disability insurance (TDI).** California became the second state to add nonindustrial disability coverage to the Social Security protection afforded to its citizens by appending Article 10 to the Unemployment Insurance Act. This became law on May 21, 1946; when the legislation took effect on December 1, 1946, this article diverted the 1% tax formerly paid by workers for unemployment insurance to a disability insurance fund. New York and New Jersey soon followed with similar programs. Two decades later, in 1969, Puerto Rico and Hawaii passed nonindustrial disability insurance laws.

Some accidents that occur are quite serious at the time but can appear rather humorous upon review.

Unique Accident

The patient was under the kitchen sink repairing a leak when the family cat came along, watched for a while, then playfully—but painfully—reached up and clawed him. Startled, the man threw his head back, cracked it on the bottom of the sink, and was knocked out cold. He came to as he was being carried out on a stretcher and explained to the attendants what had happened. One stretcher bearer laughed so hard, he relaxed his hold and the patient fell to the ground and broke his arm.

Form Approved
Budget Bureau No. 76-H0325

VETERANS ADMINISTRATION
CLAIM FOR PAYMENT OF COST OF
UNAUTHORIZED MEDICAL SERVICES

Each person, firm or institution claiming payments or reimbursements must complete this form. No carbon paper is necessary. Please use typewriter or ball point pen, and submit both copies.

1A. VETERAN'S LAST NAME – FIRST – MIDDLE INITIAL	1B. CLAIM NO.	1C. SOCIAL SECURITY NO.
Thornberg, Joey T.	c–	421-XX-4182

1D. PRESENT ADDRESS (*include zip code*)

4628 Image Street, Woodland Hills, XY 12345-1290

2. NAME AND ADDRESS OF PERSON, FIRM OR INSTITUTION MAKING CLAIM (*Leave blank if same as above*)

Gerald Practon, MD 4567 Broad Ave., Woodland Hills, XY 12345-0001

3. STATEMENT OF CIRCUMSTANCES UNDER WHICH THE SERVICES WERE RENDERED (Include diagnosis, symptoms, whether emergency existed, and reason VA facilities were not used)

Patient fell on sidewalk in front of home and suffered traumatic injury of right arm.
Symptoms: Localized pain, swelling, and bruising of right arm near elbow.
AP and lateral x-rays of right elbow show anterior dislocation right radius. Negative for fracture.
Medical care rendered in Emergency Dept. at College Hospital (99282).
Patient unable to go to VA facility as this is 60 miles away.
Treatment of closed elbow dislocation without anesthesia (23400).
Diagnosis: Anterior closed dislocation right radius (Dx code No. 832.01).

4. AMOUNT CLAIMED	*Attach bills or receipts showing services furnished, dates, and charges*
$ 237.02	attached

5. COMPLETE A OR B, AS APPROPRIATE

A. Amount claimed does not exceed that charged the general public for similar services, and payment has not been received.	B. I certify that the amount claimed has been paid and reimbursement has not been made.
Gerald Practon, MD 5/11/XX	*Joey T. Thornberg* 5/11/XX
SIGNATURE AND TITLE OF PROVIDER OF SERVICE, AND DATE	SIGNATURE OF VETERAN OR REPRESENTATIVE, AND DATE

FOR VETERANS ADMINISTRATION USE ONLY

6. ACTION ☐ APPROVED $ _____ ☐ DISAPPROVED	Treatment was provided in an emergency for a service-connected or adjunct disability, any disability of a veteran who has a total disability permanent in nature from a service-connected disability, or for any illness, injury, dental condition in the case of a veteran eligible under Chapter 31 (Vocational Rehabilitation) Title 38, U. S. Code. VA facilities were not feasibly available and delay would have been hazardous.

7. SIGNATURE, CHIEF, MEDICAL ADMINISTRATION SERVICE	8. DATE	9. ADMINISTRATION VOUCHER NO.

VA FORM
MAY 1974   10-583   SUPERSEDES VA FORM 10-583 FEB 1966 AND
WHICH WILL NOT BE USED.

Figure 15–2. Veterans Affairs Form 10-583, Claim for Payment of Cost of Unauthorized Medical Services.

State Programs

Nonindustrial disability insurance programs existed in only five states and Puerto Rico as of 2000. The law is known by a different name in each area.

State	Name of Law	Web Site
California	California Unemploy-ment Insurance Code.	www.edd.ca.gov
Hawaii	Temporary Disability Insurance Law	
New Jersey	Temporary Disability Benefits Law	www.state.nj.us
New York	Disability Benefits Law	www.web.state.ny.us
Puerto Rico	Disability Benefits Law	
Rhode Island	Temporary Disability Insurance Act	www.state.ri.us

Web sites for most of these programs also can be found at the end of this chapter.

Funding

To fund state disability insurance, a small percentage of the wage is deducted from employees' paychecks each month, or the employer may elect to pay all or part of the cost of the plan as a fringe benefit for employees. The money is then sent in quarterly installments to the state and put into a special fund.

Eligibility

To receive state disability insurance benefits, an employee must be:

▶ Employed full or part time or actively looking for work when disability begins
▶ Suffering a loss of wages because of disability
▶ Eligible for benefits depending on the amount withheld during a previous period before disability began
▶ Under the care and treatment of a physician who certifies that the employee is disabled
▶ Disabled at least 7 or 8 calendar days or hospitalized as an inpatient
▶ Filing a claim within the time limit

If the worker was employed at the time of disability, benefits are not subject to federal income tax. An employee who retires is no longer eligible for the insurance. A worker may file a claim with the state seeking exemption from program participation on religious grounds.

Types of workers not covered are employees of school districts, community college districts, and churches; state workers; federal employees; interstate railroad workers; nonprofit organization employees; and domestic workers.

Benefits

Weekly benefits are determined by the wages earned in a base period or based on a percentage of average weekly wages (Table 15–1). Benefits begin after the seventh consecutive day of disability. There is no provision under the law for hospital or other medical benefits except in Hawaii and Puerto Rico, where hospital benefits are payable under a prepaid health care program if the employee meets certain eligibility requirements.

Limited Benefits

In some states a patient may qualify for benefits if he or she is a resident of an approved alcoholic recovery facility or an approved drug-free residential facility.

Reduced Benefits

An individual may be entitled to partial benefits if he or she is receiving certain types of income:

▶ Sick leave
▶ Vacation
▶ Wages paid by employer
▶ Insurance settlement for the disability
▶ Workers' compensation benefits
▶ Unemployment benefits

Time Limits

A claim for state disability insurance should be filed within the time limit of the state laws (Table 15–1). There is usually a grace period of 7 or 8 days after the deadline. After the claim is approved, basic benefits become payable on the eighth day of disability or the first day of hospital confinement, whichever comes first. A person may continue to draw disability insurance for a maximum of 26 weeks in Hawaii, New Jersey, New York, Puerto Rico, and Rhode Island and 52 weeks in California on the same illness or injury or overlapping disabilities. An employee is also entitled to disability benefits 15 days after recovery from a previous disability or illness. For example, if a patient is discharged by the physician to return to work and is on the job 15 calendar days and then becomes ill with the same ailment, he or she may file a new claim.

| TABLE 15–1 | State Disability Information Summary | | | | |

State Disability Information Summary

State	Name of State Law	Maximum Benefit Period (wk)	Time Limit for Filing Claims	2003 Deductions From Salary (%)	Benefits
California	California Unemployment Insurance Code	52	49 days from disability	0.7	Based on earnings in a 12-month base period, which begins approximately 18 months before disability
Hawaii	Temporary Disability Insurance Law	26	90 days from disability	0.5	Based on 58% of average weekly wage
New Jersey	Temporary Disability Benefits Law	26	30 days from disability	0.5	Based on average weekly wage
New York	Disability Benefits Law	26	30 days from disability	0.5 (max. 60 cents/wk)	Based on 50% of average weekly wage (max. $170/week)
Puerto Rico	Disability Benefits Act	26	3 months from disability	0.3 employee; 0.3 employer	Based on wages earned during base year
Rhode Island	Temporary Disability Insurance Act	30	1 year from disability	1.7	Based on 4.62% of wages in the base period quarter in which wages were the highest

Medical Examinations

The claimant may be required to submit to an examination or examinations by an independent medical examiner to determine any mental or physical disability. Fees for such examinations are paid by the state department that handles disability insurance. Code 99450 for billing these medical examinations may be found in the Special Evaluation and Management Services section of Current Procedural Terminology.

Restrictions

There are many restrictions on disability insurance. A few of the major situations in which a claim could be denied are listed here.

1. Conditions covered by workers' compensation unless the rate is less than the disability insurance rate. In that case the state pays the difference between the two rates.
2. Applicants receiving unemployment insurance benefits more than a certain specified amount. *Exception:* If the applicant is on unemployment insurance and then becomes ill or injured, he or she is put on temporary disability insurance until able to go on a job interview.

3. Disabilities beginning during a trade dispute. If an employee is on strike and is injured while walking a picket line, he or she is not eligible for benefits. However, if the union is on strike and an individual member remains at home and then becomes ill or injured, he or she can claim disability and will receive benefits.
4. Confinement by court order or certification in a public or private institution as an alcoholic, drug addict, or sexual psychopath.
5. When legal custody is the cause of unemployment.
6. When the employing company has a voluntary disability plan and is not paying into a state fund.
7. Religious exemption certificate on file by employee or company with no payment being made into a state fund.
8. Pregnancy-related disability, unless the pregnancy is complicated (e.g., cases in which the patient has diabetes, varicose veins, ectopic pregnancy, or cesarean section). *Exceptions:* California, Hawaii, New Jersey, and Rhode Island have maternity benefits that may be applied for at the time the physician tells the patient to stop working.

Voluntary Disability Insurance

Persons residing and working in states that do not have state disability insurance programs may elect to contact a local private insurance carrier to arrange for coverage under a **voluntary disability insurance** plan. If these persons become ill or disabled, they receive a fixed weekly or monthly income, usually for approximately 6 months. If the disability or illness is permanent and the individual is unable to return to work, there is sometimes a small monthly income for the duration of the person's life. Some of the state laws provide that a "voluntary plan" may be adopted instead of the "state plan" if a majority of company employees consent to private coverage.

PROCEDURE: **Claims Submission**

Disability Income Claims

When the insurance billing specialist is handling disability income claim forms, he or she should note that the insured (claimant) is responsible to notify the insurance company of the disability. A proof of loss form is completed to establish disability.

The necessary facts are:

▶ Date the disability occurred
▶ Date the disabled is expected to be well enough to return to work
▶ Description of how the disability occurred
▶ Name of treating physician
▶ Explanation of how the disability prevents the insured from work

The report must show that the patient's disability meets the policy's definition of disability, or benefits will be denied. Because the definition of disability varies among policies, the critical issues are the content and wording on the claim form.

A portion of this form is usually completed by the attending physician. The following data are necessary:

▶ Medical history
▶ Dates patient became disabled
▶ Subjective symptoms (patient's own words about his or her chief complaints)
▶ Objective findings on physical examination (e.g., rashes, lacerations, abrasions, or contusions)
▶ Severity of the illness or injury (range of motion tests)
▶ Photocopies of laboratory tests, x-ray studies, or hospital discharge report
▶ Medication
▶ Treatment dates
▶ Diagnosis

▶ Prognosis (outcome of the disease or injury)
▶ Names of any other treating physician
▶ Date patient expected to return to work
▶ Description of job duties and patient's ability to perform work

Providing the information listed above helps verify the disability. In some cases the physician may wish to dictate a medical report and attach it to the claim form instead of completing a portion of the form. The insurance billing specialist must be prepared to extract data from source documents, such as medical and financial records, to complete the claim form. In such situations the physician should be asked to read the information carefully before signing the document. The patient should always be asked to sign an authorization form to release medical information. Reasons for denial of benefits often include improper choice of words or inadequate medical information.

The insurance company may request information from other places to justify payment of benefits, such as employer's records, employee's wage statements or tax forms, or the attending physician's medical records. A company representative may interview the insured if conflicting information exists.

If disability continues, additional claim forms should be completed monthly, or more frequently, by the insured and attending physician. Other sources of information may be requested; for example, records from medical specialists or Social Security records.

If the validity of the case is in question, an independent medical examiner may be asked by the insurance company to examine the disabled individual. If the claimant neglects to return claim forms, refuses telephone calls, misses appointments, or engages in questionable activities, the insurance company will discreetly engage in surveillance of the insured through the services of a professional investigation firm.

Federal Disability Claims

The Social Security Administration division called DDS has a teledictation service so the physician or psychologist can dictate the medical report over the telephone instead of completing a medical report form. The service is available at any time, including nights and weekends. A typed transcript is sent to the physician to review, sign, and return to the SSA state agency, or a report may be typed on the physician's stationery. The physician may photocopy relevant portions of the patient's chart and submit that information, but it should be legible. An authorization to release information, signed by the patient, should be on file. Copies of consultation reports and hospital summaries also are helpful. By law only data no more than 1 year old are allowed.

A medical report must include the following:

▶ Relevant medical history, past history, social history, and family history
▶ Subjective complaints (patient's symptoms)
▶ Objective findings on physical examination (e.g., results of physical or mental status examination, and blood pressure)
▶ Laboratory and x-ray findings
▶ Diagnostic studies (e.g., treadmill tests, pulmonary function tests, or electrocardiographic tracings)
▶ Diagnosis (statement of disease or injury based on signs and symptoms)
▶ Treatment prescribed, with patient's response and prognosis
▶ Medical prognosis about disability based on medical findings. A description of the individual's ability to perform work-related activities, such as standing, sitting, lifting, carrying, walking, handling objects, hearing, speaking, and traveling, is necessary. For cases of mental impairment, the statement should present the individual's capacity for understanding and remembering, sustained concentration and persistence, social interaction, and adaptation.

Veterans Affairs Disability Outpatient Clinic Claims

The processing of invoices from private physicians is a somewhat lengthy procedure as required by VA regulations and involves several steps. To keep the delay in payment to a minimum, private physicians are urged to bill the VA on a monthly basis. To ensure prompt processing, invoices should contain the following information:

1. Patient's name as shown on the ID card, VA Form 10-1174 (Fig. 15–1)
2. Patient's Social Security number
3. Condition treated, shown on every invoice, because this is the basis for approval of payment
4. Diagnosis being treated must be listed on the ID card or authorized by the statement "for any condition." Abstract the diagnosis exactly as it is stated on the ID card.
5. Treatment given and dates rendered
6. Physician's usual and customary fee for services rendered
7. Name and address of private physician and his or her Social Security or Federal Taxpayer ID number. If the ID number is assigned to a group and the physician desires to be paid individually, the VA outpatient clinic must be so advised.

Private physicians, as well as veterans, are urged to read the instructions on the ID card carefully. This is sometimes neglected and can lead to misunderstanding.

If the physician does not wish to bill the VA outpatient clinic, the patient can pay the physician and then be reimbursed, but the veteran must carefully follow the instructions on the back of the VA outpatient clinic card.

State Disability Claims

Residents of a state that provides state disability benefits may call or write to the nearest office that handles state disability insurance to obtain a claim form and insurance pamphlet. A list of offices and addresses for each state is provided in Appendix A.

In some states the claim form is in three parts and must be completed by the claimant, employer, and physician. In other states the form is in two parts and is completed by the claimant and physician (Figs. 15–3 and 15–4). In either instance the case must be substantiated by a physician before the applicant may begin receiving benefits. All information from the state disability insurance office should be read carefully and the directions followed precisely. The data requested should be provided, and the physician and patient should sign the forms. The form should be submitted within the stated time limits.

After the claim has been completed by all parties concerned, it is submitted to the nearest local office for processing. The most important items on the claim form are the following:

1. The claimant's Social Security number; without it the claim cannot be researched properly to establish wages earned in the base period.
2. The first day the patient was too sick to perform all of his or her regular work duties (item 3). This cannot be the same day the patient worked, even if the patient went home sick.
3. The last day the patient worked (item 4). List the last day the patient worked even if for only part of the day.

Note: The two dates listed in items 2 and 3 cannot be the same; for example, if the patient went home sick on October 4, that would be considered the last day worked; October 5 would be the first day the patient was unable to work.

California has been selected as the model state for examples of the different forms used in the processing of disability insurance. To establish a claim, the First Claim for Disability Insurance Form DE 2501 must be completed by both the patient (Fig. 15–3) and the attending physician (Fig. 15–4). If an extension of disability is necessary, the Physician's Supplementary Certificate Form DE 2525XX must be completed by the physician (Fig. 15–5). This accompanies the last check issued to the patient. For additional medical information that might be necessary, Forms DE 2547 and DE 2547A sometimes are sent to the attending physician for completion (Figs. 15–6 and 15–7).

CLAIM STATEMENT OF EMPLOYEE *Please read instructions on back before completing this form.*
COMPLETE *ALL* ITEMS. IF INCOMPLETE, THIS FORM WILL BE RETURNED, CAUSING A DELAY IN BENEFIT PAYMENTS

1. Print your full name:

FIRST	INITIAL	LAST
MARCIA	M.	MONROE

Other Names (including maiden, married and ethnic surnames) Used:

Your Mailing Address:

STREET ADDRESS, P.O. BOX OR RFD   APT. NO.   CITY OR TOWN   STATE AND ZIP CODE

3501 Maple Street, Woodland Hills,   XY 12345

Your Home Address: (Required if different from mailing address)
IF YOU HAVE NO STREET ADDRESS, YOU **MUST** PROVIDE SPECIFIC DIRECTIONS TO YOUR HOME

Male ☐   Female ☒   Birthdate MONTH 03 DAY 04 YEAR 1952

Do you need assistance in a language other than English? ☒ No ☐ Yes
If yes, write that language here: _____

¿Prefiere Ud. formularios escritos en español? No ☐ Sí ☐

2. **IMPORTANT:** Enter your Social Security Account Number

5	4	0		X	X		9	8	8	1

2A. If you have used another Social Security number, enter that number here

– – – – – – – – – – –

3. What was the first day you were too sick to perform all the duties of your regular or customary work, even if it was a Saturday, Sunday, holiday, or a normal day off:?

MONTH 10   DAY 10   YEAR 20xx

4. What was the last day you worked prior to your disability?

MONTH 10   DAY 09   YEAR 20xx

5. Current or Last Employer's Business Name: Telephone Number

A and B Company   (555) 487-9980

Current or Last Employer's Business Address

NUMBER AND STREET	CITY	STATE AND ZIP CODE
401 State Street	Woodland Hills,	XY 12345

6. Your occupation with this employer.   secretary   Your Badge or Payroll number: 4399

7. a. What is your usual occupation? _____ secretary

	Yes	No
b. Have you been retrained for a new occupation? If yes, please give name of that occupation:	☐	☒
8. Are you self-employed?	☐	☒
9. Did you lose any time from work because of this illness or injury during the two weeks before the last day you worked as shown in item (4) above?	☐	☒
10. Did you stop work because of sickness, injury or pregnancy? If "No," please give reason:	☒	☐
11. Have you filed for or received UNEMPLOYMENT INSURANCE benefits between the last day you worked and the first day you became disabled?	☐	☒
12. a. Has, or will your employer continue your pay by means of sick leave, pension, gift or other means?	☐	☒
b. Do you authorize the Employment Development Department to disclose benefit eligibility information to your employer to be used only for the purpose of integrating your employer's wage continuation/sick leave program with your benefits? (This information is limited to the claim effective date; the weekly and maximum benefit amounts; and the periods covered by benefit payments.)	Yes ☒	No ☐
13. Was this disability or any other disability during this claim period caused by your work? If "Yes," please provide: (a) The date of your work-caused injury: _____ and (b) The name and address of any insurance carrier from whom you are claiming or receiving Workers' Compensation benefits.	☐	☒
14. Have you recovered from your disability? If "Yes," enter date of recovery:	☐	☒
15. Have you returned to work for any day, part-time or full-time, after the beginning date of your disability as shown in item (3) above? If "Yes," please enter such dates:	☐	☒
16. At any time during your disability, were you, as a result of an arrest, confined to a jail, detention center, prison medical center or other correctional institution or any other place: If "Yes," give dates:	☐	☒

I hereby claim benefits and certify that for the period covered by this claim I was unemployed and disabled, that the foregoing statements, including any accompanying statements, are to the best of my knowledge and belief true, correct and complete. I hereby authorize my attending physician, practitioner, hospital, vocational rehabilitation counselor, employer, and California Department of Industrial Relations to furnish and disclose all facts concerning my disability and wages or earnings that are within their knowledge and to allow inspection of and provide copies of any medical, vocational rehabilitation, and billing records concerning my disability that are under their control. I understand that authorizaitons contained in this claim statement are granted for a period of five years from the date of my signature or the effective date of the claim, whichever is later. I agree that a photocopy of this authorization shall be as valid as the original.

Claim signed on:	MONTH 10	DAY 12	YEAR 20xx	Claimant's signature:	(DO NOT PRINT)	Telephone Number (555) 487-9980

▶ ▶

If your signature is made by mark (X) it must be attested by two witnesses with their addresses.

SIGNATURE-WITNESS   SIGNATURE-WITNESS

Under Section 2101 of the California Unemployment Insurance Code, it is a violation to willfully make a false statement or knowingly conceal a material fact in order to obtain the payment of any benefits, such violation being punishable by imprisonment and/or by a fine not exceeding $20,000 or both.

ADDRESS   ADDRESS

If an authorized agent is filing for benefits for an INCAPACITATED or DECEASED claimant, or a spouse is filing for a MENTALLY INCAPACITATED individual, contact the office below for the required forms and instructions.

Figure 15–3. Form DE 2501, Claim Statement of Employee. This side of the two-part form is completed by the claimant.

DOCTOR'S CERTIFICATE

Certification may be made by a licensed medical or osteopathic physician and surgeon, chiropractor, dentist, podiatrist, optometrist, designated psychologist or an authorized medical officer of a United States Government facility. Certification may also be made by a licensed nurse-midwife or nurse practitioner for the purposes of disability related to normal pregnancy or childbirth. All items on this sheet must be completed legibly.

Patient File No.	Name	Social Security Number
	MARCIA M. MONROE	540-XX-9881

17. I attended the patient for the present medical problem
    from: | MONTH DAY YEAR | MONTH DAY YEAR |

    10-12-20XX   To present   At intervals of: two visits to date

18. Are you completing this form for the sole purpose of referral or recommendation to an alcoholic recovery home or drug-free facility?
    Yes ☐   No ☒   If yes, please enter facility name and address in item #28.

19. History: cough of 2 wks duration, chest pain, 100°F

    Objective Findings/Detailed Statement of Symptoms

    Diagnosis: (REQUIRED)
    bilateral pneumonitis   bilateral pneumonitis

    ICD-9 Disease Code, Primary: (REQUIRED)   486   ICD-9 Disease Code, Secondary:

    Type of treatment and/or medication rendered to patient:
    Bed rest   Rx   antibiotic

20. Diagnosis confirmed by: **(Specify type of test or X-ray)**
    AP and lateral chest x-rays

21. Is this patient now pregnant or has she been pregnant since the date of treatment as reported above?   Yes ☐   No ☒   If "Yes," date pregnancy terminated or future EDC.

    Is the pregnancy normal?   Yes ☐   No ☐   If "No," state the abnormal and involuntary complication causing maternal disability:

22. Operation: Date performed or to be performed   DNA   Type of Operation: ICD-9 Procedutre Code: (REQUIRED)

23. Was or is patient confined as a registered bed patient in a hospital?   Yes ☐   No ☒
    If "Yes," please provide dates:
    Entered hospital on _____, 20____
    Discharged from hospital on _____, 20____

24. Has the patient at any time during your attendance for this medical problem, been incapable of performing his or her regular work as a _____ ?   Yes ☒   No ☐   If "Yes" the disability commenced on: 10-10-20XX

25. APPROXIMATE date, based on your examination of patient, disability (if any) should end or has ended sufficiently to permit the patient to resume regular or customary work. Even if considerable question exists, make SOME "estimate." This is a requirement of the Code, and the claim will be delayed if such date is not entered. Such answers as "Indefinite" or "don't know" will not suffice.   (ENTER DATE)   10-30-20XX

26. Based on your examination of patient, is this disability the result of "occupation" either as an "industrial accident" or as an "occupational disease"?
    Yes ☐   No ☒
    This should include aggravation of pre-existing conditions by occupation.

27. Have you reported this OR A CONCURRENT DISABILITY to any insurance carrier as a Workers' Compensation Claim?
    Yes ☐   No ☒   If "Yes," to whom? _____ (Name of carrier or firm)

28. Was or is patient a resident in an alcoholic recovery home or drug-free residential facility?   Yes ☐   No ☒
    If "Yes," please provide name and address:

29. Would the disclosure of this information to your patient be medically or psychologically detrimental to the patient?
    Yes ☐   No ☒

I hereby certify that, based on my examination, the above statements truly describe the patient's disability (if any) and the estimated duration thereof, and that I am a __MD__ I __GP__ licensed to practice by the State of __California__
    (TYPE OF DOCTOR)   (SPECIALTY, IF ANY)

▶ David W. Smith, MD
    PRINT OR TYPE DOCTOR'S NAME AS SHOWN ON LICENSE

▶   ORIGINAL SIGNATURE OF ATTENDING DOCTOR
    - RUBBER STAMP IS NOT ACCEPTABLE -

▶ 4567 Broad Ave., Woodland Hills, XY 12345
    NO. AND STREET   CITY   ZIP CODE

▶ C 14020   (555) 486-9002   10-19-20XX
    STATE LICENSE NUMBER   TELEPHONE   DATE OF SIGNING THIS FORM

Under Section 2116 of the California Unemployment Insurance Code, it is a violation for any individual who, with the intent to defraud, falsely certifies the medical condition of any person in order to obtain disability insurance benefits, whether for the maker or for any other person, and is punishable by imprisonment and/or a fine not exceeding twenty thousand dollars. Section 1143 requires additional administrative penalties.

Figure 15–4. Form DE 2501, Doctor's Certificate. This side of the form is completed by the attending physician. It is submitted within a set time frame, determined by the beginning date of disability, to initiate benefits. If the patient is seen by a second physician, this form is mailed to the claimant to secure the certification of a new physician or to clarify a specific claimed period of disability.

NOTICE OF FINAL PAYMENT

The information contained in your claim for Disability Insurance indicates that you are now able to work; therefore, this is the final check that you will receive on this claim.

IF YOU ARE **STILL** DISABLED: You should complete the Claimant's Certification portion of this form and contact your doctor immediately to have him/her complete the Physician's Supplementary Certificate below.

IF YOU BECOME DISABLED **AGAIN:** File a new Disability Insurance claim form.

IF YOU ARE UNEMPLOYED AND AVAILABLE FOR WORK: Report to the nearest Unemployment Insurance office of the Department for assistance in finding work and to determine your entitlement to Unemployment Insurance Benefits.

This determination is final unless you file an appeal within twenty (20) days from the date of mailing of this notification. You may appeal by giving a detailed statement as to why you believe the determination is in error. All communications regarding this Disability Insurance claim should include your Social Security Account Number and be addressed to the office shown.

CLAIMANT'S CERTIFICATION

I certify that I continue to be disabled and incapable of doing my regular work, and that I have reported all wages, Workers' Compensation benefits and other monies received during the claim period to the Employment Development Department.

ENTER YOUR SOCIAL SECURITY NUMBER *540 XX 9881*

Sign Your Name *Marcia M. Monroe*   Date signed *October 29* 20 *xx*

PHYSICIAN'S SUPPLEMENTARY CERTIFICATE

Department Use Only

1. Are you still treating patient? *Yes*   Date of last treatment *October 29* 20 *xx*

2. What present condition continues to make the patient disabled?

bilateral pneumonitis; infiltrate still present

3. Date patient recovered, or will recover sufficiently (even if under treatment) to be able to perform his/her regular and customary work *November 7* 20 *xx*   Please enter a specific or estimated recovery date.

4. Would the disclosure of this information to your patient be medically or psychologically detrimental to the patient?

Yes ☐   No ☒

I hereby certify that the above statements in my opinion truly describe the claimant's condition and the estimated duration thereof.

Date *October 29* 20 *xx*   Doctor's Signature *David W. Smith M.D.*

Phone Number *555-486-9002*

DE 2525XX Rev. 13 (3-86)   —Version en español el dorso—

Figure 15–5. Notice of Final Payment/Physician's Supplementary Certificate Form DE 2525XX. This form indicates that the period of disability is "closed" or terminated with the accompanying check, based on information in the claim records. Benefits will cease unless the reverse side of the form is completed by the claimant's physician, extending the duration of disability. This form is pink. One side of the form is in English, and the other is in Spanish.

STATE OF CALIFORNIA
EMPLOYMENT DEVELOPMENT DEPARTMENT

FOR DEPT. USE ONLY

REFER TO
↓

4920   – Our File No.
Marcia M. Monroe   – Your Patient
Secretary   – Regular or Customary Work

REQUEST FOR ADDITIONAL
MEDICAL INFORMATION

David W. Smith, MD
4567 Broad Avenue
Woodland Hills, XY 12345

The original basic information and estimate of duration of your patient's disability have been carefully evaluated. At the present time, the following additional information based upon the progress and present condition of this patient is requested. This will assist the Department in determining eligibility for further disability insurance benefits. Return of the completed form as soon as possible will be appreciated.

WM. C. SCHMIDT, M.D., MEDICAL DIRECTOR

CLAIMS EXAMINER   **DOCTOR: Please complete either Part A or B, date and sign.**

PART A   IF YOUR PATIENT HAS RECOVERED SUFFICIENTLY TO BE ABLE TO RETURN TO HIS/HER REGULAR
OR CUSTOMARY WORK LISTED ABOVE, PLEASE GIVE THE DATE, _____ 20_____.

PART B   THIS PART REFERS TO PATIENT WHO IS STILL DISABLED.

Are you still treating the patient?   YES ☒   NO ☐   ___November___ 15 , 20 _xx_
DATE OF LAST TREATMENT

What are the medical circumstances which continue to make your patient disabled?

Bilateral pneumonitis. Patient has had continual fever 100°F to 102°F,

productive cough, chest pains, and lethargy

What is your present estimate of the date your patient will be able to perform his/her regular or customary work listed above?   Date ___November 30__ 20___ xx___ .

Further Comments: _____

Would the disclosure of this information to your patient be medically or psychologically detrimental to the patient?   YES ☐   NO ☒

Date ___November___ 17   20___ xx___

David W. Smith M.D.
DOCTOR'S SIGNATURE

SE   David W. Smith, MD
ENCLOSED IS A STAMPED PREADDRESSED ENVELOPE FOR YOUR CONVENIENCE.

DE 2547 R v. 18 (8-84)

Figure 15–6. Request for Additional Medical Information Form DE 2547. This form is mailed to the physician when the normal expectancy date of the disability is reached, provided that the physician has requested a longer-than-normal duration without complications as indicated.

STATE OF CALIFORNIA

EMPLOYMENT DEVELOPMENT DEPARTMENT
P.O. Box 1529, Santa Barbara, CA 93102
(555) 963-9611

For Dept. Use Only

REFER TO

4920   - Our File No.   MEDICAL INQUIRY
Marcia M. Monroe   - Your Patient
Secretary   - Regular Work

David W. Smith, MD
4567 Broad Avenue
Woodland Hills, XY 12345

A review of the medical certificate received in conjunction with a claim for disability insurance benefits filed by your patient, named above, reveals that some additional information is needed in order to evaluate the claim properly. Your cooperation in answering the question or questions below and returning the form in the enclosed stamped and addressed envelope will be appreciated.

WM. C. SCHMIDT, MD, MEDICAL DIRECTOR

CLAIMS EXAMINER

What is the name and address of the facility that took the x-rays on this patient?

Speedy Radiology Service
4598 Main Street
Woodland Hills, XY 12345

Would the disclosure of this information to your patient be medically or psychologically detrimental to the patient: Yes ☐   No ☒

___October 24_____ 20XX   _David W. Smith MD_____
          Date   Doctor's Signature
SE   David W. Smith, MD

DE 2547A Rev. 10 (9-84)

Figure 15–7. Medical Inquiry Form DE 2547A. This form is mailed to the physician at any time during the life of the claim if any questions need to be answered or if the physician has failed to enter a prognosis date.

All follow-up correspondence should include the patient's name and Social Security number. The insurance billing specialist should promptly report any change of address, telephone number, or return-to-work date to the state disability insurance office. Patients must report any income received to the state disability insurance office because income received may affect benefits.

Conclusion

This chapter will end as it began—with a bit of levity. The following were taken from actual disability insurance application forms, completed by employees, that came across the desk of a claims adjuster.

Spelled as:	Should have been:
yellow "jonders"	yellow jaundice
"goalstones"	gallstones
"limp glands"	lymph glands
"falls teeth"	false teeth
"high pretension"	hypertension
"Pabst smear"	Pap smear
"wrecktum"	rectum

RESOURCES ON THE INTERNET

 Web sites pertaining to the law for nonindustrial disability insurance programs:
California   Unemployment   Insurance Code
www.edd.ca.gov/
Temporary Disability Benefits Law (New Jersey)
www.state.nj.us
Temporary Disability Insurance Act (Rhode Island)
www.state.ri.us
(Hawaii and Puerto Rico do not have Web sites.)

STUDENT ASSIGNMENT LIST

✔ Study Chapter 15.
✔ Answer the review questions in the *Workbook* to reinforce the theory learned in this chapter and to help prepare you for a future test.
✔ Complete the assignments in the *Workbook*. These assignments will provide you with hands-on experience in working with patient histories and completing disability insurance claim forms described in this chapter.
✔ Turn to the Glossary at the end of this textbook for a further understanding of the Key Terms used in this chapter.

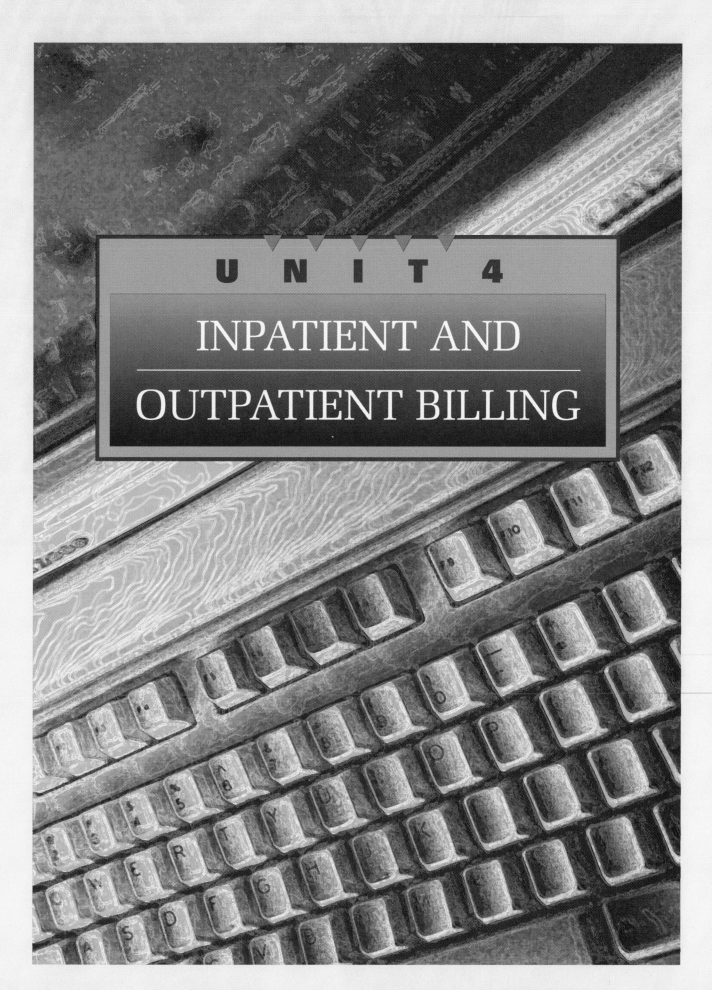

UNIT 4

INPATIENT AND

OUTPATIENT BILLING

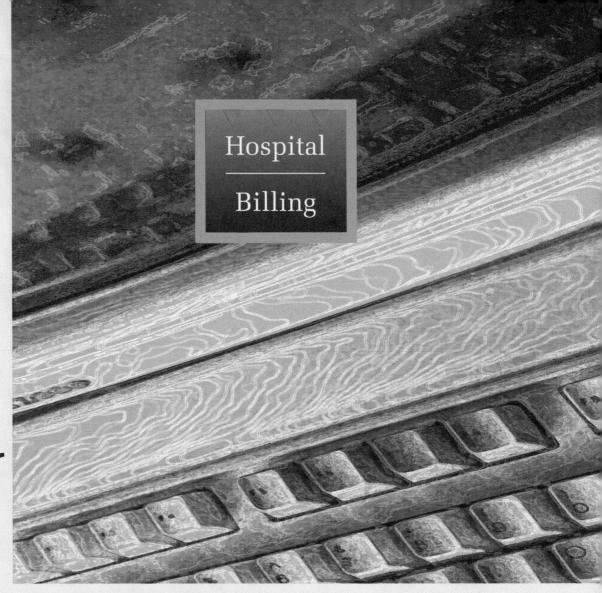

Hospital
Billing

16

CHAPTER OUTLINE

OBJECTIVES*

**After reading this chapter you
should be able to:**

■ Name qualifications
necessary to work in the
financial section of a
hospital.
■ Define appropriateness
evaluation protocols.
■ List criteria used for
admission screening.
■ Define the 72-hour rule.
■ Describe professional
review organizations and
their role in the hospital
reimbursement system.
■ Define common terms
related to hospital billing.
■ List instances of breach of
confidentiality in a hospital
setting.
■ State the role of ICD-9-CM
Volume 3 in hospital billing.
■ Identify categories in
ICD-9-CM Volume 3.
■ State reimbursement
methods made to hospitals
under managed care
contracts.
■ Explain the sequence of an
inpatient hospital stay from
billing through receipt of
payment.
■ Describe the charge
description master.
■ State when the Uniform Bill
(UB-92) claim form may and
may not be used.
■ Edit and complete insurance
claims in both hospital
inpatient and outpatient
settings to minimize their
rejection by insurance
carriers.
■ State the general guidelines
for completion of the
Uniform Bill (UB-92)
claim form.

■ Describe the history and
purpose of diagnosis-related
groups.
■ Identify how payment is
made based on
diagnosis-related groups.
■ State how payment is made
based on the ambulatory
payment classification
system.
■ Name the four types of
ambulatory payment
classifications.

KEY TERMS

admission review

ambulatory payment
classifications (APCs)

appropriateness evaluation
protocol (AEP)

capitation

case rate

charge description master
(CDM)

charges

clinical outliers

code sequence

comorbidity

cost outlier

cost outlier review

day outlier review

diagnosis-related groups
(DRGs)

DRG validation

DRG creep

elective surgery

grouper

inpatient

*International Classification
of Diseases, 9th Revision,
Clinical Modification
(ICD-9-CM)*

looping

major diagnostic categories
(MDCs)

Continued.

*Performance objectives and exercises for hands-on practical experience for this chapter
appear in the *Workbook*.

481

Patient Service Representative

Qualifications

A variety of jobs are available in the financial department and health information management (HIM) department, formerly known as the medical record department, of hospitals; therefore this chapter focuses on hospital inpatient and outpatient insurance billing and coding. Individuals who desire a position in a hospital facility business department should have knowledge and competence in the following subjects:

- ICD-9-CM diagnostic codes
- CPT and HCPCS procedure codes
- CMS-1500 insurance claim form
- Uniform Bill (UB-92) insurance claim form
- Explanation of benefits and remittance advice document
- Medical terminology
- Major health insurance programs
- Managed care plans
- Insurance claim submission
- Denied and delinquent claims

A hospital facility is larger than a clinic or private physician's office, so there is greater opportunity for advancement. An individual may be hired as an entry level coder, file clerk, or insurance verifier and advance from junior to senior clerk, insurance clerk, or patient service representative. He or she may continue to advance to an administrative position. Most hospital facilities have policies that encourage career growth by promoting jobs from within. Additional personal and physical qualifications are shown in Figure 16–1. Also refer to Chapter 1 for details on educational and training requirements and ethics and Chapter 17 for information on certification.

Primary Functions and Competencies

A generic job description for a patient service representative in a hospital business office whose primary function is to file hospital inpatient and outpatient claims with third-party payers is shown in Figure 16–1. Competencies for inpatient coding that were approved by the American Hospital Association, American Health Information Management Association, Centers for Medicare and Medicaid Services (formerly Health Care Financing Administration), and the National Center for Health Statistics are shown in Figure 16–2.

Principal Responsibilities

Because of the diversity in reimbursement methods, the insurance billing specialist must have basic knowledge of insurance programs and know how to use summary or cheat sheets, which give summaries of the contracts to correctly process each insurance claim. Accurate claim processing is essential for obtaining maximum reimbursement from the insurance company and when collecting payment from the patient. To remain an asset to employers, an insurance billing specialist must continually update his or her knowledge of coding and insurance program policies by attending seminars, workshops, classes, and in-house training. See Figure 16–1 for a list of principal responsibilities for a patient service representative.

POSITION DESCRIPTION

Title: Patient Service Representative   **Job Number: 215**
Department: Business Office   Effective Date: 3/1/00
Reports to: Patient Accounts Supervisor   Revision Date: 11/1/03

Primary Function:
To promptly file hospital inpatient and outpatient claims with third-party payers, following up in a timely and efficient manner, to ensure maximum reimbursement is received for services provided. To assist the public in obtaining full benefits from their coverage and in understanding billing procedures, always maintaining good public relations.

Principal Responsibilities:
1. Processes claims within assigned responsibility in a timely and efficient manner, performing all associated duties in order to ensure completeness and correctness of all claims information, facilitating maximum reimbursement.
   a. Analyzes, updates and corrects claim data according to established procedure.
   b. Inputs data accurately, efficiently and consistently.
   c. Performs work as scheduled, prioritizing as required for maximizing cash flow.
   d. Demonstrates thorough knowledge of third-party payers, claims requirements, UB-92 requirements by payer, computer capabilities as related to claims production, and admitting/medical records input as it affects claims.
2. Handles phone, mail and personal inquiries from and regarding patient accounts.
   a. Assists each person promptly, efficiently and courteously.
   b. Follows through on all issues identified as requiring action as a result of inquiry.
   c. Performs duties with a minimum of supervision, exhibits innovation and good judgment as well as thorough knowledge of ethical and legal billing procedures.
3. Performs related business office responsibilities as assigned by patient accounts manager.
   a. Follows hospital and department policies and procedures.
   b. Observes confidentiality in all matters.
   c. Maintains all documentation and records in accordance with federal and state regulations.
   d. Maintains good interdepartmental relations.
4. Provides coverage for A/R specialist 2 position for vacation and illness.
   a. Demonstrates knowledge of and ability to perform all duties and functions.
5. Participates in educational opportunities offered by hospital for job and personal development.
   a. Attends classes, workshops and seminars relating to billing/collection functions.
   b. Participates actively in such seminars, classes and workshops.
   c. Takes advantage of opportunities for personal growth and development as offered.
6. Takes an active role in facilitating team approach to functions within the department.
   a. Attends departmental meetings.
   b. Actively participates as team member in resolution of problems as they are identified.
   c. Analyzes current procedures, bringing suggestions for improvement to the attention of team members and supervisor for consideration.

Direction of Others:
Provides some direction to student learner. Number of persons supervised —1.

Qualifications:
High school graduation with 1–3 years experience in claims processing, business or accounting. Experience in health care field desirable.

Physical Qualifications:
These requirements may be met with the aid of mechanical devices and are those minimally necessary for safe completion of duties. They are not intended to discriminate against handicapped persons, only to ensure safe working conditions for all persons.
1. Must be able to enter data into a computer and effectively operate a 10-key adding machine.
2. Must be able to communicate in a pleasant and tactful manner to other employees and patients.
3. Must pass a pre-employment physical examination.

Working Conditions:
Normal office working conditions.

Department approval: _____ Date: _____

Administrative approval: _____ Date: _____

Human resources approval: _____ Date: _____

Figure 16–1. Job description for Patient Service Representative (hospital biller). (From Linda Goselin, *Questions and Answers: Job Descriptions Provide Guidelines for Employees/Managers: Get It in Writing,* Health Care Biller, Vol 4, No 6, Aspen Publishers, Inc., 1995.)

AMERICAN HEALTH INFORMATION MANAGEMENT ASSOCIATION
ICD-9-CM INPATIENT CODING COMPETENCIES

ICD-9-CM - International Classification of Diseases - 9th revision - Clinical Modification, Volumes 1 and 2,
Superintendent of Documents, US Government Printing Office, PO Box 371954,
Pittsburgh, PA 15250-7954, (202) 783-3238.
Volume 3, American Health Information Management Association, 919 N. Michigan Avenue,
Suite 1400, Chicago, IL 60611, (312) 787-2672.

1. Read and interpret medical record documentation to identify all diagnoses, and significant procedures that affect the current inpatient stay.

2. Assess the adequacy of medical record documentation to ensure that it supports all diagnoses and procedures assigned codes.

3. Clarify conflicting, ambiguous or non-specific information appearing in a medical record by consulting the appropriate physician.

4. Apply Uniform Hospital Discharge Data Set definitions to select the principal diagnosis, principal procedure, complications and comorbid conditions, other diagnoses and significant procedures which require coding.

5. Exclude from coding diagnoses or procedures related to an earlier episode of care which have no bearing on the current episode of care.

6. Exclude from coding nonsurgical, noninvasive procedures which carry no operative or anesthetic risk.

7. Exclude from coding information, such as symptoms or signs characteristic of the diagnosis, findings from diagnostic studies, or localized conditions, which has no bearing on the current management of the patient.

8. Apply knowledge of ICD-9-CM instructional notations and conventions to locate and assign the correct diagnostic and procedural codes and sequence them correctly.

9. Apply knowledge of current approved* ICD-9-CM coding guidelines to assign and sequence the correct diagnosis and procedure codes.

10. Apply knowledge of anatomy, clinical disease processes, and diagnostic and procedural terminology to assign accurate codes to diagnoses and procedures.

11. Select the appropriate principal diagnosis for episodes of care in which determination of the principal diagnosis is not clear-cut because the patient has multiple problems.

12. Apply knowledge of disease processes to assign non-indexed medical terms to the appropriate class in the classification system.

13. Facilitate comprehensive retrieval by recognizing when more than one code is required to adequately classify a given condition.

14. Apply knowledge of prospective payment system to confirm DRG assignment which ensures optimal reimbursement.

15. Refuse to fraudulently maximize reimbursement by assigning codes that do not conform to approved coding principles/guidelines.

16. Conduct quality assessment to ensure continuous improvement in ICD-9-CM coding and collection of quality health data.

*ICD-9-CM coding guidelines approved by the cooperating parties (American Hospital Association, American Health Information Management Association, Health Care Financing Administration, and National Center for Health Statistics) are published in *Coding Clinic for ICD-9-CM*, a quarterly publication of the Central Office on ICD-9-CM at the American Hospital Association.

January 1, 1992

Figure 16–2. ICD-9-CM Inpatient Coding Competencies. (From the American Health Information Management Association, Chicago, IL, as published in Coding Clinic for ICD-9-CM, January 1, 1992.)

HIPAA Compliance Alert
Medicolegal Confidentiality Issues

Documents

The patient's financial and medical records and any photographs are legal documents and must be kept confidential (see Chapter 3). They may not be released unless a patient has signed an authorization form to make the information public. An exception is when a medical record is subpoenaed by the court. Chapter 3 contains information on confidentiality when facsimile communication is used. When work is done in a sensitive area of a facility, document shredders should be used to destroy unwanted documents and prevent violations of confidentiality.

EXAMPLE 16-1

MEDICAL RECORD SCENARIO

An insurance billing specialist working at home has a sister who was hospitalized to undergo major surgery and wants to help his or her parents better understand the medical condition. The specialist calls a friend in the hospital billing department and asks that person to make photocopies of a document in the medical record.

COMMENT
Remember that all medical reports are confidential, so the employee must deny the request unless the sister signs a release of information that would authorize her family to have copies of the document.

EXAMPLE 16-2

FINANCIAL RECORD SCENARIO

An experienced insurance billing specialist applies for a job. At an interview, he or she presents some samples of typed insurance claims that include hospital and patient names.

COMMENT
This indicates that the prospective employee has taken data from a former employer's facility and violated the patient's confidentiality by not removing the names in the samples.

Examples 16–1 and 16–2 show breaches of confidentiality with medical and financial records.

Verbal Communication

In a hospital or office setting, verbal breaches of confidentiality may occur that could result in an insurance billing specialist being held liable and the facility being sued. New employees should be given a confidentiality orientation and asked to sign a confidentiality statement. This statement should emphasize that the employee may be subject to immediate termination in the event of a violation. Any one of the following scenarios in which the patient's right to privacy has been breached in the hospital setting may be encountered by an insurance billing specialist (Examples 16–3 through 16–6).

Computer Security

When using a computer, adhere to hospital policies with respect to the following:

▸ Use of passwords and other encryption methods
▸ Policies for composition and transmission of electronic mail
▸ Policies for use of the fax machine

EXAMPLE 16-3

A coding clerk overhears two hospital employees discussing a patient by name. Because the clerk had been working on the medical record of that patient and is now familiar with the patient's history, he or she realizes that the information being discussed is not accurate. The coding clerk then interrupts, making a comment about the patient's diagnosis.

COMMENT
Information should not be discussed with coworkers or other hospital employees and must never be related to anyone other than a person who has a valid need to provide care for the patient.

EXAMPLE 16-4

A Marilyn Monroe impersonator is discharged from the hospital after receiving plastic surgery. Over dinner at home, an insurance billing specialist relates the diagnosis and name of the surgery to his or her spouse.

COMMENT
Never discuss confidential information about patients to family or friends.

EXAMPLE 16-5

In reviewing an insurance claim before it is mailed, the insurance billing specialist realizes that he or she knows the individual who has a diagnosis that indicates a mental condition. The specialist discusses this with a coworker.

COMMENT
This is a violation because a hospital employee must never give anyone information on a patient's diagnosis.

EXAMPLE 16-6

A physician in private practice calls via cellular telephone to the billing clerk to answer a question about the diagnosis to be listed on a patient's insurance claim.

COMMENT
Cellular transmission may be intercepted by anyone with inexpensive eavesdropping equipment. In this scenario, a traditional telephone line must be used when relating confidential information about a patient's diagnosis. The physician should verify if he or she is speaking to the billing clerk.

▶ Downloading of computer data from one department to another

▶ Length of time that documents may be retained on computer hard drives by employees

▶ Procedures for deletion of confidential information

▶ Procedures for archiving of data

▶ Closing out when leaving a workstation or desk

Admission Procedures

Appropriateness Evaluation Protocols

A patient is considered an **inpatient** on admission to the hospital for an overnight stay. **Appropriateness evaluation protocols (AEPs)** must be met to certify that patients' complaints warrant admittance to the hospital. Specific criteria are used by the insurance company for admission screening. The Medicare prospective payment system (PPS) requires that all patients meet at least one severity of illness (SI) or intensity of service (IS) criterion, unless otherwise indicated, to be certified for reimbursement. Within the first 24 hours, the hospital's utilization review (UR) department analyzes the documentation on the medical record, which must reflect how the patient meets these criteria. UR is discussed in detail later in this chapter. A list of AEPs is provided in Figure 16–3.

Admitting Procedures for Major Insurance Programs

The admitting process varies according to rules set down by the patient's insurance plan. Following are basic admitting procedures and preadmission authorization requirements for the major insurance programs.

Private Insurance (Group or Individual)

It is the responsibility of the outpatient and inpatient admitting personnel to obtain complete and accurate information during initial registration of the patient. The patient must provide a current insurance card or cards. Obtain photocopies of the front and back of all cards. Some hospital facilities employ an insurance verification clerk. He or she has the responsibility of contacting the insurance company or the insured individual's employer to verify the type of insurance. The clerk also must call the insurance company to verify eligibility and benefits and determine whether prior authorization is needed.

Managed Care

There may be restrictions and various policies and procedures to follow when admitting a patient who has a managed care

---

APPROPRIATENESS EVALUATION PROTOCOL CRITERIA FOR ADMISSION CERTIFICATION

An admission may be certified if one of the following criteria is met:

SEVERITY OF ILLNESS (SI)
1. Sudden onset of unconsciousness or disorientation (coma or unresponsiveness).
2. Pulse rate <50 or >140.
3. Systolic blood pressure <80 or >200 mm Hg. Diastolic blood pressure <60 or >120 mm Hg.
4. Sudden onset of loss of sight or hearing.
5. History of persistent fever ≥ 100° F (orally) or 101° F (rectally) for more than 5 days or with white blood cell count >15,000/mm³.
6. Sudden onset of motor function loss of any body part.
7. Active, uncontrolled bleeding.
8. Electrolyte or blood gas abnormality of serum K^+: <2.5, >6.0; serum Na^+ <123, >156; CO_2 <20 mEq/L, >36 mEq/L (new findings).
9. Acute or progressive sensory, motor, circulatory, or respiratory embarrassment sufficient to incapacitate the patient (one of the IS criteria must also be met).
10. Electrocardiographic evidence of acute ischemia with suspicion of new myocardial infarction.
11. Wound dehiscence or evisceration.

INTENSITY OF SERVICE (IS)
12. Administration and monitoring of intravenous medications and/or fluid replacement (does not include tube feeding).
13. Surgery or procedure scheduled within 24 hours requiring general or regional anesthesia with use of equipment and facilities available only in a hospital.
14. Vital sign monitoring at least every 2 hours, including telemetry and bedside cardiac monitoring.
15. Use of chemotherapeutic agents that require continuous observation for a life-threatening toxic reaction.
16. Treatment in intensive/coronary care unit.
17. Administration of intramuscular antibiotics at least every 8 hours.
18. Intermittent or continuous respirator use at least every 8 hours.
19. Documentation on the medical record by the attending physician that the patient has been unsuccessfully treated as an outpatient *with* further documentation of how the patient is now to be treated as an inpatient.

Figure 16–3. Appropriateness evaluation protocol criteria for admission certification listing severity of illness and intensity of service.

---

health maintenance organization (HMO) or preferred provider organization (PPO) type of insurance. Obtain photocopies of the front and back sides of the identification card. Several types of patient admissions to the hospital are recognized by managed care plans. See Chapter 10 for further information on this subject.

Emergency Inpatient Admission

Hospital With Contract.   A patient is seen in the emergency department, and the physician determines that it is necessary to admit the patient to the hospital. The managed care program should be notified the next working day or within 48 hours to obtain an authorization number. The plan authorizes the first days of the admission automatically and approves subsequent days based on utilization review. The review organization determines the emergency status and may send written notification to the hospital and physician. The patient may have a deductible and copayment requirement. Emergency department charges are billed with charges for the inpatient stay on the Uniform Bill (UB-92) claim form. The physician's professional services for a patient seen in the emergency department are submitted on the CMS-1500 insurance claim form.

Hospital Without Contract.   The managed care program of emergency admission should be notified on the next working day to obtain an authorization number. The patient should be prepared for transfer to a contracting hospital if necessary. The patient may have the option of staying and paying the deductible, copayment, or entire bill and not file a claim with the managed care plan. The managed care plan may or may not cover any charges depending on the type of plan. However, some plans with deductibles and copayments cover certain charges.

Nonemergency Inpatient Admission

Hospital With Contract.   The patient must be referred by his or her primary care physician and obtain authorization for the length of the hospital stay. The patient may have a copayment requirement.

Hospital Without Contract.   The patient may request authorization with a noncontracted hospital; however, the patient is responsible for a higher deductible and copayment or the entire bill.

Admission to a Participating Hospital

An attending participating physician contacts the insurance plan at least 3 days before admission to give notification of a member's proposed *elective admission*. If a preadmission review is necessary, the physician is responsible for obtaining prior authorization from the review organization or the managed care contract authorization. The physician calls the hospital to relay information about the patient for admitting purposes.

Admission to a Nonparticipating Hospital

An attending physician contacts the designated review organization for admission approval in a non-emergency situation. Within 1 working day of approved requests for prior authorization, the review organization calls the physician and hospital and assigns a control number that certifies approval of the admission. The review organization furnishes the physician and hospital with an approved preadmission or referral request form.

Medicaid

A treatment authorization request form should be approved before elective admissions. For an emergency, preapproval is not necessary; however, a retroactive form is needed before the claim is billed. Photocopies of the front and back of the patient's identification card should be obtained or eligibility verified via touchtone telephone, modem, or specialized Medicaid terminal equipment. See Chapter 12 for additional information.

Medicare

Medicare patients do not need prior approval for admission to a hospital. However, their admittance should be certified by AEPs, as previously discussed in this chapter. Photocopies of the front and back of the patient's identification cards should be obtained for Medicare and any supplemental or secondary insurance policies. A *common working file* is used to verify coverage, look up information, and bill Medicare. For patients who receive both Medicare and Medicaid benefits, the claims are considered crossover claims. The claim form is processed automatically by Medicaid (in California Medi-Cal) after processing is completed by Medicare. See Chapter 11 for detailed data on the Medicare program.

TRICARE and CHAMPVA

As stated in Chapter 13, all admissions to a civilian hospital and ambulatory surgical facility require precertification. The health care finder assists with this process when a military treatment hospital is not available. Precertification should be verified; photocopies of the front and back of the patient's identification card should be obtained or eligibility verified via touchtone telephone or modem. See Chapter 13 for additional information.

Workers' Compensation

The patient does not have an insurance card in a workers' compensation case. When the patient is seen on an emergency basis, an employer's report of injury must be completed and sent to the insurance company and the state industrial accident board before a hospital or physician's insurance claim may be submitted. A case number is assigned. Appropriate information relating to the injured patient, industrial accident, insurance carrier, and employer must be obtained. The insurance adjuster must authorize admission, length of stay, and all surgical procedures for an elective admission. See Chapter 14 for further details on this subject.

Preadmission Testing

To obtain necessary diagnostic information, reduce inpatient expenses, and eliminate extra hospital days, a patient is usually sent to the hospital for **preadmission testing (PAT)** before being admitted for major surgery. Preadmission tests include diagnostic studies, such as laboratory tests, chest x-ray films, and electrocardiography. When a laboratory panel of tests is performed, each separate test must be itemized and must show the clinical benefit for each test performed based on the patient's diagnosis. In capitation cases, preadmission services are done in the physician's office and are bundled with hospital services instead of appearing as separate charges on inpatient or outpatient bills.

Medicare 72-Hour Rule

One of the most important regulations in hospital billing is compliance with the Center for Medicare and Medicaid Services' *72-hour rule,* also called the 3-day payment window rule. The Medicare rule states that if a patient receives diagnostic tests and hospital outpatient services within 72 hours of admission to a hospital (3-day payment window), then all such tests and services are combined with inpatient services. The preadmission services become part of the diagnosis-related group (DRG) payment to the hospital and may not be billed or paid separately. This is valid if the services (including emergency department services) are considered related to the reason for admission. If a hospital owns or operates a physician office that provides diagnostic or other services related to the admission within 3 days of subsequent inpatient admission, the services must be included in the DRG payment. If this rule is not followed, fraud and abuse may be considered and a penalty in the form of a fine or imprisonment may be carried out.

Exceptions to the 72-Hour Rule

The following are exceptions to the 72-hour rule:

⬤ Services provided by home health agencies, hospice, nursing facilities (NFs), and ambulance services

⬤ Physician's professional portion of a diagnostic service (the technical portion of a diagnostic service must be included in the inpatient bill)

⬤ Preadmission testing at an independent laboratory when the laboratory has no formal agreement with the health care facility

For patients with private insurance (non–Medicare) receiving tests within 24 hours of hospital admission, include such tests with inpatient billing.

HIPAA Compliance Alert

Compliance Safeguards

Problems develop when billing for the physician's office is done on a separate billing system, which makes it difficult to match the outpatient services with subsequent inpatient hospital admission billed by the hospital's system. Ideally a facility should have a computer editing program that searches for any outpatient services given within the time frame before admission, or both sides should have integrated information systems. If not, the admitting clerk must ask patients if they have received any medical service in the past 3 days. Another solution is to have a postsubmission review program that searches outpatient claims and generates a quarterly report identifying the outpatient and inpatient accounts that overlap. This can be manually reviewed; if an overpayment is found, it can be refunded to the insurance program.

Utilization Review

Each hospital should have a **utilization review (UR)** department that conducts an admission and concurrent review and prepares a discharge plan on all cases. This process determines whether admissions are justified, anticipates length of stay (LOS), and concludes the expected discharge date. If the admission is found to be necessary, it is certified.

There also are UR companies that provide utilization review and case management services for self-insured employers, third-party administrators, and insurance companies. They furnish data to the person who buys their services to achieve saving dollars, and generate reports on how much money has been saved.

Peer Review Organization

Under the PPS, responsibility for maintaining quality of care is delegated to peer review organizations, sometimes referred to as **professional review organizations (PROs).** The Peer Review Improvement Act of 1982 authorized the establishment of PROs in geographic areas across the nation. PROs are composed of licensed doctors of medicine or osteopathy actively engaged in the practice of medicine or surgery. Working under federal guidelines, these physicians evaluate other physicians about quality of professional care, as well as other factors. The PROs are responsible for the following types of review:

▶ **Admission review** for appropriateness and necessity of admissions.
▶ **Readmission review** on patients readmitted within 7 days with problems related to the first admission to determine whether the first discharge was premature or the second admission is medically necessary.
▶ **Procedure review** of diagnostic and therapeutic procedures in cases in which past abuses have been found, to determine appropriateness.
▶ **Day outlier review** of short or unusually long length of hospital stays to determine the number of days before the day outlier threshold is reached, as well as the number of days beyond the threshold. This process is done to certify necessity of admission and medical necessity of services for additional Medicare reimbursement.
▶ **Cost outlier review** of cases not eligible for day outlier review to determine the necessity of admission and the necessity and appropriateness of services rendered.
▶ **DRG validation** to find out whether the diagnostic and procedural information affecting DRG assignment is substantiated by the clinical information in the patient's chart. DRGs are discussed later in this chapter.
▶ **Transfer review** of cases involving a transfer to a distinct part or unit of the same hospital or other hospitals.

Hospitals contract with a PRO for Medicare reimbursement. If a hospital does not have a PRO contract, it will not receive payment from Medicare.

Coding Hospital Procedures

Current Procedural Terminology (CPT), Medicare's Health Care Financing Administration Common Procedure Coding System (HCPCS), and the three volumes of *International Classification of Diseases, Ninth Revision, Clinical Modification* **(ICD-9-CM)** are used to list codes on hospital insurance claims. In lieu of the books, computer software programs are available that contain the same data to locate the codes accurately, quickly, and easily. Different code books are used to code an insurance claim when a patient receives services as an outpatient or inpatient. They are the following:

▶ *Outpatient* hospital insurance claims use CPT codes for procedures and ICD-9-CM, Volumes 1 and 2, for diagnoses.
▶ *Inpatient* hospital insurance claims use ICD-9-CM, Volumes 1 and 2, for diagnoses and Volume 3 for procedures. (Some private insurance companies are requesting CPT codes.)

Chapter 4 gives basic information and instructions on how to use Volumes 1 and 2. This chapter explains the use of Volume 3. Chapter 5 gives information on CPT and HCPCS procedure codes.

Outpatient—Reason for Visit

The patient's *reason for the visit* is listed for outpatient claims rather than the patient's principal diagnosis; for example, the reason for the outpatient visit may be chest pain but anxiety could be listed as the final outpatient diagnosis.

Inpatient—Principal Diagnosis

The **principal diagnosis** is the condition that is assigned a code representing the diagnosis established after study that is chiefly responsible for the admission of the patient to the hospital. This is the most important code; therefore be sure the code for the principal diagnosis is listed first. For example, heart disease is the principal diagnosis if a patient initially comes in for heart transplantation. However, pneumonia is the principal diagnosis if the heart transplant patient goes home and then comes back to the hospital with pneumonia. Subsequent diagnostic codes should be used for any current coexisting concurrent condition (comorbidity), a condition that coexists with the principal condition, complicating the treatment and management of the principal disorder and that is documented in the record. These codes are sequenced after the principal diagnosis. Codes for conditions that were previously treated and no longer exist should not be included. A secondary diagnosis is one that may contribute to the condition, treatment, or recovery from the condition shown as the principal diagnosis. It also may define the need for a higher level of care but is not the underlying cause. The diagnostic **code sequence** (correct order) is very important in billing of hospital inpatient cases because maximum reimbursement is based on the DRGs system. This is explained in detail at the end of this chapter.

Rules for Coding Inpatient Diagnoses

There are some differences between coding diagnoses for inpatient and outpatient cases. One important difference is how *uncertain diagnoses* are coded. For inpatient cases, code all "rule out," "suspected," "likely," "questionable," "possible," or "still to be ruled out" as if it existed. For example, the physician documents upper abdominal pain, rule out cholecystitis. Assign code 575.0 (cholecystitis) for this diagnosis. This rule applies to inpatient records only.

In addition, the following rules and examples should be noted about the principal diagnosis.

▶ Codes for signs and symptoms of ICD-9-CM are not reported as principal diagnoses (Example 16–7).

EXAMPLE 16–7

PRINCIPAL DIAGNOSIS/SIGNS AND SYMPTOMS

Mr. Brown was admitted to the hospital with fever, severe abdominal pain, nausea, and vomiting.

Diagnosis: Acute appendicitis
Dx Code: 540.9 (acute appendicitis without peritonitis)
Note: Symptoms are considered integral to the condition so the condition should be coded.

▶ When two or more conditions meet the definition of principal diagnosis, either condition may be sequenced first unless otherwise indicated by the circumstances of admission or the therapy provided (Example 16–8).

EXAMPLE 16–8

TWO MEDICAL CONDITIONS

Mrs. Sanchez was admitted with acute congestive heart failure (CHF) and unstable angina. Both conditions are treated.

Diagnosis: CHF and unstable angina
Dx Code: 428.0 (CHF) or 411.1 (unstable angina)
Either code may be used.
Note: This is the focus of many compliance reviews.

▶ When a symptom is followed by a contrasting comparative diagnosis, sequence the symptom code first (Example 16–9).

Conditions that are an integral part of a documented disease process should not be coded; abnormal findings should not be coded unless the physician indicates their clinical significance.

The physician should be made aware that certain principal diagnoses are subject to 100% review by the review agency. The physician should pay special

---

EXAMPLE 16–9

SYMPTOM AS PRINCIPAL DIAGNOSIS

Miss Chan was admitted with acute epigastric abdominal pain.

Diagnosis: Epigastric abdominal pain, acute pyelonephritis versus acute gastritis.
Dx Code: 789.06 (epigastric abdominal pain)
590.10 (acute pyelonephritis)
535.00 (acute gastritis without hemorrhage)
Note: Code symptoms first followed by conditional diagnoses.

---

attention in using the following as principal diagnoses:

1. Arteriosclerotic heart disease (ASHD). This is acceptable as a diagnosis only when cardiac catheterization or open heart surgery is performed.
2. Diabetes mellitus without complications
3. Right or left bundle branch block
4. Coronary atherosclerosis

Local hospital health information management personnel should be contacted periodically to find out whether new items have been added to this list.

Coding Inpatient Procedures

ICD-9-CM Volume 3 Procedures

ICD-9-CM Volume 3, which is not used in physician's offices or outpatient hospital billing, is used for the inpatient hospital setting. This volume combines both the alphabetic and tabular lists for the classification of surgical and nonsurgical procedures and miscellaneous therapeutic and diagnostic procedures. Some editions of ICD-9-CM may contain Volumes 1, 2, and 3 in one book.

Tabular List

The tabular list is divided into chapters that relate to operations or procedures for various body systems, with the last chapter referring to miscellaneous diagnostic, therapeutic, and prophylactic procedures. Procedure codes are two digits at the category code level with one or two digits beyond the decimal point. The third and fourth digits differentiate between unilateral or bilateral, surgical approach or techniques, and among condition types (e.g., indirect and direct hernia). No alphabetic characters are used. All four digits must be listed when a three-digit code is followed by a fourth digit. Chapter categories are as follows:

Chapter 1 Operations on the Nervous System	Codes 01–05
Chapter 2 Operations on the Endocrine System	Codes 06–07

Chapter 3 Operations on the Eye   Codes 08–16
Chapter 4 Operations on the Ear   Codes 18–20
Chapter 5 Operations on the Nose,   Codes 21–29
Mouth, and Pharynx
Chapter 6 Operations on the   Codes 30–34
Respiratory System
Chapter 7 Operations on the   Codes 35–39
Cardiovascular System
Chapter 8 Operations on the Hemic   Codes 40–41
and Lymphatic System
Chapter 9 Operations on the   Codes 42–54
Digestive System
Chapter 10 Operations on the   Codes 55–59
Urinary System
Chapter 11 Operations on the Male   Codes 60–64
Genital System
Chapter 12 Operations on the   Codes 65–71
Female Genital System
Chapter 13 Obstetrical Procedures   Codes 72–75
Chapter 14 Operations on the   Codes 76–84
Musculoskeletal System
Chapter 15 Operations on the   Codes 85–86
Integumentary System
Chapter 16 Miscellaneous Diagnostic   Codes 87–99
and Therapeutic Procedures

Alphabetic Index

The Alphabetic Index is arranged by procedure (e.g., incision, excision, graft, or implant) and not anatomic site. It is used to locate the procedure that is referred to as the main term. Read any notations that appear under the main term in bold type. A main term may be followed by modifiers (e.g., a series of subterms in parentheses) that give differences in site or surgical technique (Example 16–10).

EXAMPLE 16–10

MAIN DIAGNOSTIC TERM

Amputation (cineplastic) (closed flap) (guillotine) (kineplastic) (open) 84.91

An operation named for a person is termed an *eponym.* Such names are listed both as main terms and under the main term "operation." The description of the procedure or anatomic site follows the eponym (Example 16–11).

EXAMPLE 16–11

EPONYMS

Billroth II operation (partial gastrectomy with gastro-jejunostomy) 43.7
Operation
Billroth II (partial gastrectomy with gastroduodenostomy) 43.6

PROCEDURE: Coding from Volume 3

Basic steps in coding from Volume 3 are:
1. Locate the main term (procedure) in the Alphabetical Index.
2. Read all modifiers (descriptive notations relating to the condition).
3. Obtain the code number and refer to the Tabular List (Volume 3) to verify that the code number selected matches the description of the procedure. Never code using only the Alphabetical Index because important instructions may appear in the Tabular List.
4. Note any exclusions, inclusions, remarks concerning fourth digits, colons, and any other information that may affect the choice of codes. Notice "code also" and "omit code" instructions.
5. Select the appropriate code number. Use fourth digit codes and, if necessary, apply two or more code numbers to completely describe a procedure (Example 16–12).

EXAMPLE 16–12

VOLUME 3 CODE NUMBERS

Procedure: Complete vaginal hysterectomy with bilateral salpingectomy

CODE	DESCRIPTION
68.5	Vaginal hysterectomy
66.51	Removal of both fallopian tubes at same operative episode

---

Coding Outpatient Procedures

Current Procedural Terminology

An up-to-date edition of CPT, the code book published by the American Medical Association, is used to list procedural codes on outpatient hospital insurance claims for hospital services. Chapter 5 gives basic information and instruction on how to use the code book. These codes are updated during each year. Billing software must be updated with new codes to receive maximum reimbursement.

Health Care Common Procedure Coding System

The HCPCS (pronounced "hick-picks") is used to obtain procedural codes for Medicare and some non–Medicare patients on outpatient hospital insurance claims that are not in the CPT code book (e.g., supplies, equipment rental, and drugs administered other than oral method [injectables, inhalants, and chemotherapeutics]). Chapters 5 and 11 give basic information on the three levels of this code system.

Modifiers

Refer to Chapter 5 for a detailed explanation of modifier use. Selected CPT level I modifiers that generally are used for outpatient hospital billing are:

-27 Multiple outpatient hospital E/M encounters on the same date
-50 Bilateral procedure
-52 Reduced services
-59 Distinct procedural service
-73 Discontinued outpatient procedure before anesthesia administration
-74 Discontinued outpatient procedure after anesthesia administration
-76 Repeat procedure by same physician
-77 Repeat procedure by another physician
-91 Repeat clinical diagnostic laboratory test HCPCS Level II alphanumeric modifiers

Inpatient Billing Process

The insurance billing division is often part of the hospital's business office and may be placed near the admission department, hospital cashier, or main lobby (entry and exit) of the hospital because patients need easy access. In some facilities, the financial department may be so large that it is relocated to a building at another site. The inpatient billing process involves many people and departments in the hospital. As an introduction, Figure 16–4 shows which main departments of the hospital interact as the billing process flows from beginning to end. Following are explanations of each hospital employee's role in this process.

Admitting Clerk

An admitting clerk registers the patient by interviewing and obtaining personal (demographic) and insurance information and admitting diagnosis or symptoms. There is no law requiring that a person give his or her real name on admission. High-profile individuals often give fictitious names. In some facilities, there may be a preadmission surgery form from which data are obtained for elective surgery. The admitting clerk position may be outsourced, and he or she may gather information via telephone from home for patients being admitted for elective procedures.

The patient is assigned a *patient control number* at this time. This is a unique number given for each hospital admission, and a new number is assigned for subsequent admissions. The patient's account contains this number and all charges and payments are posted to this number for the account. Copies of the admitting face sheet, which is similar to the patient registration information form, are sent to the primary care physician or surgeon's office. Registration information, copies of all authorization and signature documents, a copy of the insurance card(s), and a copy of the emergency department report if the patient is admitted through the emergency department are scanned in paperless facilities or assembled in a financial folder in facilities using a traditional system.

Insurance Verifier

An *insurance verifier,* who may work either at the hospital or from home, reads the photocopied insurance identification card and telephones the patient or physician for needed data. The insurance verifier's primary responsibility is to telephone the insurance plan to verify eligibility, predetermine coverage, and obtain authorization if necessary. In a workers' compensation case, the verifier may telephone the employer or insurance adjuster for needed data.

Attending Physician, Nursing Staff, and Medical Transcriptionist

The patient is taken to the hospital department that is providing the outpatient service or, if an inpatient, to his or her hospital room. Generally it is the attending physician's responsibility to dictate a history and physical (H&P) on admission that lists the admitting diagnosis. A medical transcriptionist transcribes the dictation into a report form. The attending physician and nurses enter daily notations on the patient's medical record as the patient receives medical

HOSPITAL BILLING PROCESS

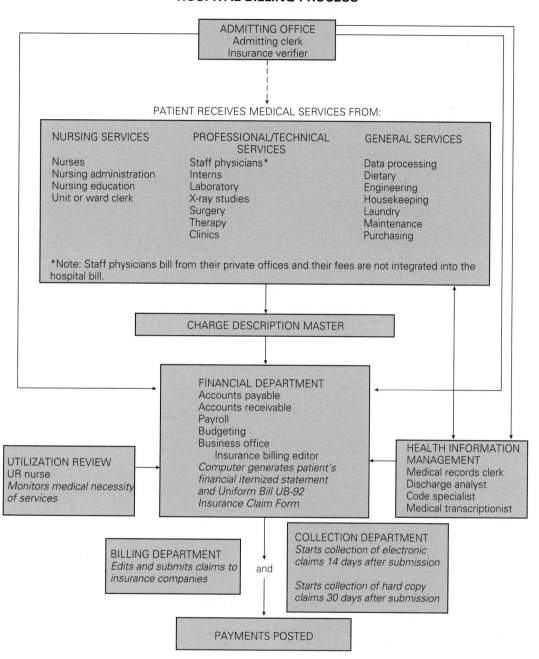

Figure 16–4. Basic flow of the hospital billing process for an inpatient.

services. A unit secretary or ward clerk inputs the physician's orders by use of a computer that electronically transmits them to other departments (e.g., pharmacy, laboratory, and radiology). A hand-held computer may be used in some hospitals. If supplies are used, stickers are removed from the supply item and scanned to record data. The attending physician supplies documentation for all medical and surgical reports, ending the patient's stay with a discharge summary that sometimes is known as a *clinical resume* or *final progress note.* This document is transcribed by the medical transcriptionist and includes

the course of treatment during the hospital stay, all diagnostic studies, consultations, admission and discharge diagnoses, operations performed, condition of patient at the time of discharge, instructions for continuing care and follow-up treatment, and time frame for postoperative office visit.

Discharge Analyst

A *discharge analyst* checks the completeness of each patient's medical record for dictated reports and signatures. He or she completes a deficiency sheet that is put on the medical record indicating any documentation deficiencies. Hospitals bill for services only after the discharge summary is completed and signed by the physician. Ideally hospital charts should be completed within 3 to 4 days, and no more than 14 days, after the patient is discharged; otherwise a cash flow problem will result. The office medical assistant can help by scheduling the physician's time so that medical records can be completed.

Charge Description Master

All services and items provided to the patient are keyed into a computer system to assist with a high volume of billing for services received by hospital patients. This may occur in one of two ways:

1. A designated person in each hospital department keys in all services and procedures using an internal code. This is referred to as *order entry*.
2. A charge sheet that has services and procedures checked off may be sent to the data processing department where a data processor keys in the information using the internal code. These services, coded with an internal code, link up in a computer system called a **charge description master (CDM)**. This is commonly referred to as a "charge master" and includes the following data:
   a. *Procedure code.* CPT and HCPCS codes appear on detail bill, outpatient bill, outpatient Uniform Bill claim form UB-92, but not usually on the inpatient UB-92 claim form.
   b. *Procedure description.* Detailed narrative of each procedure (surgery, laboratory test, and radiologic test).
   c. *Service description.* Detailed narrative of each service (evaluation and management, observation, emergency department visits, and clinical visits).
   d. *Charge.* Dollar amount for each procedure or service. This is a standard fee for the item and not the actual amount paid by a third-party payer.
   e. *Revenue code.* Three-digit code number representing a specific accommodation, ancillary service, or billing calculation related to service.

The master charge list or charge description list is a computer file unique to each hospital that accommodates the charges for items and services that may be provided to patients. The content and format of the charge master varies among facilities, but the function remains the same.

Thus charges may be easily compiled via computer from all hospital departments that furnished services to the patient. For institutional facilities (e.g., inpatient and outpatient departments, rural health clinics, chronic dialysis services, and adult day health care), each patient's data consisting of revenue codes, procedure codes, descriptions, charges, and medical record data are organized by the charge description master and printed onto a hospital Uniform Bill claim form, the UB-92.

The charge master database must be kept current and accurate to obtain proper reimbursement. It must be regularly audited; otherwise negative impacts, such as overpayment, underpayment, undercharging for services, claims rejections, fines, or penalties, may result. A committee may oversee maintenance of the charge master composed of experts in coding, billing regulations, clinical procedures, and health record documentation. Because this system often is accomplished without human intervention, there is a high risk that a single coding or mapping error could replicate and many errors could occur before identified and corrected.

Usually there is a lag time (e.g., 4 days after patient discharge) before the bill is "dropped" by the charge master to be sure that all charges have been entered.

Code Specialist

The chart is given to health information management, which is directed or managed by a Registered Health Information Administrator (RHIA). In some situations, an RHIA may act as a consultant to several hospitals and may not be employed by one hospital. This department is also composed of a discharge analyst, some code specialists, and some medical records clerks who may be Registered Health Information Technicians (RHITs). A *medical record number* is assigned at this time. The medical record number never changes (even on future admits), and all records are compiled under this number.

An HIM coder abstracts procedures and diagnoses from the medical record and assigns codes. It is possible that the coder may use an *encoder* to perform this function. As learned, an encoder is a computer software program that assigns a code to represent data. Refer to Chapter 7 for detailed information.

Coding Credentials

Accuracy of coding impacts the financial viability of acute care hospitals. The coder, whose job is highly analytical, not only should abstract information from the medical record and assign the correct code but also should guard against the most common errors of transposing numbers and leaving off fourth and fifth digits from diagnostic codes. A majority of coders in the hospital setting have credentials and have earned an Associate of Arts (AA) degree. A number of different professional organizations that offer certification for coders are mentioned in Chapter 17.

Insurance Billing Editor

The UB-92 claim form is then generated and reviewed by an insurance billing editor before it is generated or sent to the appropriate insurance company to obtain payment. Editing claims is a vital skill that is gained from hands-on experience. Information from the patient's financial data may be compared to verify insurance information. The UB-92 is considered a *summary statement* compiling all charges and is accompanied by a *detail statement,* which shows itemized charges. The detailed statement lists dates of services, codes, descriptions, and fees for individual services. The CMS-1500 claim form is used for physicians' professional outpatient claims.

A systematic approach should be established when editing a claim, and the same procedure should be used each time. This helps train the eye to notice errors or omitted information. Insurance personnel should understand coding, but in a hospital setting it is not their job to assign codes. Final code selection is done by the RHIT or, in complex cases, by the RHIA. Reviewing Blocks 42 through 47 is the most time-consuming portion of the editing process and the area that requires experience to master. This is the area where most of the errors and omissions occur. Refer to the Procedure for a suggested sequence of steps in editing a Uniform Bill (UB-92) claim form.

P R O C E D U R E : Editing a Uniform Bill (UB-92) Claim Form

---

1. Review the top left corner to see if the facility information is printed *(Blocks 1 and 5).*
2. Look to see if it is an inpatient (11X) or outpatient (13X) type of bill *(Block 4).*
3. Scan the UB-92 claim form to determine who the patient is *(Block 12),* the responsible party *(Block 38),* the insured *(Block 58),* and the patient's relationship to the insured *(Block 59).*
4. Check the birth date of the patient *(Block 14);* it should be printed in eight digits.
5. Confirm the gender of the patient *(Block 15),* comparing it with the patient's name *(Block 12).* If the patient's name could be used for either gender, verify the sex by reviewing the patient's insurance identification card, patient's medical record, or handwritten admitting record.
6. Verify the insurance information including the payer *(Block 50),* certificate, Social Security, or insurance identification number *(Block 60),* group name *(Block 61),* insurance group number *(Block 62),* employer name *(Block 65),* and employer location *(Block 66).* Blocks 50 and 60 are mandatory.
7. Confirm that data are present by reviewing the following: principal diagnostic code *(Block 67),* admitting diagnostic code *(Block 76),* and DRG number *(Block 78)* if applicable.
8. Verify that there is a principal procedure code with date *(Block 80)* and all other procedures with date(s) or service *(Block 81).* These should match the sequence and services provided and should appear in Block 43.
9. Verify that there is an attending, referring, or prescribing physician with identification number listed *(Block 82).* A physician other than the attending physician should be listed *(Block 83).*
10. Cross-check the third digit in Block 4, indicating the bill type with statement from and through dates *(Block 6),* admission date *(Block 17),* and occurrence date *(Block 32)* to see if this is the first bill. If it is not, look at the original bill so all entries are understood.
11. Inpatient: Verify the number of hospital days for semiprivate or coronary care unit (CCU) room charges *(Blocks 42 through 47).* Compare the number of units *(Block 46)* with the total number of inpatient days *(Block 7).* These should match. Look at the hour the patient was admitted *(Block 18)* and the hour of discharge *(Block 21)* if there is a discrepancy.
12. Correlate the room rates *(Block 47)* with the preceding services, making sure the per diem is based on the revenue.
13. Review all of the patient's services listed *(Block 42)* line by line. Each service listed must show a unit value *(Block 46).* Search for any revenue codes that may be used for a special type of service that may be itemized and charged separately (e.g., 274 through 279 implants or 258 through 259 special drugs).
14. Outpatient: Verify that each service described *(Block 43)* has a CPT or HCPCS code *(Block 44)* and a date of service listed *(Block 45).*
15. Check the detailed record if there is a question about a service listed. All services must be listed by hospital department.
16. Verify the total amount due by adding all amounts *(Block 47)* and comparing them with the last line item in Block 42 (001), Block 43 (Total), and final totaled amount as the last line entry in Block 47.
17. Look to see if the estimated amount due from the insurance company is calculated and shown *(Block 55).*
18. Forward the claim to the appropriate individual for an authorized signature and date *(Blocks 85 and 86).*

The claim form may go back to the health information management department after it is edited (where the coder verifies all codes) and to the contract department (where a contractor matches the bill with the insurance type). An adjustment to the account is posted, indicating the dollar amount above that which the insurance carrier will pay according to the contract. This adjustment is done after the insurance payment is received in the majority of hospitals. However, a small number of hospitals are able to write off the portion of the bill that is not covered by the insurance plan before receipt of payment. This transaction is referred to as *relieving the accounts receivable on the front end* and is desirable because the accounts receivable does not appear inflated.

Mail all claim forms to the insurance carrier for payment and retain a copy for the files. Document the patient's file with the date mailed and the address to which the insurance claim was filed. The claim may be rejected or delayed if errors are not caught, leading to slow payment or nonpayment. See Chapter 6 for a list of common reasons why claims are rejected or delayed.

Nurse Auditor

Registered nurses (RNs) work as nurse auditors and verify the doctor's orders and the medical record against each charge item on the bill. They may be onsite employees or hired offsite to come in periodically. The nurse must have clinical and financial expertise. A *clean bill* has no errors. An *under bill* has services that have been provided and not billed. An *over bill* has charged items that have not been documented in the chart. A report goes to the health information management department if a coding error or omission occurs. All such accounts have coding priority. Several types of audits follow:

▶ *Random internal audit.* This occurs continually. Blind charts are pulled and audited to maintain quality control.
▶ *Audit by request.* The patient can request an audit to verify charges.
▶ *Defense audit.* The insurance company requests an audit. The insurance auditor may or may not (but should) meet with a hospital auditor, depending on the circumstances. Charts are pulled and audited.

Reimbursement Process

Generally a hospital bill for inpatient care is much larger than the bill for services rendered in a physician's office. Individuals are admitted to hospitals for severe health problems, and many require major surgery, resulting in considerable expense to the patient. Hospitals use and maintain highly sophisticated, expensive equipment, are located in large facilities, and employ large numbers of personnel, many of whom are state licensed and specialized. Salaries and operating costs must be recovered through patient billing. The majority of hospital reimbursement is from insurance companies. However, working parents with families, elderly people, and jobless persons (even those who have insurance) have found it increasingly difficult to pay their share of the hospital bills. Consequently, accurate and timely hospital billing and good follow-up and collection techniques are in demand.

Reimbursement Methods

Growing numbers of the population are now served by a variety of managed health care programs. All of these programs operate under varying contracts, policies, and guidelines, depending on individual state and federal laws. In negotiating a reimbursement arrangement, the managed care plan administrator tries to obtain discount rates for participation by a hospital in the plan in exchange for an increased volume of patients. These programs use any one or a combination of various payment methods. Refer to Chapter 10 for definitions on types of managed care plans. A brief description of some reimbursement methods follows:

Ambulatory Payment Classifications

An outpatient classification scheme developed by Health Systems International is **ambulatory payment classifications (APCs)**. This method is based on procedures rather than diagnoses. Services associated with a specific procedure or visit are bundled into the APC reimbursement. More than one APC may be billed if more than one procedure is performed, but discounts may be applied to any additional APCs. This topic is discussed in detail at the end of this chapter.

Bed Leasing

A managed care plan leases beds from a facility (e.g., payment to the hospital of $300 per bed for 20 beds, regardless of whether those beds are used).

Capitation or Percentage of Revenue

Capitation means reimbursement to the hospital on a per-member per-month basis regardless of whether the patient is hospitalized. **Percentage of revenue** means a fixed percentage paid to the hospital to cover charges.

Case Rate

Case rate is an averaging after a *flat* rate (set amount paid for a service) has been given to certain categories of procedures (e.g., normal vaginal delivery is $1800 and cesarean section is $2300). Utilization is expected to be 80% vaginal deliveries and 20% cesarean section; therefore the case rate is $1900 for all deliveries. Specialty procedures also may be given a case rate (e.g., coronary artery bypass graft surgery or heart transplantation). *Bundled case rate* means an all-inclusive rate is paid for both institutional and professional services; for example, for coronary artery bypass graft surgery, a rate is used to pay all who provide services connected with that procedure. Bundled case rates are seen in teaching facilities in which a faculty practice plan works closely with the hospital.

Diagnosis-Related Groups

A classification system called diagnosis-related groups **(DRGs)** categorizes patients who are medically related with respect to diagnosis and treatment and are statistically similar in length of hospital stay. Medicare and some private hospital insurance payments are based on fixed dollar amounts determined by DRGs. DRGs are discussed in detail later in the chapter.

Differential by Day in Hospital

The first day of the hospital stay is paid at a higher rate (e.g., the first day may be paid at $1000 and each subsequent day at $500). Most hospitalizations are more expensive on the first day. This type of reimbursement method may be combined with a per diem arrangement.

Differential by Service Type

The hospital receives a flat per-admission reimbursement for the service to which the patient is admitted. A prorated payment may be made (e.g., 50% for intensive care and 50% medicine) if services are mixed. Service types are defined in the contract (e.g., medicine, surgery, intensive care, neonatal intensive care, psychiatry, and obstetrics).

Fee Schedule

A comprehensive listing of charges based on procedure codes, under a fee-for-service (FFS) arrangement, or discounted FFS, states fee maximums paid by the health plan within the period of the managed care contract. Usually the fee schedule is based on CPT codes. For industrial cases, whether managed care or not, this listing may be called a workers' compensation fee schedule. This document also may be known as a *fee maximum schedule* or *fee allowance schedule*.

Flat Rate

A set amount (single charge) per hospital admission is paid by the managed care plan, regardless of the cost of the actual services the patient receives.

Per Diem

Per diem is a single charge for a day in the hospital regardless of actual charges or costs incurred (e.g., a plan that pays $800 for each day regardless of the actual cost of service).

Periodic Interim Payments (PIPs) and Cash Advances

These are methods in which the plan advances cash to cover expected claims to the hospital. The fund is replenished periodically. Insurance claims may be applied to the cash advance or may be paid outside it. Generally this is done by Medicare.

Withhold

In this method, part of the plan's payment to the hospital may be withheld or set aside in a bonus pool. If the hospital meets or exceeds the criteria set down, the hospital receives its withhold or bonus; other terms used are *bonus pools, capitation, risk pools,* or *withhold pools.*

Managed Care Stop Loss Outliers

Stop loss is a form of guarantee that may be written into a contract using one of a variety of methods. The purpose is to limit the exposure of cost to a reasonable level to prevent excessive loss. Stop loss is the least understood of reimbursement issues and can leave many thousands of dollars uncollected. There are a number of different ways stop loss can be applied; each contract is different. Become familiar with each contract and the stop loss provisions in it. Following are some methods that may be encountered.

1. Case-based stop loss: This is the most common stop loss and can apply to the physician, on a smaller case basis, as well as to the individual hospital claim. For example, the hospital bill may run more than $1 million in cases of premature infants of extremely low birth weight. The contract may pay $2000 to $3000 per day, which may reimburse the hospital several hundred thousand dollars, but the hospital must absorb the excess. Stop loss provisions may pay 65% of the excess over $100,000. Thus the hospital and the insurance carrier share the loss.
2. Reinsurance stop loss: The hospital buys insurance to protect against lost revenue and receives less of a capitation fee; the amount they do not receive helps pay for the insurance. For example, after a case reaches $100,000, the plan may receive 80% of expenses in excess of $100,000 from the reinsurance company for the remainder of the year.
3. Percentage stop loss: Some managed care contracts pay a percentage of charges when the total charge exceeds $65,000.
4. Medicare stop loss: Medicare provides stop loss called *outliers* in its regulations. There are *day*

outliers for patients who remain in the hospital for long spells of illness. Medicare provides *cost outliers* for those cases in which charges exceed the DRG or $30,000. DRGs are discussed at the end of this chapter.

Some reimbursement methods that are not used very much follow:

Charges

In a managed care plan, **charges** are the dollar amount owed to a participating provider for health care services rendered to a plan member, according to a fee schedule set by the managed care plan. This is the most expensive and least desirable type of reimbursement contract, so not many of these contracts exist.

Discounts in the Form of Sliding Scale

This is a form of discount with a limit in which the percentage amount increases, based on hospital numbers. For example, a 10% reduction in charges for 0 to 500 total bed days per year with incremental increases in the discount up to a maximum percentage.

Sliding Scales for Discounts and Per Diems

Based on total volume of business generated, this is a reimbursement method in which an interim per diem is paid for each day in the hospital. For example, a lump sum is either added to or withheld from the payment due at the end of each year to adjust for actual hospital usage. This is difficult to administer because it can be done either monthly or annually.

Electronic Data Interchange

As early as the 1980s, large hospitals began submitting electronic claims for payment to third-party payers instead of printing out the UB-92 claim form; this is called electronic data interchange (EDI). The claim arrives at the insurance company the same day and receives priority for payment. This method of claim submission reduces the cost to the hospital and expedites payment. Confirmation of claim transmission and receipt is received the following day. Use of computer software assists the insurance billing editor in checking for errors before forwarding the claim to the proper claims office. This is called **scrubbing** or *cleaning the bill*. Medicare, Medicaid, group health carriers, many managed care plans, and some workers' compensation carriers mandate use of EDI. All hospital electronic billing goes through a clearinghouse where additional edits are made and claims are batched and sent electronically to insurance companies. Billing can be set up according to days or dollar amounts, typically every 30 days. If a Medicare patient remains in an acute hospital, he or she may be billed on the 60th day and not again until discharge. Refer to Chapter 7 for detailed information on this topic.

Hard Copy Billing

A printed paper copy of the UB-92 that is generated from the computer system is referred to as a hard copy. The same edits are made, and the claim is cleaned (scrubbed) before it is sent. Some insurance companies are not capable of receiving electronic claims, so billing by hard copy is mandatory. All secondary insurance companies and claims that require attachments also fit into this category.

Receiving Payment

Timeliness of payment may be included in a contract to encourage a hospital to join a plan (e.g., an additional 4% discount for paying a clean claim within 14 days of receipt), or a hospital may demand a penalty for clean claims not processed within 30 days. Some states require this payment by law.

After receipt of payment from insurance and managed care plans, the patient is sent a net bill that lists any owed deductible, coinsurance amount, and charges for services not covered under the insurance policy. Standard bookkeeping procedures are used to post entries showing payments and adjustments. Financial management for managed care programs is discussed and shown in figures in Chapter 10.

Outpatient Insurance Claims

The term **outpatient** is used when an individual receives medical service in a section or department of the hospital and goes home the same day. If an individual has an accident, injury, or acute illness, he or she may seek the services of medical personnel in the emergency department of the hospital. When seen in this department, a patient is considered an outpatient unless he or she is admitted for overnight hospital stay. Many elective surgeries are done on an outpatient surgery basis. **Elective surgery** indicates a surgical procedure that can be scheduled in advance, is not an emergency, and is discretionary on the part of the physician and patient. Elective procedures are those that are deferrable, which means that the patient will not experience serious consequences if the operation is postponed or there is failure to undergo the operation. Some insurance policies require a second opinion for elective surgery. The insurance company may not pay if the patient does not seek a second opinion and chooses to undergo surgery. See Chapter 11 for elective surgery in regard to the Medicare program. Patients may receive certain types of therapy and diagnostic testing services on an outpatient basis.

Hospital Professional Services

Although physicians make daily hospital visits to their patients, perform surgeries, discharge patients from the hospital, and are called to the hospital to provide consultations and emergency department treatment, their professional services are submitted on the CMS-1500 insurance claim form by the physician and not by the hospital billing department. Only services provided by the hospital should be submitted by the hospital unless the hospital is billing for physicians. Such hospital services include the following:

▶ Emergency department (ED) facility fee (supplies)
▶ Laboratory (technical component)
▶ Radiology (technical component)
▶ Physical and occupational therapy facility fee

Personnel who work in these departments (e.g., ED physician, pathologist, radiologist, and physical therapist) might be employees of the hospital. The hospital submits bills for professional services in that situation. The professional is billed independently if not an employee.

Using the hospital for surgical or medical consultations that could be done in a specialist's office should be avoided unless the patient physically requires admission. This necessity should be documented. If a patient is admitted for consultation only, the entire payment for hospital admission will be denied, as well as any physician fees involved.

Billing Problems

Many times, patients receive hospital bills, are stunned by the total balance due, and are unable to make sense of specific items, abbreviations, or codes on the statement. A bill should never show unexplained codes or items without descriptions. A brief hospital stay may translate into hundreds of individual charges. A patient has the right to request, examine, and question a detailed statement, as mentioned in the Patient's Bill of Rights—a nationally recognized code of conduct published by the American Hospital Association. If the bill lumps charges together under broad categories such as pharmacy, surgical supplies, and radiology and the patient requests an itemized invoice, it should be provided at no cost to the patient. In fact, consumer advocates and policies governing the Medicare program encourage consumers to scrutinize their hospital bills for mistakes. The hospital may receive a call or letter from the patient asking for an explanation of the charges if the charges seem exorbitant. Sometimes hospital billing personnel, a hospital patient representative or advocate, the attending physician, and his or her staff may be able to satisfactorily explain a confusing charge.

Some common billing errors follow:

▶ Incorrect name. Use of maiden name instead of married name

▶ Wrong subscriber. Patient's name listed in error
▶ Covered days versus noncovered days

Duplicate Statements

Duplicate billings, which may confuse the patient, can occur when a patient receives inpatient and outpatient preadmission tests or services. Perhaps a test was canceled and rescheduled, and a charge is shown for the canceled test; or several physicians may have consulted on a case, and each ordered the same test or therapy. Possibly a technician took the incorrect amount of blood or produced an unclear radiograph, submitted a charge for the service performed in error, as well as for the correct service, and thereby generated two charges for one test. These examples are hospital personnel errors; patients should not have to pay for such mistakes.

Double Billing

Another example involving a violation of Medicare policy is double billing, which results when a patient undergoes routine outpatient testing for a specific diagnosis and then develops unanticipated problems related to that diagnosis that require hospital admission. Outpatient personnel may not be aware that the patient was later admitted, and inpatient personnel may not know that the patient had undergone outpatient testing within the previous 72 hours. A hospital that bills for such services may be fined because it is in violation of the Medicare 72-hour rule. Such charges must be bundled into the inpatient DRG payment. Therefore it is imperative that the hospital billing department develop procedures to check for potential double-billing problems.

Phantom Charges

Physicians order admission procedures for each patient who enters the hospital. If a patient refuses some of these tests, the charges should be deleted from the financial records before the bill is sent out. Similarly, a patient should not be charged for refused medication. The hospital may offer a standard kit of supplies on admission or a new-mother packet when appropriate. A patient should not have to pay for supplies that he or she refuses. If a patient requests a semiprivate room but is sent to a private room because all semiprivate rooms are occupied, the patient should not be billed at the higher rate. Phantom charges may appear if a scheduled test is canceled by a physician or the patient is released early, making it imperative to check the dates and times of admission and discharge. Charges that should appear on a patient's itemized statement may be missing because the charges were transferred to the wrong patient's bill. This requires a review of the patient's medical records. The charge should be deleted from the bill when a charge cannot be accounted for by a review of the patient's medical record or by talking to the attending physician.

Hospital Billing Claim Form

Uniform Bill Inpatient and Outpatient Claim Form

In 1982 the UB-82 claim form was developed for hospital claims and was printed in green ink. A revision was issued in 1992 because it was determined that an update of this form was needed. The **Uniform Bill (UB-92) claim form** is also known as the CMS-1450. This form is considered a summary document supported by an itemized or detailed bill. It is used by institutional facilities (e.g., inpatient and outpatient departments, rural health clinics, chronic dialysis services, and adult day health care) to submit claims for inpatient and outpatient services. This claim form is printed in red ink on white paper for processing with optical scanning equipment. Figure 16–5 illustrates a completed UB-92 claim form. Dates of service and monetary values are

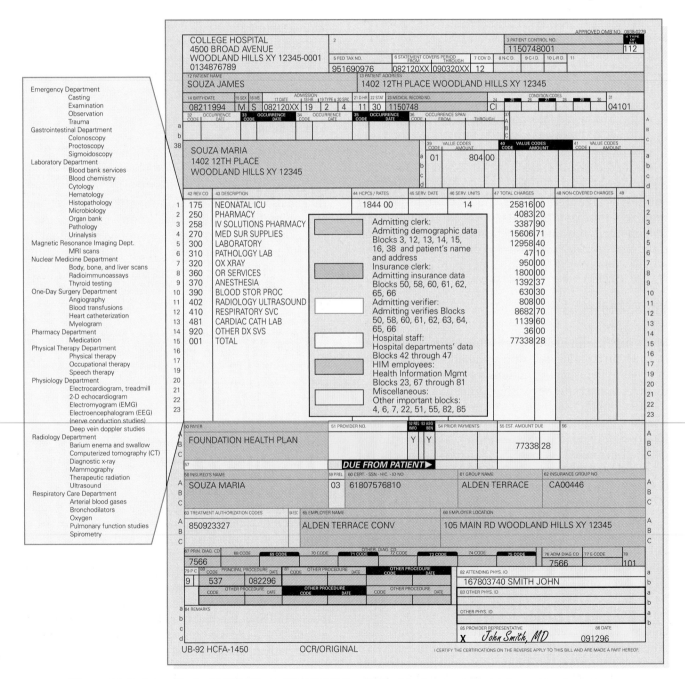

Figure 16–5. Scannable (red ink) Uniform Bill (UB-92) insurance claim form completed for an inpatient showing hospital departments that input data for hospital services. Colored blocks indicate data obtained by various hospital personnel. Job titles and the exact data each person obtains may vary from facility to facility. Block-by-block guidelines vary and may not always follow the visual guide presented here.

Patient Status Codes—cont'd

04	Discharged or transferred to an intermediate care facility
05	Discharged or transferred to another type of institution for inpatient care or referred for outpatient services to another institution
06	Discharged or transferred to home under care of organized home health service organization
07	Left against medical advice or discontinued care
08	Discharged or transferred to home under care of home intravenous therapy provider
09	Admitted as an inpatient to this hospital
10–19	Discharge to be defined at state level, if necessary
20	Expired
21–29	Expired, to be defined at state level, if necessary
30	Still a patient
31–39	Still a patient to be defined at state level, if necessary
40	Expired at home (for hospice care)
41	Expired in a medical facility such as a hospital, SNF, intermediate care facility, or freestanding hospice (for hospice care)
42	Expired, place unknown (for hospice care)
43–49	Reserved for national assignment
50	Discharged to hospice or home
51	Discharged to hospice or medical facility
52–60	Reserved for national assignment

Block 23. Medical Record Number. Enter the number assigned by the provider to the patient's medical record. **Private payers, Medicare,** and **TRICARE:** Required. **Some Medicaid programs:** May be required.

Blocks 24–30. Condition Codes. The codes help determine patient eligibility and benefits from primary or secondary insurance coverage and affect payer processing.

Condition Codes

01	Military service related
02	Condition is employment related
03	Patient is covered by insurance not reflected here
04	Patient is HMO enrollee
05	Lien has been filed
06	End-stage renal disease (ESRD) patient in first 18 months of entitlement covered by employer group health insurance
07	Treatment of nonterminal condition for hospice patient
08	Beneficiary will not provide information concerning other insurance coverage

Condition Codes—cont'd

09	Neither patient nor spouse is employed
10	Patient or spouse is employed but no employer group health plan (EGHP) coverage exists
11	Disabled beneficiary, but no large group health plan (LGHP) coverage exists
12–14	Reserved for payer use only
15	Clean claim delayed in CMS's processing system
16	SNF transition exemption
17	Patient is homeless
18	Maiden name retained
19	Child retains mother's name
20	Beneficiary requested billing
21	Billing for denial notice
22	Patient is on multiple drug regimens
23	Home caregiver is available
24	Home intravenous therapy patient also receiving home health agency (HHA) services
25	Patient is a non–U.S. resident
26	Veterans Affairs—eligible patient chooses to receive services in Medicare–certified facility
27	Patient is referred to a sole community hospital for a diagnostic laboratory test
28	Patient or spouse's EGHP is secondary to Medicare
29	Disabled beneficiary or family member's LGHP is secondary to Medicare
30	Reserved for national assignment
31	Patient is student (full-time day)
32	Patient is student (cooperative or work study program)
33	Patient is student (full-time night)
34	Patient is student (part-time)
35	Reserved for national assignment
36	General care patient is in a special unit
37	Ward accommodation at patient's request
38	Semiprivate room is not available
39	Private room is medically necessary
40	Same-day transfer
41	Partial hospitalization
42	Continuing care is not related to inpatient admission
43	Continuing care is not provided within prescribed postdischarge window
44–45	Reserved for national assignment
46	TRICARE Nonavailability Statement on file
47	Reserved for TRICARE
48	Claims submitted by a TRICARE–authorized psychiatric residential treatment center (RTC) for children and adolescents
49–54	Reserved for national assignment.
55	SNF bed is not available
56	Medical appropriateness. SNF admission was delayed more than 30 days after hospital discharge
57	SNF readmission

Continued.

Condition Codes—cont'd

58–59	Reserved for national assignment
60	Reports the stay was a day outlier
61	Requests additional payment for the stay as a cost outlier
62	Payer code indicating bill was paid under a DRG
63–65	Payer only codes
66	Provider does not wish cost outlier payment
67	Beneficiary elects not to use lifetime reserve (LTR) days
68	Beneficiary elects to use LTR days
69	Operating indirect medical education (IME) payment only
70	Self-administered epoetin (EPO) for home dialysis patient
71	Full care in dialysis unit
72	Self-care in dialysis unit
73	Self-care in dialysis training
74	Patient receiving dialysis services at home
75	Home dialysis—100% payment
76	Backup in-facility dialysis
77	Provider accepts or is obligated or required because a contractual arrangement or law to accept payment by a primary payer as payment in full
78	New coverage not implemented by HMO
79	Comprehensive outpatient rehabilitation facility (CORF) services provided offsite
80–99	Reserved for state assignment
A0	TRICARE External Partnership Program
A1	Early Periodic Screening Diagnosis Treatment/Child Health Assurance Program (EPSDT/CHAP)
A2	Physically handicapped children's program
A3	Special federal funding
A4	Family planning
A5	Disability
A6	Medicare pneumococcal pneumonia vaccine (PPV) services; influenza virus vaccine
A7	Induced abortion—danger to life
A8	Induced abortion—victim of rape or incest
A9	Second opinion surgery
B0–B9	Reserved for national assignment
C0	Reserved for national assignment
C1	Approved as billed
C2	Automatic approval as billed based on focused review
C3	Partial approval
C4	Admission or services denied
C5	Postpayment review applicable
C6	Admission preauthorization
C7	Extended authorization
C8–C9	Reserved for national assignment
D0	Change to services dates
D1	Change to charges
D2	Changes in revenue codes or HCPCS
D3	Second or subsequent interim prospective payment system bill

Condition Codes—cont'd

D4	Change in grouper input
D5	Cancel to correct health insurance claim number (HICN) or provider identification number
D6	Cancel only to repay a duplicate or Office of the Inspector General (OIG) overpayment
D7	Change to make Medicare the secondary payer
D8	Change to make Medicare the primary payer
D9	Any other change
E0	Change in patient status
E1–L9	Reserved for national assignment
M0	All-inclusive rate for outpatient services (payer-only code)
M1	Roster billed influenza virus vaccine (payer-only code)
M2	HHA payment significantly exceeds total charges (payer-only code)
M3–M9	Reserved for payer assignment
N0–W9	Reserved for national assignment
X0–Z9	Reserved for state assignment

Block 31. Reserved for national assignment.

Blocks 32–35. Occurrence Codes and Dates. Occurrence codes and dates are used to identify significant events relating to a bill that may affect payer processing (e.g., determination of liability, coordination of benefits, or administration of subrogation clauses in benefit programs). The electronic version requires an eight-character date listing year, month, and day: 20XX0328. A total of seven occurrence codes and dates may be reported on a UB-92. **Private payers** or **Medicare:** Required.

Occurrence Codes and Dates

01	Auto accident
02	No-fault insurance involved including auto accident or other
03	Accident—tort liability
04	Accident—employment related
05	Other accident
06	Crime victim
07–08	Reserved for national assignment
09	Start of infertility treatment cycle
10	Last menstrual period
11	Onset of symptoms or illness
12	Date of onset for a chronically dependent individual (CDI) (HHA claims only)
13–16	Reserved for national assignment
17	Date outpatient occupational therapy plan established or last reviewed
18	Date of retirement of patient and beneficiary
19	Date of retirement of spouse

Occurrence Codes and Dates—cont'd

20	Guarantee of payment began
21	UR notice received
22	Date active care ended
23	Date of cancellation of hospice election period
24	Date insurance denied
25	Date benefits terminated by primary payer
26	Date SNF bed became available
27	Date of hospice certification or recertification
28	Date comprehensive outpatient rehabilitation plan established or last reviewed
29	Date outpatient physical therapy plan established or last reviewed
30	Date outpatient speech pathology plan established or last reviewed
31	Date beneficiary notified of intent to bill (accommodations)
32	Date beneficiary notified of intent to bill (diagnostic procedures or treatments)
33	First day of the Medicare coordination period for ESRD beneficiaries covered by an EGHP
34	Date of election of extended care services
35	Date treatment started for physical therapy
36	Date of inpatient hospital discharge for covered transplant patient
37	Date of inpatient hospital discharge for noncovered transplant patient
38	Date treatment started for home intravenous therapy
39	Date discharged on a continuous course of intravenous therapy
40	Scheduled date of admission
41	Date of first test for preadmission testing
42	Date of discharge (hospice only)
43	Scheduled date of canceled surgery
44	Date treatment started for occupational therapy
45	Date treatment started for speech therapy
46	Date treatment started for cardiac rehabilitation
47	Date cost outlier status begins
48–49	Payer codes
50–69	Reserved for state assignment
70–99	Reserved for occurrence span codes
A0	Reserved for national assignment
A1	Birthdate—insured A
A2	Effective date—insured A policy
A3	Benefits exhausted
A4–A9	Reserved for national assignment
B0	Reserved for national assignment
B1	Birthdate—insured B
B2	Effective date—insured B policy
B3	Benefits exhausted
B4–B9	Reserved for national assignment
C0	Reserved for national assignment
C1	Birthdate—insured C
C2	Effective date—insured C policy
C3	Benefits exhausted
C4–C9	Reserved for national assignment

Occurrence Codes and Dates—cont'd

D0–D9	Reserved for national assignment
E0	Reserved for national assignment
E1	Birthdate—insured D
E2	Effective date—insured D policy
E3	Benefits exhausted
E4–E9	Reserved for national assignment
F0	Reserved for national assignment
F1	Birthdate—insured E
F2	Effective date—insured E policy
F3	Benefits exhausted
F4–F9	Reserved for national assignment
G0	Reserved for national assignment
G1	Birthdate—insured F
G2	Effective date—insured F policy
G3	Benefits exhausted
G4–G9	Reserved for national assignment
H0–I9	Reserved for national assignment
J0–L9	Reserved for national assignment
M0–Z9	See Block 36 occurrence span codes
M0	PRO/UR approved stay dates (partial approval)
M1	Provider liability—no utilization
M2	Inpatient respite days
M3–W9	Reserved for national assignment
X0–Z9	Reserved for state assignment

Block 36. Occurrence Span Codes and Dates. Enter code identifying occurrence that happened over a span of time. The electronic version requires an eight-character date listing year, month, and day (20XX0812). **Medicaid:** Complete when required. **Private payer, Medicare,** and **TRICARE:** Required.

Occurrence Span Codes and Dates

70	Qualifying stay dates (for SNF use only)
71	Prior stay dates
72	First and last visits
73	Benefit eligibility period
74	Noncovered level of care or leave of absence (LOA)
75	SNF level of care
76	Patient liability period
77	Provider liability period
78	SNF prior stay dates
79	Payer code
80–99	Reserved for state assignment

Block 37. **Internal Control Number (ICN)/Document Control Number (DCN).** Enter the ICN or DCN assigned to the original bill by the payer or the payer's intermediary. **Medicaid:** May be required depending on contract requirements. **Medi-Cal** and **private payers:** Not required. **Medicare:** Required. **TRICARE:** For reporting claim changes.

Block 38. Responsible Party Name and Address. Enter the name and address of the party responsible for the bill. **Private payers:** Required. **Medicaid, Medi-Cal, Medicare,** or **TRICARE:** Not required.

Blocks 39–41. **Value Codes and Amounts.** Enter codes that have related dollar amounts that identify monetary data required for processing claims. **Medicaid:** May be required depending on state policy. **Private payer, Medicare,** and **TRICARE:** Complete when applicable. Enter the value codes as described in the following:

Value Codes

01	Most common semiprivate room rate
02	Hospital has no semiprivate rooms
03	Reserved for national assignment
04	Inpatient professional component charges that are combined billed
05	Professional component included in charges and also billed separately to carrier
06	Medicare blood deductible amount
07	Reserved for national assignment
08	Medicare lifetime reserve amount in the first calendar year
09	Medicare coinsurance amount in the first calendar year
10	Medicare lifetime reserve amount in the second calendar year
11	Medicare coinsurance amount for second calendar year
12	Working aged beneficiary or spouse with EGHP
13	ESRD in a Medicare coordination period for an EGHP
14	No-fault insurance, including auto or other
15	Workers' compensation
16	Public health service (PHS) or other federal agency
17	Outlier amount
18	Disproportionate share amount
19	Indirect medical education amount
20	Total prospective payment system capital payment amount
21	Catastrophic
22	Supplies
23	Recurring monthly income
24	Medicaid rate code
25–29	Reserved for national assignment—Medicaid
30	Preadmission testing
31	Patient liability amount
32–36	Reserved for national assignment
37	Pints of blood furnished
38	Blood deductible pints
39	Pints of blood replaced
40	New coverage not implemented by HMO (for inpatient claims only)
41	Black lung

Value Codes—cont'd

42	Veterans affairs
43	Disabled beneficiary under age 65 with LGHP
44	Amount provider agreed to accept from primary insurer when this amount is less than total charges but greater than the primary insurer's payment
45	Accident hour
46	Number of grace days
47	Any liability insurance
48	Hemoglobin reading
49	Hematocrit reading
50	Physical therapy visits
51	Occupational therapy visits
52	Speech therapy visits
53	Cardiac rehabilitation visits
54–55	Reserved for national assignment
56	Skilled nurse—home visit hours (HHA only)
57	Home health aide—home visit hours (HHA only)
58	Arterial blood gas (PO_2/PA_2)
59	Oxygen saturation (O_2 SAT/oximetry)
60	HHA branch metropolitan statistical area (MSA)
61	Location where service is furnished (HHA and hospice)
62–65	Payer codes
66	Reserved for national assignment
67	Peritoneal dialysis
68	EPO—drug
70	Interest amount
71	Funding of ESRD networks
72	Flat rate surgery charge
73	Drug deductible
74	Drug coinsurance
75	Gramm-Rudman-Hollings reduction—for payers use only
76	Provider's interim rate
77–79	Payer codes
80–99	Reserved for state assignment
A1	Deductible payer A
A2	Coinsurance payer A
A3	Estimated responsibility payer A
A4	Covered self-administrable drugs—emergency
A5	Covered self-administrable drugs—not self administered in form and situation furnished to patient
A6	Covered self-administrable drugs—diagnostic study and other
A7–AZ	Reserved for national assignment
B0	Reserved for national assignment
B1	Deductible payer B
B2	Coinsurance payer B
B3	Estimated responsibility payer B
B4–BZ	Reserved for national assignment
C0	Reserved for national assignment
C1	Deductible payer C
C2	Coinsurance payer C
C3	Estimated responsibility payer C
C4–CZ	Reserved for national assignment
C0–D2	Reserved for national assignment
D3	Estimated responsibility patient

Value Codes—cont'd

D4–DZ	Reserved for national assignment
E0	Reserved for national assignment
EI	Deductible payer D
E2	Coinsurance payer D
E3	Estimated responsibility payer D
E4–EZ	Reserved for national assignment
F0	Reserved for national assignment
FI	Deductible payer E
F2	Coinsurance payer E
F3	Estimated responsibility payer E
F4–FZ	Reserved for national assignment
G0	Reserved for national assignment
GI	Deductible payer F
G2	Coinsurance payer F
G3	Estimated responsibility payer F
G4–GZ	Reserved for national assignment
H0–YZ	Reserved for national assignment
X0–ZZ	Reserved for national assignment

Block 42. Revenue Code. Enter a three- or four-digit code corresponding to each narrative description or standard abbreviation that identifies a specific accommodation, ancillary service, or billing calculation related to services billed. Revenue code 001 indicating a total must be the final entry on all bills. Revenue codes are an *important factor* when payment is considered by managed care contractors or private payers. Billing guidelines for revenue codes are extensive, so refer to the UB-92 *Manual* for detailed information. **Managed care:** Required because payment may be based on diagnosis, procedure, and revenue codes. For example, codes 274, 275, 276, and 278 relate to implant of a pacemaker, lens, pin, or bolt. If the correct code is not used, payment will not be made for implant item if the cost is buried in supplies. Other items to be sure to code are special drugs for chemotherapy, cardiac balloons, cardiac catheters, and so on. **Medicare:** Required. All revenue codes from 001 to 999 must be preceded with an "0." The leading "0" is added automatically for electronic claims. Basic revenue codes end in "0." Detailed revenue codes end in 1 through 9. List revenue codes in ascending order. Do not repeat revenue codes on the same claim except when required by field or for coding more than one HCPCS code for the same revenue code item. **Medi-Cal:** Not required for outpatient services except when code 0001 is used to indicate Total Charge line.

Block 43. Revenue Description. This optional block helps separate and identify descriptions of each service. The description must identify the particular service code indicated in Block 44, the HCPCS/Rates block. **Third-party payers** and

TRICARE: Required **Medicare:** Not required. **Medicaid:** May be required depending on contract.

Block 44. HCPCS/Rates/Health Insurance Prospective Payment System (HIPPS) Rate Codes. Enter the applicable CPT or HCPCS code number and modifier (applicable to ancillary services for outpatient claims), HIPPS rate code, and two-digit modifier, or the accommodation rate for inpatient claims. Dollar values must include whole dollars, the decimal, and cents (e.g., $999.99). **Medicare:** Required. **Medicaid** and **private payers:** May be required depending on contract.

Block 45. Service Date. Enter the date the service was rendered for outpatient services in eight digits (e.g., 062320XX). See the patient's itemized bill for dates. The electronic version requires an eight-character date listing year, month, and day (e.g., 20XX0128). Inpatient dates are not required in this block. **Medicare:** Required. **Medicaid** and **private payers:** May be required depending on contract.

Block 46. Service Units. Enter the number of accommodation days, ancillary units, or visits when appropriate for each revenue code. This is itemized on the patient's detail bill. **Medicare** and **private payers:** Required.

Block 47. Total Charges. Enter the total charge pertaining to the related revenue codes (Example 16–13). **Medicare** and **private payers:** Required.

Block 48. Noncovered Charges. Enter total noncovered charges for the primary payer pertaining to a particular revenue code. Personal items are not covered. **Medicaid, Medicare,** and **private payers:** Required. **Medi-Cal** and **TRICARE:** Not required.

Block 49. Unlabeled block. Reserved for national assignment.

Block 50. Payer Identification. Enter name and number identifying each payer organization from which the provider may expect some payment for the bill. Line 50A is used to report the primary payer. Line 50B is used for the secondary payer. Line 50C is used for the tertiary payer. **Medicaid, Medicare, private payers,** and **TRICARE:** Required. **Medi-Cal:** Enter "O/P MEDI-CAL" to indicate the type of claim and payer.

Block 51. Provider Number. Enter the number assigned to the provider by the payer. **Medicaid, Medicare,** and **private payers:** Required. **TRICARE:** Requires the ZIP code of the physical location of the provider plus the four-digit subidentification number.

EXAMPLE 16–13

42 REV. CD.	43 DESCRIPTION	44 HCPCS/RATES	45 SERV.DATE	46 SERV.UNITS	47 TOTAL CHARGES	48 NON-COVERED CHARGES 49	
175	Neonatal ICU	1844.00		14	25816.00		1
250	Pharmacy				4083.20		2
258	IV Solutions—Pharmacy				3387.90		3
270	Med-Sur Supplies				15606.71		4
300	Laboratory				12958.40		5
310	Pathology Lab				47.10		6
320	OX X-Ray				950.00		7
360	OR Services				1800.00		8
370	Anesthesia				1392.37		9
390	Blood/Stor-Proc				630.30		10
402	Radiology Ultrasound				808.00		11
410	Respiratory SVC			22	8682.70		12
481	Cardiac Cath Lab				1139.60		13
920	Other DX SVS				36.00		14
							15
							16
							17
							18
							19
							20
							21
							22
001	Total				77338.28		23

Block 52. **Release Information Certification Indicator.** Enter code indicating if provider has patient's signature on file permitting release of data. Y (yes); R (restricted or modified release); and N (no release). **Medicaid:** May be required depending on contract. **Medicare, private payers,** and **TRICARE:** Required. **Medi-Cal:** Not required.

Block 53. **Assignment of Benefits.** Enter Y (yes, benefits assigned) or N (no, benefits not assigned). **Private payers** and **TRICARE:** Required. **Medicaid, Medi-Cal,** and **Medicare:** Not required.

Block 54. **Prior Payments/Payers and Patient.** Enter the amount of payment received on this bill before the billing date. If payment has been received from other coverage, enter the amount on the same line as the other coverage "payer" listed in Block 50 (e.g., $100 should be entered as 100 00). *Do not* enter Medicare payments in this block; leave blank if not applicable. **Medicaid, Medi-Cal** and **Medicare:** Required.

Block 55. **Estimated Amount Due.** Enter the estimated amount due from the indicated payer according to the contract. **Medicaid, Medi-Cal, Medicare, private payers,** and **TRICARE:** Not required.

Block 56. **Untitled block.** Reserved for state assignment.

Block 57. **Untitled block.** Reserved for national assignment.

Block 58. **Insured's Name.** Enter name of the patient or insured individual in whose name the insurance is issued. If billing for an infant, use the mother's name. If billing for an organ donor, enter the recipient's name and the patient's relationship to the recipient in Block 59. Otherwise leave blank. **Medicaid, Medicare, private payers,** and **TRICARE:** Required.

Block 59. **Patient's Relationship to Insured.** Enter code number indicating relationship of the patient to the insured individual identified in Block 58. **Medicaid, Medicare, private payers,** and **TRICARE:** Required.

Patient Relationship Codes

01	Patient is the insured
02	Spouse
03	Natural child or insured has financial responsibility
	Continued

Patient Relationship Codes—cont'd

04	Natural child or insured does not have financial responsibility
05	Stepchild
06	Foster child
07	Ward of the court
08	Employee
09	Unknown
10	Handicapped dependent
11	Organ donor
12	Cadaver donor
13	Grandchild
14	Niece or nephew
15	Injured plaintiff
16	Sponsored dependent
17	Minor dependent of a minor dependent
18	Parent
19	Grandparent
20	Life partner
21–99	Reserved for national assignment

Block 60. **Certificate/Social Security Number/Health Insurance Claim/Identification Number.** Enter the insured's identification number assigned by the payer organization. Required by all programs.

Block 61. **Group Name.** Enter the group name or plan through which the health insurance coverage is provided to the insured. **Medicare** and **private payers:** Required. **Medi-Cal:** Not required. **TRICARE:** Enter the sponsor's branch of service (e.g., USAF).

Block 62. **Insurance Group Number.** Enter the insurance group number. **Private payers:** Required. **Medi-Cal** and **Medicare:** Not required. **TRICARE:** Enter the sponsor's military status and pay grade codes. **CHAMPVA:** Enter the veteran's military status code (e.g., "ACT" for active or "RET" for retired).

Block 63. **Treatment Authorization Codes.** Enter the treatment authorization request (TAR) number provided by the payer. **Medicare, private payers,** and **TRICARE:** Required. **Medi-Cal:** For services requiring a TAR, enter the 11-digit TAR Control Number. It is not necessary to attach a copy of the TAR to the claim.

Block 64. **Employment Status Code.** Enter the employment status code of the insured individual identified in Block 58. **Some Medicaid programs:** May be required. **Medi-Cal:** Not required. **Medicare** and **private payers:** Required. **TRICARE:** Enter the code that describes the employment status of the individual identified in Block 58.

Employment Status Codes

1	Employed full-time
2	Employed part-time
3	Not employed
4	Self-employed
5	Retired
6	On active military duty
7–8	Reserved for national assignment
9	Unknown

Block 65. Employer Name. Enter the employer's name for the individual listed in Block 58. **Medicaid:** May be required. **Medi-Cal:** Not required. **Medicare, private payers,** and **TRICARE:** Required.

Block 66. Employer Location. Enter the employer's location of the insured individual identified in Block 58. **Some Medicaid programs:** May be required. **Medi-Cal:** Not required. **Medicare, private payers,** and **TRICARE:** Required.

Block 67. Principal Diagnosis Code. Enter all numbers and letters of the ICD-9-CM code for the principal diagnosis, including fourth and fifth digits. Do not insert a decimal point. Required for all programs.

Blocks 68–75. Other Diagnosis Codes. Enter all numbers and letters of the ICD-9-CM codes that correspond to the patient's additional conditions that coexist at the time of admission or develop subsequently and have an effect on the treatment received or length of stay. Required for all programs. **Medi-Cal:** Not required.

Block 75. Enter DRG group number for inpatient claims.

Block 76. Admitting Diagnosis Code/Patient's Reason for Visit. Enter admitting diagnosis code, including fourth and fifth digits as stated by the physician at the time of admission for inpatient claims. For outpatient claims, enter the patient's stated reason for seeking care. Required for all programs.

Block 77. External Cause of Injury Code. If there is an external cause of injury, poisoning, or adverse effect, enter the diagnostic E code, including the third and fourth digits. **Medicare** and **private payers:** Not required.

Block 78. Unlabeled block. Reserved for state assignment.

Block 79. Procedure Coding Method Used. Enter appropriate code to identify the coding system used. **Medicaid, private payers,** and **TRICARE:** Required. **Medicare:** Not required.

Coding System Codes

1–3	Reserved for state assignment
4	CPT procedure codes
5	HCPCS codes
6–8	Reserved for national assignment
9	ICD-9-CM procedure codes

Block 80. Principal Procedure Codes and Date. Enter the procedure code for the principal procedure and date performed. The electronic version requires an eight-character date listing year, month, and day (20XX0425). **Medicaid, Medicare, private payers,** and **TRICARE:** Required.

Block 81. Other Procedure Codes and Dates. Enter one or two additional major procedure codes and dates performed to identify significant procedures other than the principal procedure and corresponding dates when procedures were performed. The electronic version requires an eight-character date listing year, month, and day (20XX0215). **Medicare, private payers,** and **TRICARE:** Required. **Medicaid:** May be required depending on contract.

Block 82. Attending Physician ID. Enter the name or provider number for the physician who has primary responsibility for the patient's care and treatment. This block is mandatory for radiologists. If the physician is a Medicaid or Medi-Cal provider, enter the state license number. Do not use a group provider number. Required by all programs.

Block 83. Other Physician ID. Enter the name or identification number of the licensed physician other than the attending physician. Required for all programs. **Medi-Cal:** On the upper line of Block 83, enter the individual nine-digit Medi-Cal provider number for the physician actually providing services. Do not use a group provider number or state license number.

Block 84. Remarks. Use this area to fulfill any reporting requirements, such as procedures that require additional information, justification for services, an emergency certification statement, or as an optional block for DRG group number for inpatient claims if not entered in Block 75. If it will not fit in this area, attach the statement to the claim. Required for all programs.

Block 85. Provider Representative Signature. Provider or authorized signer must sign and date claim. **Medicare, Medicaid, private payers,** and **TRICARE:** Required. For Medicare, a stamped signature is acceptable. For other programs, a facsimile signature may be acceptable after approval.

Block 86. Date Bill Submitted. Insert the date the claim is submitted to the insurance company or fiscal intermediary. **Medicaid, private payers,** and **TRICARE:** Required. **Medicare:** Not required.

Taking the hospital billing process a step further, Figure 16–5 illustrates which block of the UB-92 claim form is affected by the hospital department and employee. To become familiar with the UB-92 claim form, an assignment is presented in the *Workbook* asking that the 86 blocks of information be divided into six categories according to departmental input.

Diagnosis-Related Groups

History

The concept of DRGs was developed by Professors John D. Thompson and Robert B. Fetter at Yale University and tested in New Jersey from 1977 to 1979. The goal was to develop a scheme of patient classification to be used in UR.* Soon other applications were found in such areas as budgeting, planning, and reimbursement.

Because of inconsistencies and inadequacies in the original concept, a second set of DRGs was developed and has been used in New Jersey since 1982. Under the Medicare PPS, the DRGs were implemented nationwide for all hospitalizations after the Tax Equity and Fiscal Responsibility Act of 1982 (TEFRA) was passed. The purpose of a DRG-based system used for Medicare reimbursement is to hold down rising health care costs. Therefore Medicare reimbursement as a whole is expected to decrease significantly under the DRG payment system.

The Diagnosis-Related Groups System

The DRG system is a patient classification method that categorizes patients who are medically related with respect to diagnosis and treatment and who are statistically similar in length of stay. It is used to both classify past cases to measure the relative resources hospitals have expanded to treat patients with similar illnesses and to classify current cases to determine payment. This system changed hospital

reimbursement from a fee-for-service system to a lump-sum, fixed-fee payment based on the diagnoses rather than on time or services rendered. The fees were fixed by a research team, which determined a national "average" fee for each of the principal discharge diagnoses. The classifications were formed from more than 10,000 ICD-9-CM codes that were divided into 25 basic **major diagnostic categories (MDCs).** These diagnoses were assigned a specific DRG number from 001 to 511 (as of the printing of this edition) and specific values commensurate with geographic areas, types of hospitals, depreciation values, teaching status, and other specific criteria. TRICARE and other private insurance that utilize DRGs use DRG numbers 600 to 900. Most MDCs are based on a particular organ system of the body. Within MDCs, DRGs are either medical or surgical. Seven variables are responsible for DRG classifications:

▶ Principal diagnosis
▶ Secondary diagnosis (up to eight)
▶ Surgical procedures (up to six)
▶ Comorbidity and complications
▶ Age and sex
▶ Discharge status
▶ Trim points (number of hospital days for a specific diagnosis)

At the time of the initial admission review, the physician establishes a tentative diagnosis so that a tentative DRG can be assigned. The tentative DRG is assigned based on: (1) admission diagnosis; (2) scheduled procedures; (3) age; and (4) known secondary diagnoses. An individual in the Health Information Management Department obtains the pertinent patient case history information listed in the preceding and codes the principal and secondary diagnoses and operative procedure(s). Using a computer software program called a **grouper,** this information is keyed in and the program calculates and assigns the DRG payment group. The grouper is not able to consider any differences between chronic and acute conditions. **Looping** is the grouper process of searching all listed diagnoses for the presence of any comorbid condition or complication or searching all procedures for operating room procedures or more specific procedures. If any factors that affect the DRG assignment change or are added, the new information is entered and the case is assigned to the new DRG.

The following is an example of the case of a patient with chronic bronchitis who is admitted to the hospital with pneumonia; his medical record shows that he has had emphysema for many years. Refer to Figure 16–7, which lists the chronic obstructive lung disease diagnostic code as the principal diagnosis, with pneumonia as a secondary diagnosis (inaccurate DRG assignment). This entitles the hospital to receive $2723.66. However, if the pneumonia

---

*Review of hospital admissions to determine whether they are justified; this is discussed at the beginning of the chapter.

SAMPLE CASE HISTORY			
CORRECT DRG ASSIGNMENT		**INACCURATE DRG ASSIGNMENT**	
MDC 4: Respiratory System		MDC 4: Respiratory System	
Principal Diagnosis	Pneumonia (ICD9CM-486)	Principal Diagnosis	COPID (ICD9CM-496)
Secondary Diagnosis	Emphysema (ICD9CM-492.8)	Secondary Diagnosis	Pneumonia (ICD9CM-486)
Secondary Diagnosis	Chronic Bronchitis (ICD9CM-491.2)	Principal Operative Procedure	None
Principal Operative Procedure	None	Principal Operative Procedure	None
Secondary Operative Procedure	None	Secondary Operative Procedure	None
Age	69 Years	Age	69 Years
Discharge Status	Routine	Discharge Status	Routine
Sex	Male	Sex	Male
Length of Stay	15 Days	Length of Stay	15 Days
DRG	89	DRG	88
Trim Points	4–22 Days	Trim Points	3–19 Days
Rate	$3294.17	Rate	$2723.66

Figure 16–7. Case history showing correct and incorrect DRG assignment and the difference in payment between the two.

diagnostic code was listed as the principal diagnosis with two secondary diagnostic codes, emphysema and chronic bronchitis, then the hospital would be entitled to $3294.17—$570 additional reimbursement with the use of the correct DRG assignment.

A case that cannot be assigned to an appropriate DRG because of an atypical situation is called a **cost outlier.** These atypical situations are as follows:

1. **Clinical outliers:**
   a. Unique combinations of diagnoses and surgeries causing high costs. These are more common than day outliers.
   b. Very rare conditions
2. Long length of stay, referred to as *day outliers**
3. Low-volume DRGs

Inliers (hospital case falls below the mean average or expected length of stay):

1. Death
2. Leaving against medical advice (AMA)
3. Admitted and discharged on the same day

The current federal plan for outliers is the full DRG rate plus an additional payment for the services provided. An unethical practice, **DRG creep,** is to code a patient's DRG category for a more severe diagnosis than indicated by the patient's condition. This is also called upcoding.

In hospital billing, downcoding can also erroneously occur when sequencing several diagnoses (e.g., listing a normal pregnancy as the primary diagnosis for payment and complications in the secondary position when the patient remained in the hospital for an extended number of days). Additional examples are discussed in chapter 5.

The amount of payment may be increased by documenting in the patient's medical record any comorbid conditions or complications. When referring to DRGs, the abbreviation CC is used to indicate such complications or comorbidities (not the more common interpretation found in patient charting, Chief Complaint). **Comorbidity** is defined as a preexisting condition that, because of its effect on the specific principal diagnosis, will require more intensive therapy or cause an increase in length of stay by at least 1 day in approximately 75% of cases.

If a patient is admitted because of two or more conditions and the physician fails to indicate the "most resource-intensive" or "most specific" diagnosis as the principal diagnosis, the DRG assessment will be incorrect, resulting in decreased reimbursement to the health care facility (Examples 16–14 and 16–15). It is the responsibility of the attending physician to decide on a principal diagnosis based on his or her best judgment.

Both examples warrant additional payment because of comorbid conditions and complications.

The *DRG/ICD-9-CM Code Book* is a good reference and code book presented in an easy-to-use binder

---

*Day outliers are to be eliminated.

EXAMPLE 16–14

COMORBID CONDITION AND COMPLICATION

A patient has had congestive heart failure for several years and is admitted with an admitting diagnosis of chest pain and principal diagnosis of anterior wall myocardial infarction (MI). While hospitalized, the patient experiences atrial fibrillation.

Principal diagnosis:	410.1	anterior wall myocardial infarction
Comorbid condition (CC):	428.0	congestive heart failure
Complication:	427.31	atrial fibrillation

EXAMPLE 16–15

COMORBID CONDITION AND COMPLICATION

A patient has had chronic obstructive pulmonary disease (COPD) for the last 6 months and is admitted with an admitting diagnosis of chest pain and a principal diagnosis of anterior wall myocardial infarction (MI). While hospitalized, the patient experiences respiratory failure.

Principal diagnosis:	410.1	anterior wall myocardial infarction
Comorbid condition:	496	chronic obstructive pulmonary disease
Complication:	799.1	respiratory failure

and containing Volumes 1, 2, and 3 of ICD-9-CM. Sections are color-highlighted for maximum payment. Refer to Appendix B to locate publishers of ICD-9-CM code books.

Diagnosis-Related Groups and the Medical Assistant and Insurance Billing Specialist

Even though diagnosis-related groups (DRGs) affect Medicare hospital payments, stress the role of the medical assistant in a physician's office when communicating the admitting diagnosis to the hospital. This can greatly affect the DRG assignment. The medical assistant should remember the following points:

1. Give all of the diagnoses authorized by the physician, if there are more than one, when calling the hospital to admit a patient so the hospital personnel can use their expertise in listing the primary and secondary diagnoses.
2. Ask the physician to review the treatment or procedure in question when a hospital representative calls about a test, length of stay, or treatments ordered by the attending physician. The hospital needs this information to justify a higher-than-average bill to Medicare.
3. Get to know the hospital personnel on a first-name basis so that when the physician or patients have DRG-related questions, you can call on this hospital expert.

When the DRG system is implemented by other third-party payers or segments of the population other than Medicare patients, you should contact them locally to assist you. Records and hospital insurance claims must contain the correct *principal diagnosis, detailed facts to support the principal diagnosis and complications, medical data to justify all procedures performed, patient's age,* and *discharge diagnosis.*

Outpatient Classification

In late 2000 under the requirements of the Balanced Budget Act of 1997, the CMS implemented a PPS for Medicare beneficiaries. This was a move from a cost-based reimbursement system to a line-item billing system for ambulatory surgery centers and hospital outpatient services. The CMS has categorized outpatient services into an ambulatory payment classification system. Some Medicaid programs and private payers have embraced this system because of the escalation of outpatient costs.

Ambulatory Payment Classification System

Originally, ambulatory visit groups (AVGs) and then ambulatory patient groups (APGs) were developed as outpatient classification systems by Health Systems International (HSI). These groups were based on patient classifications (ICD-9-CM diagnoses, CPT and HCPCS procedures, age, and gender) rather than disease classifications. Ambulatory surgery categories (ASCs) were then adopted, replacing APGs for outpatient or 1-day surgery cases that were derived from the surgery section of the CPT. ASCs used disease and procedural coding classification systems to supply the input to the computer program to assign ASCs.

Recently the General Accounting Office (GAO) ordered Congress to begin conversion of surgical, radiologic, and other diagnostic services to an APC system effective August 1, 2000, which replaced ASCs. The more than 500 APCs are continually being modified (added to) and deleted. Because of this constant state of change, APC information is updated and released twice a year in the Federal Register.

APCs are applied to:

▶ Ambulatory surgical procedures
▶ Chemotherapy
▶ Clinic visits
▶ Diagnostic services and diagnostic tests
▶ Emergency department visits
▶ Implants
▶ Outpatient services furnished to nursing facility patients not packaged into nursing facility consolidated billing (services commonly furnished by hospital outpatient departments that nursing

facilities are not able to provide [computed tomography, magnetic resonance imaging, or ambulatory surgery])

▶ Partial hospitalization services for community mental health centers (CMHCs)
▶ Preventive services (colorectal cancer screening)
▶ Radiology, including radiation therapy
▶ Services for patients who have exhausted Part A benefits
▶ Services to hospice patient for treatment of a nonterminal illness
▶ Surgical pathology

Hospital Prospective Payment System

The development process for APCs is similar to that used for DRGs; however, the procedure code is the primary axis of classification, not the diagnosis code. The reimbursement methodology is based on median costs of services and facility cost to determine charge ratios in addition to copayment amounts. There is also an adjustment for area wage differences, which is based on the hospital wage index currently used for inpatient services. This Hospital Prospective Payment System (HOPPS) may be updated annually, not periodically. An APC group may have a number of services or items packaged within it so that separate payment cannot be obtained.

APC Status

Categories of services have payment status indicators consisting of alpha code letters or symbols. These are the following:

Category	Payment Status Indicator
Medical visits to clinic or emergency department	V
Surgical services	T
Significant procedures	S
Ancillary services	X
Acquisition of corneal tissue	F
Current drug/biological pass-through payment	G
Device pass-through payment	H
New drug/biological pass-through payment	J
Payment under another fee schedule or rate	A
Inpatient only	C
Code not used by Medicare, service not covered	E
Service is packaged into APC rate	N
New technology APCs (range 0970–0984)	#
Code unique to partial hospitalization	P

Partial hospitalization refers to a distinct and organized intensive psychiatric outpatient day treatment program designed to provide patients with profound and disabling mental health conditions an individual, coordinated, comprehensive, and multidisciplinary treatment program.

Types of APCs

The four types of APCs follow:

1. *Surgical procedure APCs.* These are surgical procedures for which payment is allowed under the PPS (e.g., cataract removal, endoscopies, and biopsies). Surgical APCs are assigned based on CPT codes.
2. *Significant procedure APCs.* These consist of nonsurgical procedures that are the main reason for the visit and account for the majority of the time and services used during the visit (e.g., psychotherapy, computed tomography and magnetic resonance imaging, radiation therapy, chemotherapy administration, and partial hospitalization). Significant procedure APCs are selected based on CPT codes.
3. *Medical APCs.* These include encounters with a health care professional for evaluation and management services. The medical APC is determined by site of service (clinic or ED), level of the E/M service (CPT code), and diagnosis from one of 20 diagnostic categories (ICD-9-CM code).
4. *Ancillary APCs.* These involve diagnostic tests or treatments not considered to be significant procedure APCs (e.g., plain x-ray film, electrocardiograms, and cardiac rehabilitation). Ancillary APCs are assigned based on CPT codes.

It is possible that multiple APCs can be used when billing for a visit. Use of CPT modifiers for hospital outpatient visits affects APC payments; therefore it is very important to accurately apply correct modifiers when applicable.

Most hospitals use a type of computer encoder program in which the CPT code is input and an APC group code number is assigned. For example, if CPT code number 99282 is input for a low level emergency department visit, the encoder assigns APC Group 610. Use of an unbundling reference book may be of help in assigning a CPT code; it is preferable to use the code that will generate the highest APC payment.

The data that hospitals submit during the first years of implementation of the APC system are vitally important to the revision of weights and other adjustments that affect payment in future years. The APC data that appear on the UB-92 claim form are shown in Figure 16–8.

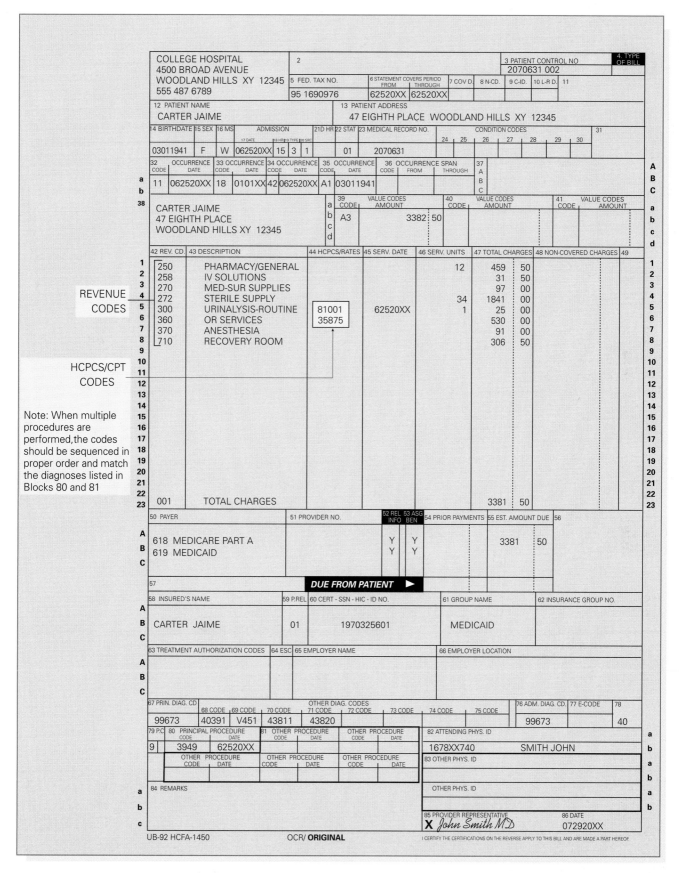

Figure 16–8. Scannable (red ink) Uniform Bill (UB-92) insurance claim form showing placement of APC data for an outpatient for submission to insurance company.

RESOURCES ON THE INTERNET

Refer to the *Federal Register* Web site for up-to-date guidelines and policies at: *www.cms.gov*

STUDENT ASSIGNMENT LIST

✔ Study Chapter 16.

✔ Answer the review questions in the *Workbook* to reinforce the theory learned in this chapter and to help prepare you for a future test.

✔ Complete the assignments in the *Workbook* to gain hands-on experience in analyzing and editing information from computer-generated UB-92 claim forms for inpatient and outpatient hospital billing. One of the assignments will assist you in further enhancing your diagnostic coding skills in relation to DRGs. These problems point out the value of coding properly in terms of proper diagnostic sequence, indicating the variance in payment.

✔ Turn to the Glossary at the end of this textbook for a further understanding of the Key Terms used in this chapter.

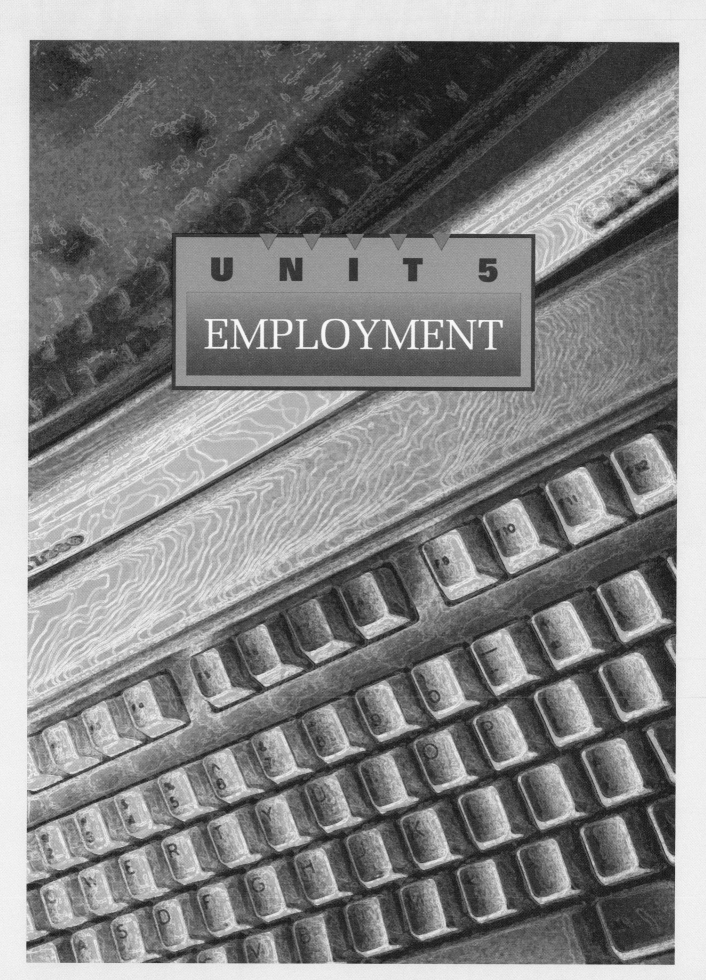

UNIT 5
EMPLOYMENT

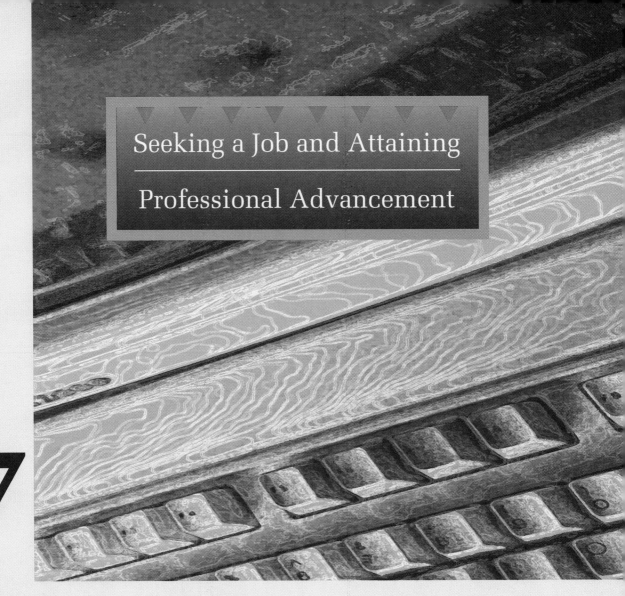

17

Seeking a Job and Attaining Professional Advancement

CHAPTER OUTLINE

- Analyze education and experience to prepare a resume.
- Identify illegal interview questions.
- Prepare responses to interview questions.
- Assess responsibilities assigned to insurance billing and coding specialists, electronic claims processors, and claims assistance professionals.
- Contact computerized job search databases for online services.
- Explore the business aspects of self-employment.
- Search online for employment opportunities.
- State types of certification and registration available to insurance billers, coders, and administrative medical assistants.

OBJECTIVES*

After reading this chapter you should be able to:

- Prepare to find a position as an insurance billing specialist, claims assistance professional, or electronic claims processor.
- Conduct a job search by listing prospective employers.
- Compose a letter of introduction to accompany the resume.

KEY TERMS

alien

application form

blind mailing

certification

Certified Coding Specialist (CCS)

Certified Coding Specialist-Physician (CCS-P)

Certified Medical Assistant (CMA)

Certified Medical Billing Specialist (CMBS)

Certified Professional Coder (CPC, CPC-A, CPC-H)

chronologic resume

claims assistance professional (CAP)

combination resume

continuing education

cover letter

electronic claims processor (ECP)

employment agency

functional resume

interview

mentor

National Certified Insurance and Coding Specialist (NCICS)

networking

portfolio

Continued.

---

*Performance objectives and exercises for hands-on practical experience for this chapter appear in the *Workbook*.

Employment Opportunities

Insurance Billing Specialist

Employment opportunities are available throughout the United States for insurance billing specialists who attain coding skills, knowledge of insurance programs, and expertise in completing insurance claims accurately. In addition to the skills necessary for performance on the job, ask yourself the following questions to determine if you need to sharpen your job-seeking techniques:

▶ Are you motivated and interested in finding a job?
▶ Can you communicate effectively in an interview?
▶ Do you enjoy good health?
▶ Are you mature?
▶ Do you have good grooming and manners?

The increase in the knowledge necessary and volume of paperwork associated with insurance claims, medical record keeping, and state and government agencies means a corresponding increase in the need for an insurance billing specialist. Because an individual can choose a number of different types of positions, this chapter provides information on each.

Examples of generic job descriptions are shown in Figures 17–1 through 17–4 to illustrate what job duties, skills, and requirements might be encountered for various insurance billing and coding positions. Job descriptions include assisting managers, supervisors, and employers in recruiting, supervising, and evaluating individuals in these positions for salary upgrades. Companies have had to modify their job descriptions to address individuals with physical impairments who may fall under the Americans with Disabilities Act.

There are two ways to work—either employed by someone or self-employed after a number of years of experience (Fig. 17–5). Some of the choices in this career field are:

▶ Insurance billing specialist
▶ Electronic claims processor
▶ Medicare or Medicaid billing specialist
▶ Claims assistance professional
▶ Coding specialist (freelance or employed)

Some hospital facilities and physicians prefer credentialed coders or insurance billers and advertise for:

▶ Certified Medical Billing Specialist (CMBS)
▶ Certified Medical Reimbursement Specialist (CMRS)
▶ Certified Professional Coder-Hospital (CPC-H or CPC)
▶ Certified Coding Specialist (CCS)
▶ Certified Coding Specialist-Physician (CCS-P)
▶ Certified Electronic Claims Processor (CECP)
▶ Certified Claims Assistance Professional (CCAP)
▶ Healthcare Reimbursement Specialist (HRS)
▶ National Certified Insurance and Coding Specialist (NCICS)
▶ Registered Medical Coder (RMC)

Becoming certified is certainly an essential goal if one seeks career advancement, and the steps to accomplish this as well as certification in other careers allied to this one are detailed at the end of this chapter.

Claims Assistance Professional

Contact local hospitals to see if they have patients who require insurance help if you wish to establish yourself as a self-employed **claims assistance professional (CAP)** (in addition to some of the aforementioned

GENERIC JOB DESCRIPTION FOR ENTRY LEVEL INSURANCE BILLING SPECIALIST

Knowledge, skills, and abilities:
1. Minimum education level consists of certificate from one-year insurance billing course, associate degree, or equivalent in work experience and continuing education.
2. Knowledge of basic medical terminology, anatomy and physiology, diseases, surgeries, medical specialties, and insurance terminology.
3. Ability to operate word processing, computer, photocopy, and calculator equipment.
4. Written and oral communication skills including grammar, punctuation, and style.
5. Ability and knowledge to use procedure code books.
6. Ability and knowledge to use diagnostic code books.
7. Ability to type or key 45 to 60 wpm.
8. Ability to work independently.
9. Certified Procedural Coder (CPC) or Certified Coding Specialist (CCS) status preferred.

Working conditions:
Medical office setting. Sufficient lighting.

Physical demands:
Prolonged sitting, standing and walking. Use of typewriter, word processor, or computer equipment. Some stooping, reaching, climbing, and bending. Occasional lifting of _____lbs. to a height of 5 feet. Hearing and speech capabilities necessary to communicate with patients and staff in person and on telephone. Vision capable of viewing computer monitors, calculators, charts, forms, text, and numbers for prolonged periods.

Salary:
Employer would list range of remuneration for the position.

Job responsibilities:	**Performance standards:**
1. Abstracts medical information from patient records.	1.1 Uses knowledge of medical terminology, anatomy and physiology, diseases, surgeries, and medical specialties. 1.2 Consults reference materials to clarify meanings of words. 1.3 Meets accuracy and production requirements adopted by employer. 1.4 Verifies with physician any vague information for accuracy.
2. Exhibits an understanding of ethical and medicolegal responsibilities related to insurance billing programs.	2.1 Observes policies and procedures related to confidentiality, medical records, release of information, retention of records, and statute of limitations for claim submission. 2.2 Meets standards of professional etiquette and ethical conduct. 2.3 Recognizes and reports problems involving fraud, abuse, embezzlement, and forgery to appropriate individuals.

Figure 17–1. Generic job description for an insurance billing specialist.

Continued.

3. Operates word processing, computer, or typewriter equipment to complete insurance claims.

3.1 Operates equipment skillfully and efficiently.
3.2 Evaluates condition of equipment and reports need for repair or replacement.

4. Follows employer's policies and procedures.

4.1 Punctual work attendance and is dependable.
4.2 Answers routine inquiries related to account balances and dates insurance forms submitted.

5. Completes and submits insurance claims accurately.

5.1 Updates insurance registration and account information.
5.2 Processes payments and posts to accounts accurately.
5.3 Handles correspondence related to insurance claims.
5.4 Reviews encounter forms for accuracy before submission to data entry.
5.5 Inserts data on insurance claims accurately.
5.6 Codes procedures and diagnoses accurately.
5.7 Telephones insurance companies with regard to delinquent claims.
5.8 Traces insurance claims.
5.9 Files appeals for denied claims.
5.10 Documents data from patients accurately.
5.11 Maintains separate insurance files.

6. Enhances knowledge and skills to keep up-to-date.

6.1 Attends continuing education activities.
6.2 Obtains current knowledge applicable to state and federal programs as they relate to insurance claim submission.
6.3 Keeps abreast of current changes in coding requirements from Medicare, Medicaid, and other third-party payers.
6.4 Assists with updating fee schedules and encounter forms with current codes.
6.5 Assists in the research of proper coding techniques to maximize reimbursement.

7. Employs interpersonal expertise to provide good working relationships with patients, employer, employees, and insurance companies.

7.1 Works with employer and employees cooperatively as a team.
7.2 Communicates effectively with patients and insurance companies regarding payment policies and financial obligations.
7.3 Executes job assignments with diligence and skill.
7.4 Assists staff with coding and reimbursement problems.
7.5 Assists other employees when needed.
7.6 Assists with giving fee estimates to patients when necessary.

Figure 17–1, cont'd

GENERIC JOB DESCRIPTION FOR
A CLAIMS ASSISTANCE PROFESSIONAL

Knowledge, skills, and abilities:
1. Minimum education level consists of certificate from one-year insurance billing course, associate degree, or equivalent in work experience and continuing education.
2. Knowledge of basic medical terminology, anatomy and physiology, diseases, surgeries, medical specialties, and insurance terminology.
3. Ability to operate typewriter, word processing, or computer equipment, as well as photocopy and calculator equipment.
4. Written and oral communication skills including grammar, punctuation, and style.
5. Ability and knowledge to use procedure code books.
6. Ability and knowledge to use diagnostic code books.
7. Ability to type or keyboard 45 to 60 wpm.
8. Ability to work independently.
9. Certified Claims Assistance Professional (CCAP) status preferred.

Working conditions:
Home office setting. Sufficient lighting and space to allow for at least 3 or more people.

Physical demands:
Prolonged sitting, standing, and walking. Use of typewriter, word processor, or computer equipment. Some stooping, reaching, climbing, and bending. Occasional lifting of _____lbs. to a height of 5 feet. Hearing and speech capabilities necessary to communicate with clients in person and on telephone. Vision capable of viewing computer monitors, calculators, charts, forms, text, and numbers for prolonged periods.

Salary:
Client would pay a percentage of reimbursement or annual salary, hourly wage, or per claim fee.

Job responsibilities:	**Performance standards:**
1. Files secondary insurance claims and maintains insurance files.	1.1 Completes accurately and submits secondary insurance claims.
2. Tracks insurance claim payments received by clients.	2.1 Maintains files and traces insurance claims for clients.
3. Exhibits an understanding of ethical and medicolegal responsibilities related to insurance billing programs.	3.1 Observes policies and procedures confidentiality of medical records, release of information, retention of records, and statute of limitations for claim submission.

Figure 17–2. Generic job description for a claims assistance professional.

Continued.

4. Knowledge of medical terminology.

5. Knowledge of procedure and diagnostic code requirements, as well as health insurance terminology.

6. Operates word processing, computer, or typewriter equipment to complete and submit secondary insurance claims.

7. Employs interpersonal expertise to provide good working relationships with clients, medical office personnel, and insurance companies.

8. Assists clients in challenging insurer's denials of payment of claims.

9. Interacts with health personnel to render additional information to appeal a denied claim and obtains payment for clients depending on terms of the health insurance policy or program.

10. Enhances knowledge and skills to keep up-to-date.

3.2 Meets standards of professional etiquette and ethical conduct.
3.3 Recognizes and reports problems involving fraud, abuse, embezzlement, and forgery to appropriate individuals.

4.1 Explains data on insurance claim forms.

5.1 Understands procedural and diagnostic codes and checks to see if correct codes were used.

6.1 Operates equipment skillfully and efficiently.
6.2 Evaluates condition of equipment and negotiates repair or replacement.

7.1 Works with clients, medical office personnel, and insurance companies with efficiency, diligence, and skill.
7.2 Communicates effectively with clients and insurance companies regarding payment policies.
7.3 Answers routine inquiries related to status of clients' accounts and dates insurance forms submitted.

8.1 Handles correspondence related to denial of insurance payment.
8.2 Telephones insurance companies and medical offices with regard to delinquent claims.

9.1 Files appeals for denied claims.

10.1 Attends continuing education activities.
10.2 Obtains current knowledge applicable to private insurance and the Medicare program related to insurance claim submission and payments.
10.3 Keeps abreast of current changes in coding requirements from Medicare, Medicaid, and other third-party payers.

Figure 17–2, cont'd

GENERIC JOB DESCRIPTION FOR
AN ELECTRONIC CLAIMS PROCESSOR

Knowledge, skills, and abilities:
1. Minimum education level consists of certificate from one-year insurance billing course, associate degree, or equivalent in work experience and continuing education.
2. Knowledge of basic medical terminology, anatomy and physiology, diseases, surgeries, medical specialties, and insurance terminology.
3. Ability to operate computer, modem, and printer, as well as photocopy and calculator equipment.
4. Written and oral communication skills including grammar, punctuation, and style.
5. Ability and knowledge to use procedure code books.
6. Ability and knowledge to use diagnostic code books.
7. Ability to key 45 to 60 wpm.
8. Ability to work independently.
9. Certified Electronic Claims Processor (CECP) status preferred.

Working conditions:
Medical office setting. Sufficient lighting.

Physical demands:
Prolonged sitting, standing and walking. Use of computer equipment. Some stooping, reaching, climbing, and bending. Occasional lifting of _____lbs. to a height of 5 feet. Hearing and speech capabilities necessary to communicate with patients and staff in person and on telephone. Vision capabilities necessary to view computer monitors, calculators, charts, forms, text, and numbers for prolonged periods.

Salary:
Employer would list range of remuneration for the position.

Job responsibilities:	**Performance standards:**
1. Acts as a link between the medical provider or facility and insurance companies.	1.1 Uses knowledge of medical terminology, anatomy and physiology, diseases, surgeries, and medical specialties.
	1.2 Understands computer applications and equipment required to convert and transmit patient billing data electronically.
	1.3 Consults reference materials to clarify meanings of words.
	1.4 Meets accuracy and production requirements adopted by employer.
	1.5 Verifies with physician any vague information for accuracy.
	1.6 Reduces volume of paperwork and variety of claim forms providers need to submit claims for payment.
2. Converts patient billing data into electronically readable formats.	2.1 Inputs data and transmits insurance claims accurately, either directly or through a clearinghouse.
	2.2 Answers routine inquiries related to account balances and dates insurance data transmitted to insurance carriers.

Figure 17–3. Generic job description for an electronic claims processor.

Continued.

2.3 Updates and maintains software applications with requirements of clearinghouses and insurance carriers.

3. Uses software that eliminates common claim filing errors, provides clean claims to insurance carriers, expedites payments to providers or facilities, and follows up on delinquent or denied claims.

3.1 Codes procedures and diagnoses accurately.
3.2 Telephones insurance companies about delinquent claims.
3.3 Traces insurance claims.
3.4 Files appeals for denied claims.

4. Exhibits an understanding of ethical and medicolegal responsibilities related to insurance billing programs and plans.

4.1 Observes policies and procedures related to confidentiality, medical records, release of information, retention of records, and statute of limitations for claim submission.
4.2 Meets standards of professional etiquette and ethical conduct.
4.3 Recognizes and reports problems involving fraud, abuse, embezzlement, and forgery to appropriate individuals.

5. Operates computer equipment to complete insurance claims.

5.1 Operates equipment skillfully and efficiently.
5.2 Evaluates condition of equipment and reports need for repair or replacement.

6. Follows employer's policies and procedures.

6.1 Must have punctual work attendance and be dependable.

7. Enhances knowledge and skills to keep up-to-date.

7.1 Attends continuing education skills activities.
7.2 Obtains current knowledge applicable to state and federal programs as they relate to transmission of insurance claims.
7.3 Keeps abreast of current changes in coding requirements from Medicare, Medicaid, and other third-party payers. Assists in the research of proper coding techniques to maximum reimbursement.

8. Employs interpersonal expertise to provide good working relationships with patients, employer, employees, and insurance companies.

8.1 Works with employer and employees cooperatively as a team.
8.2 Communicates effectively with patients and insurance companies regarding payment policies and financial obligations.
8.3 Executes job assignments with diligence and skill.
8.4 Assists staff with coding and reimbursement problems.
8.5 Assists other employees when needed.
8.6 Assists with giving fee estimates to patients when necessary.

Figure 17–3, cont'd

GENERIC JOB DESCRIPTION FOR CODERS

POSITION TITLE

Health Information/Medical Record Technician; Coder and Specialist for an acute and/or ambulatory care setting.

DEPARTMENT

Health Information/Medical Record.

JOB SUMMARY

Codes information from the medical records of patients to generate a clinical patient care database for the facility. Assures the maintenance and accuracy of diagnostic and procedural statistics for the facility, as well as optimum appropriate reimbursement from third party payers, by the timely coding of diagnoses and procedures using the required classification systems.

SPECIFIC RESPONSIBILITIES

Reviews and screens the entire medical record to abstract medical, surgical, laboratory, pharmaceutical, demographic, social and administrative data from the medical record in a timely manner.

Ensures providers that all diagnoses and procedures that may impact the facility's reimbursement are identified and attested to by the physician, if appropriate, sequenced correctly, and coded in an accurate and ethical manner for optimum reimbursement. Determines correct codes for routine, and/or new or unusual diagnoses and procedures not clearly listed in ICD-9-CM and CPT.

Consults with physicians for clarifications of clinical data when encountering conflicting or ambiguous information. Keeps abreast of regulatory changes affecting coded information required by the Health Care Financing Administration, the office of Statewide Health Planning Department, and others, as appropriate; and applies current Uniform Hospital Discharge Data Set (UHDDS) definitions for code selection.

Maintains knowledge of current information related to third-party reimbursement regulations and seeks continuing education in all phases of coding acumen.

Participates in the Coding Team's regular meetings with the objective of solving problems, brain-storming, educating physicians and others as to the coding policies and procedures of the facility, as well as promoting consistency of data collected.

Achieves a balance in quality and quantity, with a goal of maintaining both elements at a prescribed level of efficiency.

Abides by AHIMA's established code of ethical principles to safeguard the public and contribute within the scope of the profession to quality and efficiency in health care, thus promoting ethical conduct.

OTHER SPECIFIC OR POTENTIAL DUTIES/RESPONSIBILITIES FOR THIS POSITION

Identifies any loss of revenue by failure to charge for any procedures, supplies, injections, or other services, and then submits the missed charges.

Verifies all fee sheets to assure that all charges, appropriate modifiers, dates of injury, E code(s), as well as referring physicians' license numbers (when required), have been documented.

Assigns Diagnosis-Related Groups (DRGs) after identifying not only the principal diagnosis (reason for admission) but also significant complications and/or comorbidities, as well as operating room procedures following comparison of relative weights in the DRG GROUPER software, and selection of the highest reimbursement allowable among alternative principal diagnoses documented in the record.

Identifies and abstracts information from medical records for special studies and audits, internal and external.

Assists physicians, ancillary, and administrative personnel with retrieving patient care information for research, planning, and marketing projects. Answers questions regarding DRGs, as well as disease and procedure classification systems.

Figure 17–4. Generic job description for a coder. (From Stewart SP: *Generic job description for coders.* J CHIA, 1992, California Health Information Association, Fresno, CA.)

Continued.

Generates reports using a computer report-writer to retrieve coded and abstracted information from the provider's data processing system.

Orients and instructs new personnel and/or students from health information/medical record technology/administration programs, on unit operations, coding and abstracting activities.

DESCRIPTION OF SKILLS
I. TECHNICAL SKILLS REQUIRED:

A. Experience with and knowledge of instructional notations and conventions of ICD-9-CM and CPT HCPCS classification systems; and ability to follow the detailed guidelines related to their use in assigning single, and sequencing multiple, diagnosis and procedure codes for appropriate reimbursement and data collection.

B. Ability to read handwritten and transcribed documents in the medical record, interpret information, and enter complete and accurate data into an on-line computer system.

C. Comprehensive knowledge of medical diagnostic and procedural terminology required.

D. College-level understanding of disease processes, anatomy and physiology necessary for assigning accurate numeric and alpha-numeric codes.

E. Knowledge of federal, state and local government regulations and requirements which pertain to patient care information.

F. Knowledge of legalities and confidentiality issues involved with release of clinical or billing information.

G. Knowledge of third-party payer reimbursement requirements and an understanding of relative values for multimedical specialties, encounters, and procedures in acute care and ambulatory care settings.

II. DECISION-MAKING/
RESEARCH SKILLS REQUIRED:

A. Ability to query, analyze and determine the type of data needed to meet the request for information.

B. Ability to communicate technical and clinical information concerning patient care and classification systems at different levels; i.e., physicians, ancillary, and administrative personnel.

C. Ability to apply policies and procedures regarding data security and confidentiality to protect the inappropriate release of information.

D. Ability to exercise judgment with minimal supervision.

III. ORGANIZATIONAL SKILLS REQUIRED:

A. Ability to assume responsibility for compilation of clinical data related to inpatient and outpatient encounters including diagnoses, procedures, physicians and services.

B. Remains current with periodic updates of all coding manuals and guidelines in accordance with federal, state and local regulations.

C. Ability to manage time schedules, deadlines, multiple requests and priorities, and to maintain productivity.

IV. INTERPERSONAL SKILLS REQUIRED:

A. Communicates effectively, orally and in writing, with physicians, nurses and peers (both inter- and intra-departmentally) and with external organizations.

B. Communicates medical information with consideration of ethical and professional standards.

C. Upholds standards of confidentiality regarding patients, personnel and physicians.

V. EDUCATION AND
EXPERIENCE REQUIRED:

A. High school diploma.

B. Completion of an accredited program for coding certification or an accredited health information medical record technology program.
A Certified Coding Specialist (CCS), a Certified Coding Specialist —Physician (CCS-P), a Registered Health Information Technician (RHIT), or a Registered Health Information Administrator (RHIA) preferred, with current affiliation with the American Health Information Management Association.

C. Continuing education in health information management is required.

Figure 17–4, cont'd

Figure 17–5. Staff conference discussing applicants for potential interviews.

positions). Also call on small employers to see if they need assistance in explanation of their health insurance policies or enhancement of insurance benefits.

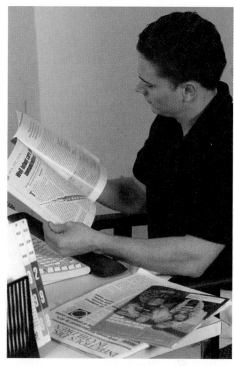

Figure 17–6. Student scanning a professional journal for job leads.

Job Search

There are several ways to seek employment. You may wish to be employed by a physician, hospital, medical facility, insurance company, or managed care organization. You may choose to be self-employed if you have had a number of years of experience or may even choose some type of combination situation. Here are suggested ways to search for a job.

1. Join a professional organization, as mentioned later in this chapter, to network with others in the same career field and to hear about job openings (Fig. 17–6). Put a notice about your availability in the chapter newsletter.

2. Attend meetings and workshops in this career field to keep up-to-date and network with others.

3. Contact the school placement personnel, complete the necessary paperwork, and leave a resume on file if you have just completed a course at a community college or trade school.

4. Spread the word to those who work in medical settings and those who might hear of openings in medical facilities, such as classmates, instructors, school counselors, relatives, and friends.

5. Contact pharmaceutical representatives, who visit physicians' offices and hospitals, for employment information or leads.

6. Visit public and private **employment agencies,** including temporary and temporary to permanent agencies. Before signing up with an agency,

ask whether the employer or applicant pays the agency fee.

7. Inquire at state and federal government offices and their employment agencies.

8. Look for part-time employment that might lead to a permanent full-time position.

9. Check bulletin boards frequently in personnel offices of hospitals and clinics for posted job offerings.

10. Go to your local medical society to see if it has a provision for supplying job leads.

11. Consult the *Yellow Pages* of the telephone directory or medical society roster for names of professional offices and hospitals to contact with an introductory telephone call or letter.

12. Send a **blind mailing** of the resume, including a cover letter, to possible prospects. A blind mailing means to send information to employers whom you do not know personally and who have not advertised for a job opening. This may result in a positive response with either a request to complete an application form or an invitation for an interview.

13. Go to the local library and look through Dun and Bradstreet's *Million Dollar Directory* and the *Middle Market Directory* for information on potential employers in many cities.

14. Visit the chamber of commerce and ask for some of their publications that contain membership directories, names of major professional employers

in specific areas, and brochures describing regional facts.

15. Subscribe to the principal newspaper of the city where employment is desired. Read help wanted ads in the classified section. Positions of interest might be listed as insurance billing specialist, reimbursement manager, insurance claims manager, insurance coordinator, insurance biller, coding/reimbursement specialist, reimbursement coordinator, coder/abstracter, electronic claims processor, and so on.

16. Telephone job hot lines of large medical clinics in your area.

17. Visit unannounced ("cold calls") at job locations.

18. Explore the Internet's World Wide Web. See Resources on the Internet at the end of this chapter.

Figure 17–7. Student doing an online job search.

Online Job Search

Because of vast communication available via the Internet's World Wide Web, newspaper and magazine classified advertisements may become resources of the past. An individual with a computer and modem can access online services. Many Web sites on the Internet incorporate text, sound, graphics, animation, and video. It is possible to locate potential employers at their Web sites who are offering jobs to health care workers by using various search engines. At some sites, you can find detailed descriptions of posted positions and locate opportunity postings by location or employer. You may be able to find and respond to a specific job of interest by delivering an online resume, attaching a cover letter, and updating your posting as often as needed. Some Web sites allow you to receive e-mailed job alerts.

There are several ways to gain access to the Internet. Your school may allow you to access the Internet on campus. Many libraries have computers with free Internet service. If you have a computer at home, you may wish to subscribe to either a commercial online service (e.g., America Online) with Internet access or an Internet service in your locale (Fig. 17–7).

Internet

Once online, go to a Web index to locate a search engine that lists different options to explore, such as Yahoo (*www.yahoo.com*), Google (*www.google.com*), Infoseek (*www.infoseek.go.com*), or Alta Vista (*www.altavista.com*). One of the resources is *Career Magazine* (*www.careermag.com/careermag/*), which lets you browse through hundreds of national job openings in a variety of fields. Check out America's Job Bank (*www.ajb.dni.us*) and E-Span Employment Database Search (*www.espan.com/*), which have job postings that you can browse according to

field, location, and career type. Go to PracticeNet (*www.practice-net.com*), which provides descriptions of medical practice opportunities. This 24-hour service names the recruiter, location, and an 800 number to contact. MedSearch America is another health employment service that posts jobs for hospitals, managed care organizations (MCOs), and pharmaceutical companies. Job seekers can send their resumes via e-mail for free online posting. Contact MedSearch online at *www.medsearch.com*

If you subscribe monthly to a commercial online service, you can network by posting a notice on a bulletin board with your resume or a note that you are looking for a particular type of position in a given locale.

Register with a computerized job search company. The firm American Computerized Employment Service (Irvine, CA),* has entered the job placement field with a trademarked system called TeleRecruiting. Job candidates may register without charge and complete an extensive profile questionnaire listing experience, skills, job-related factors, maximum commuting distance, and flex-time requirements. The firm acts as a liaison between employers and applicants. Employers use a touch tone telephone to access the computer and search for candidates. They pay an annual subscription, pay-per-search, or package search fee.

If you wish to read about career options on the Internet, obtain a book by Joyce Lain Kennedy

---

*American Computerized Employment Service, 17801 Main Street, Suite A, Irvine, CA 92714. Telephone 714-250-0221.

entitled, *Hook Up, Get Hired! The Internet Job Search Revolution,* published by John Wiley & Sons, New York.

Job Fairs

Annual community events feature job fairs at community colleges and technical trade schools or sponsored by professional associations. Job recruiters set up booths with information about their companies and available positions; however, they do not have much time to spend with each job seeker. Thus it is wise to come prepared and practice a 30-second introduction before attending. This introduction should consist of a quick overview of your career goals, experience, skills, training, education, and personal strengths. Be sure to explain what you can offer the employer. These are usually day-long events and, you may wish to investigate a number of participating employers' booths.

Go prepared by carrying a binder or folder with plenty of copies of your resume to give to the company representatives you meet. They should be neat, clean, and not folded, wrinkled, or coffee-stained. Take a pen, pencil, and notepad to obtain information. Research the employers attending so you know which ones you will visit and can appear confident, enthusiastic, interested, and knowledgeable to the job recruiter.

Take home the business card and brochure of anyone you talk to who genuinely interests you. After the fair, send that person a follow-up letter to reaffirm your interest.

Application

When visiting a potential employer, ask for an **application form** to complete and inquire if the facility keeps potential job applicants on file and for how long (Fig. 17–8). Study each question carefully before answering because the employer may evaluate the application itself to determine whether the applicant can follow instructions. Furnish as much information as possible, and if a question does not apply or cannot be answered, insert "no," "none," "NA" (not applicable), or "DNA" (does not apply). When visiting a potential employer for an application form, be sure you have prepared in advance for an interview in case an opportunity arises on that first visit.

Follow these guidelines when completing an application form:

1. Read the whole application form because some instructions may appear on the last page or last line.
2. Read the fine print and instructions: "Please print," "Put last name first," or "Complete in your own handwriting." This indicates ability to follow directions or instructions.
3. Print if your handwriting is poor, and abbreviate only when there is lack of space.
4. Complete the application in ink unless pencil is specified.
5. Refer to data from a portfolio, sample application form, or resume that has been checked for accuracy; use this information to copy onto each new application form. Be neat.
6. List correct dates of previous employment so that it will be accurate if the employer seeks verification. If a question is presented asking the reason for leaving a position, leave it blank and discuss this during the interview.
7. Name specific skills, such as procedural coding, diagnostic coding, knowledge of insurance programs, completing the CMS-1500 claim form, typing or keyboarding (number of words per minute), and speaking a second language.
8. When a question is asked about salary amount, write in "negotiable" or "flexible" and then discuss this during the interview.
9. Sign the application after completion.
10. Reread the entire form, word for word, to find any errors of omission or commission. This avoids having to apologize during an interview for a mistake.

Letter of Introduction

Individuals spend days perfecting a resume but throw together a *letter of introduction* or **cover letter** in minutes. This is a mistake. The main goal of the cover letter is to get the employer to take notice of the potential employee and resume so an interview appointment can be made. Letters should be typed, addressed to a specific person, and customized to each potential employer. If the advertisement gives a telephone number, call and ask for the name of the person doing the interviewing so the letter can include that person's name. When the name is unknown, use "Dear Sir or Madam" or "To Whom It May Concern," or a less formal "Hello" or "Good Morning."

Do not repeat everything in the resume. Begin with an attention-grabber, and get right to the point so the employer knows what you want and why. The letter should explain how the applicant's qualifications and skills would benefit the employer. Use key words that appear in the "position wanted" ad. End the letter by requesting an interview and be sure to enclose a resume. Always include a telephone number and the time of day when you are available.

Reread the letter for typos and errors in grammar, punctuation, and spelling. Avoid the use of "I" in the sentence structure (Fig. 17–9).

APPLICATION FOR POSITION / Medical or Dental Office
AN EQUAL OPPORTUNITY EMPLOYER

(in answering questions, use extra blank sheet if necessary)

No employee, applicant, or candidate for promotion, training or other advantage shall be dicriminated against (or given preference) because of race, color, religion, sex, age, physical handicap, veteran status, or national origin.

PLEASE READ CAREFULLY AND WRITE OR PRINT ANSWERS TO ALL QUESTIONS. DO NOT TYPE.

Date of application
7-2-XX

A. PERSONAL INFORMATION

Name - Last	First	Middle	Social Security No.	Area code/phone no.
Velasquez,	Jennifer	M.	3 6 1 X X 4 9 5	(555) 439-9800

Present address: Street	(Apt.#)	State	Zip	How long at this address?
1234 Martin Street, Woodland Hills		XY	12345	10 years

Previous address: **Street**   City   State   Zip
From: To:

Person to notify in case of emergency or accident - name: John Velasquez
Address: Telephone: 555-439-9800

B. EMPLOYMENT INFORMATION

For what position are you applying?:	☒Full-time ☐Part-time ☐Either	Date available for employment?:	Wage/salary expectations:
insurance biller		7-6-XX	negotiable

List hrs./days you prefer to work
M-F 8-5 PM

List any hrs./days you are not available: (Except for times required for religious practices or observances)

Can you work overtime, if necessary?
☒Yes ☐No

Are you employed now?
☐Yes ☒No

If so, may we inquire of your present employer?:☐No ☐Yes, if yes:
Name of employer:

Phone number: (   )

Have you ever been bonded?
☐Yes ☒No

If required for position, are you bondable?
☒Yes ☐No ☐Uncertain

Have you applied for a position with this office before?
☒No ☐Yes If Yes, when?:

Referred by / or where did you learn of this job?:

Can you, upon employment, submit verification of your legal right to work in the United States? ☒Yes ☐No
Submit proof that you meet legal age requirement for employment? ☒Yes ☐No

Language(s) applicant speaks or writes (if use of a language other than English is relevant to the job for which the applicant is applying: Spanish

C. EDUCATION HISTORY

	Name and address of schools attended (include current)	Dates From Thru	Highest grade/ level completed	Diploma/degree(s) obtained/areas of study
High school	ABC High School, Woodland Hills, XY	1990–1994	12	Diploma
College	Vocational-Tech School	1995		Degree/major Certificate
Post graduate	Montana State University	1995-97		Degree/major 24 credits
Other				Course/diploma/license/ certificate

Specific training, education, or experiences which will assist you in the job for which you have applied.
See résumé

Future educational plans Continuing education-preparing for certification

D. SPECIAL SKILLS

CHECK BELOW THE KINDS OF WORK YOU HAVE DONE:

		☒ MEDICAL INSURANCE FORMS	☐ RECEPTIONIST
☐ BLOOD COUNTS	☐ DENTAL ASSISTANT	☒ MEDICAL TERMINOLOGY	☒ TELEPHONES
☐ BOOKKEEPING	☐ DENTAL HYGIENIST	☐ MEDICAL TRANSCRIPTION	☒ TYPING
☒ COLLECTIONS	☐ FILING	☐ NURSING	☐ STENOGRAPHY
☒ COMPOSING LETTERS	☐ INJECTIONS	☐ PHLEBOTOMY(draw blood)	☐ URINALYSIS
☐ COMPUTER INPUT	☐ INSTRUMENT STERILIZATION	☒ POSTING	☐ X-RAY
OFFICE EQUIPMENT USED: ☒ COMPUTER	☐ DICTATING EQUIPMENT	☒ WORD PROCESSOR	☒ OTHER calculator

Other kinds of tasks performed or skills that may be applicable to position:	Typing speed 60 wpm	Shorthand speed

ORDER # 72-110 • © 1976 BIBBERO SYSTEMS, INC. • PETALUMA, CA. • (Rev. 1/95)
TO REORDER CALL TOLL FREE: (800) BIBBERO (800-242-2376) OR FAX (800) 242-9330

Mfg In U.S.A.

(PLEASE COMPLETE OTHER SIDE)

Figure 17–8. Application for Position/Medical or Dental Office form. (From Bibbero Systems, Inc., Petaluma, CA.)

E. EMPLOYMENT RECORD

LIST MOST RECENT EMPLOYMENT FIRST	May we contact your previous employer(s) for a reference? ☒Yes ☐No

	Worked performed. Be specific:
1) Employer *St. John's Outpatient Clinic*	*ins biller—see résumé*
Address: Street City State Zip code *24 Center St. Woodland Hills, XY 12345*	
Phone number *(555) 782-0155*	
Type of business *outpt hospital/clinic*	Dates Mo. Yr. Mo. Yr. From *2* *97* To *8* *2000*
Your position *ins billing specialist*	Hourly rate/salary Starting *$9/hr* Final *$11.50/hr*
Supervisor's name *Candice Johnson*	
Reason for leaving *Professional advancement*	

	Worked performed. Be specific:
1) Employer *Eastern Airlines*	
Address: Street City State Zip code *Orlando, Florida*	
Phone number *(555) 350-7000*	Dates Mo. Yr. Mo. Yr. From *1* *88* To *12* *89*
Type of business *airline transportation*	Hourly rate/salary Starting Final
Your position *receptionist*	
Supervisor's name *Gary Stevens*	
Reason for leaving *career change*	

	Worked performed. Be specific:
1) Employer	
Address: Street City State Zip code	
Phone number ( )	Dates Mo. Yr. Mo. Yr. From To
Type of business	Hourly rate/salary Starting Final
Your position	
Supervisor's name	
Reason for leaving	

F. REFERENCES — FRIENDS / ACQUAINTANCES NON-RELATED

(1) _____ *furnished upon request* _____					
Name	Address	Telephone number	(☐ Work ☐ Home)	Occupation	Years acquainted
(1) _____					
Name	Address	Telephone number	(☐ Work ☐ Home)	Occupation	Years acquainted

Please feel free to add any information which you feel will help us consider you for employment

READ THE FOLLOWING CAREFULLY, THEN SIGN AND DATE THE APPLICATION

"I certify that all answers given by me on this application are true, correct and complete to the best of my knowledge. I acknowledge notice that the information contained in this application is subject to check. I agree that, if hired, my continued employment may be contingent upon the accuracy of that information. If employed, I further agree to comply with Company/Office rules and regulations."

Signature: *Jennifer M. Velasquez* Date: *7-2-XX*

Figure 17–8, cont'd

Street Address
City, State, ZIP code
Date of letter

John Doe, MD or
Personnel Director
Street Address
City, State, ZIP code

Dear Dr. Doe:

Paragraph 1: Explain where you heard about the position and say you are writing for a position mentioned in the advertisement.

Paragraph 2: Name two or more qualifications of great interest to the prospective employer. State reasons you are interested in this specialty, location, or type of work. Mention if experienced or trained for this career field.

Paragraph 3: Refer the reader to the resume or application form enclosed.

Paragraph 4: Close the letter by asking for an interview and suggesting a date and time or that you will call for an appointment. If requesting further information about the job opening, enclose a self-addressed, stamped envelope as a courtesy. Do not end the letter with a vague statement but give the reader a specific action to take.

Sincerely yours,

(handwritten signature)

Type name

Enclosure

Figure 17–9. Suggested content for a letter of introduction to accompany a resume.

Resume

A **resume** is a data sheet designed to sell job qualifications to prospective employers. There are several formats from which to choose:

▶ **Chronologic resume** gives recent experiences first with dates and descriptive data for each job.
▶ **Functional resume** states the qualifications or skills an individual is able to perform.
▶ **Combination resume** summarizes the applicant's job skills as well as educational and employment history. The combination style is the best choice for an insurance billing specialist (Fig. 17–10).

A results-oriented resume focuses on results, not characteristics. It helps prospective employers reduce the risks that are associated with hiring because it shows what the job seeker has accomplished and his or her attitude toward work.

The ideal length for a resume is one page. It can be typed on an 8½ × 14-inch page and reduced to letter size. The resume should be keyed or typed, not handwritten, on high-quality, wrinkle-free bond off-white or white paper; single spaced internally with double spacing between main headings; and balanced spacing for all four margins. Laser-printed resumes give a professional appearance. You might want to have a longer (two-page maximum) resume on hand to offer during an interview.

Under the Civil Rights Act of 1964, enforced by the Equal Employment Opportunity Commission, information about height, weight, birth date, marital status, Social Security number, and physical condition may be omitted. Additional items to omit are salary requirements, reason for leaving jobs, date of resume preparation, date available to begin work, references, and vague references to time gaps. Questions about these items might be asked by the interviewer during an interview. Hobbies and outside interests that relate to the profession might be included. Membership or leadership positions held in professional organizations related to the medical field might be mentioned. A photograph is not necessary but might be included if it will be of value to the interviewer for recall purposes (Fig. 17–11).

The format may include the following:

▶ Title. Resume, Personal Datasheet, Biographic Sketch, or Curriculum Vitae.
▶ Heading. At the beginning of the resume, the applicant's name, address, e-mail address, and telephone and fax numbers are entered.

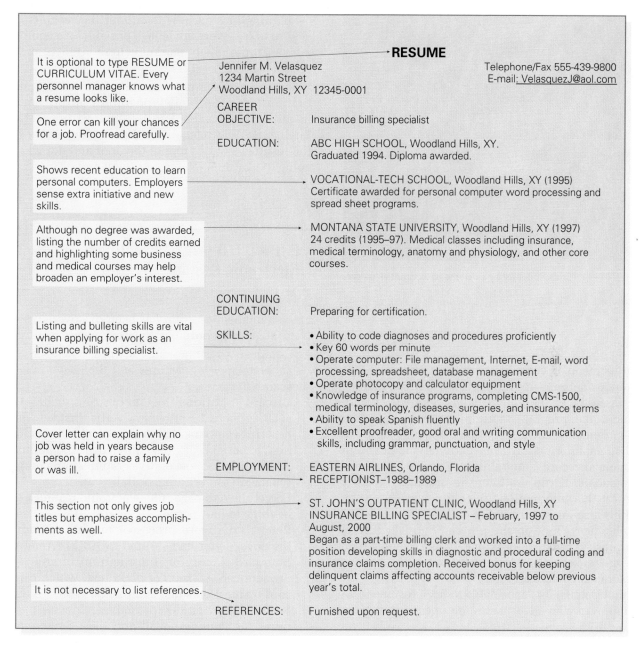

RESUME

It is optional to type RESUME or CURRICULUM VITAE. Every personnel manager knows what a resume looks like.

One error can kill your chances for a job. Proofread carefully.

Shows recent education to learn personal computers. Employers sense extra initiative and new skills.

Although no degree was awarded, listing the number of credits earned and highlighting some business and medical courses may help broaden an employer's interest.

Listing and bulleting skills are vital when applying for work as an insurance billing specialist.

Cover letter can explain why no job was held in years because a person had to raise a family or was ill.

This section not only gives job titles but emphasizes accomplishments as well.

It is not necessary to list references.

Jennifer M. Velasquez
1234 Martin Street
Woodland Hills, XY 12345-0001

Telephone/Fax 555-439-9800
E-mail: VelasquezJ@aol.com

CAREER OBJECTIVE: Insurance billing specialist

EDUCATION: ABC HIGH SCHOOL, Woodland Hills, XY. Graduated 1994. Diploma awarded.

VOCATIONAL-TECH SCHOOL, Woodland Hills, XY (1995) Certificate awarded for personal computer word processing and spread sheet programs.

MONTANA STATE UNIVERSITY, Woodland Hills, XY (1997) 24 credits (1995–97). Medical classes including insurance, medical terminology, anatomy and physiology, and other core courses.

CONTINUING EDUCATION: Preparing for certification.

SKILLS:
- Ability to code diagnoses and procedures proficiently
- Key 60 words per minute
- Operate computer: File management, Internet, E-mail, word processing, spreadsheet, database management
- Operate photocopy and calculator equipment
- Knowledge of insurance programs, completing CMS-1500, medical terminology, diseases, surgeries, and insurance terms
- Ability to speak Spanish fluently
- Excellent proofreader, good oral and writing communication skills, including grammar, punctuation, and style

EMPLOYMENT: EASTERN AIRLINES, Orlando, Florida RECEPTIONIST–1988–1989

ST. JOHN'S OUTPATIENT CLINIC, Woodland Hills, XY INSURANCE BILLING SPECIALIST – February, 1997 to August, 2000 Began as a part-time billing clerk and worked into a full-time position developing skills in diagnostic and procedural coding and insurance claims completion. Received bonus for keeping delinquent claims affecting accounts receivable below previous year's total.

REFERENCES: Furnished upon request.

Figure 17–10. Example of the combination-format resume stressing education and skills. Personal data may be excluded as a result of the Civil Rights Act of 1964, enforced by the EEOC.

▶ Summary. This may be a statement as to why the employer should be interested in this applicant. Use action words as shown in Figure 17–10 and avoid the personal pronoun.

▶ Education. Name high school, college, any business school attended, and **continuing education** classes, city and state, degree, and date received. List in reverse chronologic order. Grade average and awards or scholastic honors may be included.

▶ Professional Experience. Name all employers in reverse chronologic order with addresses, telephone numbers, and dates of employment. Include summer, full-time, part-time, and temporary jobs as well as externship and volunteer work.

▶ Skills. List typing or keyboarding words per minute, computer equipment operated, experience in medical software programs, accurate procedure and diagnostic coding, expertise in insurance claims completion and submission, knowledge of medical terminology and insurance terminology, bookkeeping (posting charges, payments, and

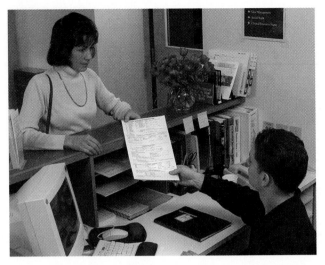

Figure 17–11. Student delivering a resume to a potential job site.

adjustments to accounts receivable journal), experience in preparing appeals for denied claims, resubmittal of delinquent claims, ability to explain insurance programs and plans (e.g., benefits, requirements, and submission of claims), ability to abstract information from patients' medical and financial records, and ability to review insurance payments. If you are fluent in another language, insert this information. Telephone and reception skills also might be mentioned.

▶ References. Type in the phrase "Furnished upon request." Prepare approximately five references on a separate sheet and be sure to contact the persons referenced *before* an interview.

▶ Final Details. It is acceptable to fax a resume to an employer who advertises a job opening but gives

Figure 17–12. Insurance billing student at an externship site.

no guidelines on how to submit the resume. It is wise to use every advantage possible in a competitive employment market where time is of the essence (Fig. 17–12).

Proofread the resume carefully for spelling, punctuation, grammar, and typographic errors. Ask a friend or professional individual with excellent English skills to read and critique it. Remember that the resume is only a foot in the door and not what is going to land that job for you—you are!

PROCEDURE : Creating an Electronic Resume

Once a medical position has been discovered, some basic steps to go online with a resume are:

1. Compose a resume using a word processor with accurate spelling features and then save in a job search file.
2. Discard traditional resume-writing techniques, such as focusing on action verbs. Instead, think descriptive nouns, such as medical biller, education, experience, skills, knowledge, and abilities.
3. Avoid the use of decorative graphics and complex typefaces, underlining, or italics.
4. Forget the one-page rule; electronic resumes may be three to four pages.
5. Refer to the word processor manual to convert the cover letter and resume to ASCII (American Standard Code for Information Interchange; pronounced AS-kee), or plain text, which can be read by most personal computers.
6. Study online guides presenting special procedures for sending e-mail and files. Some e-mail programs allow binary files to be sent, whereas others only allow ASCII text files.
7. Use the word processing software's "copy and paste" feature and enter the information into e-mail or "attach a file" to the e-mail message.
8. Do not post a letter of introduction when posting a resume to a bulletin board.
9. Upload the resume to post online using the file transfer feature of the software following the computer manual directions. The ASCII file is all that is necessary when sending the resume over an online service or from a computer to a dial direct bulletin board.

If the file is sent across the Internet, it should be doctored up in a technical form—encoded by the sender and decoded by the receiver. Take the following steps to prepare a plain ASCII text file.

PROCEDURE: Preparing a Resume in ASCII

1. Create the message using WordPerfect or Word software. Make certain all lines are no more than 65 characters in length. Put a space at the beginning of each blank line between paragraphs.
2. Proofread the resume and save it as plain ASCII text, referring to the word processing software manual for directions.
3. Log onto the bulletin board to upload the ASCII text. Go to the message menu and follow the bulletin board's directions.
4. Select or type "All" or "Resume posting" from the bulletin board's message menu for the recipient and subject.
5. Upload the resume, following the software manual's directions for the communications program being used.
6. Customize the resume by typing in additional information related to the specific job. Depending on the bulletin board, a "Message Edit" menu or the next available line will appear issuing message-editing commands.

Interview

After looking for a potential employer, preparing a resume, and completing an application, the final step in landing a job is the face-to-face interview. An **interview** is a formal consultation with questions by an employer to evaluate the qualifications of a prospective job applicant (Fig. 17–13). Make the best impression possible on the prospective employer as soon as you walk through the door. Hiring depends on positive qualities. Concentrate on good grooming and a fresh, relaxed appearance. Display a warm, positive attitude. Use proper grammar, avoid using slang, and maintain eye contact.

A female applicant should wear a clean skirt, dress, or tailored suit and nylon stockings with low-heeled pumps. A male applicant should wear a clean dark suit or sport coat, conservative necktie, white shirt, plain slacks, plain socks, and well-shined shoes. A man should avoid a lot of facial hair, long hair, earrings, and heavy after shave-lotion. A woman should have a conservative hair style, wear jewelry sparingly, and avoid heavy makeup, a low-cut neckline, a sleeveless dress, strong perfume, and dark or bright nail polish. Do not smoke or chew gum. Use a proper deodorant. Eliminate nervous habits. It has been found that when applicants have similar skills and education, the decision to hire has been based on physical appearance at the interview.

Figure 17–13. Student being interviewed for an insurance billing position.

Figure 17–14 is an example of an interview evaluation and reference investigation form. This form points out the areas an interviewer observes and how impressions are rated.

Research beforehand to know whether the salary (when offered) is acceptable. If you wish to ask questions about fringe benefits, do not appear to be overly interested in them.

Choose the right time for the interview and arrive promptly. It has been found that late Monday and Friday afternoons between 4:00 and 5:00 PM are not good times for interviews because Mondays are usually catch-up, heavily scheduled days and Fridays are getaway days. Research has proved that the likelihood of hiring the last person interviewed for a position is greater than that of hiring those interviewed first.

Role playing is a good method to use to prepare for an interview. Give a friend a list of questions to ask you, then try to answer the questions spontaneously without stumbling. Videotape or audiotape the session, if possible, to see or hear what the employer will experience.

Questions an interviewer might ask about personal life (marital status), family planning, pregnancy, provision for child care, religious preference, club memberships, height, weight, dependents, age (birth date), ethnic background, maiden name, native language, physical or psychiatric problems, spouse's employment and earnings, credit rating, and home and automobile ownership are illegal and do not have to be answered. (It is not considered discriminatory if an employer wishes to know whether an applicant smokes.) Three suggestions for handling an illegal question follow:

1. Answer the question and ignore the fact that you know it is illegal.
2. Answer with, "I think the question is not relevant to the requirements of this position."
3. Refuse to answer and contact the nearest Equal Employment Opportunity Commission (EEOC) office.

INTERVIEW EVALUATION AND REFERENCE INVESTIGATION FORM, MEDICAL or DENTAL OFFICE		SUMMARY OF EVALUATION	
		POINTS FROM APPLICATION AND INTERVIEW	
		POINTS FROM REFERENCES	
		TOTAL POINTS	
NAME OF APPLICANT	DATE	OVERALL IMPRESSION	

RATING: GOOD – 2 POINTS
FAIR – 1 POINT
POOR – 0 POINTS

POSITION APPLIED FOR:

FROM APPLICATION FOR POSITION, GAUGE APPLICANT IN FOLLOWING AREAS	GOOD	FAIR	POOR
1. STABILITY (REMAINED IN ONE PLACE OF RESIDENCE AND ONE JOB FOR A REASONABLE LENGTH OF TIME)?			
2. HEALTH?			
3. THE PROPER EDUCATIONAL BACKGROUND TO FILL THE POSITION?			
4. LEGIBLE HANDWRITING?			
5. AN EMPLOYMENT HISTORY THAT POINTS TOWARD DEPENDABILITY?			
6. LIMITATION ON WORKING HOURS?			
7. THE PROPER EXPERIENCE AND / OR SKILLS TO FILL THE POSITION?			
8. SALARY REQUIREMENT COMMENSURATE WITH POSITION?			

(Left margin labels: APPLICATION SECTION — REFERENCE)

FROM THE PERSONAL INTERVIEW – (SHOULD BE SPECIFIC QUALITIES – OBJECTIVE)			
9. SUFFICIENT CAPABILITY TO HANDLE ANY SITUATION THAT MAY ARISE WHEN ALONE IN OFFICE?			
10. AN APPROPRIATE ATTITUDE TOWARD WORK?			
11. AN APPROPRIATE VOICE, DICTION, GRAMMAR?			
12. POISE?			
13. SELF CONFIDENCE (NOT OVER-CONFIDENCE)?			
14. TACT?			
15. SUFFICIENT MATURITY FOR JOB?			
16. AN ABILITY TO EXPRESS ONESELF WELL?			
17. AN INITIATIVE OR INTEREST IN LEARNING?			
18. APPROPRIATE APPEARANCE (NEAT, CLEAN; SUITABLE TO BUSINESS)			
19. ENERGY, VITALITY AND PERCEIVED ABILITY TO HANDLE PRESSURE OF POSITION?			
20. EAGERNESS TO OBTAIN THE POSITION IN QUESTION?			
COLUMNAR TOTALS			
GRAND TOTAL			

DIRECTIONS FOR USE OF FORM:

1. Look over your ratings. A zero score on any one VITAL question should automatically eliminate applicant. Add up the total rating points and enter in the SUMMARY OF EVALUATION BLOCK in the upper right-hand corner of this page.
2. After finishing all interviews, choose the "best bets" and check their references using the reverse side of this form.
3. Enter, as above, the results of your reference check and then your overall impression. (E – Excellent, G – Good, F – Fair, P – Poor)

FORM # 72-120 © 1987 BIBBERO SYSTEMS, INC. • PETALUMA, CA. • TO REORDER CALL TOLL FREE: (800) BIBBERO (800-242-2376) OR FAX (800) 242-9330 (REV. 7/87)

Figure 17–14. Example of an Interview Evaluation and Reference Investigation form. (From Bibbero Systems, Inc., Petaluma, CA.)

NOTES:

REFERENCE INVESTIGATION			

1.

OFFICE CONTACTED	PHONE: ( )	DATE
PERSON CONTACTED		
HOW LONG HAVE YOU KNOWN THIS PERSON?		
BETWEEN WHAT DATES WAS THIS PERSON EMPLOYED BY YOU?	FROM	TO
WHAT TYPE OF WORK DID THIS PERSON DO FOR YOU?	TITLE OF POSITION:	SATISFACTORILY?
WAS THIS PERSON CONSISTENTLY COOPERATIVE?	WHAT WERE SHORTCOMINGS?	
DID THIS PERSON GET ALONG WELL WITH OTHERS?		
WAS THIS PERSON TRUSTWORTHY / DEPENDABLE?		ATTENDANCE RECORD:
WHY DID THIS PERSON LEAVE YOUR EMPLOY?		SALARY LEVEL:
WOULD YOU REHIRE THIS PERSON?		
NOTES:		
		RATING:

2.

OFFICE CONTACTED	PHONE: ( )	DATE
PERSON CONTACTED		
HOW LONG HAVE YOU KNOWN THIS PERSON?		
BETWEEN WHAT DATES WAS THIS PERSON EMPLOYED BY YOU?	FROM	TO
WHAT TYPE OF WORK DID THIS PERSON DO FOR YOU?	TITLE OF POSITION:	SATISFACTORILY?
WAS THIS PERSON CONSISTENTLY COOPERATIVE?	WHAT WERE SHORTCOMINGS?	
DID THIS PERSON GET ALONG WELL WITH OTHERS?		
WAS THIS PERSON TRUSTWORTHY / DEPENDABLE?		ATTENDANCE RECORD:
WHY DID THIS PERSON LEAVE YOUR EMPLOY?		SALARY LEVEL:
WOULD YOU REHIRE THIS PERSON?		
NOTES:		
		RATING:

3.

OFFICE CONTACTED	PHONE: ( )	DATE
PERSON CONTACTED		
HOW LONG HAVE YOU KNOWN THIS PERSON?		
BETWEEN WHAT DATES WAS THIS PERSON EMPLOYED BY YOU?	FROM	TO
WHAT TYPE OF WORK DID THIS PERSON DO FOR YOU?	TITLE OF POSITION:	SATISFACTORILY?
WAS THIS PERSON CONSISTENTLY COOPERATIVE?	WHAT WERE SHORTCOMINGS?	
DID THIS PERSON GET ALONG WELL WITH OTHERS?		
WAS THIS PERSON TRUSTWORTHY / DEPENDABLE?		ATTENDANCE RECORD:
WHY DID THIS PERSON LEAVE YOUR EMPLOY?		SALARY LEVEL:
WOULD YOU REHIRE THIS PERSON?		
NOTES:		
		RATING:

INTERVIEWER _____ DATE: _____

Figure 17–14, cont'd

Figure 17–15. Job applicant concluding an interview with an office manager.

Shake the interviewer's hand at the conclusion of the meeting (Fig. 17–15). Ask how long it will be before a job offer or denial is forthcoming, and then leave with a "thank you." If the job is offered at the interview and the applicant is not sure about accepting, ask, "How soon do you need to know?" This will allow time to think and compare job offers before making a commitment.

Portfolio

Prepare in advance for the interview by organizing a **portfolio.** Assemble letters of recommendation (from former employers, teachers, family physician, professional friends, community leaders), school diplomas or degrees, transcripts, certificates, names and addresses of references, extra copies of the resume, Social Security card, timed typing test certified by an instructor, some neatly typed insurance claim forms with evidence of coding skills, and any other items related to prior education and work experience.

Alien

Any **alien** employee must have an Employment Eligibility Verification Form I-9 on file with his or her employer. This form can be obtained by writing to the Immigration and Naturalization Service (INS) at 425 I Street, NW, Washington, DC 20536. Within 3 days of hiring an alien, the employee must show one of the following: a naturalization certification (citizen papers), an alien registration receipt card, a temporary resident receipt card, or an employment authorization card. One of these items should be in the portfolio in the event it is requested by the prospective employer during the interview.

Follow-Up Letter

Write a follow-up letter indicating thanks for the interview and restating interest in the position (Fig. 17–16). This keeps the applicant's name before the potential employer. Telephone to express continued interest in the position if no response is heard within the time frame given.

Figure 17–16. Example of a thank-you letter sent after an interview.

Street Address
City, State, ZIP code
Date of letter

John Doe, MD or
Personnel Director
Street Address
City, State, ZIP code

Dear Dr. Doe:

Thank you for spending your valuable time yesterday to interview me for the insurance billing specialist position in your clinic.

I hope that you will allow me the opportunity to prove my abilities as I feel that I am able to perform the work with expertise. Meeting your staff was most enjoyable, and it would certainly be pleasurable working with them as a team.

I am looking forward to hearing from you in the near future.

Sincerely yours,

(handwritten signature)

Type name

Self-Employment

Setting Up an Office

When an individual wishes to be his or her own boss **(self-employed),** it is usually wise to get more than 2 or 3 years of experience in the chosen career before undertaking this task. Preferably an individual should begin as an insurance billing specialist and then proceed to become an **electronic claims processor (ECP).** Some experience in public relations, as well as a strong background in insurance, is desirable for the individual who wants to work as a claims assistance professional. Outpatient hospital and physician billing experience in several specialties is vital for an outpatient coding specialist. Hospital inpatient and outpatient coding experience is necessary for a hospital coding specialist.

One must have something to offer clients when marketing and selling one's services and skills. This knowledge and expertise can only be gained with years of experience. Full-time commitment, hard work, dedication, and many long hours to obtain clients are encountered when beginning a business.

In addition, money is needed for equipment, computer software, overhead, taxes, stationery, preprinted statements, CMS-1500 claim forms, and myriad other expenses. It is vital to have sufficient funds to run the business for a period of 1 year or more. It is imperative that this be accrued before vacating a full-time job. This will help eliminate a lot of fear and anxiety over not having enough business clients. A common reason for business failure is running out of the money necessary to keep the business going. It may take a year or more to begin seeing a profit, so one must be patient.

If you work awhile before striking out independently, you will make contacts on the job that may help build clientele. Networking is extremely important when one tries to establish a successful business. Many times it is who the individual knows that may get a foot in the potential client's door. Networking may open up many opportunities.

An insurance billing specialist can work as an independent contractor to have flexible hours, work from home, and reduce a medical practice's overhead. Some communities prohibit residents from telecommuting or operating a home-based business, although most allow it with restrictions. Working at home requires self-discipline, and one must develop a schedule and stick to it. Good time management is essential. It takes additional hours to advertise, obtain clients, bill, and perform the bookkeeping tasks. Figure 17–17 is a checklist of tasks that must be done to establish a new business.

It is always wise to rent a post office box. Never use a home address because this encourages patients who might visit at inconvenient hours. In some regions, business licenses are not issued for residential areas if clients come to the door. A post office box is essential to get around this issue.

Publications available about starting your own claims processing or medical billing service are listed in Appendix B.

Finances

If an individual has had no experience or is not strong in marketing skills and small business accounting, courses may be taken to gain knowledge and instill confidence in these areas before beginning a business. Attend workshops and lectures on starting a business that are offered by financial institutions, universities, community colleges, or private institutions.

It is wise to seek the services of a lawyer, accountant, or both before legally establishing a business and making appropriate selection of the tax options involved. Establish detailed financial records from the very beginning, even if an accountant is to be hired. Obtain simplified bookkeeping software for use on the computer. Expert advice is essential and helps develop a successful business; a business could fail without it.

Establishing a business in a home may result in some deductions, so obtain the Internal Revenue Service (IRS) publication No. 587 entitled "Business Use of Your Home." Self-employment tax on net income is due each year. Quarterly estimated tax payments are required once the net income amounts to $500 or more. Keep receipts and complete records of income and expenses because these are extremely important for IRS purposes.

Paycheck stubs, copies of hours worked, and identifying data on clients must be retained for the period of time stipulated by the IRS. The following is a record retention schedule.

Bank statements: 3 years
Canceled checks: permanently
Expired contracts: 7 years
Financial statements: permanently
General correspondence: 2 years
Payroll records and summaries: 7 years
Tax returns, worksheets, and other tax documents: permanently

Keep a record of business travel expenses and document mileage. Travel log books are available at stationery stores.

Equipment

Certain items must be purchased when setting up a business at home or in a small office. Necessary equipment to consider are a computer, medical software, modem, printer, telephone answering machine, fax machine, photocopy machine, office

---

NEW BUSINESS CHECKLIST

_1. Decide what address you will use, since you may wish to obtain a post office box number instead of using your home address.

_2. Obtain a business license from the business license section of your city hall. Regulations vary in each city licensing office. You might have to obtain a home occupation permit from the planning department and have it signed by your landlord if you are renting. The city may have guidelines on hours of business, pedestrian and vehicular activity, noise, and so forth in the residential area.

_3. File a fictitious business name (Doing Business As–DBA) at the county clerk's office by obtaining the proper form for completion. If you use your given name, you do not have to file a fictitious business name.

_4. Publish the fictitious name in a local newspaper.

_5. If you have employees, contact the Internal Revenue Service (IRS) for an employer identification number and/or tax information. Obtain the booklet *Tax Guide for Small Business* No. 334 to determine business expenses that are deductible. Depending on how you set up your business, some possible tax breaks are as follows: depreciation of office equipment; declaring a room of your home as an office; subscriptions to professional publications; dues to professional associations; expenses associated with your automobile; telephone, photocopying, office supplies (stationery, books, typewriter ribbons, and so on); promotion and advertising (postage, meals with business associates, and so on); and any expenses pertaining to meetings, conventions, workshops, or seminars (registration fees, lodging, meals, transportation, parking, and so forth).

_6. If you have no employees, contact the Franchise Tax Board for the form used for estimating state withholding taxes for yourself. This must be filed quarterly. If you build up your business and have employees, obtain the proper forms and information for employees (state income tax, and state disability and unemployment insurance).

_7. Obtain the insurance that you need: health insurance, disability insurance, life insurance, liability insurance, workers' compensation (if you have employees), and so forth. Insurance is available to protect you against loss of material called "Release of Information Insurance" or "Errors and Omissions Insurance" with a "Hold Harmless" clause. You might want to consider a retirement IRA or Keogh plan.

_8. Contact the telephone company for information regarding lines for phone, fax equipment and computer modem. Inquire about custom or special calling services such as call waiting and so forth. Do this early because there is often a delay in hook-up. You might consider using your existing telephone number and switching to a business listing. This allows you to be listed in the *Yellow Pages* of your telephone directory.

_9. Open a bank account. If you want your telephone number on your checks, put the checks on hold until the telephone is confirmed. Some banks require a business license and Doing Business As documents to open an account. Take these documents with you to the bank.

_10. Order business cards, stationery, billing forms, and reference books. Design a logo for the business.

_11. Begin to advertise your business by some of the following methods: newspaper, radio, flyers, announcements, signs, word of mouth, and letters to prospects (hospitals, clinics, and physician's offices).

Additional points to consider if expanding to a location outside of a home:

_12. Check the zoning of the location at your city hall's planning department or, if you are in the county, the county's planning department. Sign a lease contingent on proper zoning and on meeting all federal, state, county, and city building safety and health requirements. Inquire about parking and sign restrictions at the planning department. Find out if you need any permits (building permit, certificate of occupancy, health permit, and so forth). City and county offices may require a sign permit for new signs and changes on old ones.

_13. If you have opened an office at a location, make a deposit for water, gas, and electricity. Rent, renovation, and janitorial or trash services must be considered.

_14. Call the assessor's office and ask to be put on the mailing list for business property tax (inventory tax).

_15. Contact the various inspectors: health, building, and safety, and sign to have all completed work inspected and the necessary permits signed off.

Figure 17–17. New business checklist. (From Diehl MO, Fordney MT: *Medical Keyboarding, Typing, and Transcribing Techniques and Procedures.* Philadelphia, Saunders, 1997.)

---

furniture, filing cabinet, and calculator. It is imperative to install a separate telephone line for clients or patients calling in. For transmitting claims electronically, a telephone line is needed to operate with the computer modem. An optional item might be a postage meter. Research equipment costs and maintenance options before purchase or lease and find out how much it costs for service contracts.

It is possible to obtain a low-interest government Small Business Administration (SBA) loan for starting a business. Loans also are available to physically challenged persons who qualify.

Insurance

Business owners find it necessary to protect income and property from unexpected loss. Workers' compensation insurance must be obtained if the business grows and employees are hired. There is a federal directive that formally exempts home offices from Occupational Safety and Health Administration (OSHA) safety inspections unless the agency learns of safety or health violations. Some types of insurance to investigate follow:

▶ Property insurance in case of fire, theft, or a disaster

▶ Disability insurance if one becomes unable to work because of illness or injury
▶ Health insurance
▶ Life insurance
▶ Business interruption insurance. (In case of fire, it would take time and money to re-create data. Backed-up data should be stored off site.)
▶ Professional liability insurance

Marketing, Advertising, Promotion, and Public Relations

Marketing refers to how a business is presented or advertised to promote sales. Marketing strategies vary depending on the section of the public that is targeted. When promoting a medical billing service, develop a well-organized marketing plan and follow basic guidelines to reach a specific target audience.

Ways to market a business and the reasons for marketing strategies are presented in Table 17–1.

Insurance billing and coding specialists market to those who will use their services in the community, such as physicians (family practitioners, surgeons, psychiatrists, psychologists, physical therapists), small hospitals, clinics, laboratories, podiatrists, and chiropractors. However, claims assistance professionals' target audience is the consumer and Medicare recipients.

Obtain figures to help convince clients that the service you are offering is better and can do more for their business than what they presently have. Save them time and money! Stress being honest, reliable, committed, efficient, and professional, and offer them something they cannot do for themselves.

Contracts or Agreements

Develop a contract or agreement when dealing with some facilities, such as an acute care hospital, whose legal department may review it before signing. This can clarify job responsibilities and help eliminate misunderstandings. Put everything in writing. A contract should define the following:

▶ Who does the coding?
▶ Will claims be filed electronically?
▶ What is the per claim processing fee?
▶ Who is responsible for rebilling?
▶ Who will handle collection procedures (follow-up telephone calls or letters)?
▶ Who pays for rebilling, photocopying of records, mailing fees, and clearinghouse charges?
▶ Under whose name will bills be sent to patients?
▶ Will the billing service phone number appear on the statement, or will a toll-free or local number be used?
▶ How will the telephone be answered?

TABLE 17–1	**Business Marketing and Strategies**
Strategy	**Reason**
Obtain professionally printed stationery and business cards.	Enhances professional image.
Pass out business cards at professional meetings.	Advertises availability and services.
Develop a business name and logo for the company.	Enables potential clients to remember you.
Ensure accuracy of all printed materials.	When items are not professionally assembled or proofread to eliminate misspelling errors, a potential client receives a negative image of the company.
Develop a professional flyer and distribute it to medical facilities and physicians' offices.	Introduces company name, advertises services, and describes benefits.
Follow up with a personal visit or telephone call.	A friendly voice and professional image offer you are available and interested.
Advertise in the journal or newsletter of the county medical society and state medical association.	Potential clients read such publications and advertisements of this nature lend to your credibility.
Place an advertisement in the newspaper or on cable television.	Circulates business within the county.
Put an ad in the *Yellow Pages*.	Solicits wider range of prospective clients.
Network with members of professional organizations.	Word of mouth advertising can be the best public relations tool, especially if done by professional peers.
Network via computer using the Internet's World Wide Web, Prodigy, CompuServe, America Online, and Genie bulletin boards for this career field.	Offers wide range of contacts.
Check with established businesses to determine whether they are overloaded with work, the owner needs a vacation, or help is needed in a temporary situation because of illness.	Present your services as a help, not a threat, to current office staff.

▶ What are the charges for coding consultation services?

▶ What are the coverage arrangements for absence or illness?

If there is any change in the terms of the agreements, write a letter outlining the new terms. Long-term contracts are preferred over short-term contracts, so put in dates of validity. Renegotiation is in order when the contract expires.

HIPAA Compliance Alert

Some contracts may include a statement on confidentiality assuring the contracting facility that all patient data will be handled in a confidential manner.

Documentation

If you are hired as a coding specialist, keep written records of the numbers of hours worked, the quantity of work done each day, and the corrections applied to the work by officials in the contracting facility or hospital. Retain any written coding guideline from the contracting facility or hospital.

Statements and Pricing

A variety of methods are used to price services, such as a percentage of reimbursement or an annual, hourly, or per claim fee. Deciding on which method depends on the type of client being served and the work to be done. Claims assistance professionals bill in 15-minute increments. Telephone other billing and insurance services, preferably outside the area, to see how they are charging because in-area competitors may be reluctant to divulge that information.

Professional Associations: Certification and Registration

More exacting professional requirements have evolved because of specialization in the allied health careers. Certification and registration are two ways of exhibiting professional standards. **Certification** is a statement issued by a board or association verifying that a person meets professional standards. **Registration** may be accomplished in two methods, as an entry in an official registry or record that lists names of persons in an occupation who have satisfied specific requirements or by attaining a certain level of education and paying a registration fee. In the latter, if there are certain requirements for registration, then an unregistered person may be prevented from working in a career for which he or she is otherwise qualified.

A number of certifications are available on a national level, depending on how you wish to specialize (Table 17–2).

Keeping Current

Membership in professional organizations helps in keeping up-to-date. Most of these associations have student as well as active and associate membership categories. You can inquire whether there is a local chapter or state organization affiliated with the national association. Benefits of belonging to a professional organization, in addition to certification and recertification, include problem solving, continuing education, and employment opportunities. Local meetings can keep you knowledgeable by providing guest speakers on topics of current interest. The newsletters and journals published by these organizations keep you abreast of current trends either as a subscriber or as a benefit when becoming a member.

Mentor

A valuable vehicle for career development is to find a **mentor** in the business. A mentor is a guide or teacher who offers advice, criticism, wisdom, guidance, and perspective to an inexperienced but promising protégé to help reach a life goal. Decide what kind of help you want, such as technical, general feedback, managerial, and so on. Then look for a mentor whose background, values, and style are similar to yours. Be willing to face criticism with a positive attitude and express gratitude when excellence is praised.

Networking

Another avenue to pursue for career development is to *network*. **Networking** is the exchange of information or services among individuals, groups, or institutions and making use of professional contacts. To do this, join as many organizations as possible because it can be difficult to keep abreast of ongoing changes in the insurance industry when you are self-employed. Many of the professional organizations publish monthly newsletters or quarterly journals, offer certification, and plan national conventions, state conferences, and regional meetings. In addition to the organizations mentioned in this chapter, some additional ones to contact are:

Health Care Management Association of Southern California

P.O. Box 27771

Santa Ana, CA 92799

Healthcare Financial Management Association (HFMA)

TABLE 17–2 Certification and Registration

Title/Abbreviation	Description to Obtain Certification or Registration	Professional Association Mailing Address	Telephone Number	Web Site	E-Mail Address
Certified Bookkeeper (**CB**)	Self-study program and employment experience; pass three tests	American Institute of Professional Bookkeepers 6001 Montrose Road, Suite 207 Rockville, MD 20852	(800) 622-0121	www.aipb.org	visit Web site
Certified Billing and Coding Specialist (**CBCS**)	High school diploma or GED and graduate from approved training program or minimum 1 yr wk exp.	National Healthcareer Association 134 Evergreen Place, 9th Floor East Orange, NJ 07018	(800) 499-9092	www.nhanow.com	info@nhanow.com
Certified Coding Associate (**CCA**) Certified Coding Specialist (**CCS**) Certified Coding Specialist-Physician (**CCS-P**)	Self-study program; pass certification examination	American Health Information Management Association (AHIMA) PO Box 97349 Chicago, IL 60690-7349	(800) 335-5535	www.ahima.org	
Certified Healthcare Billing & Management Executive (**CHBME**)	Complete comprehensive program; pass proficiency test	Healthcare Billing and Management Association (HMBA) 1550 South Coast Highway, Suite 201 Laguna Beach, CA 92651	(877) 640-4262	www.hbma.com	www.info@hbma.com
Certified Medical Administrative Assistant (**CCMA**)	High school diploma or GED and graduate from approved training program or minimum 1 yr wk exp.	National Healthcareer Association 134 Evergreen Place, 9th Floor East Orange, NJ 07018	(800) 499-9092	www.nhanow.com	info@nhanow.com
Certified Medical Assistant (**CMA**)	Graduate from accredited medical assisting program; apply to take national certifying examination	American Association of Medical Assistants (AAMA) 20 North Wacker Drive Chicago, IL 60606	(800) 228-2262	www.aama.ntl.org	visit Web site
Certified Medical Biller (**CMB**)	Pass 2-hour examination written for physician's office billers and other outpatient facilities	American Association of Medical Billers (AAMB) PO Box 44614 Los Angeles, CA 90044-0614	(323) 778-4352 Fax: (323) 778-2814	www.billers.com/aamb/page2.html	AAMB@aol.com
Certified Medical Billing Specialist (**CMBS**)	Pass 3-hour examination written for physician's office billers and other outpatient facilities	American Association of Medical Billers (AAMB) PO Box 44614 Los Angeles, CA 90044-0614	(323) 778-4352 Fax: (323) 778-2814	www.billers.com/aamb/page2.html	AAMB@aol.com

Continued.

TABLE 17-2 Certification and Registration—cont'd

Title/Abbreviation	Description to Obtain Certification or Registration	Professional Association Mailing Address	Telephone Number	Web Site	E-Mail Address
Certified Medical Billing Specialist (CMBS)	Complete 6 courses and provide evaluation of billing performance by supervisor	Medical Association of Billers (MAB) 2441 Tech Center Court, Suite 108 Las Vegas, NV 89128	(702) 240-8519 Fax: (702) 243-0359	www.physiciansWeb sites.com	mailroom@physicians Websites.com
Certified Medical Office Manager (CMOM)	Examination for supervisors or managers of small-group and solo practices	Professional Association of Health Care Office Managers (PAHCOM) 461 East Ten Mile Road Pensacola, FL 32534-9712	(800) 451-9311	www.pahcom.com	pahcom@pahcom.com
Certified Medical Practice Executive (CMPE) Nominee 1st level Certification 2nd level Fellow 3rd level	1st level - Eligible group managers join; membership/ nominee 2nd level - Complete 6 to 7 hour examination 3rd level - Mentoring project or thesis	Medical Group Management Association (MGMA), American College of Medical Practice Executives (affiliate) 104 Inverness Terrace East Englewood, CO 80112	(303) 397-7869	www.mgma.com/ acmpe	
Certified Medical Reimbursement Specialist (CMRS)	Self-study program; successfully pass 18 sections of examination	American Medical Billing Association (AMBA) 4297 Forrest Drive Sulphur, OK 73086	(580) 622-2624	www.ambanet.net/ cmrs.htm	
Certified Medical Transcriptionist (CMT)	Self-study program and successfully pass written and practical examinations offered by Medical Transcription Certification Commission (MTCC)	American Association for Medical Transcription 100 Sycamore Avenue Modesto, CA 95354-0550	(800) 982-2182	www.aamt.org	visit Web site
Certified Patient Account Technician (CPAT) Certified Clinic Account Technician (CCAT) Certified Clinic Account Manager (CCAM)	Complete self-study course; pass standard examination administered twice yearly	American Assn. of Healthcare Administrative Mgmt (AAHAM) National Certification Examination Program 11240 Waples Mill Road, Suite 200 Fairfax, VA 22030	(703) 281-4043	www.aaham.org/ aaham.cfm	debra@statmarket.com

Certification	Requirements	Organization/Address	Phone	Web site	Email
Certified Professional Coder (CPC) Certified Professional Coder-Apprentice (CPC-A) Certified Professional Coder-Hospital (CPC-H)	Independent study program; examination approximately 5 hours (CPC) and 8 hours (CPC-H) in length. No practical experience for CPC-A. Two years experience for CPC.	American Academy of Professional Coders (AAPC) 309 West 700 South Salt Lake City, UT 84101	(800) 626-CODE		
Healthcare Reimbursement Specialist (HRS)	Successfully complete open-book examination	National Electronic Biller's Alliance (NEBA) 2226-A Westborough Blvd. #504 South San Francisco, CA 94080	(650) 359-4419 Fax: (650) 989-6727	http://www.nebazone.com	mmedical@aol.com
National Certified Insurance and Coding Specialist (NCICS)	Graduate from an insurance program; sit for certification examination given by independent testing agency at many school sites across the nation	National Center for Competency Testing 7007 College Blvd., Suite 250 Overland Park, KS 66211	(800) 875-4404 Fax: (913) 498-1243	www.ncctinc.com	visit Web site
Radiology Certified Coder (RCC)	HS diploma & 1 yr FT radiology coding exp in past 4 yrs or 2 yrs FT radiology coding in past 4 yrs or apl demonstrating adequate equivalent exp.	Radiology Coding Certification Board (RCCB) Helen Tipton, Executive Director 65 Enterprise Aliso Viejo, CA 92656	(866) 227-7222 ext. 76463	www.rccb.org	helen.tipton@rccb.org
Registered Medical Assistant (RMA)	Take certification offered by the American Medical Technologist (AMT)	Registered Medical Assistant (AMT) 710 Higgins Road Park Ridge, IL 60068-5765	(847) 823-5169	www.amt1.com	amtmail@aol.com
Registered Medical Coder (RMC)	Yearly correspondence program governed by the National Coding Standards Committee and pass an examination	Medical Management Institute 1125 Cambridge Square Alpharetta, GA 30004-5724	(800) 334-5724	www.the-institute.com	bobby.carvell@ipractice.md

Two Westbrook Corporate Center, Suite 700
Westchester, IL 60154-5700

Claims assistance professionals should attend local meetings for Medicare recipients. Join local volunteer service organizations and the chamber of commerce to network with others. Contact the LEADS Club at (800) 783-3761 or The National Association of Female Executives at (800) 669-1002 for potential client leads and networking.

RESOURCES ON THE INTERNET

Job Search Resources:
Yahoo (search engine)
www.yahoo.com/
Infoseek (search engine)
www.infoseek.go.com
Alta Vista (search engine)
www.altavista.com
Career Magazine
www.careermag.com/careermag/
America's Job Bank
www.ajbb.dni.us
E-Span Employment Database Search
www.espan.com/
MedSearch
www.medsearch.com
Refer to Table 17–2 for Professional Organization Web sites.

STUDENT ASSIGNMENT LIST

✔ Study Chapter 17.
✔ Answer the review questions in the *Workbook* to reinforce the theory learned in this chapter and help prepare you for a future test.
✔ Complete the assignments in the *Workbook* to give you hands-on experience in completing an application for a position as an insurance billing specialist, preparing and typing a resume, composing a cover letter to go with the resume, having someone evaluate you during an interview, and typing a follow-up thank-you letter after being interviewed.
✔ Turn to the Glossary at the end of this textbook for a further understanding of the Key Terms used in this chapter.

A P P E N D I X A

> ## Addresses for Submitting Claims or Contacting State Insurance Commissioners and State Boards of Medical Examiners

The list of names and addresses presented here for each state has been compiled for your use in submitting insurance claim forms to state or federal programs. In addition, insurance commissioners' state offices are included if a question, problem, or complaint arises that should be resolved. Addresses for state boards of medical examiners are included in case medicolegal information is sought at a state level. State addresses for workers' compensation are given in case there is need to obtain forms and guidelines or for cases that are being settled or appealed. Insurance companies across the nation handle workers' compensation insurance; they are too numerous to include in this textbook. Federal workers' compensation district office addresses for each state may be used when submitting insurance claims for a federal worker injured while working.

The information contained in this Appendix has been reorganized so the reader can locate information quickly and easily. Look for the name of your state and then check the subheadings, which are arranged alphabetically, for the program or plan name and address.

The list of names and addresses in this Appendix has been compiled from state and federal references published in 2003. Because fiscal intermediaries (insurance carriers) for state and federal programs (e.g., CHAMPVA, Medicaid, Medicare, TRICARE) change as contracts expire, it is always wise to use the telephone directory and call to verify addresses when in doubt as to their accuracy.

ALABAMA

CHAMPVA Claim Office
CHAMPVA Center
4500 Cherry Creek Dr., S.
P.O. Box 65024
Denver, CO 80206-9024

Insurance Commissioner State Office
Insurance Commissioner
201 Monroe St., #1700 (36104)
P.O. Box 303351
Montgomery, AL 36130-3351
http://www.aldoi.org

Maternal and Child Health Program
Bureau of Family Health Services
RSA Tower, Suite 1368
201 Monroe St.
P.O. Box 303017
Montgomery, AL 36130-3017

Children's Rehabilitation Services
2129 East South Blvd.
P.O. Box 11586
Montgomery, AL 36111-0586

Medicaid Fiscal Agent
Electronic Data Systems
P.O. Box 244034
Montgomery, AL 36124
http://www.medicaid.state.al.us/

Medicare Durable Medical Equipment
Palmetto Government Benefits Administration (PGBA)
Medicare DMERC Operations
P.O. Box 100254
Columbia, SC 29202-3254
http://www.pgba.com

Medicare Fiscal Agent or Carrier
Blue Cross-Blue Shield of Alabama
Cahaba Government Benefits Administration (GBA)
P.O. Box 995
Birmingham, AL 35298
http://www.almedicare.com/

State Board of Medical Examiners
Alabama State Board of Medical Examiners
848 Washington Ave. (36104)
P.O. Box 946
Montgomery, AL 36101-0946

TRICARE Claim Office
Palmetto Government Benefits Administration (PGBA)
P.O. Box 7031
Camden, SC 29020-7031
http://www.myTRICARE.com/

Veterans Affairs Installation
Alabama Medical Centers:
  Birmingham 35233 (700 S. 19th St.)
  Montgomery 36109 (215 Perry Hill Rd.)
  Tuscaloosa 35404 (3701 Loop Rd. E.)
  Tuskegee 36083 (2400 Hospital Rd.)

Workers' Compensation Federal District Office
Office of Workers' Compensation Programs
214 North Hogan St., Suite 1006
Jacksonville, FL 32202

Workers' Compensation State Plan Office
Workmen's Compensation Division
Department of Industrial Relations
Industrial Relations Bldg.
649 Monroe St.
Montgomery, AL 36131
http://www.dir.state.al.us/wc/

ALASKA

CHAMPVA Claim Office
CHAMPVA Center
4500 Cherry Creek Dr., S.
Box 65024
Denver, CO 80206-9024

Insurance Commissioner State Office
Division of Insurance
Department of Community and Economic
 Development
P.O. Box 110805
Juneau, AK 99811-0805
http://www. labor.state.ak.us

Maternal and Child Health Program
Alaska Department of Health & Social Services
Maternal Child and Family Health
1231 Gambell St.
Anchorage, AK 99501-4627

Special Needs Services Unit
State of Alaska, Department of Health &
 Social Services, DPH, MCFH
3601 C St., Suite 934
P.O. Box 240249
Anchorage, AK 99503

Medicaid Fiscal Agent
First Health (EC)
P.O. Box 240769
Anchorage, AK 99503-0769
http://www.hss.state.ak.us/dhcs

Medicare Durable Medical Equipment
CIGNA Medicare
P.O. Box 690
Nashville, TN 37202
http://www.cignamedicare.com

Medicare Fiscal Agent or Carrier
Noridian Mutual Insurance Company
4510 13th Ave., SW
P.O. Box 6703 (claims) (58108)
Fargo, ND 58103
http://www.noridianmedicare.com

State Board of Medical Examiners
Alaska State Medical Board
550 West Seventh Avenue, Suite 1500
Anchorage, AK 99501
http://www.state.ad.us/local

TRICARE Claim Office
Palmetto Government Benefits Administration (PGBA)
P.O. Box 870001
Surfside Beach, SC 29587-8701

Veterans Affairs Installation
Alaska Veterans HC System and Regional Office
2925 De Barr Rd.
Anchorage, AK 99508-2989

Workers' Compensation Federal District Office
Office of Workers' Compensation Programs
1111 Third Ave., Suite 650
Seattle, WA 98101-3212

Workers' Compensation State Plan Office
Division of Workers' Compensation
Department of Labor & Workforce Development
1111 W. 8th St., Suite 307
P.O. Box 25512
Juneau, AK 99802-5512
http://www.labor.state.ak.us

ARIZONA

CHAMPVA Claim Office
CHAMPVA Center
4500 Cherry Creek Dr., S.
P.O. Box 65024
Denver, CO 80206-9024

Insurance Commissioner State Office
Director of Insurance
2910 North 44th St., Suite 210
Phoenix, AZ 85018-7256
http://www.state.az.us/id

Maternal and Child Health Program
CSHCN
Arizona Department of Health Services
2927 North 35th Ave., Suite 300
Phoenix, AZ 85017

Office of Women's and Children's Health
Arizona Department of Health Services
2927 North 35th Ave.
Phoenix, AZ 85017

Medicaid Fiscal Agent
Arizona Health Care Cost Containment
 System (AHCCCS)
P.O. Box 1700
Phoenix, AZ 85002-9949
http://www.ahcccs.state.az.us/

Medicare Durable Medical Equipment
CIGNA Medicare
P.O. Box 690
Nashville, TN 37202
http://www.cignamedicare.com

Medicare Fiscal Agent or Carrier
Noridian Mutual Insurance Company
4510 13th Ave., S.W.
P.O. Box 6704 (58108)
Fargo, ND 58103
http://www.noridianmedicare.com/

State Board of Medical Examiners
Arizona Medical Board
9545 E. Doubletree Ranch Rd.
Scottsdale, AZ 85258-5514
http://www.azmdboard.com

Arizona Board of Osteopathic Examiners in
  Medicine and Surgery
9535 E. Doubletree Ranch Rd.
Scottsdale, AZ 85258-5539
http://www.azosteoboard.org

TRICARE Claim Office
Except for the Yuma area:
TRICARE Central Regions 7/8
Palmetto Government Benefits Administration
P.O. Box 870026
Surfside Beach, SC 29587-8726

Yuma area:
P.O. Box 870001
Surfside Beach, SC 29587-8701

Veterans Affairs Installation
Arizona Medical Centers:
  Phoenix 85012 (650 E. Indian School Rd.)
  Prescott 86313 (500 Highway 89, North)
  Tucson 85723 (3601 S. 6th Ave.)

Workers' Compensation Federal District Office
Office of Workers' Compensation Programs
71 Stevenson St., Suite 305
P.O. Box 193769 (94119-3769)
San Francisco, CA 94105

Workers' Compensation State Plan Office
Industrial Commission of Arizona
800 W. Washington St. (85007-2922)
P.O. Box 19070
Phoenix, AZ 85005-9070

ARKANSAS

CHAMPVA Claim Office
CHAMPVA Center
4500 Cherry Creek Dr., S.
P.O. Box 65024
Denver, CO 80206-9024

Insurance Commissioner State Office
Department of Insurance
1200 W. 3rd St.
Little Rock, AR 72201-1904
http://www.state.ar.us/insurance

Maternal and Child Health Program
Section of Maternal and Child Health
Arkansas State Department of Health
4815 W. Markham, Slot 41
Little Rock, AR 72205-3867

Children's Medical Services Group
Arkansas Department of Health
P.O. Box 1437, Slot 5380
Little Rock, AR 72203

Medicaid Fiscal Agent
Electronic Data Systems (EC)
P.O. Box 8036

Little Rock, AR 72203-2501
http://www.medicaid.state.ar.us/

Medicare Durable Medical Equipment
Palmetto Government Benefits Administration (PGBA)
P.O. Box 100254
Columbia, SC 29202-3254
http://www.pgba.com/

Medicare Fiscal Agent or Carrier
Arkansas Blue Cross and Blue Shield:
  A Mutual Insurance Company
601 Gaines St.
Little Rock, AR 72202
http://www.arkmedicare.com/

State Board of Medical Examiners
Arkansas State Medical Board
2100 Riverfront Dr., Suite 200
Little Rock, AR 72202-1793
http://www.armedicalboard.org

TRICARE Claim Office
Except a small part of Arkansas in the Naval Hospital:
Millington, TN, service area:
Wisconsin Physicians Service
P.O. Box 8999
Madison, WI 53708-8999

The Millington area address is:
Palmetto Government Benefits Administration (PGBA)
P.O. Box 7031
Camden, SC 29020

Veterans Affairs Installation
Arkansas Medical Centers:
  Fayetteville 72703 (1100 N. College Ave.)
  North Little Rock 72114 (2200 Fort Roots Dr.)
  Little Rock 72205 (4300 W. 7th St.)

Workers' Compensation Federal District Office
Office of Workers' Compensation Programs
525 S. Griffin St., Room 100
Dallas, TX 75202

Workers' Compensation State Plan Office
Workers' Compensation Commission
324 Spring St.
P.O. Box 950
Little Rock, AR 72203-0950
http://www.awcc.state.ar.us

CALIFORNIA

California Medical Services
*(Known in other states as Maternal and Child Health
  Program)*
Children's Medical Services
California State Department of Health Services
714 P St., Room 323
Sacramento, CA 95814

Maternal & Child Health
California State Department of Health Services
714 P St., Room 476
Sacramento, CA 95814

CHAMPVA Claim Office
CHAMPVA Center

4500 Cherry Creek Dr., S.
P.O. Box 65024
Denver, CO 80206-9024

Insurance Commissioner State Office
Commissioner
Department of Insurance
300 Capitol Mall, Suite 1500
Sacramento, CA 95814
http://www.insurance.ca.gov

Medi-Cal Fiscal Agent
Electronic Data Systems (EC)
P.O. Box 15700
Sacramento, CA 95852-1700
http://www.medi-cal.ca.gov/
http://www.dhs.ca.gov/mcs/

Medicare Durable Medical Equipment
CIGNA Medicare
P.O. Box 690
Nashville, TN 37202
http://www.cignamedicare.com/

Medicare Fiscal Agent or Carrier
National Heritage Insurance Company
402 Otterson Dr.
Chico, CA 95928
http://www.medicarenhic.com/

State Board of Medical Examiners
Medical Board of California
1426 Howe Ave., Suite 54
Sacramento, CA 95825-3236
http://www.medbd.ca.gov

Osteopathic Medical Board of California
2720 Gateway Oaks Dr., Suite 350
Sacramento, CA 95833-3500
http://www.dca.ca.gov/osteopathic

TRICARE Claim Office
Palmetto Government Benefits Administration
TRICARE Claims
P.O. Box 870001
Surfside Beach, SC 29587-8701
http://www.myTRICARE.com

**Unemployment Compensation Disability &
State Disability Offices**
Chico
645 Salem, 95928-5576
P.O. Box 8190, 95297-8190

City of Industry (San Gabriel Valley)
17171 E. Gale Ave.,
Suite 110, 91745-1810
P.O. Box 60006, 91716-0006

Eureka
490 K St., Suite 201, 95501
P.O. Box 4986, 95502-4986

Fresno
2550 Mariposa, Room 1080A, 93721-2270
P.O. Box 32, 93702-0032

Long Beach
4300 Long Beach, Suite 600, 90807-2011
P.O. Box 469, 90801-0469

Los Angeles
221 North Figueroa St., Suite 200, 90012-2652
P.O. Box 513096, 90051-1096

Oakland
7700 Edgewater Dr., Suite 210, 94621-3018
P.O. Box 1857, 94604-1857

Redding
615 Locust St., 96099-2711
P.O. Box 991898, 96099-1898

Riverside
1190 Palmyrita Ave., Suite 100, 92507-1908
P.O. Box 59903, 92517-1903

Sacramento
5009 Broadway, 95820-1613
P.O. Box 13140, 95813-3140

San Bernardino
371 W. 3rd St., Room 101, 92401
P.O. Box 781, 92402-0781

San Diego
8977 Activity Rd., Bldg. B, Suite 200, 92126-4427
P.O. Box 120831, 92112-0831

San Francisco
745 Franklin St., Suite 300 (94102)
P.O. Box 193534, 94119-3534

San Jose
297 W. Hedding St., 95110-1628
P.O. Box 637, 95106-0637

Santa Ana
28 Civic Center Plaza, Room 735, 92701-4024
P.O. Box 1466, 92702-1466

Santa Barbara
128 E. Ortega, 93101-1631
P.O. Box 1529, 93102-1529

Santa Rosa
50 D St., Room 325, 95404-4757
P.O. Box 700, 95402-0700

Stockton
528 N. Madison St., 95202-1917
P.O. Box 201006, 95201-9006

Van Nuys (North Los Angeles)
15400 Sherman Way, Room 500, 91406
P.O. Box 10402, Van Nuys, CA 91410-0402

Woodland Hills
21210 Erwin, 91367-3714
P.O. Box 4256, 91365-4256

Veterans Affairs Installation
California Medical Centers:
  Bakersfield 93301 (1801 Westwind Dr.)
  Fresno 93703 (2615 E. Clinton Ave.)
  Livermore 94450 (4951 Arroyo Rd.)
  Loma Linda 92357 (11201 Benton St.)
  Long Beach 90822 (5901 E. 7th St.)
  Los Angeles 90012 (351 E. Temple St.)
  Martinez 94553 (150 Muir Rd.)
  Menlo Park 94025 (795 Willow Rd.)

Palo Alto 94304 (3801 Miranda Ave.)
Sacramento 95655 (10535 Hospital Way)
San Diego 92161 (3350 La Jolla Village Dr.)
San Francisco 94121 (4150 Clement St.)
Santa Barbara 93110 (4440 Calle Real)
Sepulveda 91343 (16111 Plummer St.)
W. Los Angeles 90073 (11301 Wilshire Blvd.)

Workers' Compensation Federal District Office
Office of Workers' Compensation Programs
71 Stevenson St., Suite 305 (94105)
P.O. Box 193769
San Francisco, CA 94119-3769

Workers' Compensation State Plan Offices
Department of Industrial Relations
Division of Workers' Compensation
455 Golden Gate Ave., 9th Floor
San Francisco, CA 94102

Workers' Compensation Appeals Board
http://www.dir.ca.gov

CANADA

CHAMPVA Claim Office
CHAMPVA Center
4500 Cherry Creek Dr., S.
P.O. Box 65024
Denver, CO 80206-9024

TRICARE Claim Office
Wisconsin Physician Service
P.O. Box 7985
Madison, WI 53707-7985

COLORADO

CHAMPVA Claim Office
CHAMPVA Center
4500 Cherry Creek Dr., S.
P.O. Box 65024
Denver, CO 80206-9024

Insurance Commissioner State Office
Commissioner of Insurance
1560 Broadway, Suite 850
Denver, CO 80202
http://www.dora.state.co.us/Insurance

Maternal and Child Health Program
Health Care Program for CSHCN
Division of Prevention & Intervention Services for
  Children & Youth
4300 Cherry Creek Dr., S., HPDP-WHS-A5
Denver, CO 80246-1530

Adolescent and School Health Section
Colorado Department of Public Health and Environment
4300 Cherry Creek Dr., S.
Denver, CO 80246-1530

Medicaid Fiscal Agent
Colorado Health Care Policy and Finance
  c/o Consultec
P.O. Box 30
Denver, CO 80201-0030
http://www.chcpf.state.co.us

Medicare Durable Medical Equipment
Palmetto Government Benefits Administration (PGBA)
P.O. Box 100254
Columbia, SC 29202-3254
http://www.pgba.com/

Medicare Fiscal Agent or Carrier
Noridian Mutual Insurance Company
4510 13th Ave., SW
P.O. Box 6707
Fargo, ND 58103
http://www.noridianmedicare.com/

State Board of Medical Examiners
Colorado Board of Medical Examiners
1560 Broadway, Suite 1300
Denver, CO 80220-5140
http://www.dora.state.co.us/medical

TRICARE Claim Office
Palmetto Government Benefits Administration (PGBA)
P.O. Box 870027
Surfside Beach, SC 29587-8727
http://www.myTRICARE.com

Veterans Affairs Installation
Colorado Medical Centers:
  Denver 80220 (1055 Claremont St.)
  Fort Lyon 81038 (C St.)
  Grand Junction 81501 (2121 North Ave.)
  Pueblo 81005 (1339 S. Pueblo Blvd.)

Workers' Compensation Federal District Office
Office of Workers' Compensation Programs
1999 Broadway, Suite 600
Denver, CO 80202

Workers' Compensation State Plan Office
Division of Workers' Compensation
1515 Arapahoe St., Tower 2, Suite 500
Denver, CO 80202-2117

Industrial Claims Appeal Office
1515 Arapahoe St.
Denver, CO 80202

CONNECTICUT

CHAMPVA Claim Office
CHAMPVA Center
4500 Cherry Creek Dr., S.
P.O. Box 65024
Denver, CO 80206-9024

Insurance Commissioner State Office
Director, Consumer Affairs
Department of Insurance
P.O. Box 816
Hartford, CT 06412-0816
http://www.state.ct.us/cid

Maternal and Child Health Program
Connecticut Department of Public Health
Child, Adolescent and School Health Unit
410 Capitol Ave., MS 11 MAT
P.O. Box 340308
Hartford, CT 06134-0308

MCH and CSCHN
Department of Public Health
410 Capitol Ave., MS 11MAT
P.O. Box 340308
Hartford, CT 06134-0308

Medicaid Fiscal Agent
Electronic Data Systems Corporation/Medical
  Assistance Program
P.O. Box 2941
Hartford, CT 06106
http://www.dss.state.ct.us/svcs/medical.htm

Medicare Durable Medical Equipment
HealthNow of New York
P.O. Box 6800
Wilkes-Barre, PA 18773-6800

Medicare Fiscal Agent or Carrier
First Coast Service Options
Medicare Part B
321 Research Parkway
P.O. Box 9000
Meriden, CT 06450-7148
http://www.connecticutmedicare.com

State Board of Medical Examiners
Connecticut Medical Examining Board
P.O. Box 340308
Hartford, CT 06134-0308

TRICARE Claim Office
Palmetto Government Benefits Administration (PGBA)
P.O. Box 7011
Camden, SC 29020-7011

Veterans Affairs Installation
Connecticut Health System
  Newington 06111 (555 Willard Ave.)
  W. Haven 06516 (950 Campbell Ave.)

Workers' Compensation Federal District Office
Office of Workers' Compensation Programs
JFK Federal Office Bldg., Room E-260
Boston, MA 02203

Workers' Compensation State Plan Office
Workers' Compensation Commission
21 Oak St., 4th floor
Hartford, CT 06106
http://www.state.ct.us

DELAWARE

CHAMPVA Claim Office
CHAMPVA Center
4500 Cherry Creek Dr., S.
P.O. Box 65024
Denver, CO 80206-9024

Insurance Commissioner State Office
Commissioner
Department of Insurance
841 Silver Lake Blvd.
P.O. Box 7007
Dover, DE 19904
http://www.state.de.us/inscom

Maternal and Child Health Program
CSHCN Program
Delaware Division of Public Health
P.O. Box 637, Jesse Cooper Bldg.
Dover, DE 19903

Medicaid Fiscal Agent
Medicaid Processing Unit
1901 N. Dupont Hwy (19720)
P.O. Box 907
New Castle, DE 19720
http://www.state.de.us/dhss/dss/medicaid.html

Medicare Durable Medical Equipment
HealthNow of New York
P.O. Box 6800
Wilkes-Barre, PA 18773-6800

Medicare Fiscal Agent or Carrier
Blue Cross and Blue Shield of Texas
DBA Trail Blazer Health Enterprises, Inc.
8330 LBJ Freeway, Executive Center 3
P.O. Box 660156 (75266-0156)
Dallas, TX 75266-0043
http://www.trailblazerhealth.com/

State Board of Medical Examiners
Delaware Board of Medical Practice
861 Silver Lake Blvd., Cannon Bldg., Suite 203 (19904)
P.O. Box 1401
Dover, DE 19903-1401
http://www.professionallicensing.state.de.us

TRICARE Claim Office
Palmetto Government Benefits Administration (PGBA)
P.O. Box 7011
Camden, SC 29020-7011

Veterans Affairs Installation
Medical Center
1601 Kirkwood Highway
Wilmington, DE 19805

Workers' Compensation Federal District Office
Office of Workers' Compensation Programs
Curtis Center, Suite 715 E.
170 S. Independence Mall W.
Philadelphia, PA 19106-3308

Workers' Compensation State Plan Office
Department of Labor
Division of Industrial Affairs
4425 N. Market St., 3rd Floor
Wilmington, DE 19802
http://www.delawareworks.com

DISTRICT OF COLUMBIA

CHAMPVA Claim Office
CHAMPVA Center
4500 Cherry Creek Dr., S.
P.O. Box 65024
Denver, CO 80206-9024

Insurance Commissioner State Office
Insurance Administration
810 First St., NE, Suite 701
Washington, DC 20002

Maternal and Child Health Program
Office of Maternal and Child Health
Department of Health Maternal and
 Family Health Administration
825 N. Capitol St., NE, 3rd Floor
Washington, DC 20002

Medicaid Fiscal Agent
Medicaid Assistance Administrator
825 N. Capitol St., NE, 5th Floor
Washington, DC 20002
http://dchealth.dc.gov/information/maa_outline.shtm

Medicare Durable Medical Equipment
Assigned:
AdminaStar Federal, Inc.
P.O. Box 7078
Indianapolis, IN 46207-7078
http://www.adminastar.com/

Nonassigned:
P.O. Box 7031
Indianapolis, IN 46207-7931

Medicare Fiscal Agent or Carrier
Trail Blazer Health Enterprises, Inc.
P.O. Box 660156
Dallas, TX 75266-0156
http://www.trailblazerhealth.com/

State Board of Medical Examiners
District of Columbia Board of Medicine
825 North Capitol St., NE, 2nd Floor, Room 2224
Washington, DC 20002
http://ww.dchealth.dc.gov

TRICARE Claim Office
Palmetto Government Benefits Administration (PGBA)
P.O. Box 7011
Camden, SC 29020-7011

Veterans Affairs Installation
District of Columbia Medical Center
50 Irving St., NW
Washington, DC 20422

Workers' Compensation Federal District Office
Office of Workers' Compensation Programs
800 N. Capitol St., NW, Room 800
Washington, DC 20211

Workers' Compensation State Plan Office
Department of Employment Services
Office of Workers' Compensation
1200 Upshur St., NW, 3rd Floor
Washington, DC 20011
http://www.does.ci.washington.dc.us

FLORIDA

CHAMPVA Claim Center
CHAMPVA Center
4500 Cherry Creek Dr., S.
Box 65024
Denver, CO 80206-9024

Insurance Commissioner State Office
Florida Department of Financial Services
200 E. Gaines St.

Tallahassee, Florida 32399-0300
http://www.fldfs.com/

Maternal and Child Health Program
Division of Children's Medical Services
Florida Department of Health, #SF Bin #A-13
4052 Bald Cypress Way, Bin A06
Tallahassee, FL 32399-1707

Division of Family Health Services
Department of Health
Family Health Services
Capitol Circle Office Complex
4025 Esplanade Way
Tallahassee, FL 32399-1723

Medicaid Fiscal Agent
P.O. Box 7072
Tallahassee, FL 32314-7072
http://www.fdhc.state.fl.us/medicaid/index2.shtml

Medicare Durable Medical Equipment
Palmetto Government Benefits Administration (PGBA)
P.O. Box 100254
Columbia, SC 29202-3254
http://www.pgba.com

Medicare Fiscal Agent or Carrier
First Coast Service Options
P.O. Box 2078
Jacksonville, FL 32231
http://www.floridamedicare.com/

State Board of Medical Examiners
Florida Board of Medicine, Department of Health
Medicine Quality Assurance
4052 Bald Cypress Way, BIN #C03
Tallahassee, FL 32399-3253
http://www9.myflorida.com/mqa/osteopath/os_home.html

Florida Board of Osteopathic Medicine
4052 Bald Cypress Way, SE, BIN #C06
Tallahassee, FL 32399-3253
http://www9.myflorida.com/mqa/osteopth/os_home.html

TRICARE Claim Office
Palmetto Government Benefits Administration (PGBA)
P.O. Box 7031
Camden, SC 29020-7031
http://www.myTRICARE.com

Veterans Administration Installation
Florida Medical Centers:
 Bay Pines 33744 (10000 Bay Pines Blvd., North)
 Gainesville 32608 (1601 SW Archer Rd.)
 Lake City 32025 (801 S. Marion St.)
 Miami 33125 (1201 NW 16th St.)
 Tampa 33612 (13000 Bruce B. Downs Blvd.)
 W. Palm Beach 33410 (7305 N. Military Trail)

Workers' Compensation Federal District Office
Office of Workers' Compensation Programs
214 North Hogan St., Suite 1006
Jacksonville, FL 32202

Workers' Compensation State Plan Office
Division of Workers' Compensation
Department of Labor and Employment Security

301 Forrest Bldg.
2728 Centerview Dr.
Tallahassee, FL 32399-0680

GEORGIA

CHAMPVA Claim Office
CHAMPVA Center
4500 Cherry Creek Dr., S.
P.O. Box 65024
Denver, CO 80206-9024

Insurance Commissioner State Office
Commissioner
Department of Insurance
704 W. Tower
2 Martin Luther King, Jr. Dr.
Atlanta, GA 30334
http://www.inscomm.state.ga.us

Maternal and Child Health Program
Georgia Department of Human Resources
2 Peachtree St., NW, Suite 11-206
Atlanta, GA 30303-3142

Family Health Branch
2 Peachtree St., NW, Suite 11-414
Atlanta, GA 30303-3142

Medicaid Fiscal Agent
Electronic Data Systems (EC)
P.O. Box 105013
Tucker, GA 30085
http://www.communityhealth.state.ga.us/

Medicare Durable Medical Equipment
Palmetto Government Benefits Administration (PGBA)
P.O. Box 100254
Columbia, SC 29202-3254
http://www.pgba.com/

Medicare Fiscal Agent or Carrier
Blue Cross-Blue Shield of Alabama
Cahaba Government Benefits Administration (GBA)
P.O. Box 3076
Savannah, GA 31402-3076
http://www.gamedicare.com

State Board of Medical Examiners
Georgia Composite State Board of
  Medical Examiners
2 Peachtree St., NW, 36th Floor
Atlanta, GA 30303
http://www.georgia.gov/00/home/0,2125,4802.00.html

TRICARE Claim Office
Palmetto Government Benefits Administration (PGBA)
P.O. Box 7031
Camden, SC 29020-7031
http://www.myTRICARE.com

Veterans Administration Installation
Georgia Medical Centers:
  Augusta 30904 (1 Freedom Way)
  Decatur 30033 (1670 Clairmont Rd.)
  Dublin 31021 (1826 Veterans Blvd.)

Workers' Compensation Federal District Office
Office of Workers' Compensation Programs
214 North Hogan St., Suite 1006
Jacksonville, FL 32202

Workers' Compensation State Plan Office
State Board of Workers' Compensation
270 Peachtree St., NW
Atlanta, GA 30303-1299

GUAM

Insurance Commissioner State Office
Commissioner
Department of Revenue and Taxation
Government of Guam
Bldg.13-3m, 1st Floor
Mariner Ave.
Tiyan, Barrigada, GU 96913

Maternal and Child Health Program
Department of Public Health & Social Services
Bureau of Family Health and Nursing
  Services
P.O. Box 2816
Hagatna, GU 96932

Medicare Durable Medical Equipment
CIGNA Medicare Region D DMERC
P.O. Box 690
Nashville, TN 37202

Medicare Fiscal Agent or Carrier
Noridian Mutual Insurance Company
4305 13th Ave., SW
Fargo, ND 58103

Medicare Railroad Retiree Carrier
Medicare Part B claims are handled by claim service
centers. For the address and toll-free number of the
office nearest you, call the Railroad Retirement Board
listed in your telephone directory under
U.S. Government.

State Board of Medical Examiners
Guam Board of Medical Examiners
Health Professional Licensing Office
1304 East Sunset Blvd. (96913)
P.O. Box 2816
Hagatna, GU 96932

Veterans Affairs Installation
Veterans Affairs Clinic
U.S. Naval Hospital
313 Farenholt Rd.
Agana Heights, GU 96919

Workers' Compensation State Plan Office
Worker's Compensation Commission
Department of Labor
Government of Guam
108 E St. (96913)
P.O. Box 9970
Tuyan, GU 96913

HAWAII

CHAMPVA Claim Office
CHAMPVA Center
4500 Cherry Creek Dr., S.
P.O. Box 65024
Denver, CO 80206-9024

Insurance Commissioner State Office
Commissioner
Department of Insurance
250 S. King St., 5th Floor
P.O. Box 3614
Honolulu, HI 96813-3614
http://www.hawaii.gov/insurance

Maternal and Child Health Program
Family Health Services Division
Hawaii State Department of Health
1250 Punchbowl St., Room 216
Honolulu, HI 96813

CSHCN Branch
Hawaii State Department of Health
741 Sunset Ave.
Honolulu, HI 96816

Medicaid Fiscal Agent
Hawaii Medical Service Association (EC)
P.O. Box 44500
Honolulu, HI 96804-4500
http://www.state.hi.us/dhs/

Medicare Durable Medical Equipment
CIGNA Medicare
P.O. Box 690
Nashville, TN 37202
http://www.cignamedicare.com

Medicare Fiscal Agent or Carrier
Noridian Mutual Insurance Company
P.O. Box 6712 or P.O. Box 6701
Fargo, ND 58108
http://www.noridianmedicare.com/

State Board of Medical Examiners
Hawaii Board of Medical Examiners
Department of Commerce and Consumer Affairs
1010 Richards St. (98613)
P.O. Box 3469
Honolulu, HI 96801
http://www.state.hi.us

TEMPORARY DISABILITY INSURANCE
Department of Labor & Industrial Relations
Disability Compensation Division

Hawaii
State Office Bldg.
75 Aupuni St.
Hilo, HI 96720

Kauai
State Office Bldg.
3060 Eiwa St.
Lihue, HI 96766

Maui
State Office Bldg., #2
2264 Aupuni St.
Wailuku, HI 96793

Oahu
830 Punchbowl St., Suite 210
P.O. Box 3769
Honolulu, HI 96812-3769

West Hawaii
Ashikawa Bldg.
P.O. Box 49
Kealakekua, HI 96750

TRICARE Claim Office
Palmetto Government Business Administration (PGBA)
P.O. Box 870001
Surfside Beach, SC 29587-8701
http://www.myTRICARE.com

Veterans Affairs Installation
Hawaii Medical Center and Regional Office
300 Ala Moana Blvd., Room 1352
P.O. Box 50188
Honolulu 96813-0001
  Medical Office: 808-566-1409
  Regional Office: From Oahu: 808-566-1409
  From Hawaiian neighbor islands: 800-827-1000
  From Guam: 475-8387
  From American Samoa: 11-877-285-1128

Workers' Compensation Federal District Office
Office of Workers' Compensation Programs
71 Stevenson St., Suite 305 (94105)
P.O. Box 193769
San Francisco, CA 94119-3769

Workers' Compensation State Plan Office
Disability Compensation Division
Department of Labor and Industrial Relations
830 Punchbowl St., Room 209
P.O. Box 3769
Honolulu, HI 96813

Labor and Industrial Relations Appeals Board
830 Punchbowl St., Room 404
Honolulu, HI 96813

IDAHO

CHAMPVA Claim Office
CHAMPVA Center
4500 Cherry Creek Dr., S.
P.O. Box 65024
Denver, CO 80206-9024

Insurance Commissioner State Office
Director
Department of Insurance
700 W. State St., 3rd Floor
P.O. Box 83720
Boise, ID 83720-0043
http://www.doi.state.id.us

Maternal and Child Health Program
Children's Special Health Program
Idaho Department of Health and Welfare

450 W. State St.
P.O. Box 83720
Boise, ID 83720-0036

Public Health Services
Idaho Department of Health and Welfare
450 W. State St.
P.O. Box 83720
Boise, ID 83720-0036

Medicaid Fiscal Agent
Department of Health & Welfare
P.O. Box 23
Boise, ID 83707
http://www2.state.id.us/dhw/medicaid/index.htm

Medicare Durable Medical Equipment
CIGNA Medicare
P.O. Box 690
Nashville, TN 37202
http://www.cignamedicare.com

Medicare Fiscal Agent or Carrier
CIGNA Medicare
P.O. Box 1465
Nashville, TN 37202
http://www.cignamedicare.com

Medicare Railroad Retiree Carrier
United Health Care Insurance Company
P.O. Box 10066
Augusta, GA 30999-0001

State Board of Medical Examiners
Idaho State Board of Medicine
Statehouse Mall
1755 Westgate Dr., Suite 140 (83704)
P.O. Box 83720
Boise, ID 83720-0058
http://www.born.state.id.us

TRICARE Claim Office
Northern Idaho (Benewah, Bonner, Boundary, Kootenai, Shoshone, and Latah Counties)
Foundation Health Federal Services, Inc.
Wisconsin Physician Services
TRICARE Northwest
P.O. Box 8999
Madison, WI 53708-8999

Except for six counties in Northern Idaho:
Palmetto Government Benefits Administration (PGBA)
P.O. Box 870028
Surfside Beach, SC 29587-8728
http://www.myTRICARE.com

Veterans Affairs Installation
Idaho Medical Center
500 W. Fort St.
Boise, ID 83702

Workers' Compensation Federal District Office
Office of Workers' Compensation Programs
1111 Third Ave., Suite 650
Seattle, WA 98101-3212

Workers' Compensation State Plan Office
Industrial Commission
317 Main St.

P.O. Box 83720
Boise, ID 83720-0041

ILLINOIS

CHAMPVA Claim Office
CHAMPVA Center
4500 Cherry Creek Dr., S.
P.O. Box 65024
Denver, CO 80206-9024

Insurance Commissioner State Office
Director
Department of Insurance
320 W. Washington St., 4th Floor
Springfield, IL 62767-0001
http://www.state.il.us/ins/

Maternal and Child Health Program
Office of Family Health
Illinois Department of Public Health
535 W. Jefferson St.
Springfield, IL 62702-5058

Division of Specialized Care for Children
University of Illinois at Chicago
2815 W. Washington, Suite 300
P.O. Box 19481
Springfield, IL 62794-9481

Medicaid Fiscal Agent
Department of Human Services
P.O. Box 19105
Springfield, IL 62794-9105
http://www.ins.state.il.us/

Medicare Durable Medical Equipment
Assigned:
AdminaStar Federal, Inc.
P.O. Box 7078
Indianapolis, IN 46207-7078
http://www.adminastar.com/

Nonassigned:
P.O. Box 7031
Indianapolis, IN 46207-7931

Medicare Fiscal Agent or Carrier
Wisconsin Physicians Services
1717 W. Broadway
P.O. Box 8190
Madison, WI 53713
Or
P.O. Box 1030
Marion, IL 62959
http://www.wpsic.com/

State Board of Medical Examiners
Illinois Department of Professional Regulation
100 W. Randolph St., Suite 9-300
Chicago, IL 60601
http://www.dpr.state.il.us

TRICARE Regions 2/5 Claims
Palmetto Government Benefits Administration (PGBA)
P.O. Box 7021
Camden, SC 29020-7021

Veterans Affairs Installation
Illinois Medical Centers:
  Chicago 60611 (Lakeside, 333 E. Huron St.)
  Chicago 60612 (Westside, 820 S. Damen Ave.,
   P.O. Box 8195)
  Danville 61832 (1900 E. Main St.)
  Hines 60141 (Roosevelt Rd. & 5th Ave.)
  Marion 62959 (2401 W. Main St.)
  North Chicago 60064 (3001 Green Bay Rd.)

Workers' Compensation Federal District Office
Office of Workers' Compensation Programs
230 S. Dearborn St., 8th Floor
Chicago, IL 60604

Workers' Compensation State Plan Office
Industrial Commission
100 W. Randolph St., Suite 8-200
Chicago, IL 60601
http://www.state.il.us/agency/iic

INDIANA

CHAMPVA Claim Office
CHAMPVA Center
4500 Cherry Creek Dr., S.
P.O. Box 65024
Denver, CO 80206-9024

Insurance Commissioner State Office
Commissioner
Department of Insurance
311 W. Washington St., Suite 300
Indianapolis, IN 46204-2787
http://www.state.in.us/idoi/

Maternal and Child Health Program
Children's Special Health Care Program
Indiana State Department of Health
2 N. Meridian St., Section 7-B
Indianapolis, IN 46204

State Department of Health
2 N. Meridian St., Section 7-C
Indianapolis, IN 46204

Medicaid Fiscal Agent
Family and Social Services Administration
P.O. Box 7269
Indianapolis, IN 46207
http://www.state.in.us/fssa/servicedisabl/medicaid/
  index.html

Medicare Durable Medical Equipment
Assigned:
AdminaStar Federal, Inc.
P.O. Box 7078
Indianapolis, IN 46278-7027

Nonassigned:
P.O. Box 7031
Indianapolis, IN 46207-7931

Medicare Fiscal Agent or Carrier
Part B Participating:
AdminaStar Federal, Inc.
8115 Knue Rd.
Indianapolis, IN 46250
http://www.adminastar.com/

Part B Nonparticipating:
Assigned:
AdminaStar Federal, Inc.
P.O. Box 6026
Indianapolis, IN 46206-6026

Nonassigned:
AdminaStar Federal, Inc.
P.O. Box 7073
Indianapolis, IN 46206-7073

State Board of Medical Examiners
Indiana Health Professions Bureau
402 W. Washington St., Room 041
Indianapolis, IN 46204

TRICARE Regions 2/5 Claims
Palmetto Government Benefits Administration (PGBA)
P.O. Box 7021
Camden, SC 29020-7021

Veterans Affairs Installation
Indiana Medical Centers:
  Fort Wayne 46805 (2121 Lake Ave.)
  Indianapolis 46202 (1481 W. 10th St.)
  Marion 46953 (1700 E. 38th St.)

Workers' Compensation Federal District Office
Office of Workers' Compensation Programs
1240 E. Ninth St., Room 851
Cleveland, OH 44199

Workers' Compensation State Plan Office
Worker's Compensation Board
402 W. Washington St., Room W196
Indianapolis, IN 46204
http://www.in.gov/wkcomp/index.html

IOWA

CHAMPVA Claim Office
CHAMPVA Center
4500 Cherry Creek Dr., S.
P.O. Box 65024
Denver, CO 80206-9024

Insurance Commissioner State Office
Commissioner
Division of Insurance
330 E. Maple St.
Des Moines, IA 50319-0065
http://www.iid.state.ia.us/

Maternal and Child Health Program
Family Services Bureau
Iowa Department of Public Health
321 E. 12th St., Lucas Bldg.
Des Moines, IA 50319-0075

Child Health Specialty Clinics
University of Iowa, Hospital School
100 Hawkins Dr., Room 247B CDD
Iowa City, IA 52242-1011

Medicaid Fiscal Agent
Department of Human Services
P.O. Box 14421
Des Moines, IA 50306
http://www.state.ia.us/medicalservices/medicalservices.asp

Medicare Durable Medical Equipment
CIGNA Medicare
P.O. Box 690
Nashville, TN 37202
http://www.cignamedicare.com

Medicare Fiscal Agent or Carrier
Noridian Mutual Insurance Company
P.O. Box 6712
Fargo, ND 58108
http://www.noridianmedicare.com/

State Board of Medical Examiners
Iowa Board of Medical Examiners
400 SW 8th St., Suite C
Des Moines, IA 50309-4686

TRICARE Claim Office
Palmetto Government Benefits Administration (PGBA)
P.O. Box 870029
Surfside Beach, SC 29587-8729
http://www.myTRICARE.com

Veterans Administration Installation
Iowa Medical Centers:
  Des Moines 50310 (3600 30th St.)
  Iowa City 52246 (601 Highway 6 W.)
  Knoxville 50138 (1515 W. Pleasant St.)

Workers' Compensation Federal District Office
Office of Workers' Compensation Programs
City Center Square
1100 Main St., Suite 750
Kansas City, MO 64105

Workers' Compensation State Plan Office
Division of Workers' Compensation
Department of Workforce Development
1000 E. Grand Ave.
Des Moines, IA 50319-0209
http://www.state.ia.us/iwd/wc

KANSAS

CHAMPVA Claim Office
CHAMPVA Center
4500 Cherry Creek Dr., S.
Box 65024
Denver, CO 80206-9024

Insurance Commissioner State Office
Commissioner
Department of Insurance
420 SW 9th St.
Topeka, KS 66612-1678
http://www.ink.org/public/kid

Maternal and Child Health Program
Services for CSHCN
Kansas Department of Health & Environment
1000 SW Jackson, Suite 220
Topeka, KS 66612-1274

Medicaid Fiscal Agent
Blue Cross & Blue Shield of Kansas
P.O. Box 3571
Topeka, KS 66601-3571
http://www.srskansas.org/services/HCP_index.htm

Medicare Durable Medical Equipment
CIGNA Medicare
P.O. Box 690
Nashville, TN 37202
http://www.cignamedicare.com

Medicare Fiscal Agent or Carrier
Blue Cross and Blue Shield of Kansas
1133 Topeka Ave. (66629)
P.O. Box 239
Topeka, KS 66601
http://www.kansasmedicare.com/

State Board of Medical Examiners
Kansas Board of Healing Arts
235 SW Topeka Blvd.
Topeka, KS 66603-3068

TRICARE Claim Office
Palmetto Government Benefits Administration (PGBA)
P.O. Box 870030
Surfside Beach, SC 29587-8730

Veterans Affairs Installation
Kansas Medical Centers:
  Leavenworth 66048 (4101 S. 4th St., Trafficway)
  Topeka 66622 (2200 SW Gage Blvd.)
  Wichita 67218 (5500 E. Kellogg)

Workers' Compensation Federal District Office
Office of Workers' Compensation Programs
City Center Square
1100 Main St., Suite 750
Kansas City, MO 64106

Workers' Compensation State Plan Office
Division of Workers' Compensation
Department of Human Resources
800 SW Jackson St., Suite 600
Topeka, KS 66612-1227
http://www.hr.state.ks.us/wc/html/wc.htm

KENTUCKY

CHAMPVA Claim Office
CHAMPVA Center
4500 Cherry Creek Dr., S.
Box 65024
Denver, CO 80206-9024

Insurance Commissioner State Office
Commissioner
Department of Insurance
215 W. Main St.
P.O. Box 517
Frankfort, KY 40602-0517
http://wwww.doi.state.ky.us/

Maternal and Child Health Program
Division of Adult and Child Health
Department for Health Services
275 E. Main St., HSB 2R
Frankfort, KY 40621-0001

Kentucky Commission for CSHCN
982 Eastern Parkway
Louisville, KY 40217

Medicaid Fiscal Agent
UNISYS (EC)
P.O. Box 2101
Frankfort, KY 40621-2101
http://chs.state.ky.us/dms/

Medicare Durable Medical Equipment
Palmetto Government Benefits Administration (PGBA)
P.O. Box 100254
Columbia, SC 29202-3254
http://www.pgba.com/

Medicare Fiscal Agent or Carrier
AdminaStar Federal, Inc.
8115 Knue Rd.
Indianapolis, IN 46250
http://www.adminastar.com/

State Board of Medical Examiners
Kentucky Board of Medical Licensure
Hurstbourne Office Park
310 Whittington Parkway, Suite 1B
Louisville, KY 40222-4916

TRICARE Claim Office
Palmetto Government Benefits Administration (PGBA)
P.O. Box 7021
Camden, SC 29020-7021
http://www.myTRICARE.com

Veterans Affairs Installation
Kentucky Medical Centers:
  Fort Thomas 41075 (1000 S. Ft. Thomas Ave.)
  Lexington 40502-2236 (1101 Veterans Dr.)
  Louisville 40206 (800 Zorn Ave.)

Workers' Compensation Federal District Office
Office of Workers' Compensation Programs
214 North Hogan St., Suite 1006
Jacksonville, FL 32202

Workers' Compensation State Plan Office
Department of Workers' Claims
Perimeter Park W., Bldg. C
1270 Louisville Rd.
Frankfort, KY 40601
http://labor.ky.gov/dwc/

LOUISIANA

CHAMPVA Claim Office
CHAMPVA Center
4500 Cherry Creek Dr., S.
P.O. Box 65024
Denver, CO 80206-9024

Insurance Commissioner State Office
Commissioner
Department of Insurance
950 North Fifth St.
P.O. Box 94214
Baton Rouge, LA 70804-9214
http://www.ldi.state.la.us

Maternal and Child Health Program
Children's Special Health CSHCN Program
Office of Public Health
P.O. Box 60630, Room 607
New Orleans, LA 70160

Maternal and Child Health Section
Office of Public Health
P.O. Box 60630
New Orleans, LA 70160

Medicaid Fiscal Agent
UNISYS (EC)
P.O. Box 91020
Baton Rouge, LA 70821
http://www.dhh.state.la.us/medicaid/index.htm

Medicare Durable Medical Equipment
Palmetto Government Benefits Administration (PGBA)
P.O. Box 100254
Columbia, SC 29202-3254
http://www.pgba.com/

Medicare Fiscal Agent or Carrier
Louisiana Medicare Services
P.O. Box 98501
Baton Rouge, LA 70884
http://www.lamedicare.com/

State Board of Medical Examiners
Louisiana State Board of Medical Examiners
630 Camp St.
P.O. Box 30250
New Orleans, LA 70190-0250

TRICARE Claim Office
Western two thirds, mainly west of Baton Rouge:
Wisconsin Physicians Service
P.O. Box 8999
Madison, WI 53708-8999

Eastern third of the state, including Baton Rouge and New Orleans:
Palmetto Government Benefits Administration (PGBA)
P.O. Box 7031
Camden, SC 29520-7031
http://www.myTRICARE.com

Veterans Affairs Installation
Louisiana Medical Centers:
  Alexandria 71306 (2495 Shreveport Highway 71 North, P.O. Box 69004)
  New Orleans 70112 (1601 Perdido St.)
  Shreveport 71101 (510 E. Stoner Ave.)

Workers' Compensation Federal District Office
Office of Workers' Compensation Programs
525 S. Griffin St., Room 100
Dallas, TX 75202

Workers' Compensation State Plan Office
Department of Labor
Office of Workers' Compensation
1001 N. 23rd St.
P.O. Box 94040
Baton Rouge, LA 70804-9040
http://www.laworks.net

MAINE

CHAMPVA Claim Office
CHAMPVA Center
4500 Cherry Creek Dr., S.
P.O. Box 65024
Denver, CO 80206-9024

Insurance Commissioner State Office
Bureau of Insurance
34 State House Station
Augusta, ME 04333-0034
http://www.maineinsurancereg.org

Maternal and Child Health Program
CSHCN Program
Maine Bureau of Health, Department of Human Services
State House Station #11
151 Capitol St.
Augusta, ME 04333-0011

Medicaid Fiscal Agent
Medical Claims Processing
Bureau of Medical Services
M500
Augusta, ME 04333

Medicare Durable Medical Equipment
HealthNow of New York
P.O. Box 6800
Wilkes-Barre, PA 18773-6800

Medicare Fiscal Agent or Carrier
National Heritage Insurance Company
75 Sgt. William B. Terry Dr.
Hingham, MA 02043

State Board of Medical Examiners
Maine Board of Osteopathic Licensure
2 Bangor St., 2nd Floor
142 State House Station
Augusta, ME 04333-0142

Maine Board of Licensure in Medicine
Two Bangor St.
137 State House Station
Augusta, ME 04333-0137

TRICARE Claim Office
Palmetto Government Benefits Administration (PGBA)
P.O. Box 7011
Camden, SC 29020-7011

Veterans Affairs Installation
Maine Medical Center
1 VA Center
Togus, ME 04330

Workers' Compensation Federal District Office
Office of Workers' Compensation Programs
JFK Federal Office Bldg., Room E-260
Boston, MA 02203

Workers' Compensation State Plan Office
Workers' Compensation Board
27 State House Station
Augusta, ME 04333-0027

MARYLAND

CHAMPVA Claim Office
CHAMPVA Center
4500 Cherry Creek Dr., S.
P.O. Box 65024
Denver, CO 80206-9024

Insurance Commissioner State Office
Commissioner
Insurance Administration
525 St. Paul Pl., 7th Floor
Baltimore, MD 21202-2272
http://www.mdinsurance.state.md.us/

Maternal and Child Health Program
Office of Geriatrics and CSHCN
Maryland Department of Health and Mental Hygiene
201 W. Preston St., Room 319
Baltimore, MD 21201

Maternal Health and Family Planning
Department of Health and Mental Hygiene
201 W. Preston St., Room 318
Baltimore, MD 21201

Medicaid Fiscal Agent
Health Choice
201 W. Preston St.
Baltimore, MD 21201
http://www.dhmh.state.md.us/mma/mmahome.html

Medicare Durable Medical Equipment
Assigned:
AdminaStar Federal, Inc.
P.O. Box 7078
Indianapolis, IN 46207-7078
http://www.adminastar.com/

Nonassigned:
P.O. Box 7031
Indianapolis, IN 46207-7931

Medicare Fiscal Agent or Carrier
Montgomery and Prince George's counties:
Xact Medicare Services (EC)
P.O. Box 890101
Camp Hill, PA 17089-0101

Rest of State:
Trail Blazer Health Enterprisers, LLC
8330 LBJ Freeway
Executive Center 3
P.O. Box 660595 (75266-0595)
Dallas, TX 75243

State Board of Medical Examiners
Maryland State Board of Physicians
4201 Patterson Ave., 3rd Floor
P.O. Box 2571
Baltimore, MD 21215-0095

TRICARE Claim Office
Palmetto Government Benefits Administration (PGBA)
P.O. Box 7011
Camden, SC 29020-7011

Veterans Affairs Installation
Maryland Medical Centers:
  Baltimore 21201 (Prosthetic Assessment Information
    Center, 103 E. Gay St.)
  Baltimore 21201 (10 N. Greene St.)
  Baltimore 21218 (Rehabilitation and Extended Care
    Center, 3900 Loch Raven Blvd.)
  Fort Howard 21052 (9600 N. Point Rd.)
  Perry Point 21902 (Circle Dr.)

Workers' Compensation Federal District Office
Office of Workers' Compensation Programs
800 N. Capitol St., NW, Room 800
Washington, DC 20211

Workers' Compensation State Plan Office
Workers' Compensation Commission
10 E. Baltimore St.
Baltimore, MD 21202-1641

MASSACHUSETTS

CHAMPVA Claim Center
CHAMPVA Center
4500 Cherry Creek Dr., S.
P.O. Box 65024
Denver, CO 80206-9024

Insurance Commissioner State Office
Commissioner
Division of Insurance
S. Station, 5th Floor
Boston, MA 02210-2223
http://www.state.ma.us/doi

Maternal and Child Health Program
Massachusetts Department Bureau of Family &
 Community Health
250 Washington St., 4th Floor
Boston, MA 02108-4619

Medicaid Fiscal Agent
Division of Medical Assistance
P.O. Box 45
Boston, MA 02112-0445
http://www.magnet.state.ma.us/dma/

Medicare Durable Medical Equipment
HealthNow of New York
P.O. Box 6800
Wilkes-Barre, PA 18773-6800

Medicare Fiscal Agent or Carrier
National Heritage Insurance Company
P.O. Box 1212
Hingham, MA 02044
http://www.medicarehic.com

State Board of Medical Examiners
Massachusetts Board of Registration in Medicine
560 Harrison Avenue, Suite G4
Boston, MA 02118

TRICARE Claim Office
Palmetto Government Benefits Administration (PGBA)
P.O. Box 7011
Camden, SC 29020-1294
http://www.myTRICARE.com

Veterans Affairs Installation
Massachusetts Medical Centers:
 Bedford 01730 (200 Springs Rd.)
 Boston 02130 (150 S. Huntington Ave.)
 Brockton 02301 (940 Belmont St.)
 Northampton 01053-9764 (421 N. Main St.)
 W. Roxbury 02132 (1400 VFW Pkwy)

Workers' Compensation Federal District Office
Office of Workers' Compensation Programs
JFK Federal Bldg., Room E-260
Boston, MA 02203

Workers' Compensation State Plan Office
Department of Industrial Accidents
600 Washington St., 7th Floor
Boston, MA 02111
http://www.state.ma.us/dia

MICHIGAN

CHAMPVA Claim Office
CHAMPVA Center
4500 Cherry Creek Dr., S.
P.O. Box 65024
Denver, CO 80206-9024

Insurance Commissioner State Office
Commissioner
Michigan Office of Financial and Insurance Services
611 W. Ottawa St., 2nd Floor N.
P.O. Box 30220
Lansing, MI 48933
http://www.michigan.gov/cis

Maternal and Child Health Program
CSHCS Planning Division
Michigan Department of Community Health
400 S. Pine St.
Lansing, MI 48909-7979

Michigan Department of Public Health
3423 N. Martin L. King, Jr., Blvd., Room 218
P.O. Box 30195
Lansing, MI 48909-0195

Medicaid Fiscal Agent
Medical Services Administration
P.O. Box 30043
Lansing, MI 48909
http://www.michigan.gov/mdch/

Medicare Durable Medical Equipment
Assigned:
AdminaStar Federal, Inc.
P.O. Box 7078
Indianapolis, IN 46207-7078
http://www.adminastar.com/

Nonassigned:
P.O. Box 7031
Indianapolis, IN 46207-7931

Medicare Fiscal Agent or Carrier
Wisconsin Physicians Service
8120 Penn Ave. S.
Bloomington, MN 55431
http://www.wpsic.com/

State Board of Medical Examiners
Michigan Board of Medicine
611 W. Ottawa St., 4th Floor (48933)
P.O. Box 30670
Lansing, MI 48909-8170

Michigan Board of Osteopathic Medicine and Surgery
611 W. Ottawa St., 1st Floor (48933)
P.O. Box 30670
Lansing, MI 48909-8170

TRICARE Claim Office
Palmetto Government Benefits Administration (PGBA)
P.O. Box 7021
Camden, SC 29020-7021
http://www.myTRICARE.com

Veterans Affairs Installation
Michigan Medical Centers:
  Ann Arbor 48105 (2215 Fuller Rd.)
  Battle Creek 49016 (5500 Armstrong Rd.)
  Detroit 48201 (4646 John R. St.)
  Iron Mountain 49801 (325 E. H St.)
  Saginaw 48602 (1500 Weiss St.)

Workers' Compensation Federal District Office
Office of Workers' Compensation Programs
1240 E. Ninth St., Room 851
Cleveland, OH 44199

Workers' Compensation State Plan Office
Bureau of Workers' Disability Compensation
Department of Consumer & Industry Services
7150 Harris Dr.
P.O. Box 30016
Lansing, MI 48909

MINNESOTA

CHAMPVA Claim Office
CHAMPVA Center
4500 Cherry Creek Dr., S.
P.O. Box 65024
Denver, CO 80206-9024

Insurance Commissioner State Office
Commissioner
Department of Commerce
133 E. 7th St.
St. Paul, MN 55101-2362

Maternal and Child Health Program
MCSHN
Minnesota Department of Health
85 E. Seventh Pl., Suite 400
P.O. Box 64882
St. Paul, MN 55164-0882

Medicaid Fiscal Agent
Department of Human Services (EC)
Attn: Claims
P.O. Box 64166
St. Paul, MN 55164

Medicare Durable Medical Equipment
Assigned:
AdminaStar Federal, Inc.
P.O. Box 7078
Indianapolis, IN 46207-7078
Nonassigned:
P.O. Box 7031
Indianapolis, IN 46207-7931

Medicare Fiscal Agent or Carrier
Wisconsin Physicians Services
8120 Penn Ave. S.
Bloomington, MN 55431
http://www.wpsic.com/

State Board of Medical Examiners
Minnesota Board of Medical Practice
2829 University Ave. SE, Suite 400
Minneapolis, MN 55414-3246

TRICARE Claim Office
Palmetto Government Benefits Administration (PGBA)
P.O. Box 870129
Surfside Beach, SC 29587-9729
http://www.myTRICARE.com

Veterans Affairs Installation
Minnesota Medical Centers:
  Minneapolis 55417 (One Veterans Dr.)
  St. Cloud 56303 (4801 8th St., North)

Workers' Compensation Federal District Office
Office of Workers' Compensation Programs
230 S. Dearborn St., 8th Floor
Chicago, IL 60604

Workers' Compensation State Plan Offices
Workers' Compensation Division
Department of Labor and Industry
443 Lafayette Rd. North
St. Paul, MN 55155-4319
http://www.doli.state.mn.us

Workers' Compensation Court of Appeals
25 Constitution Ave., Suite 405
St. Paul, MN 55155

MISSISSIPPI

CHAMPVA Claim Office
CHAMPVA Center
4500 Cherry Creek Dr., S.
P.O. Box 65024
Denver, CO 80206-9024

Insurance Commissioner State Office
Commissioner
Department of Insurance
1804 Walter Sillers Bldg.
P.O. Box 79
Jackson, MS 39205
http://www.doi.state.ms.us

Maternal and Child Health Program
Children and Adolescent Health
Mississippi State Health Department
570 E. Woodrow Wilson
Jackson, MS 39216

CSHCN Program
Mississippi State Health Department
2423 N. State St.
P.O. Box 1700
Jackson, MS 39215-1700

Medicaid Fiscal Agent
Electronic Data Systems
111 E. Capitol St., Suite 400 (39201)
P.O. Box 23077
Jackson, MS 38225-3076
http://www.dom.state.ms.us/

Medicare Durable Medical Equipment
Palmetto Government Benefits Administration (PGBA)
P.O. Box 100254
Columbia, SC 29202-3254
http://www.pgba.com/

Medicare Fiscal Agent or Carrier
Cahaba Government Benefits Administration (GBA)
Blue Cross and Blue Shield of Alabama
P.O. Box 23046
Jackson, MS 39225
http://www.msmedicare.com/

State Board of Medical Examiners
Mississippi State Board of Medical Licensure
1867 Crane Ridge Dr., Suite 200 B
Jackson, MS 39216

TRICARE Claim Office
Palmetto Government Benefits Administration (PGBA)
P.O. Box 7031
Camden SC 29020-7031
http://www.myTRICARE.com

Veterans Affairs Installation
Mississippi Medical Centers:
Biloxi 39531 (400 Veterans Ave.)
Jackson 39216 (1500 E. Woodrow Wilson Dr.)

Workers' Compensation Federal District Office
Office of Workers' Compensation Programs
214 North Hogan St., Suite 1006
Jacksonville, FL 32202

Workers' Compensation State Plan Office
Workers' Compensation Commission
1428 Lakeland Dr.
P.O. Box 5300
Jackson, MS 39296-5300
http://www.mwcc.state.ms.us

MISSOURI

CHAMPVA Claim Office
CHAMPVA Center
4500 Cherry Creek Dr., S.
P.O. Box 65024
Denver, CO 80206-9024

Insurance Commissioner State Office
Director of Insurance
301 W. High St., Room 630
P.O. Box 690
Jefferson City, MO 65102-0690
http://www.insurance.state.mo.us

Maternal and Child Health Program
Bureau of Special Health Care Needs
Missouri Department of Health & Senior Services
930 Wildwood Dr.

P.O. Box 570
Jefferson City, MO 65102-0570

Division of Maternal, Child & Family Health
Missouri Department of Health
930 Wildwood Dr.
P.O. Box 570
Jefferson City, MO 65102-0570

Medicaid Fiscal Agent
GTE Data Services (EC)
P.O. Box 5600
Jefferson City, MO 65102
http://www.dss.state.mo.us/dms/

Medicare Durable Medical Equipment
CIGNA Medicare
P.O. Box 690
Nashville, TN 37202
http://www.cignamedicare.com

Medicare Fiscal Agent or Carrier
Eastern Missouri:
Missouri Medicare Services
12755 Olive St. Rd., Suite 200
P.O. Box 775039 (63177)
St. Louis, MO 63141
http://www.momedicare.com/

Western Missouri:
Blue Cross and Blue Shield of Kansas
1133 SW Topeka Blvd. (66629)
P.O. Box 239
Topeka KS 66601
http://www.kansasmedicare.com

State Board of Medical Examiners
Missouri State Board of Registration for the Healing Arts
3605 Missouri Blvd. (65109)
P.O. Box 4
Jefferson City, MO 65102

TRICARE Claim Offices
St. Louis area:
Palmetto Government Benefits Administration (PGBA)
P.O. Box 7021
Camden, SC 29020-7021

Except for St. Louis area:
Palmetto Government Benefits Administration (PGBA)
P.O. Box 870130
Surfside Beach, SC 29587-9730
http://www.myTRICARE.com

Veterans Affairs Installation
Missouri Medical Centers:
  Columbia 65201 (800 Hospital Dr.)
  Kansas City 64128 (4801 Linwood Blvd.)
  Poplar Bluff 63901 (1500 N. Westwood Blvd.)
  St. Louis 63106 (915 N. Grand Blvd.)
  St. Louis 63125 (#1 Jefferson Barracks Division)

Workers' Compensation Federal District Office
Office of Workers' Compensation Programs
City Center Square
1100 Main St., Suite 750
Kansas City, MO 64105

Workers' Compensation State Plan Office
Division of Workers' Compensation
Department of Labor and Industrial Relations

3315 W. Truman Blvd.
P.O. Box 58
Jefferson City, MO 65102-0058

MONTANA

CHAMPVA Claim Office
CHAMPVA Center
4500 Cherry Creek Dr., S.
P.O. Box 65024
Denver, CO 80206-9024

Insurance Commissioner State Office
Commissioner
Department of Insurance
840 Helena Ave.
P.O. Box 4009
Helena, MT 59601-4009
http://www.sao.state.mt.us/

Maternal and Child Health Program
Children's Special Health Services
Health Resources Bureau
1218 E. 6th Ave.
Helena, MT 59620

Family and Community Health Bureau
Department of Public Health and Human Sciences
1400 Broadway, Cogswell Bldg.
P.O. Box 202951
Helena, MT 59620

Medicaid Fiscal Agent
Consultec, Inc. (EC)
P.O. Box 8000
Helena, MT 59604
http://www.dphhs.state.mt.us/hpsd/medicaid/

Medicare Durable Medical Equipment
CIGNA Medicare
P.O. Box 690
Nashville, TN 37202
http://www.cignamedicare.com

Medicare Fiscal Agent or Carrier
Blue Cross and Blue Shield of Montana, Inc.
340 N. Last Chance Gulch
P.O. Box 4310
Helena, MT 59604
http://www.medicare.bcbsmt.com/

State Board of Medical Examiners
Montana Board of Medical Examiners
Arcade Bldg., Lower Level
301 S. Park Avenue, 4th Floor
P.O. Box 200513
Helena, MT 59620-0513

TRICARE Claim Office
Palmetto Government Benefits Administration (PGBA)
P.O. Box 870127
Surfside Beach, SC 29587-9727
http://www.myTRICARE.com

Veterans Affairs Installation
Montana Centers and Regional Office:
Fort Harrison 59636 (William St. off Highway 12 W)
Miles City 59301 (210 S. Winchester)

Workers' Compensation Federal District Office
Office of Workers' Compensation Programs
1999 Broadway, Suite 600
Drawer 3558
Denver, CO 80202

Workers' Compensation State Plan Office
Employment Relations Division
Department of Labor and Industry
18050 Prospect Ave.
P.O. Box 8011
Helena, MT 59604-8011

NEBRASKA

CHAMPVA Claim Office
CHAMPVA Center
4500 Cherry Creek Dr., S.
P.O. Box 65024
Denver, CO 80206-9024

Insurance Commissioner State Office
Director
Department of Insurance
941 O St., Suite 400
Lincoln, NE 68508-3690
http://www.nol.org/home/NDOI

Maternal and Child Health Program
Division of Family Health
Nebraska Department of Health and Human Services
301 Centennial Mall S.
P.O. Box 95044
Lincoln, NE 68509-5044

Special Services for Children and Adults
Nebraska Department of Health and Human Services
301 Centennial Mall S.
P.O. Box 95044
Lincoln, NE 68509-5044

Medicaid Fiscal Agent
Health & Human Services
P.O. Box 95026
Lincoln, NE 68509-5026
http://www.hhs.state.ne.us/med/medindex.htm

Medicare Durable Medical Equipment
CIGNA Medicare
P.O. Box 690
Nashville, TN 37202
http://www.cignamedicare.com

Medicare Fiscal Agent or Carrier
Blue Cross and Blue Shield of Kansas
1133 SW Topeka Blvd. (66629)
P.O. Box 3541
Topeka, KS 66601

(Local Office)
Blue Cross and Blue Shield of Kansas
11330 Q St.
Omaha, NE 68137
http://www.kansasmedicare.com/

State Board of Medical Examiners
Nebraska Board of Medicine & Surgery
301 Centennial Mall S. (68509)
P.O. Box 94986
Lincoln, NE 68509-4986

TRICARE Claim Office
Palmetto Government Benefits Administration (PGBA)
P.O. Box 870128
Surfside Beach, SC 29587-9728
http://www.myTRICARE.com

Veterans Affairs Installation
Nebraska Medical Centers:
  Grand Island 68803 (2201 N. Broadwell Ave.)
  Lincoln 68510 (600 S. 70th St.)
  Omaha 68105 (4101 Woolworth Ave.)

Workers' Compensation Federal District Office
Office of Workers' Compensation Programs
City Center Square
1100 Main St., Suite 750
Kansas City, MO 64105

Workers' Compensation State Plan Office
Workers' Compensation Court
State Capital Bldg.
P.O. Box 98908
Lincoln, NE 68509-8908
http://www.nol.org/workcomp

NEVADA

CHAMPVA Claim Office
CHAMPVA Center
4500 Cherry Creek Dr., S.
P.O. Box 65024
Denver, CO 80206-9024

Insurance Commissioner State Office
Commissioner
Division of Insurance
1665 Hot Springs Rd., Suite 152
Carson City, NV 89706-0646
http://www.doi.state.nv.us

Maternal and Child Health Program
CHSCN
Nevada State Health Division
505 E. King St., Room 200
Carson City, NV 89710-4792

Medicaid Fiscal Agent or Carrier
Blue Cross & Blue Shield of Nevada
P.O. Box 12127
Reno, NV 89510-2127

Medicare Durable Medical Equipment
CIGNA Medicare
P.O. Box 690
Nashville, TN 37202
http://www.cignamedicare.com

Medicare Fiscal Agent or Carrier
Noridian Mutual Insurance Company
P.O. Box 6705
Fargo, ND 58108

(Blue Cross-Blue Shield of North Dakota)
5333 N. 7th St., #C-123
Phoenix, AZ 85014
http://www.noridianmedicare.com/

State Board of Medical Examiners
Nevada State Board of Medical Examiners
1105 Terminal Way, Suite 301 (89502)
P.O. Box 7238
Reno, NV 89510

Nevada State Board of Osteopathic Medicine
2860 E. Flamingo Rd., Suite G
Las Vegas, NV 89121-5208

TRICARE Claim Office
Palmetto Government Benefits Administration (PGBA)
P.O. Box 870033
Surfside Beach, SC 29587-8733
http://www.myTRICARE.com

Veterans Affairs Installation
Nevada Medical Center:
  Ely 89301 (6 Steptoe Circle)
  Las Vegas 89106 (1700 Vegas Dr.)
  Reno 89520 (1000 Locust St.)

Workers' Compensation Federal District Office
Office of Workers' Compensation Programs
71 Stevenson St., Suite 305 (94105)
P.O. Box 193769
San Francisco, CA 94119-3769

Workers' Compensation State Plan Office
Department of Business & Industry
Division of Industrial Relations
400 W. King St., Suite 400
Carson City, NE 89703

NEW HAMPSHIRE

CHAMPVA Claim Office
CHAMPVA Center
4500 Cherry Creek Dr., S.
P.O. Box 65024
Denver, CO 80206-9024

Insurance Commissioner State Office
Commissioner
Department of Insurance
56 Old Suncook Rd.
Concord, NH 03301-7317
http://www.state.nh.us/insurance

Maternal and Child Health Program
Maternal and Child Health
Department of Health and Human Services
6 Hazen Dr.
Concord, NH 03301

Bureau of Special Medical Services
New Hampshire Department of Health and
  Human Services
6 Hazen Dr.
Concord, NH 03301

Medicaid Fiscal Agent
Electronic Data Systems Federal Corporation (EC)
P.O. Box 2040
Concord, NH 03302-2040

Claims:
P.O. Box 2001
Concord, NH 03302-2201
http://www.dhhs.state.nh.us/DHHS/MEDICAIDPROGRAM/

Medicare Durable Medical Equipment
HealthNow of New York
P.O. Box 6800
Wilkes-Barre, PA 18773-6800

Medicare Fiscal Agent or Carrier
National Heritage Insurance Company
P.O. Box 1212
Hingham, MA 02043
http://www.medicarehic-com/main.htm

State Board of Medical Examiners
New Hampshire Board of Medicine
2 Industrial Park Dr., Suite 8
Concord, NH 03301-8520

TRICARE Claim Office
Palmetto Government Benefits Administration (PGBA)
P.O. Box 7011
Camden, SC 29020-7011
http://www.myTRICARE.com

Veterans Affairs Installation
New Hampshire Medical Center
718 Smyth Rd.
Manchester, NH 03104

Workers' Compensation Federal District Office
Office of Workers' Compensation Programs
JFK Federal Bldg., Room E-260
Boston, MA 02203

Workers' Compensation State Plan Office
Department of Labor
Division of Workers' Compensation
State Office Park S.
95 Pleasant Court
Concord, NH 03301

NEW JERSEY

CHAMPVA Claim Office
CHAMPVA Center
4500 Cherry Creek Dr., S.
P.O. Box 65024
Denver, CO 80206-9024

Insurance Commissioner State Office
Commissioner
Department of Insurance
20 W. State St.
P.O. Box 325
Trenton, NJ 08625-0325

Maternal and Child Health Program
Administrator MCHS-Family Health Services
State Department of Health and Senior Services
50 E. State St.
P.O. Box 364
Trenton, NJ 08625-0364

Special Child and Adult & Early Intervention Services
New Jersey State Department of Health and
 Senior Services
50 E. State St.
P.O. Box 364
Trenton, NJ 08625-0364

Medicaid Fiscal Agent
UNISYS HCFA
3705 Quaker Bridge Rd., Suite 101
P.O. Box 4808 (08650-4808)
Trenton, NJ 08619
http://www.state.nj.us/humanservices/dmahs/index.html

Medicare Durable Medical Equipment
HealthNow of New York
P.O. Box 6800
Wilkes-Barre, PA 18773-6800

Medicare Fiscal Agent or Carrier
Empire Medicare Services (Empire Blue Cross
 Blue Shield)
P.O. Box 890065
Camphill, PA 17089-0065
or
P.O. Box 69201
Harrisburg, PA 17106-9201
http://www.empiremedicare.com/

State Board of Medical Examiners
New Jersey State Board of Medical Examiners
140 E. Front St., 2nd Floor (08608)
P.O. Box 183
Trenton, NJ 08625-0183

Temporary Disability Insurance
New Jersey Department of Labor
Division of Temporary Disability Insurance
P.O. Box 387
Trenton, NJ 08625-0387
http://www.nj.gov/labor/tdi/tdiindex.html

TRICARE Claim Office
Palmetto Government Benefits Administration (PGBA)
P.O. Box 7011
Camden, SC 29020-7011

Veterans Affairs Installation
New Jersey Medical Centers:
 E. Orange 07018 (385 Tremont Ave.)
 Lyons 07939 (151 Knollkroft Rd.)

Workers' Compensation Federal District Office
Office of Workers' Compensation Programs
201 Varick St., Room 750
P.O. Box 566
New York, NY 10014-0566

Workers' Compensation State Plan Office
Department of Labor
Division of Workers' Compensation
P.O. Box 381
Trenton, NJ 08625-0381

NEW MEXICO

CHAMPVA Claim Office
CHAMPVA Center
4500 Cherry Creek Dr., S.
P.O. Box 65024
Denver, CO 80206-9024

Insurance Commissioner State Office
Superintendent
Department of Insurance
P.O. Box 1269
Santa Fe, NM 87504-1269

Maternal and Child Health Program
Children's Medical Services
Department of Health, PHD
Family Health Bureau
2040 S. Pacheco
Santa Fe, NM 87502-6110

Department of Health, PHD
Family Health Bureau
525 Camino de los Marquez, Suite 6
Santa Fe, NM 87501

Medicaid Fiscal Agent
Consultec, Inc. (EC)
1720-A Randolf Rd., S.E.
Albuquerque, NM 87106
http://www.state.nm.us/hsd/mad/Index.html

Medicare Durable Medical Equipment
Palmetto Government Benefits Administration (PGBA)
P.O. Box 100254
Columbia, SC 29202-3254

Medicare Fiscal Agent or Carrier
Oklahoma New Mexico Medicare Services
(Arkansas Blue Cross and Blue Shield)
6301 Indian School Rd. NE, #990
Albuquerque, NM 87110
http://www.oknmmedicare.com/

State Board of Medical Examiners
New Mexico Medical Board
Lamy Bldg., 2nd Floor
491 Old Santa Fe Trail
Santa Fe, NM 87501

New Mexico Board of Osteopathic Medical Examiners
2055 S. Pacheco, Suite 400
P.O. Box 25101
Santa Fe, NM 87504

TRICARE Claim Office
Palmetto Government Benefits Administration (PGBA)
P.O. Box 870032
Surfside Beach, SC 29587-8732

Veterans Affairs Installation
New Mexico Medical Center:
   Albuquerque 87108 (1501 San Pedro Dr., SE)

Workers' Compensation Federal District Office
Office of Workers' Compensation Program
525 S. Griffin St., Room 100
Dallas, TX 75202

Workers' Compensation State Plan Office
Workers' Compensation Administration
2410 Centre Ave., SE
P.O. Box 27198
Albuquerque, NM 87125-7198
http://www.state.nm.us/wca

NEW YORK

CHAMPVA Claim Office
CHAMPVA Center
4500 Cherry Creek Dr., S.
P.O. Box 65024
Denver, CO 80206-9024

Disability Benefits Bureau
See Temporary Disability Insurance

Insurance Commissioner State Office
Consumer Services Bureau
NYS Insurance Department
Agency Bldg. 1-ESP
Empire State Plaza
Albany, NY 12257
http://www.ins.state.ny.us

Consumer Services Bureau
NYS Insurance Department
65 Court St. #7
Buffalo, NY 14202
http://www.ins.state.ny.us

Maternal and Child Health Program
Division of Family and Local Health
New York State Department of Health
Corning Tower Bldg., Room 890
Albany, NY 12237-0657

Bureau of Child and Adolescent Health
New York State Department of Health
Corning Tower Bldg., Room 821
Albany, NY 12237

Medicaid Fiscal Agent
Computer Sciences Corporation (EC)
800 N. Pearl St. Albany, NY 12204
http://www.health.state.ny.us/nysdoh/medicaid/
   medicaid.htm

Medicare Durable Medical Equipment
HealthNow of New York
P.O. Box 6800
Wilkes-Barre, PA 18773-6800

Medicare Fiscal Agent or Carrier
Counties of Bronx, Columbia, Delaware, Dutchess,
Greene, Kings, Nassau, New York, Orange, Putnam,
Richmond, Rockland, Suffolk, Sullivan, Ulster, and
Westchester
Empire Blue Cross and Blue Shield (EC)
622 Third Ave.
New York, NY 10017

County of Queens
Group Health, Inc. (EC)
88 W. End Ave.
New York, NY 10023

Rest of the state:
Blue Cross and Blue Shield of Western New York, Inc.
P.O. Box 5236
Binghamton, NY 13905-5236

State Board of Medical Examiners
New York State Board for Medicine
89 Washington Avenue, West Wing, 2nd Floor
Albany, NY 12234

New York Board for Professional Medical Conduct
New York State Department of Health
433 River St., Suite 303
Troy, NY 12180-2299

Temporary Disability Insurance
Workers' Compensation Board
Disability Benefits Bureau
100 Broadway (Menands)
Albany, NY 12241

TRICARE Claim Office
Palmetto Government Benefits Administration (PGBA)
P.O. Box 7011
Camden, SC 29020-7011
http://www.myTRICARE.com

Veterans Affairs Installation
New York Medical Centers:
  Albany 12208 (113 Holland Ave.)
  Batavia 14020 (222 Richmond Ave.)
  Bath 14810 (76 Veterans Ave.)
  Bronx 10468 (130 W. Kingsbridge Rd.)
  Brooklyn 11209 (800 Poly Pl.)
  Buffalo 14215 (3495 Bailey Ave.)
  Canandaigua 14424 (400 Fort Hill Ave.)
  Castle Point 12511 (Route 9D)
  Montrose 10548 (138 Albany Post Rd.)
  New York City 10010 (423 E. 23rd St.)
  Northport 11768 (79 Middleville Rd.)
  St. Albans 11425 (179 St. & Linden Blvd.)
  Syracuse 13210 (800 Irvine Ave.)

Workers' Compensation Federal District Office
Office of Workers' Compensation Programs
201 Varick St., Room 750
P.O. Box 566
New York, NY 10014-0556

Workers' Compensation State Plan Office
Workers' Compensation Board
100 Broadway-Menands
Albany, NY 12241

NORTH CAROLINA

CHAMPVA Claim Office
CHAMPVA Center
4500 Cherry Creek Dr., S.
P.O. Box 65024
Denver, CO 80206-9024

Insurance Commissioner State Office
Commissioner
Department of Insurance
Dobbs Bldg.
430 N. Salisbury St.
P.O. Box 26387
Raleigh, NC 27611
http://www.ncdoi.net

Maternal and Child Health Program
Division of Women's and Children's Health
Department of Health and Human Services
1916 Mail Service Center
Raleigh, NC 27699-1916

Children & Youth Branch
North Carolina Department of Health and Human
  Services—Division of Public Health
1928 Mail Service Center
Raleigh, NC 27699-1928

Medicaid Fiscal Agent
Electronic Data Systems (EC)
P.O. Box 30968
Raleigh, NC 27622
http://www.dhhs.state.nc.us/dma/

Medicare Durable Medical Equipment
Palmetto Government Benefits Administration (PGBA)
P.O. Box 100254
Columbia, SC 29202-3254
http://www.pgba.com/

Medicare Fiscal Agent or Carrier
CIGNA Medicare
P.O. Box 32864
Charlotte, NC 29232
http://www.cignamedicare.com

State Board of Medical Examiners
North Carolina Medical Board
1201 Front St., Suite 100 (27609)
P.O. Box 20007
Raleigh, NC 27609-0007

TRICARE Claim Office
Palmetto Government Benefits Administration (PGBA)
P.O. Box 7021
Camden, SC 29020-7021
http://www.myTRICARE.com

Veterans Affairs Installation
North Carolina Medical Centers:
  Asheville 28805 (1100 Tunnel Rd.)
  Durham 27705 (508 Fulton St.)
  Fayetteville 28301 (2300 Ramsey St.)
  Salisbury 28144 (1601 Brenner Ave.)

Workers' Compensation Federal District Office
Office of Workers' Compensation Programs
214 North Hogan St., Suite 1006
Jacksonville, FL 32202

Workers' Compensation State Plan Office
Industrial Commission
4319 Mail Service Center
Raleigh, NC 27699-4319
http://www.comp.state.nc.us

NORTH DAKOTA

CHAMPVA Claim Office
CHAMPVA Center
4500 Cherry Creek Dr., S.
P.O. Box 65024
Denver, CO 80206-9024

Insurance Commissioner State Office
Commissioner
Department of Insurance
600 E. Blvd. Ave., 5th Floor
Bismarck, ND 58505-0320
http://www.state.nd.us/ndins

Maternal and Child Health Program
Children's Special Health Services
North Dakota Department of Human Services
Children's Special Health Services
600 E. Blvd. Ave., Dept. 325
Bismarck, ND 58505-0269

Division of Maternal and Child Health
North Dakota Department of Health
600 E. Blvd. Ave., Dept. 301
Bismarck, ND 58505-0200

Medicaid Fiscal Agent
Department of Human Services (EC)
Medical Services
600 E. Blvd. Ave., Dept. 325
Bismarck, ND 58505

Medicare Durable Medical Equipment
CIGNA Medicare
P.O. Box 690
Nashville, TN 37202
http://www.cignamedicare.com

Medicare Fiscal Agent or Carrier
Noridian Mutual Insurance Co.
4510 13th Ave., SW (58103)
P.O. Box 6706
Fargo, ND 58108
http://www.noridianmedicare.com/

State Board of Medical Examiners
North Dakota State Board of Medical Examiners
City Center Plaza
418 E. Broadway Avenue, Suite 12
Bismarck, ND 58501-4086

TRICARE Claim Office
Palmetto Government Benefits Administration (PGBA)
P.O. Box 870031
Surfside Beach, SC 29587-8731
http://www.myTRICARE.com

Veterans Affairs Installation
North Dakota Medical Center
2101 North Elm St.
Fargo, ND 58102

Workers' Compensation Federal District Office
Office of Workers' Compensation Programs
1999 Broadway, Suite 600
Denver, CO 80202

Workers' Compensation State Plan Office
Workers' Compensation Bureau
500 E. Front Ave.
Bismarck, ND 58504-5685

OHIO

CHAMPVA Claim Office
CHAMPVA Center
4500 Cherry Creek Dr., S.
P.O. Box 65024
Denver, CO 80206-9024

Insurance Commissioner State Office
Director
Department of Insurance
2100 Stella Court
Columbus, OH 43215-1067
http://www.state.oh.us/

Maternal and Child Health Program
Division of Family and Community Health Services
Ohio Department of Health
246 N. High St.
P.O. Box 1603
Columbus, OH 43216-1603

Ohio Department of Public Health
Bureau for Children with Medical Handicaps
P.O. Box 1603
Columbus, OH 43216-1603

Medicaid Fiscal Agent
P.O. Box 7965
Columbus, OH 44306
http://www.state.oh.us/odjfs/ohp/

Medicare Durable Medical Equipment
Assigned:
AdminaStar Federal, Inc.
P.O. Box 7078
Indianapolis, IN 46207-7078
http://www.adminastar.com/

Nonassigned:
P.O. Box 7031
Indianapolis, IN 46207-7931

Medicare Fiscal Agent or Carrier
Palmetto Government Benefits Administration (PGBA)
3400 Southpark Pl., #F
Grove City, OH 43123
Or
P.O. Box 182957
Columbus, OH 43218
http://www.pgba.com/

State Board of Medical Examiners
State Medical Board of Ohio
77 S. High St., 17th Floor
Columbus, OH 43215-6127

TRICARE Claim Office
Palmetto Government Benefits Administration (PGBA)
P.O. Box 7021
Camden, SC 29020-7021
http://www.myTRICARE.com

Veterans Affairs Installation
Ohio Medical Centers:
  Brecksville 44141 (10000 Brecksville Rd.)
  Chillicothe 45601 (17273 State Route 104)
  Cincinnati 45220 (3200 Vine St.)
  Cleveland 44106 (10701 E. Blvd.)
  Dayton 45428 (4100 W. 3rd St.)

Workers' Compensation Federal District Office
Office of Workers' Compensation Programs
1240 E. Ninth St., Room 851
Cleveland, OH 44199

Workers' Compensation State Plan Office
Bureau of Workers' Compensation
30 W. Spring St.
Columbus, OH 43215-2256
http://www.ohiobwc.com

OKLAHOMA

CHAMPVA Claim Office
CHAMPVA Center
4500 Cherry Creek Dr., S.
P.O. Box 65024
Denver, CO 80206-9024

Insurance Commissioner State Office
Commissioner
Department of Insurance
3814 North Santa Fe
P.O. Box 53408
Oklahoma City, OK 73118
http://www.oid.state.ok.us

Maternal and Child Health Program
Maternal and Child Health Service
Oklahoma State Department of Health
1000 NE Tenth St.
Oklahoma City, OK 73117-1299

CSHCN Director
Oklahoma Department of Health Services
P.O. Box 25352
Oklahoma City, OK 73125

Medicaid Fiscal Agent
UNISYS (HCFA)
P.O. Box 54740
Oklahoma City, OK 73154
http://www.ohca.state.ok.us/

Medicare Durable Medical Equipment
Palmetto Government Benefits Administration (PGBA)
P.O. Box 100254
Columbia, SC 29202-3254

Medicare Fiscal Agent or Carrier
Oklahoma/New Mexico Medicare Services
(Arkansas Blue Cross and Blue Shield)
Participating:
P.O. Box 24700
Oklahoma City, OK 73125

Nonparticipating:
701 NW 63rd St.
Oklahoma City, OK 73116-7693
http://www.oknmmedicare.com/

State Board of Medical Examiners
Oklahoma State Board of Medical Licensure & Supervision
5104 N. Francis Avenue, Suite C (73118)
P.O. Box 18256
Oklahoma City, OK 73118

TRICARE Claim Office
Wisconsin Physicians Service
TRICARE Northwest
P.O. Box 8999
Madison WI 53708-8999

Veterans Affairs Installation
Oklahoma Medical Centers:
  Muskogee 74401 (1011 Honor Heights Dr.)
  Oklahoma City 73104 (921 NE 13th St.)

Workers' Compensation Federal District Office
Office of Workers' Compensation Programs
525 S. Griffin St., Room 100
Dallas, TX 75202

Workers' Compensation State Plan Office
Oklahoma Workers' Compensation Court
1915 N. Stiles Ave.
Oklahoma City, OK 73105-4904

OREGON

CHAMPVA Claim Office
CHAMPVA Center
4500 Cherry Creek Dr., S.
P.O. Box 65024
Denver, CO 80206-9024

Insurance Commissioner State Office
Acting Administrator
Oregon Insurance Division
350 Winter St. NE, Room 440-2
Salem, OR 97310-3883
http://www.cbs.state.or.us/ins

Maternal and Child Health Program
Oregon Children with Special Health Care Needs
P.O. Box 574, CDRC/OHSU
Portland, OR 97207

Medicaid Fiscal Agent
Office of Medical Assistance Program (OMAP)
Claims
P.O. Box 14955
Salem, OR 97309
http://www.dhs.state.or.us/healthplan/index.html

Medicare Durable Medical Equipment
CIGNA Medicare
P.O. Box 690
Nashville, TN 37202
http://www.cignamedicare.com

Medicare Fiscal Agent or Carrier
Noridian Mutual Insurance Company
4510 13th Ave. SW (58103)
P.O. Box 6702
Fargo, ND 58108-6702
http://www.noridianmedicare.com/

State Board of Medical Examiners
Oregon Board of Medical Examiners
1500 SW First Ave., Suite 620
Portland, OR 97201-5826

TRICARE Claim Office
Wisconsin Physicians Service
TRICARE Northwest
P.O. Box 8999
Madison, WI 53708-8999

Veterans Affairs Installation
Oregon Medical Centers:
   Portland 97201 (3710 SW U.S. Veterans Hospital Rd.)
   Roseburg 97470 (913 NW Garden Valley Blvd.)

Workers' Compensation Federal District Office
Office of Workers' Compensation Programs
1111 Third Ave., Suite 650
Seattle, WA 98101-3212

Workers' Compensation State Plan Office
Department of Consumer and Business Services
Workers' Compensation Division
350 Winter St. NE, Room 27
Salem, OR 97310-3879
http://www.cbs.state.or.us.us

Workers' Compensation Board
2601 25th St. S.E., Suite 150
Salem, OR 97302-1282

PENNSYLVANIA

CHAMPVA Claim Office
CHAMPVA Center
4500 Cherry Creek Dr., S.
P.O. Box 65024
Denver, CO 80206-9024

Insurance Commissioner State Office
Commissioner
Insurance Department
1326 Strawberry Sq., 13th Floor
Harrisburg, PA 17120
http://www.insurance.state.pa.us

Maternal and Child Health Program
Division of Children and Adult Health Services
Pennsylvania Department of Health
7th Floor, Health and Welfare Bldg.
P.O. Box 90 E.
Harrisburg, PA 17108

Pennsylvania Department of Health
Division of CSCHN
Room 724, Health and Welfare Bldg.
P.O. Box 90
Harrisburg, PA 17108

Medicaid Fiscal Agent
Office of Medical Assistance Programs
P.O. Box 2675
Harrisburg, PA 17105-2675
http://www.dpw.state.pa.us/omap/dpwomap.asp

Medicare Durable Medical Equipment
HealthNow of New York
P.O. Box 6800
Wilkes-Barre, PA 18773-6800

Medicare Fiscal Agent or Carrier
HGS Administrators
P.O. Box 890418
Camp Hill, PA 17089

State Board of Medical Examiners
Pennsylvania State Board of Medicine
124 Pine St. (17101)

P.O. Box 2649
Harrisburg, PA 17105-2649

Pennsylvania State Board of Osteopathic Medicine
124 Pine St. (17101)
P.O. Box 2649
Harrisburg, PA 17105-2649

TRICARE Claim Office
Palmetto Government Benefits Administration (PGBA)
P.O. Box 7011
Camden, SC 29020-7011
http://www.myTRICARE.com

Veterans Affairs Installation
Pennsylvania Medical Centers:
   Altoona 16602 (2907 Pleasant Valley Rd.)
   Butler 16001 (325 New Castle Rd.)
   Coatesville 19320 (1400 Black Horse Hill Rd.)
   Erie 16504-1596 (135 E. 38th St.)
   Lebanon 17042 (1700 S. Lincoln Ave.)
   Philadelphia 19104 (University & Woodland Aves.)
   Pittsburgh 15215 (Delafield Rd.)
   Pittsburgh 15206 (7180 Highland Dr.)
   Pittsburgh 15240 (University Dr. C)
   Wilkes-Barre 18711 (1111 E. End Blvd.)

Workers' Compensation Federal District Office
Office of Workers' Compensation Programs
Curtis Center, Suite 715 E.
170 S. Independence Mall W.
Philadelphia, PA 19106-33008

Workers' Compensation State Plan Office
Bureau of Workers' Compensation
Department of Labor and Industry
1171 S. Cameron St., Room 324
Harrisburg, PA 17104-2501

Workers' Compensation Appeal Board
901 North 7th St., 3rd Floor S.
Harrisburg, PA 17102-0034

PUERTO RICO

CHAMPVA Claim Office
CHAMPVA Center
4500 Cherry Creek Dr., S.
P.O. Box 65024
Denver, CO 80206-9024

Insurance Commissioner State Office
Commissioner
Office of the Commission of Insurance
Fernandez Juncos Station
P.O. Box 8330
Santurce, PR 00910-8330

Maternal and Child Health Program
CSHCN Director
Puerto Rico Department of Health
Call Box 70184
San Juan, PR 00936-8184

Maternal Child Health Director
Puerto Rico Department of Health

Call Box 70184
San Juan, PR 00936-8184

Medicare Durable Medical Equipment
Palmetto Government Benefits Administration (PGBA)
(Blue Cross & Blue Shield of South Carolina)
P.O. Box 100254
Columbia, SC 29202-3254
http://www.pgba.com

Medicare Fiscal Agent or Carrier
Triple-S, Inc.
Call Box 71391
San Juan, PR 00936-1391

State Board of Medical Examiners
Puerto Rico Board of Medical Examiners
Kennedy Ave., ILA Bldg., Hogar del Obrero Portuario,
  Piso 8, Puerto Nuevo (00920)
P.O. Box 13969
San Juan, PR 00908

Temporary Disability Insurance
Department of Labor and Human Resources
Bureau of Employment Security
Disability Insurance Program
Prudencio Rivera Martinez Bldg.
505 Munoz Rivera Ave.
Hato Rey, PR 00918

TRICARE Claim Office
Wisconsin Physicians Service
P.O. Box 7985
Madison, WI 53707-7985

Veterans Affairs Installation
Puerto Rico Medical Center
10 Casia St.
San Juan, PR 00921-3201

Workers' Compensation Federal District
Office of Workers' Compensation Programs
201 Varick St., Room 750
P.O. Box 566
New York, NY 10014-0566

Workers' Compensation State Plan Office
State Insurance Fund Corporation
G.P.O. Box 365028
San Juan, PR 00936-5028

Industrial Commission
G.P.O. Box 364466
San Juan, PR 00936-4466

RHODE ISLAND

CHAMPVA Claim Office
CHAMPVA Center
4500 Cherry Creek Dr., S.
P.O. Box 65024
Denver, CO 80206-9024

Insurance Commissioner State Office
Superintendent
Insurance Division
233 Richmond St., Suite 233
Providence, RI 02903-4233

Maternal and Child Health Program
Children with Special Health Care Needs
Rhode Island Department of Health
3 Capitol Hill, Room 302
Providence, RI 02908

Medicaid Fiscal Agent
Electronic Data Systems
P.O. Box 2009
Warwick, RI 02887
http://www.dhs.state.ri.us/dhs/dheacre.htm

Medicaid Rhode Island
Medical Services Department
600 New London Ave.
Cranston, RI 02920-3037

Medicare Durable Medical Equipment
HealthNow of New York
P.O. Box 6800
Wilkes-Barre, PA 18773-6800

Medicare Fiscal Agent or Carrier
Blue Cross and Blue Shield of Rhode Island
444 Westminster St.
Providence, RI 02903-3279

State Board of Medical Examiners
Rhode Island Board of Medical Licensure & Discipline
Department of Health
Cannon Bldg., Room 205
Three Capitol Hill
Providence, RI 02908-5097

Temporary Disability Insurance
Department of Labor and Training
Temporary Disability Insurance Division
1511 Pontiac Ave., Bldg. 71-3
P.O. Box 20100
Cranston, RI 02920-0941
http://www.state.ri.us

TRICARE Claim Office
Palmetto Government Benefits Administration (PGBA)
P.O. Box 7011
Camden, SC 29020-7011
http://www.myTRICARE.com

Veterans Affairs Installation
Rhode Island Medical Center
830 Chalkstone Ave.
Providence, RI 02908

Workers' Compensation Federal District Office
Office of Workers' Compensation Programs
JFK Federal Office Bldg., Room E-260
Boston, MA 02203

Workers' Compensation State Plan Office
Department of Labor and Training
Division of Workers' Compensation
1511 Pontiac Ave.
P.O. Box 20190
Cranston, RI 02920-0942
http://www.dlt.state.ri.us/wc

Workers' Compensation Court
1 Dorrance Plaza
Providence, RI 02903

SOUTH CAROLINA

CHAMPVA Claim Office
CHAMPVA Center
4500 Cherry Creek Dr., S.
P.O. Box 65024
Denver, CO 80206-9024

Insurance Commissioner State Office
Director
Department of Insurance
1612 Marion St. (24201)
P.O. Box 100105
Columbia, SC 29202-3105

Maternal and Child Health Program
Division CSHCN
S. Carolina Department of Health & Environmental Control
1751 Calhoun St.
P.O. Box 101106
Columbia, SC 29211

Division of Children's Rehabilitative Services
Department of Health & Environmental Control
Mills/Jarrett Complex
1751 Calhoun St.
P.O. Box 101106
Columbia, SC 29211

Medicaid Fiscal Agent
Department of Human Services (EC)
Medicaid Claim Receipt
P.O. Box 1412
Columbia, SC 29202-1412

Medicare Durable Medical Equipment
Palmetto Government Benefits Administration (PGBA)
P.O. Box 100254
Columbia, SC 29202-3254

Medicare Fiscal Agent or Carrier
Medicare Part B
Blue Cross and Blue Shield of S. Carolina
DBA Palmetto Government Benefits Administration (PGBA)
P.O. Box 100190
Columbia, SC 29202-3190
http://www.pgba.com/

State Board of Medical Examiners
South Carolina State Board of Medical Examiners
Department of Labor, Licensing, and Regulation
110 Centerview Dr., Suite 202 (29210)
P.O. Box 11289
Columbia, SC 29211-1289

TRICARE Claim Office
Palmetto Government Benefits Administration (PGBA)
P.O. Box 7031
Camden, SC 29020-7031
http://www.myTRICARE.com

Veterans Affairs Installation
S. Carolina Medical Centers:
  Charleston 29401 (109 Bee St.)
  Columbia 29209-1639 (6439 Garners Ferry Rd.)

Workers' Compensation Federal District Office
Office of Workers' Compensation Programs

214 North Hogan St., Suite 1006
Jacksonville, FL 32202

Workers' Compensation State Plan Office
Workers' Compensation Commission
1612 Marion St.
P.O. Box 1715
Columbia, SC 29202-1715
http://www.wcc.state.sc.us/

SOUTH DAKOTA

CHAMPVA Claim Office
CHAMPVA Center
4500 Cherry Creek Dr., S.
P.O. Box 65024
Denver, CO 80206-9024

Insurance Commissioner State Office
Director
Division of Insurance
Department of Commerce and Regulation
118 W. Capitol Ave.
Pierre, SD 57501-2000
http://www.state.sd.us/insurance

Maternal and Child Health Program
Children's Special Health Services
South Dakota Department of Health
615 E. 4th St.
Pierre, SD 57501-3185

Office of Family Health
South Dakota Department of Health
615 E. 4th St.
Pierre, SD 57501-3185

Medicaid Fiscal Agent
Department of Social Services (EC)
Office of Medical Services/Richard F. Kneip Bldg.
700 Governors Dr.
Pierre, SD 57501-2291

Medicare Durable Medical Equipment
CIGNA Medicare
P.O. Box 690
Nashville, TN 37202
http://www.cignamedicare.com

Medicare Fiscal Agent or Carrier
Noridian Mutual Insurance Company
4510 13th Ave. SW
P.O. Box 6712 or 6707 (58108)
Fargo, ND 58103
http://www.noridianmedicare.com/

State Board of Medical Examiners
South Dakota State Board of Medical &
  Osteopathic Examiners
1323 S. Minnesota Ave.
Sioux Falls, SD 57105

TRICARE Claim Office
Palmetto Government Benefits Administration (PGBA)
P.O. Box 870131

Surfside Beach, SC 29587-9731
http://www.myTRICARE.com

Veterans' Affairs Installation
South Dakota Medical Centers:
  Fort Meade 57741 (113 Comanche Rd.)
  Hot Springs 57747 (500 N. 5th St.)
  Sioux Falls 57105 (2501 W. 22nd St.)

Workers' Compensation Federal District Office
Office of Workers' Compensation Programs
1999 Broadway, Suite 600
Denver, CO 80202

Workers' Compensation State Plan Office
Division of Labor and Management
Department of Labor
Kneip Bldg., Third Floor
700 Governors Dr.
Pierre, SD 57501-2291
http://www.sdjobs.org/dlm/dlm-home.htm

TENNESSEE

CHAMPVA Claim Office
CHAMPVA Center
4500 Cherry Creek Dr., S.
P.O. Box 65024
Denver, CO 80206-9024

Insurance Commissioner State Office
Commissioner
Department of Commerce and Insurance
500 James Robertson Parkway, 5th Floor
Nashville, TN 37243-0565
http://www.state.tn.us/commerce

Maternal and Child Health Program
CCS
North 5th Floor, Cordell Hull Bldg.
425 5th Ave.
Nashville, TN 37247-4701

Medicaid Fiscal Agent
TENN CARE
729 Church St., 3rd Floor
P.O. Box 460 (37202)
Nashville, TN 37247-6501
http://www.state.tn.us/tenncare/

Medicare Durable Medical Equipment
Palmetto Government Benefits Administration (PGBA)
P.O. Box 100254
Columbia, SC 29202-3254
http://www.pgba.com/

Medicare Fiscal Agent or Carrier
CIGNA Medicare
2 Vantage Way (37228)
P.O. Box 25226
Nashville, TN 37202
http://www.cignamedicare.com

State Board of Medical Examiners
Tennessee Board of Medical Examiners
1st Floor, Cordell Hull Bldg.
425 5th Ave. North
Nashville, TN 37247-1010

Tennessee State Board of Osteopathic Examiners
1st Floor, Cordell Hull Bldg.
425 5th Ave. North
Nashville, TN 37247-1010

TRICARE Claim Office
Palmetto Government Benefits Administration (PGBA)
P.O. Box 7031
Camden, SC 29020-7031
http://www.myTRICARE.com

Veterans Affairs Installation
Tennessee Medical Centers:
  Memphis 38104 (1030 Jefferson Ave.)
  Mountain Home 37684 (Sidney & Lamont Sts.)
  Murfreesboro 37129 (3400 Lebanon Rd.)
  Nashville 37212 (1310 24th Ave., S.)

Workers' Compensation Federal District Office
Office of Workers' Compensation Program
214 North Hogan St., Suite 1006
Jacksonville, FL 32202

Workers' Compensation State Plan Office
Workers' Compensation Division
Department of Labor & Workforce Development
710 James Robertson Parkway
Andrew Johnson Tower, 2nd Floor
Nashville, TN 37243-0665
http://www.state.tn.us/labor-wfd

TEXAS

CHAMPVA Claim Office
CHAMPVA Center
4500 Cherry Creek Dr., S.
P.O. Box 65024
Denver, CO 80206-9024

Insurance Commissioner State Office
Commissioner
Department of Insurance
333 Guadalupe St.
P.O. Box 149104
Austin, TX 78716-9104
http://www.tdi.state.tx.us

Maternal and Child Health Program
CSHCN
Texas Department of Health
1100 W. 49th St.
Austin, TX 78756-3199

Medicaid Fiscal Agent
EDS/National Heritage Insurance Company
P.O. Box 200555
Austin, TX 78720-0555
http://www.hhsc.state.tx.us/mediciad/index.html

Medicare Durable Medical Equipment
Palmetto Government Benefits Administration (PGBA)
P.O. Box 100254
Columbia, SC 29202-3254
http://www.pgba.com

Medicare Fiscal Agent or Carrier
Part B Participating:
Trail Blazer Health Enterprises
8330 LBJ Freeway
Executive Center 3
P.O. Box 660156 (75266-0156)
Dallas, TX 75243
http://www.trailblazerhealth.com/

State Board of Medical Examiners
Texas State Board of Medical Examiners
333 Guadeloupe, Tower 3, Suite 610 (78701)
P.O. Box 2018
Austin, TX 78768-2018

TRICARE Claim Office
For William Beaumont Catchment area and Cannon AFB,
New Mexico catchment area ZIP codes that
fall in Texas:
Palmetto Government Benefits Administration (PGBA)
P.O. Box 870133
Surfside Beach, SC 29587-9733
http://www.myTRICARE.com

Except William Beaumont catchment area and Cannon
AFB, New Mexico, catchment area ZIP codes that fall in
Texas:
Wisconsin Physicians Service
TRICARE Northwest
P.O. Box 8999
Madison, WI 53708-8999

Veterans Affairs Installation
Texas Medical Centers:
  Amarillo 79106 (6010 Amarillo Blvd., W.)
  Big Spring 79720 (300 Veterans Blvd.)
  Bonham 75418 (1201 E. Ninth St.)
  Dallas 75216 (4500 S. Lancaster Rd.)
  Houston 77030 (2002 Holcombe Blvd.)
  Kerrville 78028 (3600 Memorial Blvd.)
  Marlin 76661 (1016 Ward St.)
  San Antonio 78284 (7400 Merton Minter Blvd.)
  Temple 76504 (1901 Veterans Memorial Dr.)
  Waco 76711 (4800 Memorial Dr.)

Workers' Compensation Federal District Office
Office of Workers' Compensation Program
525 S. Griffin St., Room 100
Dallas, TX 75202

Workers' Compensation State Plan Office
Workers' Compensation Commission
Southfield Bldg., MS-34000 S. IH 35
Austin, TX 78704-7491
http://www.twcc.state.tx.us

UTAH

CHAMPVA Claim Office
CHAMPVA Center
4500 Cherry Creek Dr., S.
P.O. Box 65024
Denver, CO 80206-9024

Insurance Commissioner State Office
Commissioner
Department of Insurance
State Office Bldg., Suite 3110
Salt Lake City, UT 84114-6901
http://www.insurance.state.ut.us

Maternal and Child Health Program
CSHCN
Utah Department of Health
P.O. Box 144610
Salt Lake City, UT 84114-4610

Community & Family Health Services Division
Utah Department of Health
P.O. Box 142001
Salt Lake City, UT 84114-2001

Medicaid Fiscal Agent
Bureau of Medicaid Operations
P.O. Box 143106
Salt Lake City, UT 84114-3106
http://hlunix.hl.state.ut.us/medicaid/

Medicare Durable Medical Equipment
CIGNA Medicare
P.O. Box 690
Nashville, TN 37202
http://www.cignamedicare.com

Medicare Fiscal Agent or Carrier
Regency/Blue Cross and Blue Shield of Utah
2890 E. Cottonwood Parkway (84121)
P.O. Box 30270
Salt Lake City, UT 84130-0269

State Board of Medical Examiners
Utah Osteopathic Physicians and Surgeons
  Licensing Board
Heber M. Wells Bldg., 4th Floor
160 E. 300 S. (84114)
P.O. Box 146741
Salt Lake City, UT 84114-6741

Utah Physicians Licensing Board
Herber M. Wells Building, 1st Floor
160 E. 300 South
Salt Lake City, UT 84114

TRICARE Claim Office
Palmetto Government Benefits Administration (PGBA)
P.O. Box 870132
Surfside Beach, SC 29587-9732
http://www.myTRICARE.com

Veterans Administration Installation
Utah Medical Center
500 Foothill Dr.
Salt Lake City, UT 84148

Workers' Compensation Federal District Office
Office of Workers' Compensation Program
1999 Broadway, Suite 600
Denver, CO 80202

Workers' Compensation State Plan Office
Industrial Accident Division
Labor Commission
160 E. 300 S, 3rd Floor
P.O. Box 146610
Salt Lake City, UT 84114-6610

VERMONT

CHAMPVA Claim Office
CHAMPVA Center
4500 Cherry Creek Dr., S.
P.O. Box 65024
Denver, CO 80206-9024

Insurance Commissioner State Office
Commissioner
Department of Banking, Insurance, and Securities
  and Health Care Administration
89 Main St., Drawer 20
Montpelier, VT 05620-3101

Maternal and Child Health Program
Children with Special Health Care Needs
Vermont Department of Health
108 Cherry St.
P.O. Box 70
Burlington, VT 05402

Maternal and Child Health
Vermont Department of Health
108 Cherry St.
P.O. Box 70
Burlington, VT 05402-0070

Medicaid Fiscal Agent
Electronic Data Systems (EC)
P.O. Box 888
Williston, VT 05495-0888
http://www.dsw.state.vt.us/districts/HAEU/medicaid.htm

Medicare Durable Medical Equipment
HealthNow of New York
P.O. Box 6800
Wilkes-Barre, PA 18773-6800

Medicare Fiscal Agent or Carrier
National Heritage Insurance Company
75 Sgt. William B. Terry Dr.
Hingham, MA 02043
http://www.medicarehic.com

State Board of Medical Examiners
Vermont Board of Medical Practice
108 Cherry Street St.
P.O. Box 70
Burlington, VT 05402-0070

Vermont Board of Osteopathic Physiciansand
  Surgeons
26 Terrace St.
Drawer 09
Montpelier, VT 05609-1106

TRICARE Claim Office
Palmetto Government Benefits Administration (PGBA)
P.O. Box 7011
Camden, SC 29020-7011
http://www.myTRICARE.com

Veterans Affairs Installation
Vermont Medical Center
215 North Main St.
White River Junction, VT 05009

Workers' Compensation Federal District Office
Office of Workers' Compensation Programs
JFK Federal Office Bldg., Room E-260
Boston, MA 02203

Workers' Compensation State Plan Office
Department of Labor and Industry
National Life Bldg.
Drawer 20
Montpelier, VT 05620-3401
http://www.state.vt.us/labind

VIRGIN ISLANDS

CHAMPVA Claim Office
CHAMPVA Center
4500 Cherry Creek Dr., S.
P.O. Box 65024
Denver, CO 80206-9024

Insurance Commissioner State Office
Director of Insurance
Kongens Gade #18
St. Thomas, VI 00820

Maternal and Child Health Program
Clinical Care Coordinator Virgin Island
  Department of Health
Elaine Co Bldg. Complex, 2nd Floor
St. Thomas, VI 00802

Maternal and Child Health and Children with Special
  Health Care Needs
3012 Vitraco Mall
Estate Golden Rock
Christiansted
St. Croix, VI 00820-4320

Medicare Durable Medical Equipment
Palmetto Government Benefits Administration (PGBA)
(Blue Cross & Blue Shield of S. Carolina)
P.O. Box 100254
Columbia, SC 29202-3254
http://www.pgba.com/

Medicare Fiscal Agent or Carrier
Medicare/Triple-S, Inc.
Call Box 71391
San Juan, Puerto Rico 00936-1391

Medicare Railroad Retiree Carrier
Medicare Part B Claims are handled by claim service
centers. For the address and toll-free number of the
office nearest you, call the Railroad Retirement Board
listed in your telephone directory under U.S. Government.

State Board of Medical Examiners
Virgin Islands Board of Medical Examiners
Department of Health
48 Sugar Estate, 2nd Floor
St. Thomas, VI 00802

Veterans Affairs Installation
For information on VA benefits, call 800-827-1000

Workers' Compensation Federal District Office
Office of Workers' Compensation Programs
201 Varick St., Room 750
P.O. Box 566
New York, NY 10014-0566

Workers' Compensation State Plan Office
Department of Labor
Workers' Compensation Division
3012 Vitraco Mall, Golden Rock
Christiansted
St. Croix, VI 00820-4666

VIRGINIA

CHAMPVA Claim Office
CHAMPVA Center
4500 Cherry Creek Dr., S.
Box 65024
Denver, CO 80206-9024

Insurance Commissioner State Office
Commissioner, Bureau of Insurance
State Corporation Commission
1300 E. Main St.
P.O. Box 1157
Richmond, VA 23218
http://www.state.va.us/scc

Maternal and Child Health Program
Office of Family Health Services
1500 E. Main St., Suite 104
Richmond, VA 23219

CSHCN Program
VA Department of Health Office of Family Health Services
1500 E. Main St., Room 138
Richmond, VA 23218

Medicaid Fiscal Agent
HCFA
P.O. Box 27444
Richmond, VA 23261-7444
http://www.dmas.state.va.us/

Medicare Durable Medical Equipment
Assigned:
AdminaStar Federal, Inc.
P.O. Box 70778
Indianapolis, IN 46207-7078
http://www.adminastar.com/

Nonassigned:
P.O. Box 7031
Indianapolis, IN 46207-7931

Medicare Fiscal Agent or Carrier
Trail Blazer Health Enterprises
P.O. Box 650208
Dallas, TX 75265-0208
or
P.O. Box 26463
Richmond, VA 23261
http://www.trailblazerhealth.com/

State Board of Medical Examiners
Virginia Board of Medicine
6603 W. Broad St., 5th Floor
Richmond, VA 23230-1717

TRICARE Claim Offices
Certain Northern Virginia ZIP codes located near the Washington, DC, area and a few ZIP codes in the northeast part of West Virginia:
Palmetto Government Benefits Administration (PGBA)

P.O. Box 7011
Camden, SC 29020-7011
http://www.myTRICARE.com

Most of Virginia:
Palmetto Government Benefits Administration (PGBA)
P.O. Box 7021
Camden, SC 29020-7021
http://www.myTRICARE.com

Veterans Affairs Installation
Virginia Medical Centers:
  Hampton 23667 (100 Emancipation Dr.)
  Richmond 23249 (1201 Broad Rock Rd.)
  Salem 24153 (1970 Roanoke Blvd.)

Workers' Compensation Federal District Office
Office of Workers' Compensation Programs
800 N. Capitol St., NW, Room 800
Washington, DC 20211

Workers' Compensation State Plan Office
Workers' Compensation Commission
1000 DMV Dr. (23220)
P.O. Box 1794
Richmond, VA 23220
http://www.vwc.state.va.us

WASHINGTON

CHAMPVA Claim Office
CHAMPVA Center
4500 Cherry Creek Dr., S.
Box 65024
Denver, CO 80206-9024

Insurance Commissioner State Office
Commissioner of Insurance
Office of the Commissioner of Insurance
14th Ave. and Water St.
P.O. Box 40255
Olympia, WA 98504-0255
http://www.insurance.wa.gov

Maternal and Child Health Program
Maternal and Child Health
Washington State Department of Health
P.O. Box 47880
Olympia, WA 98504-7880

CSHCN Program
Washington State Department of Health
Community and Family Health
P.O. Box 47880
Olympia, WA 98504-7880

Medicaid Fiscal Agent
Division of Program Support
P.O. Box 9248
Olympia, WA 98507-9248

Medicare Durable Medical Equipment
CIGNA Medicare
P.O. Box 690
Nashville, TN 37202
http://www.cignamedicare.com

Medicare Fiscal Agent or Carrier
Noridian Mutual Insurance Company
4510 13th Ave. SW
P.O. Box 6700 (58108)
Fargo, ND 58103
http://www.noridianmedicare.com/

State Board of Medical Examiners
Washington Medical Quality Assurance Commission
1300 SE Quince St. (98501)
P.O. Box 47866
Olympia, WA 98504-7866

Washington State Board of Osteopathic Medicine and
 Surgery
Washington State Department of Health
310 Israel Road SE, Tumwater, (98501)
P.O. Box 47869
Olympia, WA 98504-7869

TRICARE Claim Office
Wisconsin Physicians Service
TRICARE Northwest
P.O. Box 8929 or P.O. Box 8999
Madison, WI 53708-8929 (8999)

Veterans Affairs Installation
Washington Medical Centers:
  Seattle 98108 (1660 S. Columbian Way)
  Spokane 99205 (4815 N. Assembly St.)
  Tacoma 98493 (9600 Veterans Dr., SW, American Lake)
  Walla Walla 99362 (77 Wainwright Dr.)

Workers' Compensation Federal District Office
Office of Workers' Compensation Programs
1111 Third Ave., Suite 650
Seattle, WA 98101-3212

Workers' Compensation State Plan Office
Board of Industrial Insurance Appeals
2430 Chandler Court, SW
P.O. Box 42401
Olympia, WA 98504-2401

Department of Labor and Industry
7273 Linderson Way SW
P.O. Box 44001
Olympia, WA 98504-4001
http://www.wa.gov/lni

WEST INDIES

CHAMPVA Claim Office
CHAMPVA Center
4500 Cherry Creek Dr., S.
P.O. Box 65024
Denver, CO 80206-9024

TRICARE Claim Office
Wisconsin Physicians Service
P.O. Box 7985
Madison, WI 53707-7985

WEST VIRGINIA

CHAMPVA Claim Office
CHAMPVA Center
4500 Cherry Creek Dr., S.

P.O. Box 65024
Denver, CO 80206-9024

Insurance Commissioner State Office
Commissioner
Department of Insurance
1124 Smith St.
P.O. Box 50540
Charleston, WV 25301
http://www.state.wv.us/insurance

Maternal and Child Health Program
Office of Maternal and Child Health
West Virginia Department of Health
350 Capitol St., Room 427
Charleston, WV 25301-3714

Children's Specialty Care Division
Office of Maternal, Child & Family Health
350 Capitol St., Room 427
Charleston, WV 25301-3714

Medicaid Fiscal Agent
Department of Health and Human Resources
Capitol Complex Bldg. 6-350
Capitol St., Suite 251
Charleston, WV 25301

Medicare Durable Medical Equipment
Assigned:
AdminaStar Federal, Inc.
P.O. Box 7078
Indianapolis, IN 46207-7078
http://www.adminastar.com/

Nonassigned:
P.O. Box 7031
Indianapolis, IN 46207-7931

Medicare Fiscal Agent or Carrier
Palmetto Government Benefits Administration (PGBA)
3400 Southpark Pl., #F
Grove City, OH 43123
or
P.O. Box 182957
Columbus, OH 43218
http://www.pgba.com/

State Board of Medical Examiners
W. Virginia Board of Medicine
101 Dee Dr.
Charleston, WV 25311

W. Virginia Board of Osteopathy
334 Penco Rd.
Weirton, WV 26062

TRICARE Claim Offices
Palmetto Government Benefits Administration (PGBA)
P.O. Box 7021
Camden, SC 29020-7021
http://www.myTRICARE.com

Veterans Affairs Installation
W. Virginia Medical Centers:
  Beckley 25801 (200 Veterans Ave.)
  Clarksburg 26301 (1 Medical Center Dr.)
  Huntington 25704 (1540 Spring Valley Dr.)
  Martinsburg 25401 (Route 9)

Workers' Compensation Federal District Office
Office of Workers' Compensation Programs
Curtis Center, Suite 715 E.
170 S. Independence Mall W.
Philadelphia, PA 19106-3308

Workers' Compensation State Plan Office
Bureau of Employment Programs
Workers' Compensation Division
4700 MacCorkle Ave., SE (25304)
Executive Offices
P.O. Box 3824
Charleston, WV 25338-3824
http://www.state.wv.us/BEP/wc

Workers' Compensation Appeal Board
104 Dee Dr.
P.O. Box 2628
Charleston, WV 25329

WISCONSIN

CHAMPVA Claim Office
CHAMPVA Center
4500 Cherry Creek Dr., S.
P.O. Box 65024
Denver, CO 80206-9024

Insurance Commissioner State Office
Commissioner
Office of the Commissioner of Insurance
121 E. Wilson St. (53702)
P.O. Box 7873
Madison, WI 53702

Maternal and Child Health Program
Wisconsin Department of Health & Family Services
Division of Public Health
BFCH/CSHCN
P.O. Box 2659
Madison, WI 53701-2659

Medicaid Fiscal Agent
Electronic Data Systems (EC)
6406 Bridge Rd.
Madison, WI 53784-0002
http://www.dhfs.state.wi.us/medicaid/

Medicare Durable Medical Equipment
Assigned:
AdminaStar Federal, Inc.
P.O. Box 7027
Indianapolis, IN 46207-7027
http://www.adminastar.com/

Nonassigned:
P.O. Box 7031
Indianapolis, IN 46207-7931

Medicare Fiscal Agent or Carrier
Wisconsin Physicians Service
Insurance Corporation
1717 Broadway (53713)
P.O. Box 1787
Madison, WI 53701
http://www.wpsic.com/

State Board of Medical Examiners
Wisconsin Medical Examining Board
Department of Regulation & Licensing
1400 E. Washington Ave., Room 178 (53703)
P.O. Box 8935
Madison, WI 53708-8935

TRICARE Claim Office
Palmetto Government Benefits Administration (PGBA)
P.O. Box 7021
Camden, SC 29020-7021
http://www.myTRICARE.com

Veterans Affairs Installation
Wisconsin Medical Centers:
 Madison 53705 (2500 Overlook Terrace)
 Milwaukee 53295 (5000 W. National Ave.)
 Tomah 54660 (500 E. Veterans St.)

Workers' Compensation Federal District Office
Office of Workers' Compensation Programs
230 S. Dearborn St., 8th Floor
Chicago, IL 60604

Workers' Compensation State Plan Office
Labor and Industry Review Commission
P.O. Box 8126
Madison, WI 53708

Workers' Compensation Division
Department of Workforce Development
201 E. Washington Ave., Room C100 (53703)
P.O. Box 7901
Madison, WI 53707-7901
http://www.dwd.state.wi.us/wc

WYOMING

CHAMPVA Claim Office
CHAMPVA Center
4500 Cherry Creek Dr., S.
P.O. Box 65024
Denver, CO 80206-9024

Insurance Commissioner State Office
Commissioner
Department of Insurance
Herschler Bldg.
122 W. 25th St., 3rd Floor E.
Cheyenne, WY 82002-0440

Maternal and Child Health Program
Maternal and Child Health
Division of Public Health
Hathaway Bldg., Room 465
Cheyenne, WY 82002-0480

CSHCN Manager
Division of Public Health
Hathaway Bldg., 4th Floor, Room 467
Cheyenne, WY 82002-0480

Medicaid Fiscal Agent
ACS
P.O. Box 547
Cheyenne, WY 82003

Medicare Durable Medical Equipment
CIGNA Medicare
P.O. Box 690
Nashville, TN 37202
http://www.cignamedicare.com

Medicare Fiscal Agent or Carrier
Noridian Mutual Insurance Company
4510 13th Ave., SW
P.O. Box 6708 (58108-6708)
Fargo, ND 58103
http://www.noridianmedicare.com/

State Board of Medical Examiners
Wyoming Board of Medicine
Colony Bldg., 2nd Floor
211 W. 19th St.
Cheyenne, WY 82002

TRICARE Claim Office
Palmetto Government Benefits Administration (PGBA)
P.O. Box 870126
Surfside Beach, SC 29587
http://www.myTRICARE.com

Veterans Affairs Installation
Wyoming Medical Centers:
　Cheyenne 82001 (2360 E. Pershing Blvd.)
　Sheridan 82801 (1898 Fort Rd.)

Workers' Compensation Federal District Office
Office of Workers' Compensation Programs
1999 Broadway, Suite 600
Denver, CO 80202

Workers' Compensation State Plan Office
Workers' Safety & Compensation Division
Department of Employment
Herschler Bldg. E.
122 W. 25th St.
Cheyenne, WY 82002
http://wydoe.state.wy.us/wscd

APPENDIX B

Reference List of Audiotapes, Books, Newsletters, Periodicals, Software, and Videotapes

Entries are listed as follows: Title, edition if any, comments if any (in parentheses), author (in parentheses), date of publication or production where appropriate, and publisher. Look through the subject matter headings on this page, review entries within the sections you select, note the name of the publisher or manufacturer, and then find it under "Name and Addresses of Resources" at the end of this Appendix.

INDEX

RESOURCE LIST

AUTOMATION
See *Electronic Data Interchange*

BILLING
See also *Fees, Reimbursement, Charges*

Newsletters
The Health Care Biller: The Communication Network for America's Health Care Biller (paperback), Aspen Publishers, Inc.
Codetrends (monthly publication), Medical Association of Billers

Reference Guides
Health Care Billing & Collections: Forms, Checklists & Guidelines (looseleaf), Aspen Publishers, Inc.

CERTIFICATION
Certification Study Guide for CPAM/CCAM Exams. American Guild of Patient Account Management
Certified Coding Specialist Certification Guide. American Health Information Management Association
Certified Professional Coder/CPC-Hospital Outpatient. Independent Study Programs. American Academy of Professional Coders
Certified Professional Coder Examination Study Guide. American Academy of Professional Coders
CPC Exam Prep Program (Doris Ramirez), Professional Practice Builders

CHARGES
See *Fees, Reimbursement, Charges*

CLAIMS ASSISTANCE PROFESSIONALS
Books
Medical Claims Processing (self-employment book), (Clement and Associates), Entrepreneur
PROClaimer Analyst Newsletter (monthly), Strategic Decisions Plus

CODING
Books, Diagnostic and Procedural
Adams' Guide to Coding and Reimbursement (Wanda Adams), 1998, Elsevier/Mosby

Ambulatory Facility Coding (Catalog #214), Medical Business Resource Center

Annual Hospital Version, The Educational Annotation of ICD-9-CM, Volumes 1, 2, 3 (updated annually), Channel Publishing, Ltd.

Annual Physician Version, The Educational Annotation of ICD-9-CM, Volumes 1 and 2 (updated annually), Channel Publishing, Ltd.

Chiropractic Code Book (excerpts from CPT, HCPCS, and ICD-9-CM with RVUs, updated annually), Chart-Care Solutions

Coder's Desk Reference (updated annually), Ingenix Publishing Group

Coding and Payment Guide for the Physical Therapist, CPT, HCPCS Level II, ICD-9-CM, Ingenix Publishing Group

Coding for Quality, CPT Coding for Outpatient Surgery, a Comprehensive Guide (updated periodically), Health-care Management Advisors, Inc.

Common Orthopedic Procedures and Diagnostic Codes, A Reference Guide, American Academy of Orthopaedic Surgeons

Compendium of ICD-9-CM for Ob-Gyn, Cardiology, Neurology, Ophthalmology, Urology, Orthopedics, Commission on Professional Hospital Activities

Complete Coding Tutor (updated annually), Ingenix Publishing Group

CPT-4 Teaching Manual, American Academy of Pediatrics

CPT and HCPCS Coding Made Easy! A Comprehensive Guide to CPT and HCPCS Coding for Health Care Professionals, 2001, Practice Management Information Corporation

CPT Coding Tool (updated annually), Practice Management Information Corporation

CPT Coding, E & M, RBRVS (Catalog #201), Medical Business Resource Center

CPT Coding—Operative Reports (Catalog #204), Medical Business Resource Center

CPT Coding—Paraprofessional, HCPCS (Catalog #203), Medical Business Resource Center

CPT Coding—Surgical (Catalog #202), Medical Business Resource Center

CPT Guidebook, American Academy of Orthopaedic Surgeons

CPT Handbook for Psychiatrists (Chester W. Schmidt, Jr.), American Psychiatric Press, Inc.

CPT, ICD-9, and HCPCS, Coding Illustrated: The Eyeball; Lower Face; Skeletal Structures and Definitions; Soft Tissue; Peripheral Vascular System; Uterus. Tubes, and Ovaries; Nonpregnant, 1999, Ingenix Publishing Group

Current Procedural Terminology (CPT), (available in computer software, magnetic tape, published annually), American Medical Association

Diagnosis Coding, American College of Emergency Physicians

Diagnostic & Statistical Manual of Mental Disorders (DSM-IV), American Psychiatric Press, Inc.

Easy Coder (This code book is available for the following specialties: cardiology, dermatology, ears/nose/throat, family practice, internal medicine, obstetrics/gynecology, ophthalmology, orthopedics, psychiatry, and urology), Unicor Medical, Inc.

E/M Coding Made Easy, 1998, Practice Management Information Corporation

ENT Diagnosis Code, CPT, ICD-9-CM Diagnosis and Procedures, William J. Hunt

Evaluation and Management Coding and Documentation Guide, Ingenix Publishing Group

Generic Hospital ICD-9-CM, Volumes 1, 2, 3 (paperback, updated annually), Channel Publishing, Ltd.

Getting Paid for What You Do, Coding for Optimal Reimbursement (Gary M. Knaus), 1997, McGraw-Hill Healthcare Management Group

Laboratory Cross Coder, Ingenix Publishing Group

ICD-9 Chart, Effective CPT Coding for Rheumatology Practices, American College of Rheumatology

ICD-9-CM Code Book, Volumes 1, 2, & 3, HCIA Inc.

ICD-9-CM Coding for Physicians Offices (Billie C. Bradford), McGraw-Hill Healthcare Management Group

ICD-9-CM Coding Made Easy! A Comprehensive Coding Guide for Health Care Professionals (updated annually), Practice Management Information Corporation

ICD-9 Coding Utility for Medical Billing (software program), KFC Medical Systems, Inc.

ICD-9-CM, Volumes 1 and 2 (for physicians); Volume 3 (for hospitals), (updated annually), Ingenix Publishing Group

ICD-9-CM Diagnosis Coding Advisor (updated annually), Ingenix Publishing Group

ICD-9-CM, International Classification of Diseases, 9th Revision, Clinical Modification (color coded, updated annually), (Context Software Systems), McGraw-Hill Healthcare Management Group

ICD-9-CM International Classification of Diseases, 9th Revision, Clinical Modification, Volumes 1 and 2, Volumes 1, 2 and 3, or Binder Version or Hardbound Version, Practice Management Information Corporation

ICD-9-CM to CPT Radiology Cross Code, R. B. Holt

ICD-9-CM Coding Handbook (Faye Brown), 2000, American Hospital Association

ICD-9-CM Coding in a SNAP (alphabetical listing of over 1700 commonly used diagnosis codes, updated annually), (Ann G. Uniack), Skilled Nursing Assessment Programs (SNAP)

ICD-9 Coding—Introduction (Catalog #211), Medical Business Resource Center

ICD-9 Coding—Late Effects, V Codes (Catalog #212), Medical Business Resource Center

ICD-9 Coding—Special Tables, E Codes (Catalog #213), Medical Business Resource Center

ICD-10, The International Statistical Classification of Diseases and Related Health Problems, Tenth Revision, Volume 1 (World Health Organization), 1992, distributed by Ingenix Publishing Group

ICD-10 Made Easy, 1999, Ingenix Publishing Group

Interventional Radiology Coder (This company publishes code books for ambulatory surgery procedures, emergency services, and laboratory tests), Medical Learning Incorporated

The Interventional Radiology Coding User's Guide (updated annually), The Society of Cardiovascular and Interventional Radiology

Introduction to Coding (Catalog #200), Medical Business Resource Center

Key Questions in Cardiopulmonary Coding, American Health Consultants, Inc.

Key Questions in Medicare Coding, American Health Consultants, Inc.

Key Questions in Oncology Coding, American Health Consultants, Inc.

Key Questions in Orthopaedic Coding, American Health Consultants, Inc.

Key Questions in Surgical Coding, American Health Consultants, Inc.

Medical Terminology—Basic (Catalog #229/230), Medical Business Resource Center

Medical Terminology—Body Systems (Catalog #231), Medical Business Resource Center

Medical Terminology—Body Systems II (Catalog #232), Medical Business Resource Center

Modifiers Made Easy (published annually), Ingenix Publishing Group

National Correct Coding Guide (updated annually), Ingenix Publishing Group

National Correct Coding Primer (Part B News), United Communications Group

Orthopaedic ICD-9-CM Expanded, American Academy of Orthopaedic Surgeons

Post Binder Hospital Version, The Educational Annotation of ICD-9-CM, Volumes 1, 2, 3 (updated annually), Channel Publishing, Ltd.

Principles of CPT Coding, 2001, American Medical Association

Principles of ICD-9-CM Coding, 2003, American Medical Association

Procedure Coding, American College of Emergency Physicians

Soft Cover Hospital Version, The Educational Annotation of ICD-9-CM, Volumes 1, 2, 3, (updated annually), Channel Publishing, Ltd.

Soft Cover Physician Version, The Educational Annotation of ICD-9-CM, Volumes 1 and 2 (soft cover), Channel Publishing, Ltd.

Specialty Coding Manuals, Medical Management Institute

Ingenix Coding and Payment Guide (books are available for the following specialties: podiatry services, radiology services, and behavioral health science), Ingenix Publishing Group

Ingenix Coding Companion (books are available for the following specialties: cardiology, general surgery, obstetrics/gynecology, ophthalmology, orthopedics, otorhinolaryngology), Ingenix Publishing Group

Ingenix Color-Coded Annotated ICD-9-CM Code Book, Ingenix Publishing Group

Ingenix Guide to APC and ASC Groups, St. Anthony/ Ingenix Publishing Group

Ingenix ICD-9-CM Code Book for Home Health Services, Nursing Homes & Hospices, Ingenix Publishing Group

Ingenix ICD-9-CM Code Book for Physician Compliance, Combined Volumes 1 and 2, in 3-hole binder with indexes and color coded for maximum reimbursement, Ingenix Publishing Group

Ingenix Medicare Reimbursement Guide for Radiology Services: The Coding, Billing and Coverage Guide, Ingenix Publishing Group

Ingenix Updatable ICD-9-CM Code Book, Ingenix Publishing Group

Ingenix Updatable ICD-9-CM Code Book for Outpatient Services, Ingenix Publishing Group

Ingenix Updatable ICD-9-CM Code Book for Physician Compliance, Ingenix Publishing Group

Using CPT for Cardiothoracic Reimbursement: A Manual for Surgeons and Insurance Billing Specialists, Society of Thoracic Surgeons

Code Cards

"Code-Its" (compiled list of most common ICD-9-CM codes in each specialty. Request specialty—family practice, cardiology, ears/nose/throat, obstetrics/gynecology, urology, pediatrics, podiatry, cardiovascular surgery, ophthalmology, laminated cards), Karen Zupko & Associates

Code Journals

CPT Assistant (four issues), American Medical Association

Code Hotlines

Hotlines for Coding and Billing, St. Anthony's Hotline, (703) 836-9471, Ingenix Publishing Group

Code Newsletters

AAPC News, American Academy of Professional Coders

Clinical Coding and Reimbursement (published annually), Ingenix Publishing Group

The Coding Connection, Group Health Management Corporation

Coding News, Unicor Medical, Inc.

How to Get Paid (features Medicare, coding, and third-party payer information, monthly), Opus Communications

Physicians Payment Update (includes center section specific to coding strategies), American Health Consultants, Inc.

Reimbursement Updated, Ingenix Publishing Group

Ingenix Coding and Reimbursement (newsletters for the following: behavior health services, cardiovascular, ear/nose/throat and allergy, general surgery, non-physician practitioner, obstetrics/gynecology, ophthalmology, orthopaedics, pediatrics, physicians, radiology), Ingenix Publishing Group

Ingenix Hospital Fast Payment Report Newsletter, Ingenix Publishing Group

Ingenix ICD-9-CM Coding for Reimbursement, Ingenix Publishing Group

Code Research and Review Services

Ingenix Operative Report and Coding, Research and Review Service, Ingenix Publishing Group

Code Software

Alpha II ICD-9 Coder, Unicor Medical, Inc.

Claims Editor, Context Software Systems, Inc.

Code Master Plus, Code Master Corporation

CODELINK, Context Software Systems, Inc.

Codelink for Ophthalmology (Context Software Systems), McGraw-Hill Healthcare Management Group

Codelink for Oral & Maxillofacial Surgery (Context Software Systems), McGraw-Hill Healthcare Management Group

Codelink for Orthopaedics (Context Software Systems), McGraw-Hill Healthcare Management Group

Codelink Software (CPT, HCPCS, and ICD-9-CM codes), (Context Software Systems), McGraw-Hill Healthcare Management Group

Codemanager (CPT, HCPCS, ICD-9-CM codes, CCI Edits, and Stedman's Medical Dictionary), American Medical Association

Code-Search, Diagnostic Data, Inc.

Diagnostic ICD-9-Code Software (Context Software Systems), McGraw-Hill Healthcare Management Group

ICD-9-CM (floppy disk), American Medical Association

ICD-9-CM Volume I Software and HCPCS Level II Software, Opus Communications

InfoCoder (ICD-9-CM encoder), Channel Publishing, Ltd.

MCSS CPT and HCPCS Software (ADP Business Assessments), MedSmart

MCSS CPT and ICD-9 and HCPCS Software (ADP Business Assessments), MedSmart

MCSS CPT and ICD-9 Software (ADP Business Assessment), MedSmart

MCSS ICD-9 Software (ADP Business Assessment), MedSmart

Medcoder Idea Planners, Inc.

Medical Code Software System MCSS Automated Code Finder (searches CPT, ICD-9, and HCPCS), MCSS CPT Software (ADP Business Assessments), MedSmart

Omnicode and ICD Coder, SRC Systems

QuickCODE, Dr. P's Software, Inc.

RBRVS FEECALC (calculates physicians' payments under the Medicare RBRVS fee schedule, upgraded periodically), United Communications Group

Surgical Cross Coder (CPT and ICD-9 Codes), Ingenix Publishing Group

COLLECTIONS

Successful Billing and Collection Handbooks, Conomikes Reports, Inc.

Newsletters

Health Care Collector (monthly), Aspen Publishers, Inc. How to Get Paid, Opus Communications

Software

Appeal Solutions (450 appeal letters), 1998, Appeal Solutions

COMPLIANCE

See also *Fraud and Abuse*

Compliance Guide to Electronic Health Records, A Practical Reference to Legislation, Codes, Regulations, and Industry Standards, 2001, Faulkner & Gray, Inc.

Health Care Fraud and Abuse, 2000, American Medical Association

HIPAA: A Guide to Health Care Privacy and Security Law, (Lisa Boyle and David Mack, updated periodically), Aspen Publishers

Medicare Billing Compliance Guide (updated annually), Ingenix Publishing Group

Medicare Billing Compliance Reference Manual (updated annually), Ingenix Publishing Group

Medicare Rules and Compliance Regulations, 1999, Medical Management Institute

National Correct Coding Guide (updated annually), Ingenix Publishing Group

The National Correct Coding Manual (updated annually), Medical Management Institute

Ingenix Complete Guide to Part B Billing Compliance, Ingenix Publishing Group

DELINQUENT AND DENIED CLAIMS

Collections from Insurance Carriers

Collections Made Easy! A Comprehensive Guide for Medical and Dental Professionals (Michael J. Berry), Practice Management Information Corporation

DIAGNOSIS-RELATED GROUPS

Ingenix Clinical Coder, Ingenix Publishing Group

Ingenix DRG Optimizer, Ingenix Publishing Group

Ingenix DRG Working Guidebook, Ingenix Publishing Group

DIAGNOSTIC AND PROCEDURE HANDBOOKS FOR TERMINOLOGY (DPT)

These medical books may be of some assistance as references for researching medical terminology when doing diagnostic and procedural coding.

Diagnostic Procedures Handbook Including Keyword Index (Franklin A. Michota, Jr., MD), 2001, Lexi-Comp

The Merck Manual of Diagnosis and Therapy, Merck Sharp and Dohme Research Laboratories, 1999, distributed by MedSmart

DICTIONARIES AND GLOSSARIES

Dorland's Illustrated Medical Dictionary, 2000, Elsevier/W. B. Saunders

Health Insurance Terminology: A Glossary of Health Insurance Terms, Health Insurance Association of America

Stedman's Medical Dictionary, 2000, Lippincott Williams & Wilkins

Taber's Cyclopedic Medical Dictionary (Clayton L. Thomas, editor), 2001, F. A. Davis Company

DISABILITY BENEFIT PROGRAMS

Booklets and Pamphlets

Obtain from the state disability programs for the following states: California, Hawaii, New Jersey, New York, Puerto Rico, Rhode Island. See Appendix A for state addresses.

Newsletters

Unemployment Insurance Reports With Social Security (weekly), Commerce Clearing House, Inc.

Disability Income Insurance

Disability Income Insurance: An Overview of Income Protection Insurance, Health Insurance Association of America

DOCUMENTATION, MEDICAL

Documentation and Reimbursement for Physician Offices (Lynn Kuehn and LaVonne Wieland), 1999, American Health Information Management Association

Medical Documentation, Streamlining an Essential Clinical Process, Ingenix Publishing Group

Physician Documentation for Reimbursement (Gabrielle M. Kotoski and Melinda S. Stegman), 1994, Aspen Publishers, Inc.

EDUCATION AND TRAINING

Audiocassette Tapes

Individual Health Insurance, Parts A and B, Group Life & Health Insurance, Parts A, B, and C, Long-Term Care, Health Insurance Association of America

Books

Basic CPT/HCPCS Coding (Sherri A. Mallett), 2000, American Health Information Management Association

Basic ICD-9-CM Coding (Lou Ann Schraffenberger), 2000, American Health Information Management Association

Basic ICD-9-CM for Physician Office Coding (Anita Hazelwood and Carol Venable), 2001, American Health Information Management Association

Basic Keyboarding for the Medical Office Assistant (Edna Moss), 1999, Delmar Publishers, Inc.

Case Study Workbook (for advanced coder), (Patricia Morin-Spatz), 2001, MedBooks

Coding Curriculum Guide, American Health Information Management Association

Coding Skills for the Medical Assistant (Joy Renfro), 1993, American Association of Medical Assistants

Coding Workbook for the Physician's Office (published annually), (Alice G. Covell), Delmar Publishers, Inc.

Complete Coding Tutor 2001, Ingenix Publishing Group

CP "Teach," Instructors Manual (published annually), (Patricia Morin-Spatz), MedBooks

CP "Teach," Workbook (published annually), (Patricia Morin-Spatz), MedBooks

CP "Teach" Expert Coding Made Easy! Textbook (published annually), (Patricia Morin-Spatz), MedBooks

CPT: Beyond the Basics (self-study, four lessons), (Gail I. Smith), 2000, American Health Information Management Association

CPT Coding Workbook for the Student, Medical Learning Incorporated

CPT/HCPCS for Physician Office Coding (Therese M. Jorwic), 2000, American Health Information Management Association

Glencoe Medical Insurance Coding Workbook (Nenna L. Bayes, Joanne Valerius, and Cindy Keller), 2001, Glencoe/McGraw-Hill

ICD-9-CM: Beyond the Basics (self-study, four lessons), (Ellen Anderson and Toula Nichols), American Health Information Management Association

Intermediate CPT/HCPCS for Physician Office Coding (Donna M. Didier), 2000, American Health Information Management

Med-Index Self-Tests (Coding Instructions), Ingenix Publishing Group

Module II, The Advanced Coder, California Health Information Association

Multispecialty Medical Coding Workbook (updated annually), (Sandra Soerries), Soerries Enterprises

Step-by-Step Medical Coding (Carol J. Buck), 2003, Elsevier/W. B. Saunders

Steps to Coding with ICD-9-CM for Long Term Care, 2000, California Health Information Association

Steps to Coding with ICD-9-CM Module I, The Beginning Coder, California Health Information Association

Courses

See also *Videotapes; Workshops and Seminars*

CPT-4 Clinic: Basic Procedural Coding, Ingenix Publishing Group

Electronic Medical Claims, Strategic Decisions Plus

Evaluation and Management Training (2-hour training session), (Sandra Soerries), Soerries Enterprises

ICD-9-CM Clinic: Basic Diagnostic Coding, Ingenix Publishing Group

Multispecialty Medical Coding Workbook (updated annually), (Sandra Soerries), Soerries Enterprises

Physician Reimbursement Clinic: Managing Payment, Billing & Coding in the RBRVS Era, St. Anthony/Ingenix Publishing Group

S.O.S. for the Medical Office (12-hour training session), (Sandra Soerries), Soerries Enterprises

Ingenix Basic ICD-9-CM Coding: Self-Directed Training for the Physician Office Professional (four audiocassette tapes and workbook), Ingenix Publishing Group

The 3-in-1 Coding Workshop: ICD-9-CM, CPT and HCPCS Level II, Ingenix Publishing Group

ELECTRONIC DATA INTERCHANGE

Books

Automated Medical Payments Directory (updated annually), Faulkner & Gray, Inc.

Compliance Guide to Electronic Health Records, A Practical Reference to Legislation, Codes, Regulations, and Industry Standards, 2001, Faulkner & Gray, Inc.

Claims Processing Bulletin Board Service

Claims Wizard Software, Info Alliance

Computer Bulletin Board for Claims Professionals, Info Alliance

Electronic Medical Claims Presentation Manual, Strategic Decisions Plus

Health Care Software Sourcebook, Aspen Publishers, Inc.

ETHICS

See also Law and Ethics

Code of Medical Ethics, Current Opinions with Annotations, 2001, American Medical Association

FEES, REIMBURSEMENT, CHARGES

"Fees on Disk" Software (specialties: cardiology, dermatology, family/general practice, internal medicine, ob/gyn/surgery), HealthCare Consultants of America, Inc.

Health Care Billing and Collections Forms, Checklists and Guidelines (Health and Administration Development Group), 1997, Aspen Publishers, Inc.

Health Care Financial Transactions Manual (Thomas C. Fox, Carol Colborn, Carl Krasik, and Joseph W. Metro) (revised periodically), West Group

"Medirisk Physician Fee Schedules," (reports are available for 30 specialties and all geographic regions), Ingenix Publishing Group

Physician Fee Analyzer Plus, Ingenix Publishing Group

Physicians Fee & Coding Guide, A Comprehensive Fee and Coding Reference (updated annually), (James R. Lyle and Hoyt W. Torras), HealthCare Consultants of America, Inc.

Physicians' Fee Reference (available in book and on disk, updated annually), Wasserman Medical Publishers Limited

Physician Fees, A Comprehensive Guide for Fee Schedule Review and Management (updated annually), Practice Management Information Corporation

Reimbursement Manual for the Medical Office (a comprehensive guide to coding, billing and fee management), (James R. Davis), 2001, Practice Management Information Corporation

Reimbursement Strategies, Master the Payment Cycle Today, Ingenix Publishing Group

RVP Fees: Primary Care (software program), McGraw-Hill Healthcare Management Group

RVP Fees: Version 3.1 (software program), McGraw-Hill Healthcare Management Group

What Are My Fees? A Physician's Guide to the Complete Local Medicare Fee Schedule, McGraw-Hill Healthcare Management Group

What Are My Fees? A Physician's Guide to the Complete National Medicare Fee Schedule (Cambridge Health Economics Group), McGraw-Hill Healthcare Management Group

FRAUD AND ABUSE

See also Videotapes

"Consumer Fraud—Medicare and Home Medical Equipment" (pamphlet 1992:332.525), United States Government Printing Office

Health Care Fraud and Abuse, A Physician's Guide to Compliance, 2000, American Medical Association

Health Care Fraud and Abuse (revised annually), (Paul P. Cacioppo), West Group

HCFA COMMON PROCEDURE CODING SYSTEM (HCPCS)

HCPCS Common Proceduring Coding System (non–CPT-4 portion). Order document number 01706000307-3 from US Government Printing Office

HCPCS, HCFA Common Procedure Coding System, spiral bound version or binder version, (annual publication), Practice Management Information Corporation

HCPCS Level II Code Book (updated annually), Wasserman Medical Publishers, Limited

HCPCS Level II Codes (published annually), Ingenix Publishing Group

HCPCS Level II, National Codes (published annually), (Context Software Systems), McGraw-Hill Healthcare Management Group

HCPCS, Medicare's National Level II Codes, Ingenix Publishing Group

Ingenix HCPCS Report Newsletter, Ingenix Publishing Group

HEALTH INSURANCE

Books

The Business of Insurance, 1993, Health Insurance Association of America

From Patient to Payment: Insurance Procedures for the Medical Office (Rhoda Collins), 1998, Glencoe/McGraw-Hill

Glencoe Medical Insurance (Cindy Keller, Nenna L. Bayes, and Joanne Valerius), 2001, Glencoe/McGraw-Hill

Mastering the Reimbursement Process (L. Lamar Blount and Joanne M. Waters), 2001, American Medical Association

Understanding Medical Insurance: A Step by Step Guide (JoAnn C. Rowell), 2004, Delmar Publishers, Inc.

HEALTH MAINTENANCE ORGANIZATIONS/ PREFERRED PROVIDER ORGANIZATIONS

See *Managed Care*

HOSPITAL INSURANCE CLAIMS

APC Claims Auditor (updated annually), Ingenix Publishing Group

APC Payment Manual (updated annually), Ingenix Publishing Group

APC Reference Manual (updated annually), Ingenix Publishing Group

APC Pocket Guide (updated annually), Ingenix Publishing Group

Complete Guide to APCs (updated annually), Ingenix Publishing Group

DRG Compliance Auditor (updated annually), Ingenix Publishing Group

DRG Companion (updated annually), Ingenix Publishing Group

DRG Guidebook (updated annually), Ingenix Publishing Group

Hospital Chargemaster Guide (updated annually), Ingenix Publishing Group

Outpatient Procedures Resource Book (updated annually), Ingenix Publishing Group

UB-92 Editor (updated annually), Ingenix Publishing Group

Newsletter

Health Care Biller (monthly), Aspen Publishers, Inc.

INSURANCE DIRECTORIES

Health Insurance Carrier Directory, A Comprehensive Guide to Insurance Carriers & Claims Processing, binder or spiral-bound versions (annual publication), Practice Management Information Corporation

Insurance Directory (updated annually), Ingenix Publishing Group

Physicians' Insurance Reference (updated annually), Wasserman Medical Publishers, Limited

LAW AND ETHICS

See also *Ethics*

Books

Glencoe Law & Ethics for Medical Careers (Karen Judson and Sharon Blesie Hicks), 1999, Glencoe/McGraw-Hill

Health Care Fraud and Abuse (revised annually), (Paul P. Cacioppo), West Group

Law, Liability & Ethics for Medical Office Personnel (Myrtle R. Flight), Delmar Publishers, Inc.

Medicolegal Forms with Legal Analysis, American Medical Association

Newsletters

In Confidence (6 issues/year), American Health Information Management Association

Patient Confidentiality, Alphabetical Guide to the Release of Medical Information (updated annually), Ingenix Publishing Group

Software

Black's Law Dictionary (electronic edition, 3.5" or 5.25" disks), (Henry Campbell Black), West Group

MANAGED CARE

Conomikes Managed Care Handbook, Conomikes Associates, Inc.

CPT Guidebook for Managed Care, 1997, Ingenix Publishing Group

Criteria for Participating in Managed Care Systems, How to Evaluate a Managed Care System Contract, American Medical Association

Doctors Resource Service (DRS) (publication, videocassette, audiocassette, mailed every 6 weeks), American Medical Association

HMO/PPO Directory (published annually), Medical Economics Publishing

The Managed Care Handbook, A Comprehensive Guide to Preparing Your Practice for the Managed Care Revolution, Practice Management Information Corporation

Managed Care Organizer (system for referencing plan contracts and requirements, monitoring plan utilization, providing in-plan referrals, tracking referrals, and calculating and comparing plan profitability), Ingenix Publishing Group

Managed Care Resource Guide (quarterly), Managed Care Information Center

The Managed Health Care Handbook (Peter R. Kongsvedt), 2001, Aspen Publishers, Inc.

Managing Managed Care for the Physician's Office (Carol K. Richards), 1991, American Association of Medical Assistants

Negotiating Managed Care Contracts (Medical Management Institute), 1994, McGraw-Hill Health Care Management Group

The Physician's Guide to Managed Care (David B. Nash), 1994, Aspen Publishers, Inc.

Physician's Guide to Managed Care, A Comprehensive Guide to Managed Competition, Managed Care, and Global Budgeting (James R. Lyle and Hoyt W. Torras), 1993, HealthCare Consultants of America, Inc.

Newsletters

CCH Monitor, The Newsletter of Managed Care (biweekly), Commerce Clearing House, Inc.

CCH Pulse, The Health Care Reform Newsletter (bimonthly), Commerce Clearing House, Inc.

Physician's Managed Care Report (monthly), American Health Consultants, Inc.

MEDICAID
Bulletins

Obtain from State Intermediary. See Appendix A for the address in your state.

CD-ROM

The Medicare and Medicaid Guide, Volumes 1 to 5 updated weekly and CD-ROM updated monthly, Commerce Clearing House, Inc.

The Medicare/Medicaid Library (CD-ROM monthly subscription with modem access to bulletin board service, which contains updates to Federal Register), Information Handling Services (IHS) Regulatory Products

Newsletters

California Medi-Cal Guide (monthly), *Commerce Clearing House, Inc.*

MEDICAL MANAGEMENT

Managing Medical Office Personnel, A Comprehensive Guide to Personnel Management in the Medical Practice, 2001, Practice Management Information Corporation

Newsletters

Conomikes Reports on Medical Practice Management (monthly), Conomikes Associates, Inc.

The Doctor's Office (monthly), Opus Communications

Journal of CHIA (includes articles on coding, reimbursement, and legal issues; directed to hospitals and ambulatory surgery centers, monthly), California Health Information Association

Medical Office Manager, Medical Office Manager

The Physician's Advisory (monthly), Advisory Publications

Physician's Marketing & Management (monthly), American Health Consultants, Inc.

Uncommon Sense (monthly), Practice Performance Publishing, Inc.

MEDICARE
Books

Commerce Clearing House and the American Medical Association Physicians' Medicare Guide (every other month), Commerce Clearing House, Inc.

Complete Guide to Medicare Coverage Issues (updated annually), Ingenix Publishing Group

Guide to RBRVS for Primary Care Physicians (also other RVS fee guides and insurance publications), HealthCare Consultants of America, Inc.

Key Questions in Medicare Coding, American Health Consultants

Make Medicare Work For You (updated to include RBRVS) (James R. Lyle and Hoyt W. Torras), 1992, HealthCare Consultants of America, Inc.

Medicare at a Glance: How Carriers Scrutinize Your Procedural Coding, Ingenix Publishing Group

Medicare Billing Compliance Guide (published annually), Ingenix Publishing Group

The Medicare Coverage Issues Manual (Denise L. Knaus), McGraw-Hill HealthCare Management Group

Medicare RBRVS: The Physicians' Guide Book, 2003, American Medical Association

Medicare Rules & Regulations, Volumes 1 through 8 (updated as necessary), (Context Software Systems, Inc.), McGraw-Hill HealthCare Management Group

Medicare Rules & Regulations, A Survival Guide to Policies, Procedures and Payment Reform, 2001, Practice Management Information Corporation

The Medicare Survival Guide (Denise L. Knaus), McGraw-Hill HealthCare Management Group

Part B Answer Book, Medicare Billing Rules from A to Z (updated quarterly), United Communications Group

Part B Pocket Billing Guide (updated quarterly), United Communications Group

The ProSTAT Guide to Medicare (Philip L. Bear), Ingenix Publishing Group

Ingenix Color-Coded Medicare Coverage Manual (with color-coded prompts), Ingenix Publishing Group

Ingenix Complete Guide to Medicare Coverage Issues, Ingenix Publishing Group

Ingenix Complete Guide to Part B Billing and Compliance, Ingenix Publishing Group

Ingenix Guide to Ambulatory Surgery Center Payment Groups, Ingenix Publishing Group

Ingenix Medicare Billing Compliance Guide, Ingenix Publishing Group

Ingenix Medicare Billing and Compliance Source Book,
Ingenix Publishing Group
Ingenix Medicare Correct Coding and Payment Manual,
Ingenix Publishing Group
Ingenix Medicare Outpatient Reference Manual, Ingenix
Publishing Group
*Ingenix Medicare Reimbursement Guide for Radiology
Services. The Coding, Billing and Coverage Reference,*
Ingenix Publishing Group

Bulletins

Obtain from State Intermediary. See Appendix A to
obtain the address for your state.

CD-ROM

The Medicare and Medicaid Guide, Volumes 1 through
5 updated weekly and CD-ROM updated monthly,
Commerce Clearing House, Inc.
The Medicare/Medicaid Library, IHS Regulatory Products

Newsletters

Conomike's Medicare Hotline (monthly), Conomike's
Reports, Inc.
Medicare Review (monthly), Shannon Publications, Inc.
Part B News (bimonthly), United Communications Group
Physicians' Medicare Guide Newsletter (every other
month), Commerce Clearing House, Inc.

PREFERRED PROVIDER ORGANIZATIONS

See *Managed Care*

REIMBURSEMENT

See Fees, Reimbursement, Charges

RELATIVE VALUE STUDIES

Relative Value Studies with Regard to Radiology (write
for information), American College of Radiology
*Resource Based Relative Value Scale (RBRVS), Physi-
cians Fee Schedule,* Addendum E, page 63852, Federal
Register, Stock No. 069-001-00063-7, December 2, 1993,
United States Government Printing Office
Ingenix Complete RBRVS, (updated annually), Ingenix
Publishing Group
Ingenix Relative Values for Physicians, Ingenix Pub-
lishing Group

SELF-EMPLOYMENT

Audiotapes

Electronic Medical Claims Marketing Strategies, Strategic
Decisions Plus

Books

Health Service Businesses on your Home-Based PC
(Rick Benzel), (may be purchased from Oxford
Medical Systems), Windcrest/McGraw-Hill
Independent Medical Coding (Donna Avila-Weil and
Rhonda Regan), 1999, Rayve Productions, Inc.

Magazines

Home Office Computing (monthly), Home Office Computing

Marketing

Brochure Collection (24 sample pieces), Strategic Decisions Plus

Newsletter

PRO Claimer Analyst (monthly), Strategic Decisions
Plus

Software

Eazy Quote, Strategic Decisions Plus
PowerLeads for Medical Claims Businesses, InfoAlliance

TRICARE

Bulletins

Obtain from State Intermediary. See Appendix A for
the address in your state.

Newsletters

Understanding CHAMPUS, Volume 1 (updated as
needed), Commerce Clearing House, Inc.

VIDEOTAPES

"Beginning ICD-9-CM," 2-hour videotape, binder, and
workbook, Channel Publishing, Ltd.
"The Case for Case Management," Health Insurance
Association of America
"Coding for Quality," ICD-9-CM Level 1 (26 video-
tapes); Introduction to CPT (3 videotapes), Healthcare
Management Advisors, Inc.
"E & M Coding & Documentation," ChartCare Solutions
"Fighting Fraud," Health Insurance Association of
America
"ICD-10" (HealthMarket International), Medical Learning
Incorporated
"Medicare Part B: Putting an End to Fraud & Abuse,"
8 minutes, Blue Shield of California
"Protecting Tomorrow: Long-Term Care," Health Insur-
ance Association of America
*"Understanding Limiting Charges, Benefits of Medicare
Part B Beneficiaries,"* 8 minutes, Blue Shield of
California

WORKERS' COMPENSATION

*Healthcare Management Guidelines Return-to-Work
Planning* (Milliman and Robertson, Inc.), distributed
by Ingenix Publishing Group
*Official California Workers' Compensation Medical Fee
Schedule* (California Medical Fee Schedule), State of
California

WORKSHOPS AND SEMINARS

American Health Information Management Association
Conomikes Reports, Inc.
Medical Management Institute
Medical Management Information Services, Inc.
The Reimbursement Manager Training Program (RMTP),
Ingenix Publishing Group
Ingenix Seminars
    Advanced Cardiovascular Coding
    Ambulatory Surgery Coding Clinic
    Ambulatory Training Series
    Cardiovascular Coding Workshop
    CPT-4 Hospital Clinic
    Emergency Medicine Workshop
    Ob/Gyn Coding Workshop
    Ophthalmology Coding Workshop
    Orthopaedic Coding Workshop
    Physician Billing & Reimbursement
    Radiology Coding & Reimbursement
    Three-In-One Coding Clinic
United Communications Group
See also *Education and Training Courses,* which offer
prior approval and continuing education units.

NAMES AND ADDRESSES OF RESOURCES

Advisory Publications
P.O. Box 551, Norristown, PA 19404
(610) 941-4488 or (888) 941-4488
www.smartpracticemanagement.com

American Academy of Orthopaedic Surgeons
6300 N. River Road, Rosemont, IL 60018-4226
Phone: (800) 346-AAOS, (800) 626-6726, or
  (708) 823-7186
Fax: (708) 823-8125
www.aaos.org

American Academy of Pediatrics
141 N.W. Point Boulevard, P.O. Box 927, Elk Grove
  Village, IL 60009-0927
(800) 433-9016 or (708) 228-5005
www.aap.org

American Academy of Professional Coders
309 West 700 South, Salt Lake City, UT 84101
(800) 626-CODE
www.aapc.com

American Association of Medical Assistants
20 N. Wacker Drive, Suite 1575, Chicago, IL 60606
(800) 228-2262
www.aama-natl.org

American College of Emergency Physicians
P.O. Box 619911, Dallas, TX 75261
(800) 798-1822
www.acep.org

American College of Radiology RVS
1891 Preston White Drive, Reston, VA 22090

American College of Rheumatology
60 Executive Park South, Suite 150 Atlanta, GA 30329
(404) 633-3777

**American Guild of Patient Account Management,
  National Certification Examination Program**
1101 Connecticut Avenue, NW, Suite 700,
  Washington, DC 20036

American Health Consultants, Inc.
3525 Piedmont Road, NE, Bldg. 6, Suite 400, (30305),
  P.O. Box 740060, Department 1203, Atlanta,
  GA 30374-9822
www.ahcpub.com/online.html

**American Health Information Management
  Association,**
Books and publications:
233 North Michigan Avenue, Suite 2150
Chicago, IL 60601-5519
(312) 233-1100 or (800) 335-5535
Certification information:
Attention: AHIMA Coordinator, Professional
  Examination Service
475 Riverside Drive, New York, NY 10115
(212) 870-3136
www.ahima.org

American Medical Association
515 N. State Street, P.O. Box 10946, Chicago,
  IL 60610-0946
(800) 621-8335
www.amapress.com

American Psychiatric Press, Inc.
1400 K Street, NW, Washington, DC 20005
(800) 368-5777
www.appi.org

**American Society for Parenteral and Enteral
  Nutrition**
8630 Fenton Street, Suite 412, Silver Spring,
  MD 20910-3805
(301) 587-6315

Appeal Solutions
703 Blue Oak, Lewisville, TX 75067
(888) 399-4925

Aspen Publishers, Inc.
7201 McKinney Circle (21704) P.O. Box 990, Frederick,
  MD 21705-9727
Phone: (800) 638-8437
www.aspenpub.com

Blue Shield of California, Fraud & Abuse Unit
P.O. Box 2807, Chico, CA 95927
(916) 896-7055

California Health Information Association
5108 E. Clinton Way, Suite 113, Fresno, CA 93727-0538
(800) 247-8907

California Medical Fee Schedule
Department 05445, P.O. Box 39000, San Francisco,
  CA 94139

Channel Publishing, Ltd.
4750 Longley Lane, Suite 110, Reno, NV 89502
(800) 248-2882
www.channelpublishing.com

ChartCare Solutions
7803 N. 12th Avenue, Phoenix, AZ 85021
(800) 449-1272
www.chirocode.com

Code Master Corporation
10 South Riverside Plaza, Chicago, IL 60611

Commerce Clearing House, Inc.
4025 West Peterson Avenue (60646), P.O. Box 5490,
  Chicago, IL 60680-9882
(800) 835-5224
www.cch.com

**Commission on Professional Hospital Activities
  (CPHA)**
P.O. Box 1809, Ann Arbor, MI 48106
(313) 769-6511

Conomikes Associates, Inc.
151 Kalmus Drive, Suite B150, Costa Mesa,
  CA 92626-9627
(800) 421-6512
www.conomikes.com

Context Software Systems, Inc.
241 S. Frontage Road, Suite 38, Burr Ridge,
  IL 60521
(800) 783-3378 or (708) 654-8800

F. A. Davis Company/Publishers
1915 Arch Street, Philadelphia, PA 19103
(800) 323-3555
www.fadavis.com

Delmar Publishers, Inc.
5 Maxwell Drive, P.O. Box 8007, Clifton Park,
  NY 12065-3003
(800) 347-7707
www.DelmarHealth.com

DiagnostIC Data, Inc.
20 Balfour Drive, West Hartford, CT 06117
(800) 999-6405
www.diagdata.com

Dr. P's Software, Inc.
3525 S. National, Suite 110, Springfield,
  MI 65807

Elsevier/Mosby
11830 Westline Industrial Drive, St. Louis,
  MO 63146
Phone: (800) 633-6699
Fax: (314) 432-1380
www.elsevier.com

Elsevier/W. B. Saunders
625 Walnut St., Philadelphia, PA 19106
Phone: (800) 523-1649
Fax: (215) 238-8369
www.elsevier.com

Entrepreneur
6001 D Landerhaven, Cleveland, OH 44124

Faulkner & Gray, Inc.
11 Penn Plaza, 17th floor, New York,
  NY 10117-0373
(800) 535-8403

Glencoe, Macmillan/McGraw-Hill
P.O. Box 508, Columbus, OH 43216
(800) 334-7344
www.glencoe.com

Group Health Management Corporation
P.O. Box 12929, Tucson, AZ 85732

HCIA Inc.
300 East Lombard Street, Baltimore, MD 21202
(800) 568-3282
www.solution.com

HealthCare Consultants of America, Inc.
1054 Claussen Road, Augusta, GA 30907
Phone: (888) 738-7494 or (706) 738-2078
Fax: (706) 722-9869
www.hcca.com

Healthcare Management Advisors, Inc.
1091-C Cambridge Square, Atlanta, GA 30201-1844
(800) 875-8HMA
www.hma.com

Health Insurance Association of America
1021 F Street, NW, Suite 500, Washington DC
  20004-1204
(202) 824-1600
www.hiaa.org

Health Market International
4885 Lone Oak Court, Ann Arbor, MI 48108
(313) 665-1360

Dr. R. B. Holt
2182 E. Sublette Place, Sandy, UT 84093-1056

Home Office Computing
P.O. Box 51344, Boulder, CO 80321-1344

William J. Hunt, MD
3540 Forest Hill Boulevard, West Palm Beach,
  FL 33406

Idea Planners, Inc.
2075 San Marino Way, North, Clearwater, FL 34623

InfoAlliance
6701 Seybold, Suite 219, Madison, WI 53719

**Information Handling Services (IHS) Regulatory
  Products**
6160 S. Syracuse Way, Englewood, CO 80110
(800) 525-5539 or (303) 267-0543
www.ihshealth.com

Ingenix Publishing Group
5225 Wiley Post Way, Suite 500 (84116-2889), P.O. Box
  27116, Salt Lake City, UT 84152-6180
Phone: (800) 464-3649
Fax: (801) 983-4033
www.ingenixonline.com

Ingenix Seminars
5224 Juliette Street, Springfield, VA 22151
(800) 632-0123
www.ingenix.com

KFC Medical Systems, Inc.
713 St. Louis Avenue, Long Beach, CA 90804

Lexi-Comp
Hudson, OH
(800) 837-LEXI
www.lexi.com

Lippincott Williams & Wilkins
530 Walnut Street, Philadelphia, PA 19106-3621
(800) 777-2295
www.LWW.com

Managed Care Information Center
3100 Highway 138, Wall Township, NJ 07719-1442

McGraw-Hill Healthcare Management Group
1221 Avenue of the Americas, New York, NY 10020

MedBooks
101 West Buckingham Road, Richardson, TX 75081
(800) 443-7397
www.medbooks.com

Medical Business Resource Center
1221 E. Osborn Road, Suite 101, Phoenix, AZ 85014

Medical Economics Publishing
5 Paragon Drive, Montvale, NJ 07645
(800) 432-4570
www.memag.com

Medical Learning Incorporated
245 East Sixth Street, Suite 502, St. Paul, MN 55101
Phone: (800) 252-1578
Fax: (612) 224-4694
www.medlearn.com

Medical Management Information Services, Inc.
6475 E. Pacific Coast Highway, Suite 409 (90802),
  P.O. Box 33-409, Long Beach, CA 90801

Medical Management Institute
11405 Old Roswell Road, Alpharetta, Georgia 30004
(800) 334-5724
www.institute.md and *www.codingbooks.com*

Medical Office Manager
P.O. Box 500845, Atlanta, GA 31150

MedSmart
1590 S. Milwaukee Avenue, Suite 212, Libertyville,
  IL 60048

Opus Communications
100 Hoods Lane, P.O. Box 1168, Marblehead,
  MA 01945
(800) 650-6787
www.hcmarketplace.com

Oxford Medical Systems
230 Nortland Boulevard, Suite 223, Cincinnati, OH
  45246

Practice Management Information Corporation
4727 Wiltshire Boulevard, Los Angeles, CA 90010
(800) MED-SHOP
medicalbookstore.com

Practice Performance Publishing, Inc.
2508 E. Willow, Suite 302, Long Beach,
  CA 90806
Professional Practice Builders
2000 Ticonderoga Drive, San Mateo, CA 94402
(415) 573-0109
Rayve Productions, Inc.
(800) 852-4890
Shannon Publications, Inc.
Northcreek Place 1, 9441 LBJ Freeway, Suite 510,
  Box 2, Dallas, TX 75243-9940
(800) 578-4888
Skilled Nursing Assessment Programs (SNAP)
P.O. Box 574, San Anselmo, CA 94979
Phone: (415) 454-5752
Fax: (415) 453-6029
**The Society of Cardiovascular and Interventional
  Radiology**
10201 Lee Highway, Suite 500, Fairfax, VA 22030
(703) 691-1805
www.scvir.org
Society of Thoracic Surgeons
401 N. Michigan Avenue, Chicago, IL 60611-4267
(312) 644-6610
www.sba.com
Soerries Enterprises
8318 S. Outer Belt Road, Oak Grove, MO 64075
(816) 690-8996
SRC Systems
14785 Omicron Drive, Texas Research Park,
  San Antonio, TX 78245-3201
**State of California, Department of
  Industrial Relations, Division of Workers'
  Compensation**
455 Golden Gate Avenue, Room 5182, San Francisco,
  CA 94102

Strategic Decisions Plus
P.O. Box 2108, Silverthorne, CO 80498
Unicor Medical, Inc.
4160 Carmichael Road, Suite 101, Montgomery,
  AL 36106
(800) 825-7421 or (205) 260-8150
www.unicormed.com
United Communications Group
11300 Rockville Pike, Suite 1100 (20852), P.O. Box
  90608, Washington, DC 20077-7637
(800) 929-4824
United States Government Printing Office
Superintendent of Documents, Washington, DC 20402
www.pueblo.gsa.gov
Wasserman Medical Publishers, Limited
3036 S. 92nd Street, P.O. Box 27365, West Allis,
  WI 53227
(800) 669-3337
www.medfees.com
West Group
620 Opperman Drive, P.O. Box 64526, Eagan,
  MN 55123-1396
(800) 328-9352
www.westgroup.com
Windcrest/McGraw-Hill
Blue Ridge Summit, PA 17294-0850
Karen Zupko & Associates
980 N. Michigan Avenue, #1325, Chicago, IL 60611
(312) 642-5616
www.karenzupko.com

APPENDIX C

Medi-Cal

CHAPTER OUTLINE

OBJECTIVES*

- Define key terms and abbreviations inherent to Medi-Cal.
- Identify the patient's Medi-Cal benefits identification card and list important information to obtain from the card.
- Describe the point-of-service device and state how it relates to the recipient's eligibility and share of cost.
- List important information to obtain from the patient's Medi-Cal identification card.
- State how to verify a patient's Medi-Cal eligibility.
- Explain how to identify patients covered by Medi-Cal prepaid health plans.
- Understand the benefits and nonbenefits of Medi-Cal.
- Explain when it is necessary to use and how to complete a Treatment Authorization Request Form.
- List basic Medi-Cal claim procedure guidelines.
- State how to collect information and process claim forms for Medi-Cal patients who have additional coverage.
- Explain how to minimize the number of insurance forms rejected because of improper completion.
- Identify the Medi-Cal time limit for submitting claims.
- Identify when an OOY Medi-Cal claim will be accepted by the fiscal intermediary.

---

*Performance objectives and exercises for hands-on practical experience for this appendix appear in the *Workbook*.

■ Edit the Uniform Bill (UB-92) Outpatient Claim Form.

■ Explain entries shown on a Remittance Advice Details document.

■ Identify information on a Resubmission Turnaround Document.

■ State when to use and how to complete a Claims Inquiry Form.

KEY TERMS

Medi-Cal terms are used when reading updates to the program policy manuals, which are available via the Internet or in hard copy by annual subscription. However, abbreviations are used rather than complete terms or phrases during lectures and in some publications about the Medi-Cal program. Therefore study both thoroughly. In addition to the key terms given in Chapter 12 used for Medicaid and Other State Programs, the following key terms and abbreviations are emphasized for study from Appendix C that are specific to the Medi-Cal program.

accounts receivable (A/R) transaction

Aid to the Blind (AB)

Aid to Families with Dependent Children (AFDC)

Aid to the (permanently) Disabled (ATD)

automated eligibility verification system (AEVS)

benefits identification card (BIC)

California Children's Services (CCS)

Child Health and Disability Prevention Program (CHDP)

claim control number (CCN)

claims and eligibility real-time software (CERTS)

Claims Inquiry Form (CIF)

Comprehensive Perinatal Services Program (CPSP)

computer media claims (CMC)

County Medical Services Program (CMSP)

Department of Health Services (DHS)

durable medical equipment (DME)

Electronic Data Systems (EDS) Corporation

electronic funds transfer (EFT)

eligibility verification confirmation (EVC)

Genetically Handicapped Persons Program (GHPP)

medically indigent (MI)

medically needy (MN)

nursing facility (NF)

Old Age Survivors, Health and Disability Insurance (OASHDI) Program

point-of-service (POS) device or network

presumptive eligibility (PE)

Provider Telecommunications Network (PTN)

Remittance Advice Details (RAD)

Resubmission Turnaround Document (RTD)

share of cost (SOC)

Treatment Authorization Request (TAR) form

Voice Drug TAR System (VDTS)

For the history of Medicaid and basic knowledge about how the welfare system works, read Chapter 12 before reading Appendix C. As mentioned in Chapter 12, in California the Medicaid program is known as Medi-Cal and became effective on March 1, 1966. Medi-Cal is administered by the California State **Department of Health Services (DHS),** a department of the California State Human Relations Agency. The information in this appendix is a brief overview of the Medi-Cal program with basic guidelines for most regions in California. For additional current detailed information on policies and procedures supplied by the current fiscal intermediary, refer to either an updated *Medi-Cal Provider Manual for Medical Services* or go online to obtain the information at *www.medi-cal.ca.gov*.

Types of Medi-Cal Plans

Managed Care Plans

The Medi-Cal program has evolved into health care plans (HCPs) that fall into one of several managed care plan (MCP) models:

▶ MCP: County Organized Health System (COHS)
▶ MCP: Fee-for-Service/Managed Care (FFS/MC)
▶ MCP: Geographic Managed Care (GMC)
▶ MCP: Prepaid Health Plan (PHP)
▶ MCP: Primary Care Case Management (PCCM)
▶ MCP: Special Projects
▶ MCP: Two-Plan Model

Individuals covered under these plans must seek treatment from facilities contracted under the MCP, except in emergencies. Otherwise services will not be reimbursed by Medi-Cal. If service is not available through contracted facilities and the patient seeks care outside of the plan, a denial letter from the health plan must accompany the Medi-Cal claim.

Descriptions of Managed Care Plans

The *MCP: County Organized Health System (COHS)* is a local agency created by a county board of supervisors to contract with the Medi-Cal program. Enrolled recipients choose their health care provider from among all COHS providers.

The *MCP: Fee-for-Service/Managed Care (FFS/ MC)* program requires specific Medi-Cal recipients to enroll in state-contracted FFS/MC Networks (FFS/MCN) administered by selected rural counties. Enrollees may select a primary care provider (PCP) who will manage their health care. The PCP provides primary care services and referrals for all necessary specialty services through an ongoing patient–physician relationship. The county is paid a case management fee for creating the provider network, establishing enrollee outreach services, and monitoring use.

The *MCP: Geographic Managed Care (GMC)* program model was established to provide medical and dental care for Medi-Cal recipients in specified aid code categories for a capitated fee. Each county may have different guidelines as to the delivery of the dental care; that is, a recipient either may choose between various dental MCPs or may receive dental care on a fee-for-service basis.

The *MCP: Prepaid Health Plan (PHP)* was established to allow Medi-Cal recipients to enroll in health maintenance organizations (HMOs) as an alternative to the Medi-Cal fee-for-service program. PHPs are required to render, on a capitated at-risk basis, all basic Medi-Cal covered benefits. PHPs provide case management, prevention, and health maintenance services. These plans have membership services and member grievance procedures. PHPs render care to privately insured individuals as well as Medi-Cal recipients.

The *MCP: Primary Care Case Management (PCCM)* program contractors case manage medical care for a voluntarily enrolled population of Medi-Cal recipients. PCCM plans are capitated for most outpatient services. Prior approval requests must be obtained for noncapitated services that require authorization under the fee-for-service program, with the exception of acute inpatient facility psychiatric services and Adult Day Health Care (ADHC) services. PCCM contractors also assume an additional responsibility to arrange and authorize inpatient services, which are reimbursed fee-for-service by Medi-Cal. Contracts participate in program savings through a savings sharing agreement with the DHS.

The *MCP: Special Projects* are new managed care county programs or pilot projects to extend coordinated, competent care to identified populations. These special projects are designed to improve recipients' health status and avoid unnecessary costs.

With the *MCP: Two-Plan Model,* the DHS contracts with two managed care plans in each of 12 California counties to provide medical services to most Medi-Cal recipients in each county. Each county offers both a local initiative plan and a commercial plan. Local initiative plans are operated by a locally developed comprehensive managed care organization. Commercial plans are operated by nongovernmental managed health care organizations. Medi-Cal recipients may enroll in either plan.

Medi-Cal Eligibility

Individuals in the following groups are entitled to benefits under the Medi-Cal program:

▶ Californians who qualify for **Old Age Survivors, Health and Disability Insurance (OASHDI) program**
▶ **Aid to Families with Dependent Children (AFDC)**
▶ **Aid to the Blind (AB)**
▶ **Aid to the (permanently) Disabled (ATD)**
▶ **Medically needy (MN)** people whose incomes are above the assistance level but who are unable to provide mainstream medical care and are eligible as **medically indigent (MI).**

Share of Cost

Some medically needy patients have a dollar amount (liability) to meet each month called **share of cost (SOC).** This is the amount of money that must be paid by the patient each month before any Medi-Cal benefits will begin.

Identification Card

The State of California Department of Health Services issues a plastic **benefits identification card (BIC)** to each Medi-Cal recipient when the individual is declared eligible for benefits (Fig. C–1). County welfare departments may issue paper Medi-Cal cards in exceptional cases for temporary use (e.g., retroactive eligibility). A person may have a Medi-Cal card, but this does not indicate proof of eligibility.

Eligibility Verification

It is the provider's responsibility to verify that the person to receive care is eligible during the month service is rendered and is the individual to whom the card was issued. Eligibility, which is verified at the first of the month, is valid for the entire month of service. Inspect the card and look for the following key points.

▶ The recipient's identification number may be numeric or alphanumeric.

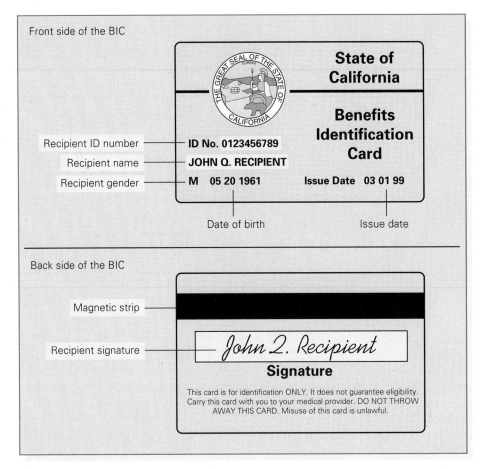

Front side of the BIC

State of
California

Benefits
Identification
Card

Recipient ID number — ID No. 0123456789

Recipient name — JOHN Q. RECIPIENT

Recipient gender — M   05 20 1961

Issue Date   03 01 99

Date of birth

Issue date

Back side of the BIC

Magnetic strip

Recipient signature — *John 2. Recipient*

Signature

This card is for identification ONLY. It does not guarantee eligibility.
Carry this card with you to your medical provider. DO NOT THROW
AWAY THIS CARD. Misuse of this card is unlawful.

Figure C–1. Medi-Cal sample plastic benefits identification card. This is a white card with blue letters on the front and black letters on the back.

▶ The issue date on the card must match the issue date on the recipient's master file accessed through the Medi-Cal point-of-service network.

▶ The recipient's date of birth on the card must match the recipient's date of birth on the recipient's master file, accessed through the point-of-service network.

▶ The recipient's signature located on the back of the BIC is used to verify the recipient's identification. This should be compared with the signature on a valid California driver's license, a California identification card issued by the Department of Motor Vehicles, another acceptable picture identification card, or another credible document of identification.

Verification Methods

Methods by which to verify eligibility and perform SOC and Medi-Service transactions are listed in the following:

▶ **Point-of-service (POS)** device. This is a piece of equipment interfaced with an analog telephone line. It has swipe card capabilities, or data may be manually input. It is used to identify recipient eligibility, obtain SOC liability status, key in SOC

payment toward balance, reserve Medi-Services, perform Family PACT (planning, access, care, and treatment) client eligibility transactions, and submit pharmacy or CMS-1500 insurance claims.

▶ An **eligibility verification confirmation (EVC)** number on a printout from the POS device verifies that an inquiry was received and eligibility information was transmitted. The insurance billing specialist should keep the eligibility verification confirmation number in the recipient's file and use it as proof of eligibility for the entire month. When a Medi-Cal recipient is limited to receive certain medical services, a restriction message is returned from the Medi-Cal host computer after verification of eligibility. Document that the services relate to the applicable restriction (e.g., date of service and name of provider who prescribed limited services). Never bill Medi-Cal for the SOC that a patient pays. Instead enter the amount paid into the POS system and indicate the amount on the CMS-1500 claim form. This will let the Medi-Cal fiscal intermediary know that the patient has paid and clear the SOC, allowing the recipient to become eligible for Medi-Cal benefits. Figure C–2 illustrates SOC and Medi-Service printouts from the POS device.

POS DEVICE

STRIPE SIDE

POS DEVICE: SHARE OF COST PRINTOUT

EDS TRAINING 3213 PROSPECT PARK TERMINAL

XX-02-15
01:44:35

PROVIDER NUMBER:
HSC3017XX

TRANSACTION TYPE: SHARE OF COST

RECIPIENT ID:
607357101

YEAR AND MONTH OF BIRTH:
1964-10

DATE OF ISSUE:
XX-02-01

DATE OF SERVICE:
XX-02-15

CASE NUMBER:

PROCEDURE CODE:
90945

PATIENT APPLIED AMOUNT:
$50.00

TOTAL BILLED AMOUNT:
$100.00

LAST NAME: JOHNSO.
AMOUNT DEDUCTED: $50.00
SHARE OF COST HAS BEEN MET.

POS DEVICE: MEDI-SERVICE PRINTOUT

EDS 10050 OLSON DRIVE TERMINAL T309006

XX-02-15
17:16:36

PROVIDER NUMBER:
HSC3017XX

TRANSACTION TYPE: MEDI-SERVICES

RECIPIENT ID:
607357101

YEAR AND MONTH OF BIRTH:
1966-12

DATE OF ISSUE:
XX-02-01

DATE OF SERVICE:
XX-02-15

PROCEDURE CODE:
A2000

LAST NAME: JOHNSO. MEDI SVC
RESERVATION APPLIED.

Figure C–2. Point-of-service device and two examples of printouts: Share of cost and Medi-Service.

▶ **Claims and eligibility real-time software (CERTS).** This is computer software that allows providers to electronically verify recipient eligibility, clear SOC liability, reserve Medi-Services, perform Family PACT client eligibility transactions, and submit pharmacy or CMS-1500 claims by use of a personal computer. Both a modem and telephone line are necessary. An EVC number on a printout from the software verifies that an inquiry was received and eligibility information was transmitted.

▶ **Computer software.** This may be existing software modified by a vendor or a vendor-supplied software package capable of performing the transactions. An EVC number verifies that an inquiry was received and eligibility information was transmitted.

▶ **Automated eligibility verification system (AEVS).** This is an interactive voice response system allowing providers to access recipient eligibility, clear SOC, or reserve a Medi-Service. A touch-tone telephone is necessary. An EVC number verifies that an inquiry was received and eligibility information was transmitted. However, this system is not able to perform SOC or Medi-Service transactions.

Receipt of an EVC number does not guarantee claim payment. Carefully review all information returned with the eligibility response to ensure that services are covered under the recipient eligibility.

Medi-Cal Benefits

The basic medical benefits provided under Medi-Cal include the following:

▶ Physician services
▶ Inpatient or outpatient hospital services in any approved hospital
▶ Laboratory and x-ray services
▶ Nursing home services
▶ Home health care
▶ Private duty nursing
▶ Outpatient clinic services
▶ Dental services (through Delta Dental, called Denti-Cal)
▶ Hearing aids
▶ Drugs and medical supplies
▶ Optometric services and eye appliances
▶ Physical therapy and other diagnostic, preventive, or rehabilitative services and equipment
▶ Medicare deductible and premium payment. Medi-Cal also pays the full deductible under Medicare Part A and buys into Medicare Part B by paying the monthly premiums for those who are older than 65, disabled, or blind. These persons are called Medicare/Medi-Cal recipients (see Chapter 11).
▶ Obstetric services. The **Comprehensive Perinatal Services Program (CPSP)** offers a wide range of services to pregnant Medi-Cal recipients from conception through 60 days after the month of delivery.

In addition to maternity services, certified providers may be reimbursed for nutritional, psychosocial, and health education services; case coordination; client orientation; and vitamin and mineral supplements. A federal or state program designed to ease access to prenatal care is called **presumptive eligibility (PE).** It allows the provider to offer immediate temporary coverage for prenatal care to low-income pregnant women pending a formal Medi-Cal application.

Medi-Services

Medi-Services are certain services supplied by chiropractors, psychologists, acupuncturists, podiatrists, occupational therapists, speech pathologists, and audiologists. Most recipients eligible for Medi-Cal are allowed two Medi-Services per calendar month.

Prior Approval

Telecommunications Networks

The **Provider Telecommunications Network (PTN)** is an automated voice-response system that allows the provider to use the telephone to obtain checkwrite, claim, and prior authorization (TAR) information for services rendered through the Medi-Cal program, **County Medical Services Program (CMSP), Child Health and Disability Prevention (CHDP) Program, California Children's Services (CCS),** and **Genetically Handicapped Persons Program (GHPP).** If a provider chooses to use the PTN, it must be the primary source of checkwrite (issuing of Medi-Cal payment check), claim, and TAR information. Providers are automatically enrolled in the PTN and assigned a seven-digit provider identification number (PIN) that must be used to access the PTN on a touch-tone telephone.

Treatment Authorization Request

Certain procedures and services require prior approval from the Medi-Cal field office consultant. The approval process is begun by either completing a **Treatment Authorization Request (TAR) form** 50-1 (Fig. C–3) or accessing the Medi-Cal Web site via the Internet to electronically transmit an e-TAR.

To find out whether a particular service requires a TAR, refer to the *Medi-Cal Provider Manual for Medical Services* or go to the Medi-Cal Web site at *www.medi-cal.ca.gov*. Find the TAR benefit and nonbenefit list that indicates what services require a TAR or are not a benefit. Some, but not all, of the TAR–required services are as follows:

▶ Long-term care facility services
▶ Some vision services
▶ Inpatient hospital services
▶ Home health agency services

① STATE USE ONLY

SERVICE CATEGORY

3

TYPEWRITER ALIGNMENT
Elite Pica

① CONFIDENTIAL PATIENT INFORMATION
1A FOR F.I. USE ONLY

C C N

TREATMENT AUTHORIZATION REQUEST
STATE OF CALIFORNIA DEPARTMENT OF HEALTH SERVICES

F.I. USE ONLY
40 41
42 43

TYPEWRITER ALIGNMENT
Elite Pica

(PLEASE TYPE) FOR PROVIDER USE 2A (PLEASE TYPE)

VERBAL CONTROL NO. 1B

TYPE OF SERVICE REQUESTED ②
DRUG [X] OTHER

REQUEST IS RETROACTIVE?
[ ] YES [X] NO

IS PATIENT MEDICARE ELIGIBLE?
[ ] YES [X] NO

PROVIDER PHONE NO.
(555) 555-1111
AREA

32A PATIENT'S AUTHORIZED REPRESENTATIVE (IF ANY) ENTER NAME AND ADDRESS
•
•
•

③ PROVIDER NO.
HSC12345F

PLEASE TYPE YOUR NAME AND ADDRESS HERE

PROVIDER NAME AND ADDRESS 2B

SMITH, SUSAN MD
727 ELM BLVD
ANYTOWN, CA 90101

30 83

FOR STATE USE

33 PROVIDER; YOUR REQUEST IS:
1 [ ] APPROVED AS REQUESTED [ ] DENIED [ ] DEFERRED
2 [ ] APPROVED AS MODIFIED (ITEMS MARKED BELOW AS AUTHORIZED MAY BE CLAIMED) [ ] JACKSON VS RANK PARAGRAPH CODE

BY John Doe
MEDI-CAL CONSULTANT

NAME AND ADDRESS OF PATIENT
PATIENT NAME (LAST, FIRST, M. I.)
④ APPLEGATE, NANCY

MEDI-CAL IDENTIFICATION NO.
⑤ 253971060 CD/HECKT

⑥

REVIEW COMMENTS INDICATOR

I.D. # DATE
34 01 35 08 20 XX 44

STREET ADDRESS
1515 RIVER ROAD

SEX AGE DATE OF BIRTH
⑦ F 32 ⑧ 06 18 65

CITY, STATE, ZIP CODE
SACRAMENTO, CA 95822

8A PATIENT STATUS:
[X] HOME [ ] BOARD AND CARE
[ ] SNF/ICF [ ] ACUTE HOSPITAL

COMMENTS/ EXPLANATION

PHONE NUMBER
AREA
(555) 545-1123

DIAGNOSIS DESCRIPTION:
ENDOMETRIOSIS

8B ICD-9-CM DIAGNOSIS CODE
617.9

MEDICAL JUSTIFICATION:
8C VISTA HOSPITAL - 1200 MAPLE ST., ANYTOWN, CA

UNCONTROLLABLE ENDOMETRIOSIS

RETROACTIVE AUTHORIZATION GRANTED IN ACCORDANCE WITH SECTION 51003 (B)
36 [ ]1 [ ]2 [ ]3 [ ]4 [ ]5 [ ]6

	AUTHORIZED YES	NO	APPROVED UNITS	SPECIFIC SERVICES REQUESTED	UNITS OF SERVICE	PROCEDURE OR DRUG CODE	QUANTITY	CHARGES
1	⑨ [X]		⑩ 3	⑩A DAYS: 3 HOSPITAL DAYS REQUESTED	⑩B	⑪	⑫ 3	$ ⑫A
2	13 [X]		14 1	HYSTERECTOMY	1	15 5815070	16 1	$ 1300.00
3	17		18			19	20	$
4	21		22			23	24	$
5	25		26			27	28	$
6	29		30			31	32	$

TO THE BEST OF MY KNOWLEDGE, THE ABOVE INFORMATION IS TRUE, ACCURATE AND COMPLETE AND THE REQUESTED SERVICES ARE MEDICALLY INDICATED AND NECESSARY TO THE HEALTH OF THE PATIENT.

Susan Smith MD 8-10-XX
39A SIGNATURE OF PHYSICIAN OR PROVIDER TITLE DATE

AUTHORIZATION IS VALID FOR SERVICES PROVIDED
37 FROM DATE 38 TO DATE
09 01 XX 09 30 XX

TAR CONTROL NUMBER
39B OFFICE SEQUENCE NUMBER PI
12 61240229 0

NOTE: AUTHORIZATION DOES NOT GUARANTEE PAYMENT. PAYMENT IS SUBJECT TO PATIENT'S ELIGIBILITY. BE SURE THE IDENTIFICATION CARD IS CURRENT BEFORE RENDERING SERVICE. SEND TO FIELD SERVICES (F.I. COPY)

SEE YOUR PROVIDER MANUAL FOR ASSISTANCE REGARDING THE COMPLETION OF THIS FORM.

50-1 12/87

Figure C–3. Example of a Medi-Cal Treatment Authorization Request form completed by a primary care physician for preauthorization of a professional service.

▶ Chronic hemodialysis services
▶ Some transportation services
▶ Some **durable medical equipment (DME)**, medical supplies, or prosthetic/orthotic appliances
▶ Hearing aids
▶ Some pharmacy services
▶ Some surgical procedures

Response to a form-generated TAR takes 10 to 15 days, but an e-TAR has a quicker response time. Once an e-TAR is submitted, it is electronically routed to the appropriate field office for a decision (adjudication). Providers can return to the Web site to check TAR status (approved, denied, or deferred). A TAR Transmittal Form MC3020 may be completed to help track submitted TARs or to appeal a TAR. Check with the field office to determine if and when faxed TARs will be accepted, because policies vary from one office to another.

If the request for hospitalization of a patient is approved, a copy of the approved TAR should be faxed or sent to the hospital before admission of the patient. In some cases it is not possible to obtain a TAR in advance of hospital admission or initiation of a treatment program. Authorization may be obtained by telephone or fax in these cases. Call the local department of health services field office to receive approval, and then complete and submit a TAR Form 50-1 to the field office, indicating that it was already authorized by including:

▶ Date authorized
▶ Name of person who gave authorization
▶ Approximate time of day at which authorization was given
▶ Verbal number stated by the field office

Do not bill the fiscal intermediary with the verbal TAR number.

A **Voice Drug TAR System (VDTS)** is also available and linked to the Medi-Cal Drug Units to permit the processing of TARs after completion of a recording. VDTS can *only* be used to request *urgent* and *initial* drug TARs, inquire about the status of previously entered drug TARs, or inquire whether a patient is receiving continual care with a drug.

PROCEDURE: Completing a Treatment Authorization Request Form 50-1

The following item numbers and descriptions correspond to Figure C–3.

1. Leave blank.
1A. The fiscal intermediary inserts a **claim control number (CCN)** in this box.
1B. Verbal Control Number is generally left blank unless this number is obtained by telephone.

2. Enter an "X" in the appropriate boxes to show Drug or Other, Retroactive Request, or Medicare eligibility status.
2A. Enter the provider's area code and telephone number.
2B. Enter the provider's name and complete address.
3. Enter the nine-digit Medi-Cal rendering provider number. When requesting authorization for an elective hospital admission, the hospital provider number must be entered in this box. The hospital name may be placed in the Medical Justification area.
4. Enter the patient's last name, first name, middle initial, address, and telephone number.
5. Enter the recipient's Medi-Cal identification number from the BIC. The county code and aid code must be entered above this box. Do not use any characters (dashes, hyphens, or special characters) in the remaining blank positions of the Medi-Cal ID field or in the Check Digit box (Fig. C–4).
6. Insert the letter P to indicate pending if the patient's Medi-Cal eligibility is not yet established and the Medi-Cal number is unknown.
7. Use a capital M for male or F for female, obtained from the BIC. Enter the patient's age in the AGE box.
8. Enter the recipient's date of birth in six-digit format. If not available, enter the year of the recipient's birth preceded by "0101."
8A. Patient's status: Enter an X if patient is an inpatient in a **nursing facility** Level A (NF-A) or nursing facility Level B (NF-B). Enter the name of the facility in the Medical Justification area of the form.

Figure C–4. Block 5 of the Treatment Authorization Request (50-1) form. Leave check digit block blank. This example shows placement of the county code and aid code on the form above block 5.

8B. Diagnosis: Enter the description of the diagnosis and its code from the diagnostic code book.

8C. Medical justification: Provide sufficient supporting information for the consultant to determine whether the service is medically justified. Attach documentation if necessary. Enter name of the hospital or nursing facility Level A or B. Requests by nonmedical providers must include the name and telephone number of the prescriber (placed in the lower left corner of this box).

9. Leave blank. Consultant will indicate if the service line item is authorized.

10. Approved Units. Leave blank. Consultant will indicate the number of times the procedure, item, or days have been authorized.

10A. Specific Services Requested: Indicate the name of the procedure, item, or service requested.

10B. Units of Service: Leave blank.

11. Enter the procedure code (five-digit CPT with two-digit modifier or five-character HCPCS when necessary). When requesting hospital days, the stay must be requested on the first line of the TAR with the provider entering the word "DAY(S)."

12. Enter the number of times a procedure or service is requested or the number of hospital days requested.

12A. Indicate the dollar amount of the provider's usual and customary charge for the service(s) requested.

13–32. Additional TAR lines 2 through 6.

32A. Enter the name and address of the patient's authorized representative, representative payee, conservator over the person, legal representative, or other representative handling the recipient' s medical and personal affairs, if applicable.

33–36. Leave blank. Consultant's determination and comments will be entered in this section. The TAR must show the consultant's signature. Comments and Explanation lines: List the approved procedures or any further information the provider must submit with the CMS-1500 claim.

37–38. Leave blank. Consultant will indicate valid dates of authorization.

39A. Signature of physician or provider: the provider or authorized representative must sign and date the form.

39B. Leave blank. Medi-Cal field office consultant will enter a two-digit prefix and a one-digit suffix to the preprinted eight-digit number. This 11-digit number must be entered on the CMS-1500 claim form when the service is billed, indicating prior authorization has been obtained. PI means pricing information and is to be left blank. *Do not attach a copy of the TAR to the CMS-1500 claim form.*

40–43. Leave blank.

Claim Procedure

Fiscal Intermediaries

Two fiscal intermediaries are contracted by the state of California to receive and audit claims for payment of medical services and make payments to providers of services. When the contract expires, these intermediaries may change, but at present they are (1) **Electronic Data Systems (EDS) Corporation** in Sacramento, California, for hospital billing and outpatient professional services and (2) Delta Dental (formerly California Dental Services) for dental services under Denti-Cal. Refer to Appendix A for the address of EDS.

Copayment

Current law requires Medi-Cal recipients to make a nominal copayment for most outpatient services, some emergency department services, and some prescribed drugs. Copayment is never necessary for the following:

▶ Any person 18 years of age or younger
▶ Any woman receiving perinatal care
▶ Any child in AFDC foster care
▶ Any person who is an inpatient in a health facility (e.g., hospital, skilled nursing facility or intermediate care facility)
▶ Any service for which payment by Medi-Cal is $10 or less
▶ Emergency services or family planning services and supplies; the health care provider has the option to collect or not collect copayment at the time at which emergency service is rendered. Figure C–5 lists the services subject to copayment, copayment fees, and exclusions.

Time Limit

Medi-Cal claims must be submitted within 6 months from the end of the month of service to be reimbursed at 100% of the Medi-Cal maximum allowable. To be eligible for full reimbursement on late claims, one of the approved billing limit exception codes (1-8 or A) shown in the provider manual must be used in Field 22 of the CMS-1500 claim form. Claims submitted more than 6 months after the month of service are reimbursed at the following reduced rates.

100%	1–6 months after the month of service
75%	7–9 months after the month of service
50%	10–12 months after the month of service
0%	Over 1 year from the month of service

MEDI-CAL COPAYMENT CRITERIA

Services Subject to Copayment	Copay-ment Fee	Exceptions to Fee
NONEMERGENCY SERVICES PROVIDED IN AN EMERGENCY ROOM A nonemergency service is defined as "any service not required for alleviation of severe pain or in the immediate diagnosis and treatment of severe medical conditions which, if not immediately diagnosed and treated, would lead to disability or death." Such services provided in an emergency room are subject to copayment.	$5.00	1. Persons age 18 or under. 2. Any woman during pregnancy and the postpartum period (through the end of the month in which the 60-day period following termination of pregnancy ends) 3. Persons who are inpatients in a health facility (hospital, skilled nursing facility or intermediate care facility)
OUTPATIENT SERVICES Physician, optometric, chiropractic, psychology, speech therapy, audiology, acupuncture, occupational therapy, podiatric, surgical center, hospital or outpatient clinic, physical therapy.	$1.00	4. Any child in AFDC-foster care 5. Any service for which the program's payment is $10 or less
DRUG PRESCRIPTIONS Each drug prescription or refill.	$1.00	6. Any hospice patient 7. Family planning services and supplies

Figure C–5. Medi-Cal copayment criteria.

An Over-One-Year (OOY) claim may be submitted with appropriate documentation or justification attached using exception code 8 for one of the following reasons:

▶ Retroactive eligibility
▶ Court order
▶ State of administrative hearing
▶ County error
▶ Department of Health Services approval
▶ Reversal of decision on appealed TAR
▶ Medicare or other health coverage

Helpful Billing Tips

When submitting an insurance claim for surgical procedures performed, the Medi-Cal global fee includes the preoperative visit 7 days before surgery, the surgical procedure, and the postoperative care (0, 10, 30, or 90 days). This differs from standard surgical and Medicare global package policies.

Medi-Cal and Other Coverage

Medi-Cal and Private Insurance

Medi-Cal is considered the payer of last resort, and the physician must bill all other insurance carriers first and then Medi-Cal. Have the patient sign an assignment of benefits form for the other insurance. After payment is received from the other insurance carrier, include a copy of the other insurance EOB when submitting the Medi-Cal claim.

Medi-Cal and Medicare

Outpatient claims for recipients eligible for both Medicare and Medi-Cal coverage must always be billed to Medicare before Medi-Cal. These claims may be referred to as *crossover claims* because after being processed by Medicare, claims are automatically crossed over to the Medi-Cal fiscal intermediary for final processing unless 100% of the claim was paid by Medicare. The claim *must be assigned* or it will not be crossed over. Hardcopy billing instructions for Medicare Part B crossover claims are different from the instructions for submitting standard Medicare or Medi-Cal claims. When submitting a crossover claim, enter an "X" in both the Medicaid and Medicare boxes of Block 1 on the CMS-1500 claim form to identify the claim as a crossover. Enter the Medicare claim number from the identification card in Block 1a. Include the Medi-Cal recipient identification number in either Block 9a or Block 32, depending on the circumstances of the case (Fig. C–6). The Medi-Cal provider identification number appears in Block 31.

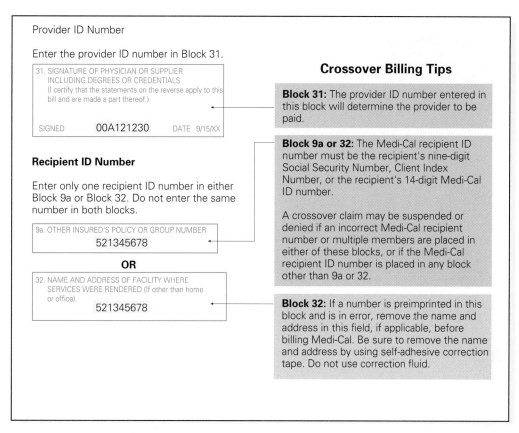

Figure C–6. Medicare and Medi-Cal crossover billing tips for completing the CMS-1500 insurance claim form.

Medi-Cal and TRICARE

Bill TRICARE first if a Medi-Cal patient is also covered by TRICARE. Then bill Medi-Cal and attach the TRICARE Summary Payment Voucher to the claim form (see Chapter 13).

Computer Media Claims

The **computer media claims (CMC)** system permits submission of Medi-Cal claims via telecommunication through magnetic tape or diskette and modem. A variety of computer software formats are acceptable. The *Medi-Cal CMC Technical Manual* and the Medi-Cal Web site at *www.medi-cal.ca.gov* contains the latest specifications to update existing systems.

Health Insurance Claim Form CMS-1500

Complete an CMS-1500 claim form and mail it to the fiscal intermediary in the blue and white envelope provided by EDS after verifying Medi-Cal eligibility using one of the aforementioned methods.

Instructions for Completing the CMS-1500 Claim Form for the Medi-Cal Program

Refer to these OCR guidelines and the Medi-Cal template shown in Figure C–7.

Top of Form. Do not type to the right of the bar code because the fiscal intermediary inserts a claim number in that space.

Block 1. Check Medicaid box for Medi-Cal claims.

Block 1a. Enter the Medi-Cal number in the left portion of the block. Do not enter dashes or other special characters in this block.

Block 2. Enter the last name, first name, and middle initial of the patient as shown on the patient's identification card. Do not use any punctuation.

Block 3. Enter the patient's birth date using six digits and indicate gender.

Block 4. Complete only if the patient has not been issued an identification card and is covered under another person (e.g., infant younger than 2 months of age); otherwise leave blank.

Block 5. Enter the patient's mailing address and residential telephone number.

Block 6. Generally, leave blank. Check "child" for a claim submitted for a child younger than 2 months of age using the mother's identification card.

APPROVED OMB 0936-006

PLEASE
DO NOT
STAPLE
IN THIS
AREA

HEALTH INSURANCE CLAIM FORM

6 Digits

1. MEDICARE	MEDICAID	CHAMPUS	CHAMPVA	GROUP HEALTH PLAN (SSN or ID)	FECA BLK LUNG (SSN)	OTHER	1a. INSURED'S I.D. NUMBER	(FOR PROGRAM IN ITEM 1)
☐ (Medicare #)	☒ (Medicaid #)	☐ (Sponsor's SSN)	☐ (VA File #)	☐	☐	☐ (ID)	MEDI-CAL ID NUMBER	

2. PATIENT'S NAME (Last Name, First Name, Middle Initial)	3. PATIENT'S BIRTH DATE MM DD YYYY	SEX	4. INSURED'S NAME (Last Name, First Name, Middle Initial)
PATIENT'S COMPLETE NAME	DATE OF BIRTH M☐ SEX F☐		MOTHER'S NAME FOR NEWBORN

5. PATIENT'S ADDRESS (No., Street)	6. PATIENT RELATIONSHIP TO INSURED	7. INSURED'S ADDRESS (No., Street)
PATIENT'S COMPLETE ADDRESS	Self ☐ Spouse ☐ Child ☐ Other ☐	N/A

CITY	STATE	8. PATIENT STATUS N/A	CITY	STATE
PATIENT'S CITY	ST	Single ☐ Married ☐ Other ☐	N/A	N/A

ZIP CODE	TELEPHONE (include Area Code)		ZIP CODE	TELEPHONE (include Area Code)
PATIENT'S ZIP	( )PATIENT'S PHONE	Employed ☐ Full-Time Student ☐ Part-Time Student ☐	N/A	( )N/A

9. OTHER INSURED'S NAME (Last Name, First Name, Middle Initial)	10. IS PATIENT'S CONDITION RELATED TO:	11. INSURED'S POLICY GROUP OR FECA NUMBER
N/A		N/A

a. OTHER INSURED'S POLICY OR GROUP NUMBER	a. EMPLOYMENT? (CURRENT OR PREVIOUS)	a. INSURED'S DATE OF BIRTH MM DD YYYY	SEX
N/A	☐ YES ☐ NO	N/A	M☐ F☐

b. OTHER INSURED'S DATE OF BIRTH MM DD YYYY	SEX	b. AUTO ACCIDENT?	PLACE (State)	b. EMPLOYER'S NAME OR SCHOOL NAME
N/A	M☐ N/A F☐	N/A ☐ YES ☐ NO N/A	N/A

c. EMPLOYER'S NAME OR SCHOOL NAME	c. OTHER ACCIDENT?	c. INSURANCE PLAN NAME OR PROGRAM NAME
N/A	N/A ☐ YES ☐ NO	N/A

d. INSURANCE PLAN NAME OR PROGRAM NAME	10d. RESERVED FOR LOCAL USE	d. IS THERE ANOTHER HEALTH BENEFIT PLAN?
N/A	PATIENT'S SHARE OF COST	OTHER COVERAGE/DOLLAR AMOUNT ☐ YES ☐ NO If yes, return to and complete item 9 a-d.

READ BACK OF FORM BEFORE COMPLETING AND SIGNING THIS FORM.
12. PATIENT'S OR AUTHORIZED PERSON'S SIGNATURE I authorize the release of any medical or other information necessary to process this claim. I also request payment of government benefits either to myself or to the party who accepts assignment below.

SIGNED   N/A   DATE   N/A

13. INSURED'S OR AUTHORIZED PERSON'S SIGNATURE I authorize payment of medical benefits to the undersigned physician or supplier for services described below.

SIGNED   EVC Number

14. DATE OF CURRENT: MM DD YYYY ◀ ILLNESS (First symptom) OR INJURY (Accident) OR PREGNANCY (LMP)	15. IF PATIENT HAS HAD SAME OR SIMILAR ILLNESS GIVE FIRST DATE MM DD YYYY	16. DATES PATIENT UNABLE TO WORK IN CURRENT OCCUPATION MM DD YYYY TO MM DD YYYY
DATE OF ONSET	N/A	FROM N/A TO

17. NAME OF REFERRING PHYSICIAN OR OTHER SOURCE	17a. I.D. NUMBER OF REFERRING PHYSICIAN	18. HOSPITALIZATION DATES RELATED TO CURRENT SERVICES MM DD YYYY TO MM DD YYYY
NAME OF REFERRING PROVIDER	REFERRING PROVIDER NUMBER	FROM FROM DOS TO THRU DOS

19. RESERVED FOR LOCAL USE	20. OUTSIDE LAB? $ CHARGES
REMARKS/EMERGENCY CERTIFICATION STATEMENT	OUTSIDE LAB ☐ YES ☐ NO N/A | N/A

21. DIAGNOSIS OR NATURE OF ILLNESS OR INJURY (RELATE ITEMS 1,2,3 OR 4 TO ITEM 24E BY LINE)	22. MEDICAID RESUBMISSION CODE ORIGINAL REF. NO.
1. PRIMARY ICD 9-CM 3. N/A	MEDICARE STATUS ZONE N/A
2. SECONDARY ICD 9-CM 4. N/A	23. PRIOR AUTHORIZATION NUMBER TAR CONTROL NUMBER 11-digit

24. A DATE(S) OF SERVICE From MM DD YYYY To MM DD YYYY	B Place of Service	C Type of Service	D PROCEDURES, SERVICES, OR SUPPLIES (Explain Unusual Circumstances) CPT/HCPCS | MODIFIER	E DIAGNOSIS CODE	F $ CHARGES	G DAYS OR UNITS	H EPSDT Family Plan	I EMG	J COB	K RESERVED FOR LOCAL USE
DATE OF SERVICE FROM DATE OF SERVICE	POS N/A		PRO-CEDURE CODE MOD N/A	N/A	SERVICE CHARGES	Q U A N T I T Y	F P / C H D P	E M E R C E R T	B I L L I N G L I M I T	RENDERING PROVIDER NUMBER
6 Digits										

25. FEDERAL TAX I.D. NUMBER SSN EIN	26. PATIENT'S ACCOUNT NO.	27. ACCEPT ASSIGNMENT? (For govt. claims, see back)	28. TOTAL CHARGE	29. AMOUNT PAID	30. BALANCE DUE
N/A ☐ ☐	PATIENT ACCOUNT NUMBER	☐ YES ☐ NO N/A	$ TOTAL CHARGES	$ TOTAL DEDUCTIONS	$ NET AMT BILLED

31. SIGNATURE OF PHYSICIAN OR SUPPLIER INCLUDING DEGREES OR CREDENTIALS (I certify that the statements on the reverse apply to this bill and are made a part thereof.)	32. NAME AND ADDRESS OF FACILITY WHERE SERVICES WERE RENDERED (if other than home or office)	33. PHYSICIAN'S, SUPPLIER'S BILLING NAME, ADDRESS, ZIP CODE AND PHONE #
SIGNATURE OF PROVIDER OR PERSON AUTHORIZED	FACILITY PROVIDER NUMBER	PROVIDER NAME ADDRESS CITY, STATE, ZIP PROVIDER PHONE NUMBER
SIGNED DATE		MEDI-CAL PROVIDER # GRP# N/A

(APPROVED BY AMA COUNCIL ON MEDICAL SERVICE 8/88)   PLEASE PRINT OR TYPE   FORM HCFA (12 90) FORM OCWP 1500   FORM RRB 1500

REORDER FROM STANDARD REGISTER FORM NO HC0901B-2

CARRIER

PATIENT AND INSURED INFORMATION

PHYSICIAN OR SUPPLIER INFORMATION

Figure C–7. CMS-1500 claim form illustrating Medi-Cal required fields.

Block 7. blank.

Block 8. Leave blank.

Blocks 9, 9a, 9b, 9c, and 9d. Leave blank; for crossover claims, list the Medi-Cal identification number in Block 9a or in Block 32.

Block 10a. Check "yes" if applicable; otherwise leave blank.

Block 10b. Leave blank.

Block 10c. Leave blank.

Block 10d. Enter the amount of the patient's SOC for the procedure, service, or supply. Do not enter a decimal point (.) or dollar sign ($); for example, $95.00 should be shown as 9500.

Blocks 11, 11a, 11b, and 11c. Leave blank.

Block 11d. Check "Yes" if recipient has other health coverage (OHC); otherwise leave blank. OHC includes private insurance carriers, PHPs, and HMOs. Eligibility under Medicare or Medi-Cal MCP is NOT considered Other Health Coverage. If OHC has paid, enter the amount in the right side of this block (e.g., $50.00 should be shown as 5000).

Block 12. Leave blank.

Block 13. No signature required; however, the EVC number may be entered here.

Block 14. Complete if applicable.

Blocks 15 and 16. Leave blank.

Block 17. Enter complete name and degree of referring physician, when applicable.

Block 17a. Enter the Medi-Cal nine-digit provider number or state license number (not UPIN) of the referring provider or nonphysician practitioner working under the supervision of a physician.

Block 18. Enter dates of hospital confinement and discharge as six digits if service is related to inpatient hospitalization.

Block 19. Enter remarks or a statement certifying the claim includes emergency services.

Block 20. Leave blank if not applicable. Check "Yes" if the claim includes fees for outside laboratory tests and state in Block 19 that a specimen was sent to an unaffiliated laboratory.

Block 21. List up to two diagnostic codes (primary and secondary).

Block 22. Medicare status codes are required for Charpentier claims. In all other circumstances, these codes are optional. The Medicare status codes are:

Code Explanation

0	Younger than 65, does not have Medicare coverage
*1	Benefits exhausted
*2	Utilization committee denial or physician noncertification
*3	No prior hospital stay
*4	Facility denial
*5	Noneligible provider
*6	Noneligible recipient
*7	Medicare benefits denied or cut short by Medicare intermediary
8	Noncovered services
*9	PSRO denial
*L	Medi/Medi Charpentier (rebill): Benefit limitations
*R	Medi/Medi Charpentier (rebill): Rates
*T	Medi/Medi Charpentier (rebill): Both rates and benefit limitations

Note: A permanent injunction (*Charpentier* v. *Belshe [Coye/Kizer]*) filed December 29, 1994, allows providers to rebill Medi-Cal for supplemental payment for Medicare/Medi-Cal Part B services, excluding physician services (e.g., G0001 venipuncture or laboratory tests). All Charpentier rebilled claims must have been first processed as Medi/Medi crossover claims.

Block 23. Enter the 11-digit TAR control number, if applicable.

Block 24A. Enter date of service, using six digits.

Block 24B. Enter POS code (refer to Figure 6–4.)

Block 24C. Leave blank.

Block 24D. Enter the appropriate CPT/HCPCS code for each procedure, service, or supply and applicable modifier without a hyphen.

Block 24E. Leave blank.

Block 24F. Enter the fee for each listed service from the fee schedule. Do not enter dollar signs or decimal points. Always include cents.

Block 24G. Each service must be listed on separate lines (no date ranging). Indicate that each service was performed one time by listing "1" in this block.

Block 24H. Enter code for family planning (FP) or CHDP services. Leave blank if not applicable.

---

*Documentation required.

Code Description

1 Family planning/ster-
ilization (sterilization
consent form must be
attached)

2 Family planning/other

3 CHDP screening re-
lated

Block 24I. Enter an "X" if the claim includes emergency services taking place in a hospital emergency department, and attach an emergency certification statement or enter a statement in Block 19.

Block 24J. Enter code that corresponds with billing limit exception and include the required documentation (see Medi-Cal provider manual).

Block 24K. Enter the nine-digit Medi-Cal provider number of the rendering provider if part of a group practice or different from the billing provider number in Block 33.

Block 25. Leave blank.

Block 26. Enter the patient's account number assigned by the physician's accounting system. Do not use dashes or slashes.

Block 27. Leave blank.

Block 28. Enter total charges for services listed in Block(s) 24F.

Block 29. Enter only the payment on claim if applicable (e.g., SOC).

Block 30. Enter balance due on claim (Block 28 less Block 29).

Block 31. Type the provider's name and show the signature of the physician or the physician's representative above or below the name. Enter the six-digit date the form was prepared. On crossover claims, enter the provider number.

Block 32. Enter only the facility's nine-digit provider number. Do not include the name and address of the facility. For crossover claims, list the Medi-Cal identification number here and in Block 9a.

Block 33. Enter the name and address of the physician or group billing for services and the individual or group nine-character Medi-Cal provider number in the PIN# area as shown in Figure C–8.

To delete specific information from Blocks 24A through K on the CMS-1500 claim form, draw a thin black line through the entire line but do not

```
33. PHYSICIAN'S, SUPPLIER'S BILLING NAME, ADDRESS, ZIP
    CODE AND PHONE #
    COLLEGE CLINIC
    4567 BROAD AVENUE
    WOODLAND HILLS XY 12345 0001
    013 486 9002
PIN#        ZZR12005F          GRP#
```

Figure C–8. Block 33 of the CMS-1500 insurance claim form indicating the location for insertion of an individual or group nine-character Medi-Cal provider number.

obliterate. Enter the correct information on another line. Use white paper tape or dry line tape to block out and correct a typed error in all other blocks. There is no need to write "See Attachments" because the equipment stamps the same assigned claim number on all accompanying sheets until the equipment recognizes another bar code. Keep the small printout from the POS device for the physician's records and, in general, do not use this receipt as an attachment. If for some reason the printout is sent to the fiscal intermediary, attach it to a standard-size sheet of paper, noting the EVC number in Block 13.

Uniform Bill (UB-92) Outpatient Claim Form

The Uniform Bill (UB-92) claim form is used by institutional facilities (e.g., inpatient and outpatient departments, rural health clinics, chronic dialysis services, and adult day health care) to submit claims for outpatient services.

Instructions for Completing the UB-92 Claim Form

When editing a computer-generated UB-92 claim form, refer to basic Medi-Cal block-by-block information about completion of the UB-92 claim form in Chapter 16. Figure 16–5 shows a completed UB-92 claim form; however, because Medi-Cal guidelines vary from the block-by-block illustration shown, refer to the block-by-block Medi-Cal instructions in that chapter. Outpatient claims are submitted in an orange envelope, and inpatient claims are submitted in a red envelope provided the by the EDS.

After Claim Submission

Remittance Advice Details

A Remittance Advice Details (RAD), formerly known as Explanation of Benefits and Remittance Advice (EOB/RA), accompanies all Medi-Cal payment vouchers (checks) sent to the physician. Five categories of adjudicated claims appear on an RAD:

1. Adjustments
2. Payments or approvals
3. Denials
4. Suspends
5. Accounts receivable (A/R) transactions.

Some categories of adjudicated claims are shown in Chapter 12, Figure 12–8 illustrating the Medicaid resolution process.

Electronic RADs are transmitted via computer to providers who have individual agreements with the fiscal intermediary. The State Controller's Office also sends a hard copy of the RAD.

Providers receiving RADs should reconcile each claim transaction to their records. Claim payments are posted as credits to the patient's financial accounting record card. Negative adjustments are posted as debits to the patient's financial accounting record card. Each claim being reported, or not reported, must be accounted for, the necessary follow-up performed, and all the rules governing timelines followed.

Adjustments

When overpayments or underpayments occur, an adjustment is initiated and two lines appear on the RAD. The first line indicates a "take back" of the original payment (original CCN); the second line reflects the correct payment of the claim (new CCN). The net amount between the two lines is the adjustment. CCNs are assigned to identify and track claims as they move through the claims processing system.

Approvals or Payments

If an original claim or a previously denied claim is approved for payment, it is listed on the RAD. If a reduction in the billed amount is warranted, the explanation will be given by means of a three-digit code.

Electronic Funds Transfer

Through **electronic funds transfer (EFT),** providers may have their payments deposited directly into their bank accounts, and paper warrants will not be generated. However, the provider will receive an RAD document. This system will be phased in to enrollees, so keep abreast of the latest information through Medi-Cal bulletins.

Denials

Denial of claims is shown only on the RAD. Review denied claims to ensure they are correct. If a physician believes that the claim was incorrectly denied, he or she should submit a Claims Inquiry Form (CIF) for reconsideration of the claim. Until the claim is resubmitted for processing, it is no longer in the system. When the claim is resubmitted, it will be given a new CCN and be processed as a new claim in the system. For translations of the RAD codes and billing tips on how to correct denied claims, refer to the *Medi-Cal Provider Manual for Medical Services.*

Suspends

A claim requiring special handling or correction of errors is placed in temporary suspense and may be referred to as a *suspend*. Claims in suspense for 30 days or more are listed. Suspends should be referenced to determine whether an RTD was issued. There are several general explanation codes for suspended claims. Such a listing does not explain the reason but lets the physician know that the claim was received by the fiscal intermediary. *Do not send CIFs for claims that have been temporarily suspended.*

Accounts Receivable Transactions

An **A/R transaction** is a miscellaneous transaction as a result of a cost settlement, state audit, or refund check received by the fiscal intermediary. A three-digit code indicates the reason for the A/R transaction. A/R transactions show when it is necessary to recover funds from a provider or, in certain situations, to pay funds to a provider. The A/R system is used in financial transactions pertaining to:

▶ Recoupment of interim payments
▶ Withholds against payments to providers according to state instructions
▶ Payments to providers according to state instructions

Amounts may be either positive or negative amounts that correspond to the increase or decrease in the amount of the Medi-Cal voucher (check). An adjustment may be initiated by the provider, fiscal intermediary, or the state. Some adjustments refer to previously paid claims that may be adjusted if an error in payment occurred. A/R transactions are posted to the appropriate suspense account.

Resubmission Turnaround Document

The fiscal intermediary sends a **Resubmission Turnaround Document (RTD),** the RTD 65-1, to providers when the submitted claim form has questionable or missing information. This document eliminates the need for providers to resubmit the entire claim form to correct a limited number of errors. The RTD must be completed and returned to the fiscal intermediary by the date specified on the RTD.

PROCEDURE: Completing the Resubmission Turnaround Document

Part A of the RTD describes the information that requires correction, and part B corrects the suspended claim. To complete an RTD, either type or hand write the correct data on the appropriate line in the Correct Information section of Part B. The data should be entered exactly as required on the claim form (e.g., no dashes, all dates in six-digit format). If a line is correct, it is not necessary to repeat the data; leave blank that line of the Correct Information section. Providers must return Part B of the RTD to the fiscal intermediary, but *do not* mail RTDs in the same envelope with claims. Refer to the *Medi-Cal Medical Services Provider Manual* for the address. Figure C–9 shows a correctly completed RTD, and the following item numbers and descriptions correspond to the figure. The top of the form contains instructions for completing the form.

1. Information block: The name of the claim form box in question.
2. Submitted information: Questionable or missing information on the claim as entered into the Medi-Cal system.
3. Service code: Procedure code, medical supply code, or drug code for the services under inquiry.
4. Error code: See Item 7. RTD error codes are *not* the same as the remittance advice denial codes. Note that 0012 indicates that "the number given on the claim as the TAR control number is not numeric or has an incorrect number of digits."
5. Beginning date of service: Date the service was rendered.
6. Corrected information: If the information in Item 2 should be corrected, the correct information may be noted here for the provider's records. The actual correction of the information that is sent to the fiscal intermediary is entered in Item 21.
7. Error description: This is the full explanation of the code that appears in Item 4. Compare this with your copy of the claim to assist you in identifying the error; the error description will be helpful.
8. Provider's name and address.
9. Provider's identification number.
10. Final notice: This is for the fiscal intermediary's use only.
11. Date of notice.
12. Number of pages in RTD.
13. Service date(s) and provider reference number.
14. Preprinted information that identifies the patient, Medi-Cal identification number, medical records number, total charges, and specific CCN.
15. Correspondence reference number: leave blank.
16. Provider's identification number.
17. Provider's name.
18. Patient's Medi-Cal identification number entered by the provider on the original claim.
19. Patient's name.
20. For fiscal intermediary's use only.
21. Enter correct information (Part B of the RTD) in the numbered box that corresponds with the error line in the Information Block (Item 1 in Part A). If the information in Part A is correct, leave the corresponding line blank. When entering correct information, enter all characters (numbers and letters) exactly as they would be entered on the claim. Corrected information on the RTD must be the same alphabetic or numeric format required on the claim form (e.g., date of birth: June 6, 1968, would be entered 060668). Claims cannot be processed if the corrected information is not accurate or is not shown in the required format.
22. Signature. All RTDs must be signed and dated by the provider or an authorized representative.
23. Blocks 1 through 6 are no longer used.

Claims Inquiry Form

A **Claims Inquiry Form (CIF)** 60-1 is used when tracing a claim, resubmitting a claim after a denial, or requesting an adjustment for underpaid or overpaid claims (Fig. C–10). This form also may be used to request SOC reimbursement for a previously paid claim, but such cases must be submitted separately. CIFs should be submitted within six months of the date of the RAD and mailed in a black and white envelope provided by the EDS.

Providers wishing to refund an incorrect payment may complete a CIF, noting the overpayment, and forward the refund to the fiscal intermediary. Attach a photocopy of the RAD. It should be mentioned that if an overpayment is received and an insurer presses the provider of service for a refund, the insurance plan can always recoup the money requested from the next check. This happens frequently with refunds owed to Medicare, Medicaid, and other government payers.

For denial and adjustment requests, complete a CIF and attach a legible copy of the corrected claim form, a copy of the RAD on which the claim is listed, and any other pertinent information.

A CIF may be used to trace claims submitted to the fiscal intermediary more than 45 days previously that have not appeared on the RAD as approved or denied and that are not indicated on the most recent RAD as suspended. When submitting a tracer, leave the CCN box blank.

RESUBMISSION TURNAROUND DOCUMENT

INSTRUCTIONS: Listed in Section "A" are error(s) found on the original claim. To expedite payment, type the correct information in the numbered Box of Section "B" that corresponds to numbered line in Section "A", sign and date the form, and return Section "B" (bottom portion) to F.I. Please respond promptly as the claim cannot be paid unless your corrections are received by October 30, 1999. See your provider manual for assistance regarding the completion of this form.

INFORMATION BLOCK	SUBMITTED INFORMATION	SERVICE CODE	ERROR CODE	BEG DOS - PATIENT NAME - COR INFO
TAR CONTROL NUMBER A1123456789			0012	XX/08/01 Smith, Mike
(1)	(2)	(3)	(4)	(5) (6)

(7) ERROR DESCRIPTION

0012 - THE NUMBER GIVEN ON THE CLAIM AS THE TAR CONTROL NUMBER IS NOT NUMERIC OR HAS AN INCORRECT NUMBER OF DIGITS

PROVIDER NAME AND ADDRESS

(9) PROVIDER NUMBER XXXXXXXX   FINAL NOTICE (10)

ABC PROVIDER
123 ANY STREET
ANYTOWN, CA 95000
(8)

(11) DATE August 30, 20XX   PAGE 1 (12) OF 1

SERVICE DATE(S) / PROVIDER REFERENCE NO. August 15, 20XX (13)

RETAIN THIS PORTION

PATIENT NAME (14)	MEDI-CAL ID NUMBER	MEDICAL RECORDS NO.	TOTAL CHARGES	CLAIM CONTROL NUMBER
SMITH, MIKE	1234567899	123455	$1575.00	0170626097022

DETACH AND RETURN TO APPROPRIATE F.I.

DO NOT STAPLE IN BAR AREA

CORRESPONDENCE REFERENCE NUMBER - F.I. USE ONLY (15)

4

PROVIDER NUMBER
XXXXXXXX (16)   FINAL NOTICE AUGUST 30, 1999

PROVIDER NAME
ABC PROVIDER (17)

PATIENT MEDI-CAL ID NO.
1234567899 (18)

PATIENT NAME
SMITH, MIKE (19)

This is to certify that the correct information is true, accurate and complete and that the provider has read, understands, and agrees to be bound by and comply with the statements and conditions contained on the back of this form.

(22)
Signature of provider or person authorized by provider to bind provider by above signature to statements and conditions contained on this form.   DATE

F.I. USE ONLY

CCN 0170626097022   CLAIM TYPE   PAGE 1 OF PAGES 1

SUBMITTED INFORMATION A1123456789   ERROR CODE 0012   LINE 01   FIELD 012

(20)

CORRECT INFORMATION MUST BE ENTERED ON THE SAME LINE AS THE ERROR SHOWN IN SECTION "A"

CORRECT INFORMATION

LABEL
☐ 1 (21) 11234567899
☐ 2
☐ 3
☐ 4
☐ 5
☐ 6

IF SPECIFICALLY REQUESTED, PLACE LABEL IN THE BOX INDICATED BELOW. THIS SPACE MAY ALSO BE USED FOR COMMENTS.

1	2 (23)	3
4	5	6

B

Figure C–9. Completed Medi-Cal Resubmission Turnaround Document Form 65-1.

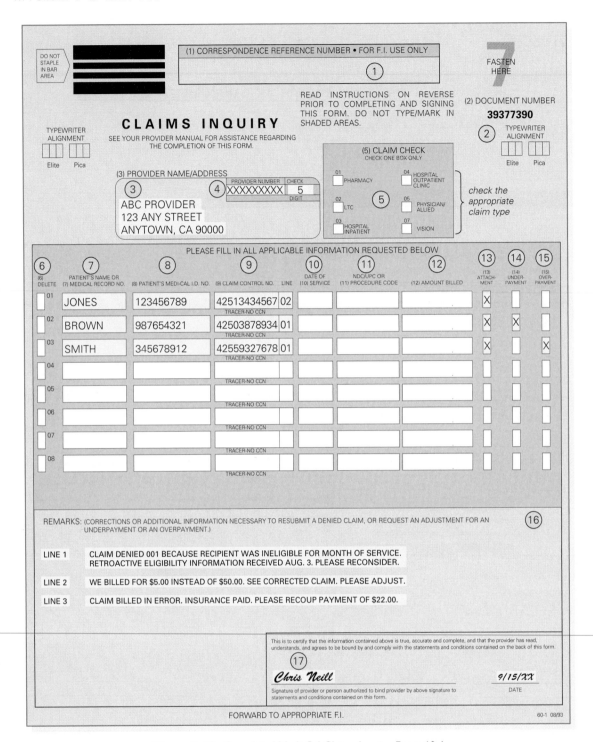

Figure C–10. Completed Medi-Cal Claims Inquiry Form 60-1.

As many as eight claims may be listed on a single CIF when tracing. Do not attach claim copies or any other documentation to a tracer. The CIF request for tracing a claim will automatically review the recipient's history and generate a response letter showing the results of the review. Based on the information in the letter, a CIF may be resubmitted for denial reconsideration, adjustment, or proof of previous timely submission.

PROCEDURE: Completing the Claims Inquiry Form

Each line on the CIF corresponds to a single line on the CMS-1500 claim form. Complete the lines on the CIF according to the type of inquiry you wish to make. Adjustment and denial reconsideration requests may be combined on one CIF. Tracer requests must be submitted separately.

The correct number of characters must be entered in the spaces provided on the form. Any time a reference is made to a claim previously adjudicated, be certain to indicate the previous CCN and attach a copy of the corrected claim and RAD. *Do not* submit CIFs for claims that are listed under the Suspends heading on the RAD. Each numbered item refers to the numbers on the CIF (see Fig. C–10).

1. Correspondence reference number: Leave blank. The fiscal intermediary will assign a number.
2. Document number: A preprinted number identifying the CIF.
3. Provider's name and address: Enter provider's name, street address, city, state, and ZIP code.
4. Provider's number: Enter the nine-character provider identification number, plus optional check digit, assigned by the Department of Health Services.
5. Claim type: Enter an "X" in the box indicating the claim type. Check only one box.
6. Delete: Enter an "X" to delete the entire line. Enter the correct billing information on another line.
7. Patient's name or medical record number: Enter up to the first 10 letters of the patient's last name or the first 10 characters of the patient's medical record number.
8. Patient's Medi-Cal identification number: Enter the recipient's identification number that appears on the RAD showing adjudication of that claim.
9. CCN: Enter the 13-digit number assigned by the fiscal intermediary to the claim line in question. This may be found on the RAD. If this line is blank, the inquiry will be considered a tracer request.
10. Date of service: Enter the date in six-digit format (e.g., 0606XX), on which the service was rendered. For consecutive date ranges (block-billed claims), enter the "From" date of service.
11. NDC/UPC or procedure code: Enter the appropriate procedure code, modifier, and drug or supply code if applicable. Codes of less than 11 digits should be left-justified. *Long-term care and inpatient providers may leave this box blank.*
12. Amount billed: Enter the amount originally billed, using the two boxes to the right of the decimal point to reflect cents.
13. Attachment: Enter an "X" when attaching documentation and when resubmitting a denied claim. All CIFs should have attachments except when submitting a tracer.
14. Underpayment: Enter an "X" for an underpayment adjustment of a paid claim. *Do not* mark if the claim was denied.

15. Overpayment: Enter an "X" if all or part of the claim was overpaid. *Do not* mark if the claim was denied.
16. Remarks: Use this area to state the reason for submitting a CIF and include the corresponding line number if listing multiple claim lines on the CIF.
17. Signature: The provider or an authorized representative must sign the CIF.

Appeal Process

A provider with a grievance or complaint about payment of claims must direct this grievance or complaint to the fiscal intermediary *within* 90 days of the action causing the grievance or complaint. The appeal is subject to automatic denial if the 90-day limit is not met. Appeals must be submitted using the Appeal Form 90-1 (Fig. C–11) and should include legible copies of supporting documentation (e.g., claim forms, RADs, CIFs, and TARs). Appeals are sent in a lavender envelope provided by the EDS. The fiscal intermediary will send an acknowledgment within 15 days of receipt and make a decision within 30 days from the date of the acknowledgment. If the appealed claim is approved for reprocessing, it will appear on a RAD. A subsequent appeal may be made if the provider is not satisfied with the decision. Judicial remedy no later than 1 year after receipt of the decision may be undertaken if the provider is still not satisfied with the decision.

PROCEDURE: Completing an Appeal Form

Each numbered item refers to the numbers on the Appeal Form shown in Figure C–11.

1. Appeal reference number: Leave blank. The fiscal intermediary will assign a number.
2. Document number: A preprinted number is used when requesting information about the status of an appeal.
3. Provider's name and address: Enter the provider's name, street address, city, state, and ZIP code.
4. Provider's number: Enter the nine-character provider's identification number, plus check digit, assigned by the Department of Health Services. Appeal acknowledgment may be delayed without the correct provider number.
5. Claim type: Enter an X in the box indicating the claim type. Check only one box.
6. Statement of appeal: This is for information purposes only.

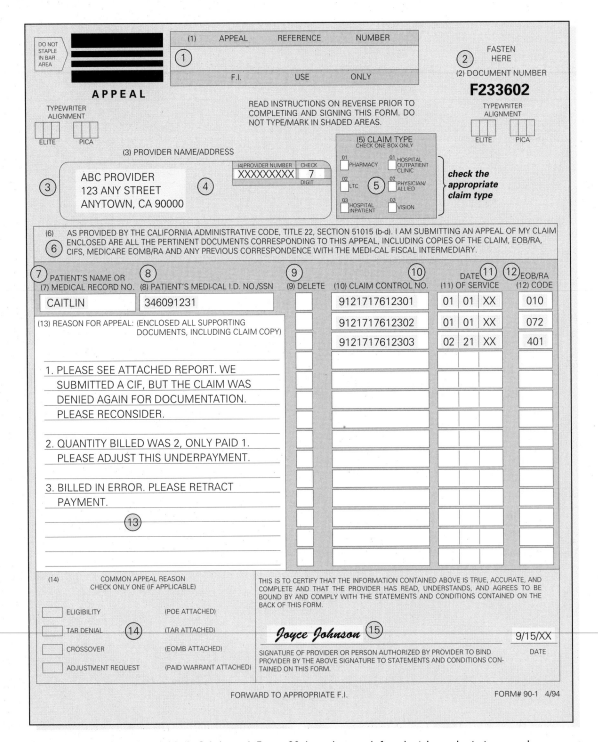

Figure C–11. Completed Medi-Cal Appeal Form 90-1 to be used for denial resubmissions, underpayment reconsiderations, and overpayment returns.

7. Patient's name or medical record number: Enter up to the first 10 letters of the patient's last name or the first 10 characters of the patient's medical record number.

8. Patient's Medi-Cal identification number and Social Security Number (SSN): Enter the recipient's identification number that appears on the plastic BIC or paper Medi-Cal card.

9. Delete: Enter an "X" to delete the corresponding line. Enter correct billing information on another line.

10. CCN: For adjudicated claims, enter the 13-digit number assigned by the fiscal intermediary to the claim line in question. This number appears on the RAD. When appealing a non-adjudicated claim (e.g., a traced claim that

could not be located), the CCN field is not required.

11. Date of service: Enter the date the service was rendered in six-digit format (0102XX). For claims billed in a "From-Through" format, enter the "From" date of service.

12. RAD code or EOB/RA code: Enter the RAD message code for the claim line (e.g., 010, 072, or 401) when appealing an adjudicated claim.

13. Reason for appeal: Indicate the specific reason for filing an appeal. Remember to attach all supporting documentation.

14. Common appeal reason: Check one of the boxes if applicable. Include a copy of the claim and supporting documents (e.g., TAR or RAD). Box 13 may be left blank if this box is used.

15. Signature: The provider or an authorized representative must sign.

RESOURCES ON THE INTERNET

Federal Register
http://www.archives.gov
Medicaid
http://www.cms.gov/Medicaid
Medi-Cal
http://www.medi-cal.ca.gov

STUDENT ASSIGNMENT LIST

✔ Study Chapter 12 and Appendix C.

✔ Answer the self-study review questions in the *Workbook* to reinforce the theory learned in these portions of the text and help prepare you for a future test.

✔ Complete the assignments in the *Workbook* to give you experience abstracting from case histories, posting to financial accounting record cards, and completing forms pertinent to the Medi-Cal program.

✔ Turn to the Glossary at the end of this textbook for a further understanding of the Key Terms used in this chapter.

Glossary

Chapter number(s) is shown in parentheses after each term.

Abuse (1): Incidents or practices, not usually considered fraudulent, that are inconsistent with accepted sound medical business or fiscal practices.

Accident (14): An unexpected happening causing injury traceable to a definite time and place.

Accidental death and dismemberment (15): An insurance policy provision that protects the insured if he or she suffers loss of sight or loss of limb(s) or death by accident.

Accounts receivable (9): The total amount of money owed for professional services rendered.

Accounts receivable (A/R) transaction (C): A miscellaneous Medi-Cal accounting transaction that results from cost settlements, state audits, or refund checks received by the fiscal intermediary.

Active duty service member (ADSM) (13): An active member of the United States government military services (e.g., Army, Navy, Air Force, Marines, or Coast Guard).

Actual charge (5): A physician's actual fee for his or her service at the time the insurance claim is submitted to the insurance company or government payer.

Acute (3): A medical condition that runs a short but relatively severe course.

Adjudication (14): The final determination of the issues involving settlement of an insurance claim, also known as *a claim settlement.*

Admission review (16): A review for appropriateness and necessity of admissions.

Advance beneficiary notice (ABN) (11): An agreement given to the patient to read and sign before rendering a service if the participating physician thinks that it may be denied for payment because of medical necessity or limitation of liability by Medicare. The patient agrees to pay for the service; also known as a *waiver of liability agreement or responsibility statement.*

Adverse effect (4): An unfavorable, detrimental, or pathologic reaction to a drug that occurs when appropriate doses are given to humans for prophylaxis (prevention of disease), diagnosis, and therapy.

Age analysis (9): The procedure of systematically arranging the accounts receivable, by age, from the date of service.

Aid to the Blind (AB) (C): A group that is entitled to benefits under the Medi-Cal program.

Aid to Families with Dependent Children (AFDC) (C): A group that is entitled to benefits under the Medi-Cal program.

Aid to the (permanently) Disabled (ATD) (C): A group that is entitled to benefits under the Medi-Cal program.

Alien (17): An individual belonging to another country or people; a foreigner.

Allowable charge (13): An amount on which TRICARE figures the patient's cost-share for covered care. This is based on 75% to 80% of the *allowable* charge.

Ambulatory payment classifications (APCs) (16): A system of outpatient hospital reimbursement based on procedures rather than diagnoses.

American Health Information Management Association (AHIMA) (1): A national professional organization for promoting the art and science of medical record management and improving the quality of comprehensive health information for the welfare of the public.

American Medical Association (AMA) (1): A national professional society of physicians.

Ancillary services (10): Supportive services other than routine hospital services provided by the facility, such as x-ray films and laboratory tests.

Appeal (8): A request for a review of an insurance claim that has been underpaid or denied by an insurance company to receive additional payment.

Applicant (2): A person applying for insurance coverage.

Application form (17): A request form to be completed with pertinent data when applying for employment.

Appropriateness evaluation protocol (AEP) (16): Nineteen criteria for admission under the prospective payment system, separated into two categories: severity and intensity of illness. To allow a patient admission to an acute care facility, one criterion from each category must be met.

Approved charges (11): A fee that Medicare decides the medical service is worth, which may or may not be the same as the actual amount billed. The patient may or may not be responsible for the difference.

Armed Services Disability (15): A disability occurring or aggravated while the patient is in military service.

Assignment (2, 11): A transfer, after an event insured against, or an individual's legal right to collect an amount payable under an insurance contract. For Medicare, an agreement in which a patient assigns to the physician the right to receive payment from the fiscal intermediary.

Under this agreement, the physician must agree to accept 80% of the allowed amount as payment in full once the deductible has been met. For TRICARE, providers who accept assignment agree to accept 75% or 80% of the TRICARE allowable charge as the full fee, collecting the deductible and 20% or 25% of the allowable charge from the patient. With other carriers, accepting assignment means that, in return for payment of the claim, the provider accepts the terms of the contract between the patient and carrier. The provider also accepts the payment from the carrier as payment in full with no balance billing of the patient.

Attending physician (3): A medical staff member who is legally responsible for the care and treatment given to a patient.

Audit trail (7): A paper trail or path left by a transaction when it is processed.

Authorized provider (13): A physician or other individual authorized provider of care or a hospital or supplier approved by TRICARE to provide medical care and supplies.

Automated eligibility verification system (AEVS) (C): An interactive voice-response system in the Medi-Cal program that allows providers to access recipient eligibility, clear share of cost, or reserve a Medi-Service.

Automatic stay (9): A court order that goes into effect once a bankruptcy petition is filed; all other legal actions are halted, such as attachments and foreclosures.

Back up (7): A duplicate data file: tape, CD-ROM, disk, or ZIP disk used to record data; it may be used to complete or redo the operation if the primary equipment fails.

Balance (9): An amount owed on a credit transaction; also known as the outstanding or unpaid balance.

Bankruptcy (9): A condition under which a person or corporation is declared unable to pay debts.

Batch (7): A group of claims for different patients from one office submitted in one computer transmission.

Beneficiaries (13): Individuals entitled to receive insurance policy or government program health care benefits. Also known as *participants, subscribers, dependents, enrollees,* or *members.*

Benefit period (11, 15): A period of time for which payments for Medicare inpatient hospital benefits are available. A benefit period begins the first day an enrollee is given inpatient hospital care (nursing care or rehabilitation services) by a qualified provider and ends when the enrollee has not been an inpatient for 60 consecutive days. In workers' compensation cases the maximum amount of time that benefits will be paid to the injured or ill person for the disability. For disability insurance, it is the maximum amount of time that benefits will be paid to the injured or ill person for a disability.

Benefits identification card (BIC) (C): A Medi-Cal identification card.

Benign tumor (4): An abnormal growth that does not have the properties of invasion and metastasis and is usually surrounded by a fibrous capsule; also called a *neoplasm.*

Bilateral (5): When coding surgical procedures, this term refers to both sides of the body.

Bit (7): A binary digit, either a 1 or 0.

Blanket contract (2): Comprehensive group insurance coverage through plans sponsored by professional associations for their members.

Blanket position bond (1): Insurance that provides coverage for all employees regardless of job title, in the event of a financial loss to the employer by the act of an employee.

Blind mailing (17): To send a resume with cover letter to possible prospects whom the individual does not know personally and who have not advertised for a job opening.

Bonding (1): An insurance contract by which, in return for a stated fee, a bonding agency guarantees payment of a certain sum to an employer in the event of a financial loss to the employer by the act of a specified employee or by some contingency over which the employer has no control.

Breach of confidential communication (3): "Breach" means breaking or violation of a law or agreement. In the context of the medical office it means the unauthorized release of information about the patient.

Buffing (10): A physicians justifying the transference of sick, high-cost patients to other physicians in a managed care plan.

Bug (7): An error in a program.

Bundled codes (5): To group more than one component (service or procedure) into one CPT code.

By report (BR) (14): A report must be submitted with the claim when the notation BR follows the procedure code description. This term is sometimes seen in workers' compensation fee schedules.

Byte (7): The number of bits used to represent one character.

California Children's Services (CCS) (C): A state program for disabled children.

Capitation (2, 10, 16): A system of payment used by managed care plans in which physicians and hospitals are paid a fixed, per capita amount for each patient enrolled over a stated period of time, regardless of the type and number of services provided; reimbursement to the hospital on a per-member/per-month basis to cover costs for the members of the plan. Capitation also can mean a set amount to be paid per claim.

Carrier-direct system (7): Electronic transmission of insurance claims from the physician to the insurance company.

Carve outs (10): Medical services not included within the capitation rate as benefits of a managed care contract and may be contracted for separately.

Case rate (16): An averaging after a flat rate is given to certain categories of procedures.

Cash flow (1, 9): In a medical practice, the amount of *actual* cash generated and available for use by the medical practice within a given period of time.

Catastrophic cap (13): The maximum dollar amount that a member has to pay under TRICARE or CHAMPVA in any fiscal year or enrollment period for covered medical bills.

Catchment area (13): In the TRICARE program, an area, defined by ZIP codes, that is approximately 40 miles in radius surrounding each United States military treatment facility.

Categorically needy (12): Aged, blind, or disabled individuals or families and children who meet financial eligibility requirements for Aid to Families with Dependent Children, Supplemental Security Income, or an optional state supplement.

Centers for Medicare and Medicaid Services (CMS) (11): Formerly known as the Health Care Financing Administration (HCFA), CMS divides responsibilities among three divisions: the Center for Medicare Management, the Center for Beneficiary Choices, and the Center for Medicaid and State Operations.

Central processing unit (CPU) (7): The brains of a computing device controlling the internal memory that directs the flow and processing of information.

Certification (17): A statement issued by a board or association verifying that a person meets professional standards.

Certified Coding Specialist (CCS) (17): A title received by a person after appropriate training and by passing a certification examination administered by the American Health Information Management Association for hospital-based coding.

Certified Coding Specialist-Physician (CCS-P) (17): A title received by a person after appropriate training and by passing a certification examination administered by the American Health Information Management Association for physician-based coding.

Certified Medical Assistant (CMA) (17): A title received by a person after appropriate training and by passing a certification examination administered by the American Association of Medical Assistants, Inc.

Certified Professional Coder (CPC) (17): A title received by a person after appropriate training and by passing a certification examination administered by the American Academy of Professional Coders.

CHAMPVA (2, 13): The Civilian Health and Medical Program of the Department of Veterans Affairs, a program for veterans with total, permanent, service-connected disabilities or surviving spouses and dependents of veterans who died of service-connected disabilities.

Charge description master (CDM) (16): A computer program that is linked to various hospital departments and includes procedure codes, procedure descriptions, service descriptions, fees, and revenue codes; also known as *charge master.*

Charges (16): The dollar amount a hospital bills an outlier case based on the itemized bill.

Chief complaint (CC) (3, 4): A patient's statement describing symptoms, problems, or conditions as the reason for seeking health care services from a physician.

Child Health and Disability Prevention (CHDP) Program (C): A state health and disability prevention program for children.

Chronic (3): A medical condition persisting over a long period of time.

Chronologic resume (17): A data sheet that outlines experience and education by dates.

Churning (1, 10): Physicians' seeing a high volume of patients—more than medically necessary—to increase revenue. May be seen in fee-for-service or managed care environments.

Civil Service Retirement System (CSRS) (15): A program for federal employees hired before 1984.

Claim (2): A bill sent to an insurance carrier requesting payment for services rendered; also known as *encounter record.*

Claim control number (CCN) (C): A number assigned by the Medi-Cal fiscal intermediary on a Treatment Authorization Request and used for reference when processing the request.

Claims assistance professional (CAP) (1, 17): A practitioner who works for the consumer and helps patients organize, complete, file, and negotiate health insurance claims of all types to obtain maximum benefits, as well as tell patients what checks to write to providers to eliminate overpayment.

Claims and eligibility real-time software (CERTS) (C): Computer software that allows Medi-Cal providers to electronically verify recipient eligibility, clear share of cost liability, reserve Medi-Services, perform Family PACT (planning, access, care, treatment) client eligibility transactions, and submit pharmacy or CMS-1500 claims using a personal computer.

Claims examiner (14): In industrial cases, a representative of the insurer who authorizes treatment and investigates, evaluates, and negotiates the patient's insurance claim and acts for the company in the settlement of claims; also known as *claims adjuster, claim representative,* and *claims administrator.*

Claims Inquiry Form (CIF) (C): A Medi-Cal form used for tracing a claim, resubmitting a claim after a denial, or when requesting an adjustment for underpaid or overpaid claims.

Claims-review type of foundation (10): A type of foundation that provides peer review by physicians to the numerous fiscal agents or carriers involved in its area.

Clean claim (6): A completed insurance claim form submitted within the program time limit that contains all the necessary information without deficiencies so it can be processed and paid promptly.

Clearinghouse (7): A third-party administrator (TPA) that receives insurance claims from the physician's office, performs software edits, and redistributes the claims electronically to various insurance carriers.

Clinical outliers (16): Cases that cannot adequately be assigned to an appropriate DRG owing to unique combinations of diagnoses and surgeries, very rare conditions, or other unique clinical reasons. Such cases are grouped together into clinical outlier DRGs and therefore are considered *outliers.*

Closed panel program (10): A form of HMO that limits the patient's choice of personal physicians to those doctors practicing in the HMO group practice within the geographic location or facility. A physician must meet very narrow criteria to join a closed panel.

Code sequence (16): The correct order of diagnostic codes (1, 2, 3, 4) when submitting an insurance claim that affects maximum reimbursement. Other factors affecting maximum reimbursement are accurate diagnostic code selection and linking the proper service or procedures provided to the patient.

Coinsurance (2): A cost-sharing requirement under a health insurance policy providing that the insured will assume a percentage of the costs for covered services; for Medicare, after application of the yearly cash deductible, the portion of the reasonable charges (20%) for which the beneficiary is responsible.

Collateral (9): Any possession, such as an automobile, furniture, stocks, or bonds, that secures or guarantees the discharge of an obligation.

Collection ratio (9): The relationship between the amount of money owed and the amount of money collected in reference to the doctor's accounts receivable.

Combination code (4): A code from one section of the procedural code book combined with a code from another section that is used to completely describe a procedure performed; in diagnostic coding, a single five-digit code used to identify etiology and secondary process (manifestation) or complication of a disease.

Combination resume (17): A data sheet that combines specific dates or work experience with educational skills.

Comorbidity (3, 16): An ongoing condition that exists along with the condition for which the patient is receiving treatment; in regard to DRGs, a preexisting condition that, because of its presence with a certain principal diagnosis, will cause an increase in length of stay by at least 1 day in approximately 75% of cases. Also known as *substantial comorbidity.*

Competitive Medical Plan (CMP) (2): A state licensed health plan similar to a health maintenance organization (HMO) that delivers comprehensive, coordinated services to voluntarily enrolled members on a prepaid capitated basis. CMP status may be granted by the federal government for the enrollment of Medicare beneficiaries into managed care plans, without having to qualify as an HMO.

Compliance program (3): A management plan composed of policies and procedures to accomplish uniformity, consistency, and conformity in medical record keeping that fulfills official requirements.

Complication (4): A disease or condition arising during the course of, or as a result of, another disease modifying medical care requirements; for DRGs, a condition that arises during the hospital stay that prolongs the length of stay by at least 1 day in approximately 75% of cases. Also known as *substantial complication.*

Comprehensive (C) (3): A term used to describe a level of history or physical examination.

Comprehensive code (5): A single procedural code that describes or covers two or more CPT component codes that are bundled together as one unit.

Comprehensive Perinatal Services Program (CPSP) (C): A program that offers a wide range of services to pregnant Medi-Cal recipients.

Comprehensive type of foundation (10): A type of foundation that designs and sponsors prepaid health programs or sets minimum benefits of coverage.

Compromise and release (C and R) (14): An agreement arrived at, whether in or out of court, for settling a workers' compensation case after the patient has been declared permanent and stationary.

Computer billing (9): Producing statements via a computer system.

Computer media claims (CMC) (C): A system that permits submission of Medi-Cal claims via telecommunication through magnetic tape or diskette and modem.

Concurrent care (3): The provision of similar services (e.g., hospital visits) to the same patient by more than one physician on the same day. Usually there is the presence of a separate physical disorder.

Conditionally renewable (2): An insurance policy renewal provision that grants the insurer a limited right to refuse to renew a health insurance policy at the end of a premium payment period.

Confidential communication (1): A privileged communication that may be disclosed only with the patient's permission.

Confidentiality (1): The state of treating privately or secretly, and not disclosing to other individuals or for public knowledge, the patient's conversations or medical records.

Consultation (3): Services rendered by a physician whose opinion or advice is requested by another physician or agency in the evaluation or treatment of a patient's illness or suspected problem.

Consultative examiner (CE) (15): A physician who is paid a fee to examine or test a person for disability under either the SSDI or SSI program.

Consulting physician (3): A provider whose opinion or advice about evaluation or management of a specific problem is requested by another physician.

Continuing education (17): Formal education pursued by a working professional and intended to improve or maintain professional competence.

Continuity of care (3): When a physician sees a patient who has received treatment for a condition and is referred by the previous doctor for treatment of the same condition.

Contract (2): A legally enforceable agreement when relating to an insurance policy; for workers' compensation cases, an agreement involving two or more parties in which each is obligated to the other to fulfill promises made. (The contract exists between the physician and the insurance carrier.)

Conversion factor (5): The dollars and cents amount that is established for one unit as applied to a procedure or service rendered. This unit is then used to convert various procedures into fee-schedule payment amounts by multiplying the relative value unit by the conversion factor.

Cooperative care (13): A term used when a patient is seen by a civilian physician or hospital for services cost-shared by TRICARE.

Coordination of benefits (13): Two insurance carriers working together and coordinating the payment of their benefits, so that there is no duplication of benefits paid between the primary and secondary insurance carriers. In TRICARE, the coordination of the payment of TRICARE benefits with the payment of benefits made by the double coverage plan, so that there is no duplication of benefits paid between the double coverage plan and TRICARE. Likewise applied to disability programs.

Copayment (copay) (10): A patient's payment (e.g., 20% of a bill or flat fee of $10 per visit) of a portion of the cost at the time the service is rendered. Also referred to as *coinsurance.*

Correct coding initiative (CCI) (11): Federal legislation that attempts to eliminate unbundling or other inappropriate reporting of procedural codes for professional medical services rendered to patients.

Cost-of-living adjustment (15): A disability insurance provision to increase monthly benefits.

Cost outlier (16): A typical case that has an extraordinarily high cost when compared with most discharges classified to the same DRG.

Cost outlier review (16): A review by a Professional Review Organization (PRO) for the necessity of a patient's hospital admission and to determine whether all services rendered were medically necessary. Cost outlier cases are recognized only if the case is not eligible for day outlier status.

Cost-share (13): The portion of the allowable charges (20% or 25%) after the deductible has been met that the TRICARE patient is responsible for.

Counseling (3): A discussion between the physician and a patient, family, or both concerning the diagnosis, recommended studies or tests, prognosis, risks, and benefits of treatment, treatment options, patient and family education, and so on.

County Medical Services Program (CMSP) (C): A county program for medical services.

Cover letter (17): A letter of introduction prepared to accompany a resume when seeking a job.

Covered services (12): Specific services and supplies for which Medicaid will provide reimbursement; these consist of a combination of mandatory and optional services stated in the plan

CPT (5): See *Current Procedural Terminology.*

Credit (9): 1. From the Latin *credere,* meaning "to believe" or "to trust"; trust in regard to financial obligation. 2. Accounting; entry reflecting payment by a debtor (patient) of a sum received on his or her account.

Credit card (9): A card issued by an organization and devised for the purpose of obtaining money, property, labor, or services on credit.

Creditor (9): A person to whom money is owed.

Critical care (3): In reference to coding professional services, this phrase relates to intensive care provided in a variety of acute life-threatening conditions requiring constant bedside attention by a physician.

Crossover claim (11): A bill for services rendered to a patient receiving benefits simultaneously from Medicare and Medicaid or from Medicare and a Medigap plan. Medicare pays first and then determines the amounts of unmet Medicare deductible and coinsurance to be paid by the secondary insurance carrier. The claim is automatically transferred (electronically) to the secondary insurance carrier for additional payment; also known as *claims transfer.*

Current Procedural Terminology (CPT) (5): A reference procedural code book using a five-digit numerical system to identify and code procedures established by the American Medical Association.

Customary fee (5): The amount that a physician usually charges the majority of her or his patients.

Cycle billing (9): A system of billing accounts at spaced intervals during the month based on breakdown of accounts by alphabet, account number, insurance type, or date of first service.

Day outlier review (16): A review of potential day outliers (short or unusually long length of hospital stay) to determine the necessity of admission and number of days before the day outlier threshold is reached, as well as the number of days beyond the threshold. The PRO determines the certification of additional days.

Day sheet (2): A register for recording daily business transactions (charges, payments, or adjustments); also known as *daybook, daily log,* or *daily record sheet.*

Debit card (9): A card permitting bank customers to withdraw from any affiliated automated teller machine (ATM) and make cashless purchases from funds on deposit without incurring revolving finance charges for credit.

Debt (9): A legal obligation to pay money.

Debtor (9): A person owing money.

Debug (7): To remove errors from a software program or the computer itself.

Deductible (2, 10): A specific dollar amount that must be paid by the insured before a medical insurance plan or government program begins covering health care costs.

Defense Enrollment Eligibility Reporting System (DEERS) (13): An electronic database used to verify beneficiary eligibility for those individuals in the TRICARE programs.

Delinquent claim (8): An insurance claim submitted to an insurance company, for which payment is overdue.

Denied claim (8): An insurance claim submitted to an insurance company in which payment has been rejected owing to a technical error or because of medical coverage policy issues.

Department of Health Services (DHS) (C): Medi-Cal is administered by this state department, which is a department of the California State Human Relations Agency.

Deposition (14): The process of taking sworn testimony from a witness out of court. This is usually done by an attorney.

Detailed (D) (3): A term used to describe a level of history or physical examination.

Diagnosis-related groups (DRGs) (16): A patient classification system that categorizes patients who are medically related with respect to diagnosis and treatment and statistically similar in length of hospital stay. Medicare hospital insurance payments are based on fixed dollar amounts for a principal diagnosis as listed in DRGs.

Diagnostic cost groups (DCGs) (11): A system of Medicare reimbursement for HMOs with risk contracts in which enrollees are classified into various DCGs on the basis of each beneficiary's prior 12-month hospitalization history.

Diagnostic creep (16): Coding that is inappropriately altered to obtain a higher payment rate. Also known as *coding creep, DRG creep,* or *upcoding.*

Digital fax claim (6): An insurance claim sent to the insurance carrier via facsimile but never printed on paper. The fax is encoded while in electronic form via an optical code reader and electronically entered into the claims processing system.

Dingy claim (6): Dingy claims happen when the Medicare contractor cannot process a claim for a particular service or bill type because of the type of software program used to transmit the claim; it may be incompatible with the receiving system. The claims are held until the necessary system changes are implemented to pay the claim correctly.

Direct referral (10): Certain services in a managed care plan may not require preauthorization. The authorization request form is completed and signed by the physician and handed to the patient (e.g., obstetrical care or dermatology) to be done directly.

Dirty claim (6): A claim submitted with errors or one that requires manual processing to resolve problems or is rejected for payment.

Disability Determination Services (DDS) (15): A state Social Security division office that assesses a case for disability benefits.

Disability income insurance (2, 15): A form of health insurance that provides periodic payments to replace income when the insured is unable to work as a result of illness, injury, or disease—not as a result of a work-related accident or condition.

Disabled (11): For purposes of enrollment under Medicare, individuals younger than 65 years of age who have been entitled to disability benefits under the Social Security Act or the railroad retirement system for at least 24 months are considered disabled and are entitled to Medicare.

Discount (9): A reduction of a normal charge based on a specific amount of money or a percentage of the charge.

Disenrollment (10): A member's voluntary cancellation of membership in a managed care plan.

Documentation (3): A chronologic detailed recording of pertinent facts and observations about a patient's health as seen in chart notes and medical reports; entries in the medical record such as prescription refills, telephone calls, and other pertinent data. For computer software, a user's guide to a program or piece of equipment.

Double indemnity (15): A feature in some life and disability insurance policies that provides for twice the face amount of the policy to be paid if death results to the insured from accidental causes.

Downcoding (5): This occurs when the coding system used by the physician's office on a claim does not match the coding system used by the insurance company receiving the claim. The insurance company computer system converts the code submitted to the closest code in use, which is usually down one level from the submitted code, generating decreased payment.

Down time (7): The period during which a computer is malfunctioning or not operating correctly.

DRG creep (16): See *diagnostic creep.*

Dun message (9): A message or phrase to inform or remind a patient about a delinquent account.

Durable medical equipment (DME) (C): A billing phrase used to specify medical supplies, devices, and equipment to Medicare and Medi-Cal fiscal intermediaries for reimbursement.

Durable medical equipment (DME) number (6): A group or individual provider number used when submitting bills for specific medical supplies, devices, and equipment to the Medicare fiscal intermediary for reimbursement.

E codes (4): A classification of ICD-9-CM coding used to describe environmental events, circumstances, and conditions as the external cause of injury, poisoning, and other adverse effects. E codes are also used in coding adverse reactions to medications.

Early and Periodic Screening, Diagnosis, and Treatment (EPSDT) (12): The EPSDT program covers screening and diagnostic services to determine physical or mental defects in recipients younger than age 21 years and health care, treatment, and other measures to correct or ameliorate any defects and chronic conditions discovered. In New York, this is called the Child Health Assurance Program (CHAP).

Elective surgery (16): A surgical procedure that may be scheduled in advance, is not an emergency, and is discretionary on the part of the physician and patient.

Electronic claim (6): An insurance claim submitted to the insurance carrier via a central processing unit (CPU), tape diskette, direct data entry, direct wire, dial-in telephone, digital fax, or personal computer download or upload.

Electronic claims processor (ECP) (7, 17): An individual who converts insurance claims to standardized electronic format and transmits electronic insurance claims data to the insurance carrier or clearinghouse to help the physician receive payment. Sometimes referred to as *electronic claims professional.*

Electronic claim submission (ECS) (7): Insurance claims prepared on a computer and submitted via modem (telephone lines) to the insurance carrier's computer system. Also called *electronic media claims (EMC).*

Electronic data interchange (EDI) (7): The process by which understandable data items are sent back and forth via computer linkages between two or more entities that function alternatively as sender and receiver.

Electronic Data Systems (EDS) Corporation (C): The Medi-Cal fiscal intermediary in the state of California.

Electronic funds transfer (EFT) (C): A paperless computerized system enabling funds to be debited, credited, or transferred, eliminating the need for personal handling of checks.

Electronic mail (e-mail) (7): Transmitting, receiving, storing, and forwarding of text, voice messages, attachments, or images by computer from one person to another.

Electronic signature (2): An individualized computer access and identification system (e.g., a series of numbers, letters, electronic writing, voice, computer key, and fingerprint transmission [biometric system]) accepted by both parties to show intent, approval of, or responsibility for computer document content.

Eligibility (2): Qualifying factors that must be met before a patient receives benefits (medical services) under a specified insurance plan, government program, or managed care plan.

Eligibility verification confirmation (EVC) (C): A reference number on a printout from the Medi-Cal point-of-service device that verifies that an inquiry was received and eligibility information was transmitted.

Emancipated minor (2): A person younger than 18 years of age who lives independently, is totally self-supporting, and possesses decision-making rights.

Embezzlement (1): A willful act by an employee of taking possession of an employer's money.

Emergency (13): A sudden and unexpected medical condition, or the worsening of a condition, that poses a threat to life, limb, or sight and requires immediate treatment to alleviate suffering (e.g., shortness of breath, chest pain, or drug overdose).

Emergency care (3): Health care services provided to prevent serious impairment of bodily functions or serious dysfunction to any body organ or part. Advanced life support may be necessary. Not all care provided in an emergency department of a hospital can be termed "emergency care."

Employer identification number (EIN) (6): An individual's federal tax identification number issued by the Internal Revenue Service for income tax purposes.

Employment agency (17): A business organization that refers job applicants to potential employers.

Encounter form (2, 7): See *multipurpose billing form.*

Encryption (7): To assign a code to represent data. This is done for the purpose of security.

End-stage renal disease (ESRD) (11): Individuals who have chronic kidney disease requiring dialysis or kidney transplant are considered to have ESRD. To qualify for Medicare coverage, an individual must be fully or currently insured under Social Security or the railroad retirement system or be the dependent of an insured person. Eligibility for Medicare coverage begins with the third month after beginning a course of renal dialysis. Coverage may commence sooner if the patient participates in a self-care dialysis training program or receives a kidney transplant without dialysis.

Eponym (3): The name of a disease, anatomical structure, operation, or procedure, usually derived from the name of a place where it first occurred or a person who discovered or first described it.

Ergonomic (14): Science and technology that seeks to fit the anatomic and physical needs of the worker to the workplace.

Established patient (3): An individual who has received professional services within the past 3 years from the physician or another physician of the same specialty who belongs to the same group practice.

Estate administrator (9): One who takes possession of the assets of a decedent, pays the expenses of administration and the claims of creditors, and disposes of the balance of an estate in accordance with the statutes governing the distribution of decedents' estates.

Estate executor (9): One who takes possession of the assets of a decedent, pays the expenses of administration and the claims of creditors, and disposes of the balance of an estate in accordance with the decedent's will.

Ethics (1): Standards of conduct generally accepted as a moral guide for behavior by which an insurance billing or coding specialist may determine the appropriateness of his or her conduct in a relationship with patients, the physician, co-workers, the government, and insurance companies.

Etiology (4): The cause of disease; the study of the cause of a disease.

Etiquette (1): Customs, rules of conduct, courtesy, and manners of the medical profession.

Exclusion(s) (2, 15): Provisions written into the insurance contract denying coverage or limiting the scope of coverage.

Exclusive provider organization (EPO) (2, 10): A type of managed health care plan that combines features of HMOs and PPOs. It is referred to as exclusive because it is offered to large employers who agree not to contract with any other plan. EPOs are regulated under state health insurance laws.

Expanded problem focused (EPF) (3): A phrase used to describe a level of history or physical examination.

Explanation of benefits (EOB) (8): A document detailing services billed and describing payment determinations; also known in Medicare, Medicaid, and some other programs as a *remittance advice.* In the TRICARE program, it is called a *summary payment voucher.*

Explanation of Medicare benefits (EOMB): See *remittance advice.*

Expressed contract (2): A verbal or written agreement.

Extended (2): To carry forward the balance of an individual financial accounting record.

External audit (3): A review done after claims have been submitted (retrospective review) of medical and financial records by an insurance company or Medicare representative to investigate suspected fraud or abusive billing practices.

Extraterritorial (14): State laws effective outside the state by either specific provision or court decision. In workers' compensation cases, benefits under the state law that apply to a compensable injury of an employee hired in one state but injured outside that state.

Facility provider number (6): A facility's (hospital, laboratory, radiology office, nursing facility) provider number to be used by the facility to bill for services, or by the performing physician to report services done at that location.

Facsimile (3): An electronic process for transmitting graphic and written documents over telephone lines.

Family history (FH) (3): A review of medical events in the patient's family, including diseases that may be hereditary or place the patient at risk.

Federal Employees' Compensation Act (FECA) (14): An Act instituted in 1908 providing benefits for on-the-job injuries to all federal employees.

Federal Employees Retirement System (FERS) (15): A program for federal employees hired after 1984 or those hired before 1984 who switched from CSRS to FERS.

Fee for service (10): A method of payment in which the patient pays the physician for each professional service performed from an established schedule of fees.

Fee schedule (5, 9, 14): A list of charges or established allowances for specific medical services and procedures. See also *Relative value studies (RVS).*

File (7): A collection of related data stored under a single title.

Financial accounting record (2, 9): An individual record indicating charges, payments, adjustments, and balances owed for services rendered; also known as *ledger.*

Fiscal agent (12): An organization under contract to the state to process claims for a state Medicaid program; insurance carrier handling claims from physicians and other suppliers of service for Medicare Part B; sometimes also referred to as *fiscal intermediary.*

Fiscal intermediary (FI) (11, 13): An organization under contract to the government that handles claims under Medicare Part A from hospitals, skilled nursing facilities, home health agencies, or providers of medical services and supplies. For TRICARE and CHAMPVA, the insurance company that handles the claims for care received within a particular state or country. Also known as *fiscal agent, fiscal carrier,* and *claims processor.*

Formal referral (10): An authorization request (telephone, fax, or completed form) required by the managed care organization contract to determine medical necessity and grant permission before services are rendered or procedures performed.

Format (7): The organization or appearance of data.

Foundation for medical care (FMC) (2, 10): An organization of physicians sponsored by a state or local medical association concerned with the development and delivery of medical services and the cost of health care.

Fraud (1): An intentional misrepresentation of the facts to deceive or mislead another.

Functional resume (17): A data sheet that highlights qualifications and skills.

Future purchase option (15): See *cost-of-living adjustment.*

Garnishment (9): A court order attaching a debtor's property or wages to pay off a debt.

Gatekeeper (10): In the managed care system, this is the physician who controls patient access to specialists and diagnostic testing services.

Genetically Handicapped Persons Program (GHPP) (C): A state program for genetically disabled children.

Gigabyte (7): A computer storage capacity that holds approximately 1 billion bytes or characters.

Global surgery policy (5): A Medicare policy relating to surgical procedures in which preoperative and postoperative visits (24 hours before [major] and day of [minor]), usual, intraoperative services, and complications not requiring additional trips to the operating room are included in one fee.

Group provider number (6): A number assigned to a group of physicians submitting insurance claims under the group name and reporting income under one name; used instead of the individual's physician's number (PIN) for the performing provider.

Grouper (16): The computer software program that assigns DRGs of discharged patients using the following information: patient's age, sex, principal diagnosis, complications/comorbid conditions, principal procedure, and discharge status.

Guaranteed renewable (2, 15): A clause in an insurance policy that means the insurance company must renew the policy as long as premium payments are made. However, the premium may be increased when it is renewed. These policies may have age limits of 60, 65, or 70 years or may be renewable for life.

Guarantor (2): An individual who promises to pay the medical bill by signing a form agreeing to pay or who accepts treatment, which constitutes an expressed promise.

Hard copy (7): A printout from a printer via computer.

Hardware (7): The physical components of a computer system (e.g., display screen or hard disk).

Health benefits advisor (HBA) (13): An individual at military hospitals or clinics who is there to help TRICARE beneficiaries obtain medical care through the military and through TRICARE.

Health Care Financing Administration (HCFA) (11): See *Centers for Medicare and Medicaid Services (CMS).*

Healthcare Common Procedure Coding System (HCPCS) (5): The CMS's Common Procedure Coding System. A three-tier national uniform coding system developed by the Centers for Medicare and Medicaid Services (CMS), formerly HCFA, used for reporting physician or supplier services and procedures under the Medicare program. Level I codes are national CPT codes, Level II codes are HCPCS national codes used to report items not covered under CPT, and Level III codes are HCPCS regional or local codes used to identify new procedures or items for which there is no national code. Pronounced "hick-picks."

Health Care Finder (HCF) (13): A health care professional, generally a registered nurse, who is located at TRICARE Service Centers to act as a liaison between military and civilian providers, verify eligibility, determine availability of services, coordinate care, facilitate the transfer of records, and perform first-level medical review.

Health insurance (2): A contract between the policyholder or member and insurance carrier or government program to reimburse the policyholder or member for all or a portion of the cost of medical care rendered by health care professionals; generic term applying to lost income arising from illness or injury; also known as *accident and health insurance* or *disability income insurance.*

Health Insurance Claim Form (CMS-1500) (6): Now known as CMS-1500. A universal insurance claim form developed and approved by the American Medical Association Council on Medical Service and the Centers for Medicare And Medicaid Services. It is used by physicians and other professionals to bill outpatient services and supplies to TRICARE, Medicare, and some Medicaid programs, as well as some private insurance carriers and managed care plans.

Health maintenance organization (HMO) (2, 10): The oldest of all prepaid health plans. A comprehensive health care financing and delivery organization that provides a wide range of health care services with an emphasis on preventive medicine to enrollees within a geographic area through a panel of providers. Primary care physician "gatekeepers" are usually reimbursed via capitation. In general, enrollees do not receive coverage for the services from providers who are not in the HMO network, except for emergency services.

Hearing (15): The second level of the appeal process for an individual applying for SSDI or SSI. This is a hearing before an administrative law judge who had no part in the initial or reconsideration disability determination.

High complexity (HC) (3): A phrase used to describe a type of medical decision making when a patient is seen for an E/M service.

High risk (2): A high chance of loss.

History of present illness (HPI) (3): A chronologic description of the development of the patient's present illness from the first sign or symptom or from the previous encounter to the present.

Hospice (11): A public agency or private organization primarily engaged in providing pain relief, symptom management, and supportive services to terminally ill patients and their families in their own homes or in a home-like center.

Hospital insurance (11): Known as Medicare Part A. A program providing basic protection against the costs of hospital and related after-hospital services for individuals eligible under the Medicare program.

Implied contract (2): A contract between physician and patient not manifested by direct words but implied or deduced from the circumstance, general language, or conduct of the patient.

In-area (10): Within the geographic boundaries defined by an HMO as the area in which it will provide medical services to its members.

Incomplete claim (6): Any Medicare claim missing necessary information; such claims are identified to the provider so they may be resubmitted.

Indemnity (2): Benefits paid to an insured while disabled; also known as *reimbursement.*

Independent medical evaluator (IME) (14): Physicians who make examinations of individuals, independent of the attending physician, and render an unbiased opinion about the degree of disability of a worker. IMEs are appointed by the referee or appeals board at state expense.

Independent (or Individual) Practice Association (IPA) (2, 10): A type of HMO in which a program administrator contracts with a number of physicians who agree to provide treatment to subscribers in their own offices. Physicians are not employees of the MCO and are not paid salaries. They receive reimbursement on a capitation or fee-for-service basis; also referred to as a *medical capitation plan.*

Injury (14): In a workers' compensation policy, this term signifies any trauma or damage to a body part or disease sustained, arising out of, and in the course of employment, including injury to artificial members and medical braces of all types.

Inpatient (16): A term used when a patient is admitted to the hospital for overnight stay.

Input (7): That which goes into a computer memory bank.

Inquiry (8): See *tracer.*

In situ (4): A description applied to a malignant growth confined to the site of origin without invasion of neighboring tissues.

Insurance adjuster (14): An individual at the workers' compensation insurance carrier overseeing an industrial case, authorizing diagnostic testing and medical treatment, and communicating with the provider of medical care.

Insurance balance billing (9): A statement sent to the patient after his or her insurance company has paid its portion of the claim.

Insurance billing specialist (1): A practitioner who carriers out claims completion, coding, and billing responsibilities and may or may not perform managerial and supervisory functions; also known as an *insurance claims processor* or *reimbursement specialist.*

Insured (2): An individual or organization protected in case of loss under the terms of an insurance policy.

Intelligent character recognition (ICR) (6): Same as *optical character recognition.*

Interactive transaction (7): Back and forth communication between user and computer.

Interface (7): The point at which two different systems are linked (e.g., computer to printer or modem).

Intermediate care facilities (ICFs) (11): Institutions furnishing health-related care and services to individuals who do not require the degree of care provided by acute care hospitals or nursing facilities.

Internal review (3): The process of going over financial documents before and after billing to insurance carriers to determine documentation deficiencies or errors.

International Classification of Diseases, Ninth Revision, Clinical Modification (ICD-9-CM) (4, 16): A diagnostic code book that uses a system for classifying diseases and operations to facilitate collection of uniform and comparable health information. A code system to replace this is ICD-10, which is being modified for use in the United States.

Internet (7): A large interconnected message-forwarding system linking academic, commercial, government, and military computer networks all over the world.

Interview (17): Meeting an individual face to face for evaluating and questioning a job applicant.

Intoxication (4): A diagnostic coding term that relates to an adverse effect rather than a poisoning when drugs such as digitalis, steroid agents, and so on are involved.

Invalid claim (6): Any Medicare claim that contains complete, necessary information but is illogical or incorrect (e.g., listing an incorrect provider number for a referring physician). Invalid claims are identified to the provider and may be resubmitted.

Italicized code (4): A diagnostic code in ICD-9-CM, Volume 1 Tabular list, that may never be sequenced as the principal diagnosis.

Itemized statement (9): A detailed summary of all transactions of a patient's account: dates of service, detailed charges, payments (copayments and deductibles), date the insurance claim was submitted, adjustments, and account balance.

Keypad (7): A device, separate or part of the keyboard, that contains keys to control mathematical functions.

Kilobyte (7): An expression for standard quantity measurement of disk or computer storage capacity.

Late effect (4): An inactive residual effect or condition produced after the acute phase of an illness or injury has ended.

Ledger card (2, 9): See *financial accounting record.*

Lien (9, 14): A claim on the property of another as security for a debt. In litigation cases, it is a legal promise to satisfy a debt owed by the patient to the physician out of any proceeds received on the case.

Limiting charge (11): A percentage limit on fees, specified by legislation, that nonparticipating physicians may bill Medicare beneficiaries above the fee schedule amount.

List service (listserv) (1): An online computer service run from a Web site where questions may be posted by subscribers.

Local area network (LAN) (7): An interlink of multiple computers contained within a room or building that allows sharing of files and devices such as printers.

Long-term disability insurance (15): A provision to pay benefits to a covered disabled person as long as he or she remains disabled, up to a specified period exceeding 2 years.

Looping (16): The automated grouper (computer software program that assigns DRGs) process of searching all listed diagnoses for the presence of any comorbid condition or complication, or searching all procedures for operating room procedures or other specific procedures.

Lost claim (8): An insurance claim that cannot be located after sending it to an insurer.

Low complexity (LC) (3): Phrase used to describe a type of medical decision making when a patient is seen for an E/M service.

Major diagnostic categories (MDCs) (16): A broad classifications of diagnoses. There are 83 coding system-oriented MDCs in the original DRGs and 23 body system-oriented MDCs in the revised set of DRGs.

Major medical (2): A health insurance policy designed to offset heavy medical expenses resulting from catastrophic or prolonged illness or injury.

Malignant tumor (4): An abnormal growth that has the properties of invasion and metastasis (e.g., transfer of diseases from one organ to another). The word "carcinoma" (CA) refers to a cancerous or malignant tumor.

Managed care organizations (MCOs) (10): A generic term applied to a managed care plan. May apply to EPO, HMO, PPO, integrated delivery system, or other weird arrangement. MCOs are usually prepaid group plans, and physicians are typically paid by the capitation method.

Manual billing (9): Processing statements by hand; may involve typing statements or photocopying the patient's financial accounting record and placing it in a window envelope, which then becomes the statement.

Maternal and Child Health Program (MCHP) (2, 12): A state service organization to assist children younger than 21 years of age who have conditions leading to health problems.

Medicaid (MCD) (2, 12): A federally aided, state-operated and -administered program that provides medical benefits for certain low-income persons in need of health and medical care. California's Medicaid program is known as *Medi-Cal.*

Medi-Cal (12): California's version of the nationwide program known as Medicaid. See *Medicaid.*

Medical necessity (3, 11): The performance of services and procedures that are consistent with the diagnosis in accordance with standards of good medical practice, performed at the proper level, and provided in the most appropriate setting. Medical necessity must be established (via diagnostic or other information presented on the individual claim under consideration) before the carrier may make payment.

Medical record (3): Written or graphic information documenting facts and events during the rendering of patient care.

Medical report (3): A permanent, legal document (letter or report format) that formally states the consequences of the patient's examination or treatment.

Medical service order (14): An authorization given to the physician, either written or verbal, to treat the injured or ill employee.

Medically indigent (MI) (C): See *medically needy.*

Medically (or psychologically) necessary (13): Medical or psychologic services considered appropriate care and generally accepted by qualified professionals to be reasonable and adequate for the diagnosis and treatment of illness, injury, pregnancy, and mental disorders, or that are reasonable and adequate for well-baby care.

Medically needy (MN) (12, C): Persons in need of financial assistance or whose income and resources will not allow them to pay for the costs of medical care; also called *medically indigent* in some states.

Medicare (M) (2, 11): A nationwide health insurance program for persons age 65 years and older and certain disabled or blind persons regardless of income, administered by HCFA. Local Social Security offices take applications and supply information about the program.

Medicare/Medicaid (Medi-Medi) (2, 11): Refers to an individual who receives medical or disability benefits from both Medicare and Medicaid programs; sometimes referred to as a *Medi-Medi case* or *crossover.*

Medicare Part A (11): Hospital benefits of a nationwide health insurance program for persons age 65 years and older and certain disabled individuals regardless of income, administered by CMS. Local Social Security offices take applications and supply information about the program.

Medicare Part B (11): Medical insurance of a nationwide health insurance program for persons age 65 years and older and certain disabled individuals regardless of income, administered by CMS. Local Social Security offices take applications and supply information about the program.

Medicare Part C (11): Medicare + Choice plans offer a number of health care options in addition to those available under Medicare Part A and Part B. Plans may include health maintenance organizations, fee-for-service plans, provider-sponsored organizations, religious fraternal benefit societies, and Medicare medical savings accounts.

Medicare Secondary Payer (MSP) (11): The primary insurance plan of a Medicare beneficiary that must pay for any medical care or services first before Medicare is sent a claim.

Medicare Summary Notice (MSN) (11): A document received by the patient explaining amount charged, Medicare approved, deductible, and coinsurance for medical services rendered.

Medigap (MG) (11): A specialized supplemental insurance policy devised for the Medicare beneficiary that covers the deductible and copayment amounts typically not covered under the main Medicare policy written by a nongovernmental third-party payer. Also known as *Medifill.*

Megabyte (7): Computer storage capacity in which one megabyte is equal to 1000 kilobytes (1024 characters).

Member (2): Person covered under an insurance program's contract, including: (1) the subscriber or contract holder who is the person named on the membership identification card; and (2) in the case of (a) two-person coverage, (b) one adult-one child coverage, or (c) family coverage (eligible family dependents enrolled under the subscriber's contract).

Memory (7): Storage in computer.

Mentor (17): Guide or teacher who offers advice, criticism, wisdom, guidance, and perspective to an inexperienced but promising protégé to help reach a life goal.

Military treatment facility (MTF) (13): All uniformed service hospitals or health clinics; also known as *military hospitals* or *uniformed service hospitals.*

Modem (7): A MOdulator DEModulator unit, a device that converts data into signals for telephone transmission and then (at the receiving end) back again into data.

Moderate complexity (MC) (3): A phrase used to describe a type of medical decision making when a patient is seen for an E/M service.

Modifier (5): In CPT coding, a two-digit add-on number placed after the usual procedure code number to indicate a procedure or service has been altered by specific circumstances. The two-digit modifier may be separated by a hyphen. In HCPCS Level II coding, one-digit or two-digit add-on alpha characters, placed after the usual procedure code number (Example G–1).

EXAMPLE G–1

27372-51 (typed on one line)
OR
73100-RT

Mouse (7): A device used to input computer data.

Multipurpose billing form (7): An all-encompassing billing form personalized to the practice of the physician, it may be used when a patient submits an insurance billing; also called *charge slip, communicator, encounter form, fee ticket, patient service slip, routing form, superbill,* and *transaction slip.*

Multiskilled health practitioner (MSHP) (1): An individual cross-trained to provide more than one function, often in more than one discipline. These combined functions can be found in a broad spectrum of health-related jobs, ranging in complexity including both clinical and administrative functions. The additional skills added to the original health care worker's job may be of a higher, lower, or parallel level. The terms *multiskilled, multicompetent,* and *cross trained* can be used interchangeably.

National alphanumeric codes (11): Alphanumeric codes developed by CMS, formerly HCFA. See *Healthcare Common Procedure Coding System (HCPCS).*

National Certified Insurance and Coding Specialist (NCICS) (17): An insurance and coding certification that is awarded by an independent testing agency, the National Center for Competency Testing (NCCT).

National provider identifier (NPI) (6): A Medicare lifetime 10-digit number issued to providers. When adopted, it will be recognized by Medicaid, Medicare, TRICARE, and CHAMPVA programs and eventually may be used by private insurance carriers.

Netback (9): Evaluating a collection agency's performance by taking the amount of monies collected and subtracting the agency's fees.

Networking (17): Exchanging information or services among individuals, groups, or institutions and making use of professional contacts.

New patient (NP) (3): An individual who has not received any professional services from the physician or another physician of the same specialty who belongs to the same group practice within the past 3 years.

No charge (NC) (9): Waiving the entire fee owed for professional care.

Nonavailability Statement (NAS) (13): When the uniformed services hospital cannot provide the inpatient care and the patient lives in a certain ZIP code near a military hospital, the patient must obtain this statement, signed by the commanding officer, before getting nonemergency inpatient care at a civilian hospital. INAS means inpatient nonavailability statement.

Noncancellable clause or policy (2, 15): An insurance policy clause that means the insurance company cannot increase premium rates and must renew the policy until the insured reaches the age stated in the contract. Some disability income policies have noncancellable terms.

Nondisability (ND) claim (14): A claim for an on-the-job injury that requires medical care but does not result in loss of working time or income.

Nonexempt assets (9): One's total property (in bankruptcy cases) not falling in the exemption category; including money, automobile equity, and property, more than a specified amount, depending on the state in which the person lives.

Nonparticipating physician (nonpar) (11): A provider who does not have a signed agreement with Medicare and has an option about assignment. The physician may not accept assignment for all services or has the option of accepting assignment for some services and collecting from the patient for other services performed at the same time and place.

Nonparticipating provider (nonpar) (2, 13): A provider who decides not to accept the determined allowable charge from an insurance plan as the full fee for care. Payment goes directly to the patient in this case, and the patient is usually responsible to pay the bill in full.

Nonprivileged information (1): Information consisting of ordinary facts unrelated to the treatment of the patient. The patient's authorization is not required to disclose the data unless the record is in a specialty hospital or in a special service unit of a general hospital, such as the psychiatric unit.

Not elsewhere classifiable (NEC) (4): This term is used in the ICD-9-CM diagnostic coding system when the code lacks the information necessary to code the term in a more specific category.

Not otherwise specified (NOS) (4): Unspecified. Used in ICD-9-CM numeric code system for coding diagnoses.

Nursing facility (NF) (1, C): A specially qualified facility that has the staff and equipment to provide skilled nursing care and related services that are medically necessary to a patient's recovery; formerly known as a *skilled nursing facility.*

Occupational illness (or disease) (14): An abnormal condition or disorder caused by environmental factors associated with employment. It may be caused by inhalation, absorption, ingestion, or direct contact.

Occupational Safety and Health Administration (OSHA) (14): A federal agency that regulates and investigates safety and health standards in work locations.

Old Age Survivors, Health and Disability Insurance (OASHDI) Program (C): A group that is entitled to benefits under the Medi-Cal program.

Optical character recognition (OCR) (6): A device that can read typed characters at very high speed and convert them to digitized files that can be saved on disk. Also known as *intelligent character recognition (ICR).*

Optionally renewable (2): An insurance policy renewal provision in which the insurer has the right to refuse to renew the policy on a date and may add coverage limitations or increase premium rates.

Ordering physician (3): The physician ordering non-physician services for a patient (e.g., diagnostic laboratory tests, pharmaceutical services, or durable medical equipment) when an insurance claim is submitted by a non-physician supplier of services. The ordering physician also may be the treating or performing physician.

"Other" claims (6): Medicare claims not considered "clean" claims that require investigation or development on a prepayment basis to determine if Medicare is the primary or secondary carrier.

Other health insurance (OHI) (13): Health care coverage for TRICARE beneficiaries through an employer, an association, or a private insurer. A student in the family may have a health care plan through school.

Outpatient (16): A patient who receives services in a health care facility, such as a physician's office, clinic, urgent care center, emergency department, or ambulatory surgical center and goes home the same day.

Output (7): Information transferred from internal memory storage to external storage.

Overpayment (8): Money paid over and above the amount due by the insurer or patient.

Paper claim (6): An insurance claim submitted on paper, including those optically scanned and converted to an electronic form by the insurance carrier.

Partial disability (15): A disability from an illness or injury that prevents an insured person from performing one or more of the functions of his or her regular job.

Participating physician (10): 1. A physician who contracts with an HMO or other insurance company to provide services. 2. A physician who has agreed to accept a plan's payments for services to subscribers (e.g., some Blue plans). Eighty percent of practicing American physicians are participating physicians.

Participating physician (par) (11): A physician who agrees to accept payment from Medicare (80% of the approved charges) plus payment from the patient (20% of approved charges) after the $100 deductible has been met.

Participating provider (par) (2, 13): One who accepts TRICARE assignment. Payment in this case goes directly to the provider. The patient must still pay the cost-share outpatient deductible and the cost of care not covered by TRICARE. See *assignment.*

Partnership program (13): A program that lets TRICARE–eligible individuals receive inpatient or outpatient treatment from civilian providers of care in a military hospital or from uniformed services providers of care in civilian facilities.

Password (7): A combination of letters and numbers that each individual is assigned to access computer data.

Past history (PH) (3): A patient's past experiences with illnesses, operations, injuries, and treatments.

Patient registration form (2): A questionnaire designed to collect demographic data and essential facts about medical insurance coverage for each patient seen for professional services; also called *patient information form.*

Peer review (8): The review of a patient's case by one or more physicians using federal guidelines to evaluate another physician in regard to the quality and efficiency of medical care. This is done to discover overutilization or misutilization of a plan's benefits.

Peer review organization (PRO) (11): A state-based group of practicing physicians paid by the federal government to review hospital care of Medicare patients to determine appropriateness and quality of care.

Pending claim (6): An insurance claim held in suspense because of review or other reason. These claims may be cleared for payment or denied.

Per capita (10): See *capitation.*

Percentage of revenue (16): The fixed percentage of the collected premium rate that is paid to the hospital to cover services.

Per diem (16): A single charge for a day in the hospital regardless of any actual charges or costs incurred.

Permanent and stationary (P & S) (14): A phrase used when a workers' compensation patient's condition has become stabilized and no improvement is expected. It is only after this declaration that a case can be rated for a compromise and release.

Permanent disability (PD) (14): An illness or injury (impairment of the normal use of a body part) expected to continue for the lifetime of the injured worker that prevents the person from performing the functions of his or her regular occupation, therefore impairing his or her earning capacity.

Personal bond (1): Insurance that provides coverage for those who handle large sums of money during business transactions.

Personal insurance (2): An insurance plan issued to an individual (or his or her dependents). Also known as *individual contract.*

Petition (14): A formal written request commonly used to indicate an appeal; also means any request for relief other than an application.

Phantom billing (1): Billing for services not performed.

Physical examination (PE) (3): Objective inspection or testing of organ systems or body areas of a patient by a physician.

Physically clean claim (6): Insurance claims with no staples or highlighted areas. The bar code area has not been deformed.

Physician provider group (PPG) (10): A physician-owned business that has the flexibility to deal with all forms of contract medicine and still offer its own packages to business groups, unions, and the general public.

Physician's fee profile (4): A compilation of each physician's charges and the payments made to him or her over a given period of time for each specific professional service rendered to a patient.

Ping-ponging (1): Excessive referrals to other providers for unnecessary services.

Point-of-service (POS) device or network (C): A piece of equipment interfaced with an analog telephone line used to identify Medi-Cal recipient eligibility, obtain share of cost liability status, key in share of cost payment toward balance, reserve Medi-Services, perform Family PACT (planning, access, care, and treatment) client eligibility transactions, and submit pharmacy or CMS-1500 insurance claims.

Point-of-service (POS) option (13): Individuals under the TRICARE program can choose to get TRICARE–covered nonemergency services outside the prime network of providers without a referral from the primary care manager and without authorization from a health care finder.

Point-of-service (POS) plan (2, 10): A managed care plan in which members are given a choice as to how to receive services, whether through an HMO, PPO, or fee-for-service plan. The decision is made at the time the service is needed (e.g., "at the point of service"); sometimes referred to as *open-ended HMOs, swing-out HMOs, self-referral options,* or *multiple option plans.*

Poisoning (4): A condition resulting from an overdose of drugs or chemical substances or from the wrong drug or agent given or taken in error.

Portfolio (17): A compilation of items that represents a job applicant's skills.

Position-schedule bond (1): Insurance that provides coverage for a designated job title rather than a named individual.

Post (2): A record or transfer financial entries, debit or credit, to an account (e.g., daysheet, financial account record [ledger], bank deposit slip, check register, or journal).

Preadmission testing (PAT) (16): Treatment, tests, and procedures done 48 to 72 hours before admission of a patient into the hospital. This is done to eliminate extra hospital days.

Preauthorization (2, 13): A requirement of some health insurance plans to obtain permission for a service or procedure before it is done and to see whether the insurance program agrees it is medically necessary.

Precertification (2): To find out whether treatment (surgery, tests, or hospitalization) is covered under a patient's health insurance policy.

Predetermination (2): To determine before treatment the maximum dollar amount the insurance company will pay for surgery, consultations, postoperative care, and so forth.

Preferred provider organization (PPO) (2, 10): A type of health benefit program in which enrollees receive the highest level of benefits when they obtain services from a physician, hospital, or other health care provider designated by their program as a "preferred provider." Enrollees may receive substantial, although reduced, benefits when they obtain care from a provider of their own choosing who is not designated as a "preferred provider" by their program.

Premium (2, 11): The cost of insurance coverage paid annually, semiannually, or monthly to keep the policy in force. In the Medicare program, monthly fee that enrollees pay for Medicare Part B medical insurance. This fee is updated annually to reflect changes in program costs.

Prepaid group practice model (10): A plan under which specified health services are rendered by participating physicians to an enrolled group of persons, with fixed periodic payments made in advance, by or on behalf of each person or family. If a health insurance carrier is involved, it contracts to pay in advance for the full range of health services to which the insured is entitled under the terms of the health insurance contract. Such a plan is one form of a *health maintenance organization.*

Presumptive eligibility (PE) (C): A federal/state program designed to ease access to prenatal care offering immediate temporary coverage to low-income women pending a formal Medi-Cal application.

Prevailing charge (5): A fee that is most frequently charged in an area by a specialty group of physicians. The top of this range establishes an overall limitation on the charges that a carrier, which considers prevailing charges in reimbursement, will accept as reasonable for a given service without special justification.

Primary care manager (PCM) (13): A physician who is responsible for coordinating and managing all the TRICARE beneficiary's health care unless there is an emergency.

Primary care physician (PCP) (10): A physician (e.g., family practitioner, general practitioner, pediatrician, obstetrician/gynecologist, or general internist) who oversees the care of patients in a managed health care plan (HMO or PPO) and refers patients to see specialists (e.g., cardiologists, oncologists, or surgeons) for services as needed. Also known as a *gatekeeper.*

Primary diagnosis (4): Initial identification of the condition or chief complaint for which the patient is treated for outpatient medical care.

Principal diagnosis (4, 16): A condition established after study that is chiefly responsible for the admission of the patient to the hospital.

Prior approval (12): The evaluation of a provider request for a specific service to determine the medical necessity and appropriateness of the care requested for a patient. Also called *prior authorization* in some states.

Privileged information (1): Data related to the treatment and progress of the patient that can be released only when written authorization of the patient or guardian is obtained.

Problem focused (PF) (3): A phrase used to describe a type of medical decision making when a patient is seen for an E/M service.

Procedure code numbers (5): Five-digit numeric codes that describe each service the physician renders to a patient.

Procedure review (16): A review of diagnostic and therapeutic procedures to determine appropriateness.

Professional Association of Health Care Office Managers (PAHCOM) (17): A nationwide organization dedicated to providing a strong professional network for health care office managers.

Professional component (PC) (5): That portion of a test or procedure (containing both a professional and technical component) that the physician performs (e.g., interpreting an electrocardiogram [ECG], reading an x-ray, or making an observation and determination using a microscope).

Professional courtesy (9): A discount or exemption from charges given to certain people at the discretion of the physician rendering the service. It is rarely used in current medicine.

Professional review organizations (PROs) (16): Groups of licensed physicians and osteopaths engaged in the practice of medicine or surgery in a particular area, formed to ensure adequate review of the services provided by the various medical specialties and subspecialties in the area, as well as providing DRG validation, a group of physicians working with the government to review cases for hospital admission and discharge under government guidelines. Also known as *peer review.*

Program (7): See *software.*

Prompt (7): A list of items displayed on a CRT from which the typist can choose the function to be performed. Also known as *menu.*

Prospective payment system (PPS) (11): A method of payment for Medicare hospital insurance based on diagnosis-related groups (DRGs) (a fixed dollar amount for a principal diagnosis).

Prospective review (3): The process of going over financial documents before billing is submitted to the insurance company to determine documentation deficiencies and errors.

Provider identification number (PIN) (6): A carrier-assigned number that every physician uses who renders services to patients when submitting insurance claims.

Provider Telecommunications Network (PTN) (C): An automated voice-response system that allows the provider to use the telephone to obtain checkwrite, claim, and prior authorization information for services rendered through the Medi-Cal program and several other state programs.

Quality assurance program (13): A plan that continually assesses the effectiveness of inpatient and outpatient care in the TRICARE and CHAMPVA programs.

***Qui tam* action (11):** An action to recover a penalty, brought by an informer in a situation in which one portion of the recovery goes to the informer and the other portion to the state or government.

Random access memory (RAM) (7): Allows data to be stored randomly and retrieved directly by specifying the address location.

Read-only memory (ROM) (7): Data stored in ROM can be read but not changed. It usually contains a permanent program.

Readmission review (16): A review of patients readmitted to a hospital within 7 days with problems related to the first admission, to determine whether the first discharge was premature or the second admission is medically necessary.

Reasonable fee (5, 11): A charge is considered reasonable if it is deemed acceptable after peer review even though it does not meet the *customary* or *prevailing* criteria. This includes unusual circumstances or complications requiring additional time, skill, or experience in connection with a particular service or procedure. In Medicare, the amount on which payment is based for participating physicians.

Rebill (resubmit) (8): To send another request for payment for an overdue bill to either the insurance company or patient.

Recipient (12): A person certified by the local welfare department to receive the benefits of Medicaid under one of the specific aid categories; an individual certified to receive Medicare benefits.

Reconsideration (15): The first level of appeal process for an individual applying for SSDI or SSI. It is a complete review of the claim by a medical or psychologic consultant or disability examiner team who did not take part in the original disability determination.

Referral (3): The transfer of the total or specific care of a patient from one physician to another. In managed care, a request for authorization for a specific service.

Referring physician (3): A physician who sends the patient for testing or treatment noted on the insurance claim when it is submitted by the physician performing the service.

Regional office (RO) (15): A Social Security state office.

Registered Medical Assistant (RMA) (17): A title earned by completing appropriate training and passing a registry examination administered by the American Medical Technologists (AMT).

Registered Medical Coder (RMC) (17): A registered title awarded after completion of coursework given by the Medical Management Institute (MMI) with recertification requirements.

Registration (17): Entry in an official registry or record that lists names of persons in an occupation who have satisfied specific requirements or by attaining a certain level of education and paying a registration fee.

Reimbursement (9): Repayment; the term used when insurance payment is pending.

Reimbursement specialist (1): See *insurance billing specialist*.

Rejected claim (6, 8): An insurance claim submitted to an insurance carrier that is discarded by the system because of a technical error (omission or erroneous information) or because it does not follow Medicare instructions. It is returned to the provider for correction or change so that it may be processed properly for payment.

Relative value studies (scale) (RVS) (5): A list of procedure codes for professional services and procedures that are assigned unit values that indicate the relative value of one procedure over another.

Relative value unit (RVU) (11): A monetary value assigned to each service based on the amount of physician work, practice expenses, and the cost of professional liability insurance. These three RVUs are then adjusted according to geographic area and used in a formula to determine Medicare fees.

Remittance advice (RA) (8, 11): A document detailing services billed and describing payment determination issued to providers of the Medicare or Medicaid program; also known in some programs as an *explanation of benefits*.

Remittance Advice Details (RAD) (C): A document that accompanies all Medi-Cal payment vouchers (checks) sent to providers of medical services.

Residual benefits (15): A term used in disability income insurance for disability that is not work related. It is the payment of partial benefits when the insured is not totally disabled.

Resource-based relative value scale (RBRVS) (11): A system that ranks physician services by units and provides a formula to determine a Medicare fee schedule.

Respite care (11): A short-term hospice inpatient stay for a terminally ill patient to give temporary relief to the person who regularly assists with home care of a patient.

***Respondeat superior* (1):** "Let the master answer." Refers to a physician's liability in certain cases for the wrongful acts of his of her assistant(s) or employee(s).

Resubmission Turnaround Document (RTD) (C): A document that the Medi-Cal fiscal intermediary sends to providers when a claim form has questionable or missing information.

Resume (17): A summary of education, skills, and work experience, usually in outline form.

Retrospective review (3): The process of going over financial documents after billing an insurance carrier to determine documentation deficiencies and errors.

Review (8): To look over a claim to assess how much payment should be made.

Review of systems (ROS) (3): An inventory of body systems obtained through a series of questions used to identify signs or symptoms that the patient might be experiencing or has experienced.

Running balance (2): An amount owed on a credit transaction; also known as *outstanding* or *unpaid balance*.

Scrubbing (16): The process in which computer software checks for errors before a claim is submitted to an insurance carrier for payment; also known as *edit check* or *cleaning the bill*.

Second-injury fund (14): See *subsequent injury fund*.

Secondary diagnosis (4): A second reason to the primary diagnosis for an office or hospital encounter that may contribute to the condition or define the need for a higher level of care but is not the underlying cause. There may be more than one secondary diagnosis.

Secured debt (9): A debt (an amount owed) in which a debtor pledges certain property (collateral), in a written security agreement, to the repayment of the debt.

Self-employment (17): Working for oneself, with direct control over work, services, and fees.

Self-referral (10): A patient in a managed care plan that refers himself or herself to a specialist. The patient may be required to inform the primary care physician.

Sequelae (14): Diseased conditions after, and usually resulting from, a previous disease.

Service area (10): The geographic area defined by an HMO as the locale in which it will provide health care services to its members directly through its own resources or arrangements with other providers in the area.

Service benefit program (13): A program (e.g., TRICARE) that provides benefits without a contract guaranteeing the indemnification of an insured party against a specific loss; there are no premiums. TRICARE Standard is considered a service benefit program.

Service-connected injury (13): Injury incurred by a service member while on active duty.

Service retiree (13): An individual who is retired from a career in the armed forces; also known as a *military retiree*.

Share of cost (12, C): The amount the patient must pay each month before he or she can be eligible for Medicaid. Also known as *liability* or *spend down*.

Short-term disability insurance (15): A provision to pay benefits to a covered disabled person as long as he or she remains disabled, up to a specified period not exceeding 2 years.

Skip (9): A debtor who has moved and neglected to give a forwarding address (e.g., skipped town).

Slanted brackets (4): A symbol used with a diagnostic code in ICD-9-CM, Volume 2, Alphabetic Index, indicating the code may never be sequenced as the principal diagnosis.

Social history (SH) (3): An age-appropriate review of a patient's past and current activities (e.g., smoking, diet intake, and alcohol use).

Social Security Administration (SSA) (15): Administers SSDI and SSI programs for disabled persons.

Social Security Disability Insurance (SSDI) (15): Entitlement program for disabled workers or self-employed individuals.

Social Security number (SSN) (6): An individual's tax identification number issued by the federal government.

Soft copy (7): That which is displayed on a CRT screen.

Software (7): Instructions (programs) necessary to make hardware perform a specific task.

Sponsor (13): For the TRICARE program, the service person (active duty, retired, or deceased) whose relationship makes the patient (dependent) eligible for TRICARE.

Staff model (10): The type of HMO in which the health plan hires physicians directly and pays them a salary.

Star symbol (5): A symbol (*) that appears next to certain procedure code numbers indicating special guidelines to be followed when using those surgical codes.

State disability insurance (SDI) (2, 15): See *unemployment compensation disability*.

State license number (6): A number issued to a physician who has passed the state medical examination indicating his or her right to practice medicine in the state where issued.

Statute of limitations (9): A time limit established for filing lawsuits; may vary from state to state.

Stop loss (10, 16): An agreement between a managed care company and a reinsurer in which absorption of prepaid patient expenses is limited; or limiting losses on an individual expensive hospital claim or professional services claim; form of reinsurance by which the managed care program limits the losses of an individual expensive hospital claim.

Straightforward (SF) (3): Phrase used to describe a type of medical decision making when a patient is seen for an E/M service.

Subpoena (3): "Under penalty." A writ that commands a witness to appear at a trial or other proceeding and give testimony.

Subpoena duces tecum (3): "In his possession." A subpoena that requires the appearance of a witness with his or her records. Sometimes the judge permits the mailing of records and the physician is not necessary to appear in court.

Sub rosa films (14): Videotapes made without the knowledge of the subject; used to investigate suspicious claims in workers' compensation cases.

Subscriber (2): The contract holder covered by an insurance program or managed care plan, who either has coverage through his or her place of employment or has purchased coverage directly from the plan or affiliate. This term is used primarily in Blue Cross and Blue Shield plans.

Subsequent injury fund (SIF) (14): A special fund that assumes all or part of the liability for benefits provided to a worker because of the combined effect of a work-related impairment and a preexisting condition; also known as *second-injury fund*.

Summary payment voucher (13): The document the fiscal agent sends to the provider or beneficiary, showing the service or supplies received, allowable charges, amount billed, the amount TRICARE paid, how much deductible has been paid, and the patient's cost-share.

Supplemental benefits (15): Disability insurance provisions that allow benefits to the insured to increase the monthly indemnity or receive a percentage of the policy premiums if an individual keeps a policy in force for 5 or 10 years or does not file any claims.

Supplemental Security Income (SSI) (11, 12): A program of income support for low-income aged, blind, and disabled persons established by Title XVI of the Social Security Act.

Supplementary medical insurance (SMI) (11): Part B—medical benefits of Medicare program.

Surgical package (5): Unstarred surgical procedure code numbers include the operation; local infiltration, digital block, or topical anesthesia; and normal, uncomplicated postoperative care. This is referred to as a "package," and one fee covers the whole package.

Suspended claim (8): An insurance claim that is processed by the insurance carrier but held in an indeterminate (pending) state about payment either because of an error or the need for additional information.

Technical component (5): That portion of a test or procedure (containing both a technical and a professional component) that pertains to the use of the equipment and the operator who performs it (e.g., ECG machine and technician, radiography machine and technician, and microscope and technician).

Temporary disability (TD) (14, 15): The recovery period after a work-related injury during which the employee is unable to work and the condition has not stabilized; a schedule of benefits payable for the temporary disability.

Temporary disability insurance (TDI) (15): See *unemployment compensation disability*.

Tertiary care (10): Services requested by a specialist from another specialist (e.g., neurosurgeons, thoracic surgeons, and intensive care units).

Third-party liability (14): Third-party liability exists if an entity is liable to pay the medical cost for injury, disease, or disability of a person hurt during the performance of his or her occupation and the injury is caused by an entity not connected with the employer.

Third-party subrogation (14): The legal process by which an insurance company seeks from a third party, who has caused a loss, recovery of the amount paid to the policyholder.

Total disability (15): A term that varies in meaning from one disability insurance policy to another. An example of a liberal definition might read, "The insured must be unable to perform the major duties of his or her specific occupation."

Total, permanent service-connected disability (13): A total permanent disability incurred by a service member while on active duty.

Tracer (8): An inquiry made to an insurance company to locate the status of an insurance claim (e.g., claim in review, claim never received, and so forth).

Transfer review (16): Review of transfers to different areas of the same hospital that are exempted from prospective payment.

Treating or performing physician (3): A provider who renders a service to a patient.

Treating practitioner (3): A nurse practitioner, clinical nurse specialist, or physician assistant who furnishes a consultation or treats a Medicare beneficiary for a specific medical problem and uses the results of a diagnostic test in the management of the beneficiary's specific medical problem.

Treatment Authorization Request (TAR) form (C): A Medi-Cal form that must be completed by a provider for certain procedures and services that require prior approval.

TRICARE (2): A three-option managed health care program offered to spouses and dependents of service personnel with uniform benefits and fees implemented nationwide by the federal government.

TRICARE Extra (13): A PPO–type of TRICARE option in which the individual does not have to enroll or pay an annual fee. On a visit-by-visit basis, the individual may seek care from an authorized network provider and receive a discount on services and reduced cost-share (copayment).

TRICARE for Life (13): A health care program that offers additional TRICARE benefits as a supplementary payer to Medicare for uniformed service retirees, their spouses, and survivors age 65 or older.

TRICARE Prime (13): A voluntary HMO–type option for TRICARE beneficiaries.

TRICARE Service Center (13): An office staffed by TRICARE Health Care Finders and beneficiary service representatives.

Turfing (10): Transferring the sickest, high-cost patients to other physicians so the provider appears as a low-utilizer in a managed care setting.

Two-party check (8): A check that is made out to the physician and the patient by the maker.

Unbundling (5): The practice of using numerous CPT codes to identify procedures normally covered by a single code; also known as *itemizing, fragmented billing, exploding,* or *à la carte medicine*; billing under Medicare Part B for nonphysician services to hospital inpatients furnished to the hospital by an outside supplier or another provider.

Under the new law, unbundling is prohibited, and all non-physician services provided in an inpatient setting will be paid as hospital services.

Unemployment compensation disability (UCD) (2, 15): Insurance that covers off-the-job injury or sickness and is paid for by deductions from a person's paycheck. This program is administered by a state agency and is sometimes also known as *state disability insurance (SDI)* or *temporary disability insurance (TDI).*

Uniform Bill (UB-92) claim form (16): A Uniform Bill insurance claim form developed by the National Uniform Billing Committee for hospital inpatient billing and payment transactions.

Unique provider identification number (UPIN) (6): A number issued by the Medicare fiscal intermediary to each physician who renders medical services to Medicare recipients; used for identification purposes on the CMS-1500 claim form.

Unsecured debt (9): Any debt (amount owed) that is not secured or backed by any form of collateral.

Upcoding (5): Deliberate manipulation of CPT codes for increased payment.

Urgent care (13): Medically necessary treatment that is required for illness or injury that would result in further disability or death if not treated immediately.

Usual, customary, and reasonable (UCR) (5): A method used by insurance companies to establish their fee schedules in which three fees are considered in calculating payment: (1) the usual fee is the fee typically submitted by the physician; (2) the customary fee falls within the range of usual fees charged by providers of similar training in a geographic area; and (3) the reasonable fee meets the aforementioned criteria or is considered justifiable because of special circumstances. UCR uses the conversion factor method of establishing maximums; the method of reimbursement used under Medicaid by which state Medicaid programs set reimbursement rates using the Medicare method or a fee schedule, whichever is lower.

Utilization review (UR) (10, 16): A process, based on established criteria, of reviewing and controlling the medical necessity for services and providers' use of medical care resources. Reviews are carried out by allied health personnel at predetermined times during the hospital stay to assess the need for the full facilities of an acute care hospital. In managed care systems, such as an HMO, reviews are done to establish medical necessity, thus curbing costs. Also called *utilization* or *management control.*

V codes (4): A subclassification of ICD-9-CM coding used to identify health care encounters that occur for reasons other than illness or injury and to identify patients whose injury or illness is influenced by special circumstances or problems.

Verbal referral (10): A primary care physician informs the patient and telephones to the referring physician that the patient is being referred for an appointment.

Veteran (13): Any person who has served in the armed forces of the United States, especially in time of war; is no longer in the service; and has received an honorable discharge.

Veterans Affairs (VA) disability program (15): A program for honorably discharged veterans who file claim for a service-connected disability.

Veterans Affairs (VA) outpatient clinic (2, 15): A clinic where medical and dental services are rendered to veterans who have service-related disabilities.

Video display terminal (VDT) (7): A television-like screen attached to a computer or word processing terminal; also known as a *cathode ray tube (CRT).*

Virus (7): A destructive program that attaches and copies itself to other programs in a computer system. Some viruses destroy programs and data after a precise lapse of time.

Voice Drug TAR System (VDTS) (C): A Medi-Cal telecommunication system for processing urgent and initial drug Treatment Authorization Requests, to inquire about the status of previously entered drug TARs, or to inquire whether a patient is receiving continual care with a drug.

Volume performance standard (VPS) (11): The desired growth rate for spending on Medicare Part B physician services, set each year by Congress.

Voluntary disability insurance (15): A majority of employees of an employer voluntarily consent to be covered by an insured or self-insured disability insurance plan instead of a state plan.

Waiting period (WP) (14, 15): For disability insurance, the initial period of time when a disabled individual is not eligible to receive benefits even though unable to work; for workers' compensation, the days that must elapse before workers' compensation weekly benefits become payable.

Waiver of premium (15): A disability insurance policy provision that an employee does not have to pay any premiums while disabled. Also known as *elimination period.*

Withhold (10): A portion of the monthly capitation payment to physicians retained by the HMO until the end of the year to create an incentive for efficient care. If the physician exceeds utilization norms, he or she will not receive it.

Workers' Compensation Appeals Board (WCAB) (14): The board that handles workers' compensation liens and appeals.

Workers' compensation (WC) insurance (2, 14): A contract that insures a person against on-the-job injury or illness. The employer pays the premium for his or her employees.

Work hardening (14): An individualized program of therapy using simulated or real job duties to build up strength and improve the worker's endurance to be able to work up to 8 hours per day. Sometimes work site modifications are instituted to get the employee back to gainful employment.

Write-off (9): Assets or debts that have been determined to be uncollectable and therefore are adjusted off the accounting books as a loss.

Yo-yoing (1): Calling patients back for repeated and unnecessary follow-up visits.

Index

Note: Page numbers set in italics indicate figures, page numbers followed by *t* indicate tables.